OBESITY IN EUROPE 91

Obesity in Europe 91 represents the edited proceedings of the 3rd European Congress on Obesity, held in Nice, France, 30 May – 1 June 1991

OBESITY IN EUROPE 91

Proceedings of the 3rd European Congress on Obesity

Edited by

G. Ailhaud,
B. Guy-Grand,
M. Lafontan and
D. Ricquier

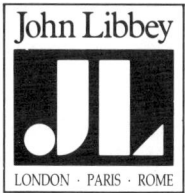

John Libbey
LONDON · PARIS · ROME

British Library Cataloguing in Publication Data
Obesity in Europe 91
  I. Ailhaud, G.
  616.3

ISBN: 0 86196 273 7
ISSN: 0955-6389

Published by

John Libbey & Company Ltd, 13 Smiths Yard, Summerley Street, London SW18 4HR, England.
Telephone: 081-947 2777: Fax 081-947 2664
John Libbey Eurotext Ltd, 6 rue Blanche, 92120 Montrouge, France.
John Libbey - C.I.C. s.r.l., via Lazzaro Spallanzani 11, 00161 Rome, Italy

© 1992 John Libbey & Company Ltd. All rights reserved.
Unauthorised duplication contravenes applicable laws.
Printed and Bound in Great Britain by
Hartnolls Limited, Bodmin, Cornwall.

Table of Contents

Chapter 1	Development of adipose tissue from dormant preadipocytes to adipocytes and from BAT to WAT **Gérard AILHAUD**	1
Chapter 2	Human obesities: chaos or determinism? **Claude BOUCHARD**	7
Section I	**Multifaceted aspects of human obesity**	**15**
Chapter 3	Self-reported intake as a measure for energy intake: a validation against doubly labelled water **K.R. WESTERTERP, W.P.H.G. VERBOEKET-VAN de VENNE, G.A.L. MEIJER and F. ten HOOR**	17
Chapter 4	Effect of a very low calorie diet on muscle bioenergetics at rest and during excercise: 31-P nuclear magnetic resonance study **V. ŠTICH, M. HÁJEK, A. HORSKÁ, V. HAINER, J. VĚTVICKA, J. HRDINA and M. KUNEŠOVÁ**	23
Chapter 5	Increased metabolic efficiency in a subset of obese patients **M. WECK, S. FISCHER, H. KARST, R. NOACK, W. LEONHARDT, K. FÜCKER and M. HANEFELD**	29
Chapter 6	The effect of weight loss on erythrocyte membrane function in patients with morbid obesity **Yishai LEVY, Nizar ELIAS, Uri COGAN and Daniel YESHURUN**	35
Section II	**Neuro-endocrine regulation of food intake**	**39**
Chapter 7	Fat intake, fat digestion and the satiety signal for fat intake **Charlotte ERLANSON-ALBERTSSON and Jie MEI**	41
Chapter 8	Absence of complete caloric compensation following mild deprivation at the end of the dark phase in lean female rats **Mary Lisa SASSANO, Francoise J. SMITH and L. Arthur CAMPFIELD**	47
Chapter 9	Intracerebroventricular injection of monosodium glutamate (MSG) stimulates food intake in Long-Evans rats **A. STRICKER-KRONGRAD, B. BECK, J.P. MAX, J.P. NICOLAS and C. BURLET**	51
Chapter 10	Stress related overeating, d-fenfluramine and neuroendocrine responses in the ageing rat **Francoise LACOUR, Denis RAVEL, Bernard KERDELHUÉ, Joseph ESPINAL and Jacques DUHAULT**	55
Chapter 11	Evaluation of the action of a non-absorbable fat on appetite and energy intake in lean, healthy males **Victoria J. BURLEY and John E. BLUNDELL**	63

Chapter 12	The effect of myco-protein on hunger, satiety and subsequent food consumption **W.H. TURNBULL, D. BESSEY, J. WALTON and A.R. LEEDS**	67
Chapter 13	Buspirone and food intake in women volunteers in relation to the menstrual cycle **Elizabeth GOODALL, Mary WHITTLE, John COOKSON and Trevor SILVERSTONE**	71

Section III   Genetics of obesity in animal models and humans   75

Chapter 14	Genetics of obesity in animal models and in humans **Paul TRAYHURN**	77
Chapter 15	Losses of total body fat and of abdominal adipose tissue and the response of plasma lipoproteins to aerobic excercise training in identical twins **Jean-Pierre DESPRÉS, Sital MOORJANI, Paul J. LUPIEN, Angelo TREMBLAY, André NADEAU, Germain THÉRIAULT and Claude BOUCHARD**	81
Chapter 16	Recessive inheritance of a major gene for human obesity? Analysis of the Danish adoption study **Thorkild I.A. SØRENSEN, Claus HOLST and Albert J. STUNKARD**	85
Chapter 17	Glucose transporter (Glut 1) as a possible candidate gene for obesity **Jolanta U. WEAVER, Peter G. KOPELMAN and Graham A. HITMAN**	89
Chapter 18	White adipocytes from young obese Zucker rats maintain excessive lipogenic enzyme activity in long term culture **Véronique BRIQUET-LAUGIER, Annie QUIGNARD-BOULANGE, Isabelle DUGAIL, Bernadette ARDOUIN, Xavier LE LIEPVRE and Marcelle LAVAU**	95
Chapter 19	Development of thyroxine 5′monodeiodinase activity in brown adipose tissue of young Zucker rats **V. MARIE, F. DUPUY and R. BAZIN**	101

Section IV   Epidemiological aspects of obesity   107

Chapter 20	Obesity in Europe – some epidemiological observations **J.C. SEIDELL**	109
Chapter 21	Variations of the body mass index in the French population from 0 to 87 years **M.F. ROLLAND-CACHERA, T.J. COLE, M. SEMPÉ, J. TICHET, C. ROSSIGNOL and A. CHARRAUD**	113
Chapter 22	The relation of obesity and fat distribution to blood lipid levels **Berit Lilienthal HEITMANN**	121
Chapter 23	Body fat distribution and breast cancer. Preliminary results from a case-control study in women from Southern Italy **Renato BORRELLI, Emilia DE FILIPPO, Luca SCALFI, Gelsomina BUGLIONE, Franco CONTALDO, Achille MARONE, Valerio PARISI, Franco CREMONA, Francesco SCOGNAMIGLIO, Raffaele PALAIA, Fulvio RUFFOLO and Marco SALVATORE**	125
Chapter 24	Weight changes among 13,097 adult Finns over six years **M. KORKEILA, J. KAPRIO, A. RISSANEN, M. KOSKENVUO and K. HEIKKILÄ**	129
Chapter 25	Relationships of fasting plasma insulin to anthropometry and blood lipids in European subjects: influence of gender **M. CIGOLINI, J.C. SEIDELL, J.P. DESLYPERE, J. CHARZEWSKA, B.M. ELLSINGER, L. ZAMBELLI, M.G. ZENTI and F. CONTALDO**	135

| Section V | Management of obesity | 139 |

Chapter 26	Fat cell adrenergic receptors: from molecular approaches to therapeutic strategies Max LAFONTAN, Jean-Sébastien SAULNIER-BLACHE, Christian CARPENE, Dominique LANGIN, Jean GALITZKY, Maria PORTILLO, Dominique LARROUY and Michel BERLAN	141
Chapter 27	Identification and analysis of an adipose specific enhancer Reed A. GRAVES, Peter TONTONOZ, Susan R. ROSS and Bruce M. SPIEGELMAN	155
Chapter 28	The management of obesity John F. MUNRO and Nicola COLLEDGE	163
Chapter 29	Factors influencing completion and attrition in a weight control programme R. RICHMAN, C.M. BURNS, K. STEINBECK and I. CATERSON	167
Chapter 30	Increased resting respiratory quotient. A predictor of weight-relapse in post-obese women Paolo M. SUTER, Yves SCHUTZ and Eric JEQUIER	173
Chapter 31	Contribution of low intensity exercise training to treatment of abdominal obesity. Importance of "metabolic fitness" Jean-Pierre DESPRÉS, Denis PRUD'HOMME, Angelo TREMBLAY and Claude BOUCHARD	177
Chapter 32	Long term result of surgical treatment of obesity with vertical banded gastroplasty A. LAURENT-JACCARD, C. WYSS, P. BURCKHARDT and A. JAYET	183
Chapter 32	Treatment of abdominal obese men with testosterone Per MÅRIN, Sten HOLMÄNG*, Göran HOLM, Lars JÖNSSON and Per BJÖRNTORP	188

| Section VI | Obesity and related disorders | 189 |

Chapter 34	Obesity and related disorders H. DITSCHUNEIT	191
Chapter 35	Normal feedback inhibition of insulin secretion by insulin but reduced metabolic clearance rate of the hormone in obese subjects A.J. SCHEEN, M. CASTILLO, G. PAOLISSO, B. JANDRAIN and P.J. LEFEBVRE	201
Chapter 36	Does hyperinsulinaemia increase the adrenocortical androgen secretion in obese hirsute women J. LÉONET and J. KOLANOWSKI	207
Chapter 37	Microalbuminuria in the non-diabetic obese patient P. VALENSI, M. BUSBY, M.E. COMBES and J.R. ATTALI	213
Chapter 38	Possible relationship between proteinuria and obesity A. SAIBENE, F. CAVIEZEL, F. ZILLI, L. GIANOLLI, F. DOSIO and G. POZZA	217
Chapter 39	Radiological osteoarthrosis, subjective symptoms and clinical findings in the extremity joints of severely obese and control subjects T. RÖNNEMAA, H. ALARANTA and T. AALTO	221
Chapter 40	Disturbances in respiratory function in obese subjects J. RAISON, D. CASSUTO, E. ORVOEN-FRIJA, M.F. DORE, J. ROCHEMAURE and B. GUY-GRAND	227

Section VII CNS-Periphery relationships — 231

Chapter 41 New aspects of the physiopathology of obesity and insulin resistance in rodents — 233
B. JEANRENAUD, I. CUSIN, C. GUILLAUME-GENTIL,
F. ASSIMACOPOULOS-JEANNET, J. TERRETTAZ
and F. ROHNER-JEANRENAUD

Chapter 42 Caloric regulation in liver-transplanted rats — 237
C. LARUE-ACHAGIOTIS, A. MICHEL, J. BERNARBÉ, J. BOILLOT and
J. LOUIS-SYLVESTRE

Chapter 43 Control of cephalic thermogenic phase of feeding — 241
J. LEBLANC, P. DIAMOND, M. GRIGGIO, A. NADEAU and D. RICHARD

Chapter 44 Does insulin play a role in cephalic postprandial thermogenesis? — 249
Laurent BRONDEL, Geneviève VAILLANT, Michel GUIGUET
and Marc FANTINO

Chapter 45 The influence of meal composition on plasma serotonin and
norepinephrine concentrations — 255
I. BLUM, Y. VERED, E. GRAFF, Y. GROSSKOPF, R. DON, A. HARSAT
and O. RAZ

Chapter 46 Glucocorticoid hormone effects on visceral adipose tissue metabolism
and distribution — 259
M. REBUFFÉ-SCRIVE, A. MOYER and J. RODIN

Chapter 47 Increased pancreatic islet blood flow in obese Zucker rats — 263
Nadia ATEF, Alain KTORZA, Luc PICON and Luc PENICAUD

Section VIII Enzymatic and metabolic regulation of adipose tissue — 267

Chapter 48 The role of gut hormones in the adipose tissue metabolism of lean and
genetically obese (ob/ob) mice — 269
J. OBEN, R. ELLIOTT, L. MORGAN, J. FLETCHER and V. MARKS

Chapter 49 Activation of multiple insulin effectors in white adipose tissue in 1 week
VMH-lesioned rats — 273
Béatrice COUSIN, Karen AGOU, Anne Françoise BURNOL,
Armelle LETURQUE, Jean GIRARD and Luc PENICAUD

Chapter 50 Late expression of the α_2-adrenergic mediated antilipolysis during adipocyte
differentiation of hamster preadipocytes — 277
Jean Sébastien SAULNIER-BLACHE, Michèle DAUZATS,
Danielle DAVIAUD, Danielle GAILLARD, Gérard AILHAUD,
Raymond NÉGREL and Max LAFONTAN

Chapter 51 *In situ* investigations of adipose tissue metabolism — 281
Peter ARNER

Chapter 52 Anti-obesity action of ICI D7114 is associated with the appearance of active
brown adipose tissue in adult dogs — 289
B.R. HOLLOWAY, O. CHAMPIGNY, O. BLONDELL, D. RICQUIER,
R.M. MAYERS and M.G. BRISCOE

Chapter 53 Fatty acid-binding protein (FABP) in rat brown adipose tissue — 293
Asim K. DUTTA-ROY, Yiming HUANG and Paul TRAYHURN

Section IX Control of energy expenditure — 297

Chapter 54 Swedish obese subjects, SOS. An intervention study of obesity — 299
Lars SJÖSTRÖM

Chapter 55	Psychological and behavioural determinants of regional fat deposition **Judith RODIN**	307
Chapter 56	Effect of longterm overfeeding on energy expenditure **Angelo TREMBLAY, Jean-Pierre DESPRÉS, Germain THÉRIAULT and Claude BOUCHARD**	319
Chapter 57	Meal-induced thermogenesis in lean and obese prepubertal children **Claudio MAFFEIS, Yves SCHUTZ and Leonardo PINELLI**	323
Chapter 58	Energy expenditure determines weight loss independent of BMI, RMR, FFM or nitrogen conservation: a VLCD study **A. COXON, S. KREITZMAN, P. JOHNSON and W. MORGAN**	327
Chapter 59	Increased energy expenditure and carbohydrate oxidation in post-obese women on a high-carbohydrate diet. Mediation by the sympathetic nervous system **A. ASTRUP, B. BUEMANN, N.J. CHRISTENSEN, J. MADSEN and F. QUAADE**	333
Chapter 60	Are sex hormones involved in resting metabolic rate and glucose-induced thermogenesis? **Greet VANSANT, Luc Van GAAL and Ivo De LEEUW**	337

Section X Cellular and molecular biology in the analysis of obesity   341

Chapter 61	Cellular and molecular biology in the analysis of obesity **Daniel RICQUIER**	343
Chapter 62	Identification of a marker of the preadipose state as a component of the extracellular matrix **Azeddine IBRAHIMI, Sylvie BARDON, Bénédicte BERTRAND, Gérard AILHAUD and Christian DANI**	347
Chapter 63	Adrenergic regulation of differentiation and proliferation in brown adipocyte cultures **Jan NEDERGAARD, Myriam NÉCHAD, Stefan REHNMARK, David HERRON, Anders JACOBSSON, Pertti KUUSELA, Pere PUIGSERVER, Josef HOUSTEK, Gennady BRONNIKOV and Barbara CANNON**	355
Chapter 64	The Siberian hamster as a new model to study the hormonal regulation of brown adipocyte differentiation and uncoupling protein expression **Susanne KLAUS, Anne-Marie CASSARD, Martin KLINGENSPOR and Daniel RICQUIER**	363
Chapter 65	Mitochondrial DNA variants in relation to body fat **France T. DIONNE, Josée TRUCHON, Lucie TURCOTTE, Angelo TREMBLAY, Jean-Pierre DESPRÉS and Claude BOUCHARD**	369

Section XI Adipose tissue metabolism and regional distribution   375

Chapter 66	Psychosocial factors and fat distribution **Per BJÖRNTORP**	377
Chapter 67	Plasma glucagon levels in upper body obesity. Glucagon–lipid interactions **Luc Van GAAL, Greet VANSANT and Ivo De LEEUW**	389
Chapter 68	Changed adipose tissue distribution after treatment of Cushing's syndrome **Lars LÖNN, Henry KVIST, Lars SJÖSTRÖM and I. ERNEST**	393
Chapter 69	Lactate production in subcutaneous adipose tissue in lean and obese man **P.-A. JANSSON, U. SMITH and P. LÖNNROTH**	397

Chapter 70	Epinephrine-induced glycerol release in subcutaneous adipose tissue measured by microdialysis in patients with android obesity **Herwig H. DITSCHUNEIT, Marion FLECHTNER-MORS and Hans DITSCHUNEIT**	401
Chapter 71	Vasoactive substances in human adipose tissue biopsies **D.L. CRANDALL, H.E. HERZLINGER, P. CERVONI, T.M. SCALEA and J.G. KRAL**	405
Chapter 72	Site differences in the regulation of adipose tissue lipolysis in men **P. MAURIÈGE, J.P. DESPRÉS, D. PRUD'HOMME, M.C. POULIOT, A. TREMBLAY and C. BOUCHARD**	411

Section XII Psychosocial aspects of human obesity — 415

Chapter 73	Psychosocial aspects of obesity: pathogenetic and therapeutic importance **B. GUY-GRAND and M. LE BARZIC**	417
Chapter 74	Body size, age, ethnicity, attitudes and weight loss **Pippa CRAIG and Ian CATERSON**	421
Chapter 75	Fear and loathing of obesity: the rise of dieting in childhood **Andrew J. HILL**	427
Chapter 76	Counterregulation as a function of cognitive restraint? **M.S. WESTERTERP-PLANTENGA, E. VAN DEN HEUVEL, L. WOUTERS and F. TEN HOOR**	431
Chapter 77	Cognitive control of eating behaviour disinhibition of control, and successful weight reduction **Joachim WESTENHOEFER and Volker PUDEL**	437
Chapter 78	Lipolytic regulation during mental stress **Anders WENNLUND, Hans WAHRENBERG, Jan BOLINDER and Peter ARNER**	441

Indexes

Author Index	447
Subject Index	451

Foreword

The *Third European Congress on Obesity* took place in Nice, France, 30 May to 1 June 1991. Following the first two successful meetings in Stockholm (1988) and Oxford (1989), it was impressive to note both a growing attendance and the increasing importance of areas as diverse as psychophysiology, control of food intake, pharmacology and molecular biology. It is our opinion that several original reports have indicated new research directions and have paved the way to major breakthroughs.

The rapid publication of these proceedings is due to a successful combination of efficient authors, professional publisher and ... impatient editors.

We have benefitted greatly from the help of major donors, sponsors and contributors (who are listed separately in the acknowledgements) and we wish to thank all of the 1034 participants for a pleasant, scientifically stimulating and, we believe, rather informal Third Congress.

Gérard AILHAUD
Bernard GUY-GRAND
Max LAFONTAN
Daniel RICQUIER

Acknowledgements

The Organizing Committee gratefully acknowledges the generosity of the many supporting institutions who contributed to the success of the ECO91 meeting:

Major Donors

Eli Lilly International Corporation
Institut de Recherches Internationales Servier (IRIS)

Sponsors

Ardix Médical
France Glace Findus
ICI Pharmaceuticals
Merck, Sharp & Dohme-Chibret
Parke-Davis International
Pierre Fabre Santé
Sandoz Nutrition

Contributors

Clarins
F. Hoffman-La Roche International
L'Oréal
Merck, Sharp & Dohme International
Nutra-Sweet
Pfizer International
SmithKline Beecham Pharmaceuticals
Société Générale des Eaux Minérales Vittel
Sopad Nestlé
The Upjohn Company
Weight Watchers France

Chapter 1

Development of Adipose Tissue from Dormant Preadipocytes to Adipocytes and from BAT to WAT

Gérard AILHAUD
Centre de Biochimie du CNRS (UMR 134), Université de Nice-Sophia Antipolis, UFR Sciences, Parc Valrose, 06108 Nice Cédex 2, France

Summary

The various molecular events taking place *in vitro* during the differentiation of adipose precursor cells from established clonal lines have been extensively investigated. These studies have allowed us to demonstrate that dormant preadipocytes are present *in vivo* in various species, including man. Analysis *in vitro* of the signalling pathways required for terminal differentiation of preadipocytes to adipocytes has been performed; it led us to postulate that hyperplasia of adipose tissue is due to a few hormonal signals which are required at the same time above threshold levels. The existence of distinct adipose precursor cells for BAT and WAT is supported by recent reports, as well as the likely transformation of brown adipocytes into white adipocytes. A few strategies which can be envisioned to control adipose tissue mass at the cell level are briefly discussed.

Introduction

The acquisition of new fat cells from embryonic to adult life has received wide experimental support both in rodents and humans. Morphological differentiation of fat tissue takes place during the second trimester of gestation in both male and female foetuses[22]. First noticeable in the head and neck, it is present in the main adipose deposits at about 28 weeks[4,21]. In man as in other species like pig, the emergence of fat globules is tightly coupled to neovascularization of the tissue and leads to the formation of mature adipocytes able to respond to lipolytic hormones[15,23]. These observations indicate that the various biological signals required for complete adipose cell differentiation are already present in the human foetus. In that respect, it is worth pointing out that "differentiation" as applied to adipose precursor cells can have distinct meanings, and that this can lead to confusion.

From a developmental perspective, all adipose precursor cells are differentiated (or determined) as they are not progenitors of any other cell type. From a chronological perspective, adipose cell differentiation is characterized *in vitro* by a sequence of events during which fibroblast-like cells from established clonal lines become committed and acquire early markers, but do not yet contain triacylglycerol (defined as preadipocytes). Terminal differentiation of preadipocytes refers to accumulation of lipid droplets coupled to the acquisition of various late markers, among which is glycerol-3-phosphate dehydrogenase (GPDH) required for triacylglycerol synthesis.

Another important point with respect to human embryos are the relationships between brown adipose tissue (BAT) and white adipose tissue (WAT), as it is commonly accepted that

BAT and WAT are present in newborns. Thus, at the cell level, the existence of a single or distinct adipoblast raises an interesting issue if one considers in adult rodents the postulated role of BAT in diet-induced thermogenesis. At the cell level (vide infra), adipose differentiation is a multistep process. The establishment from mice and hamster of clonal lines of adipose precursor cells (i.e. preadipocyte cell lines)[1] has allowed us to gain some insights into this process in vitro: (i) precursor cells (adipoblasts) are unipotential, leading to the formation of adipose cells only, (ii) emergence of early markers is coupled to growth arrest, leading to the formation of preadipocytes, (iii) emergence of late markers, including lipid accumulation, is coupled to a limited growth resumption of early marker-expressing cells (defined as terminal differentiation), leading to the formation of adipocytes, and (iv) growth hormone (GH), triiodothyronine (T_3) and insulin are required for the expression of late markers only[3].

Status of differentiation-specific markers in vivo

So far, the most specific markers of adipose cells in mice are pOb24 as early marker, aP2 and adipsin as late markers. pOb24 mRNA encodes for a protein homologous to the alpha-2 chain of human collagen VI[16], aP2 mRNA encodes for a 14 kDa protein which binds fatty acids[29] whereas adipsin mRNA encodes for a secreted protease having complement D activity[28]. The relative proportion of various differentiation-specific mRNAs has been examined in mouse adipose deposits. The results, obtained with the epididymal and inguinal fat tissues, have shown that the bulk of pOb24 mRNA, mainly localized in adipose tissue, is present in the stromal-vascular cells whereas it is only present at a low level in mature adipocytes. In contrast, late mRNA markers (GPDH, aP2) and even more so very late mRNA markers (adipsin) are mainly distributed in mature adipocytes. Beta-actin mRNA, the proportion of which does not change during the differentiation of Ob17 cells, equally distributes between both fractions[3]. Therefore cells having expressed early markers are present in the stromal-vascular compartment of adipose tissue. The existence of pOb24-positive cells has been also directly assessed in adipose tissues of very old mice; this result is striking as the formation of new fat cells should be quite limited at that age. Therefore cells that can be considered as dormant preadipocytes are indeed present in the various adipose deposits of very old mice. We have therefore suggested that the critical clue to understanding the terminal differentiation process of fat cells from precursor cells in vivo is the delicate balance between growth arrest leading to dormant, partly differentiated cells present throughout life and a situation whereby these cells resume a limited proliferation and differentiate irreversibly into mature fat cells. This balance will depend upon the differential sensitivity of dormant cells to respond to a given set of mitogenic–adipogenic stimuli (vide infra). In other words, this hypothesis relies on the concept of polyclonality developed in the case of primary cultures of rat stromal-vascular cells grown and differentiated in serum-supplemented medium[10,11,14,17,30]. According to this concept, as a function of age, the adipose deposits contain a lower number but an increasing proportion of clones of preadipocyte cells having a decreasing sensitivity to respond to hormonal signals. However, it is important to point out that dormant cells, which may remain unresponsive in vivo, can become responsive in vitro under appropriate conditions. This appears to be the case, in serum-free chemically-defined medium, for stromal-vascular cells of abdominal fat tissue from middle-aged as well as old men and women[14]. This conclusion brings a molecular basis to previous studies which showed that rodents and man keep the ability to produce new fat cells late during adult life.

Taken together, these various observations underline the importance of identifying the panoply of biological signals which are required for terminal differentiation of preadipocytes.

Signalling pathways involved in the terminal differentiation of preadipocytes

Using serum-free, chemically-defined culture conditions, arachidonic acid has been characterized as being the main adipogenic factor present in foetal bovine serum[12]. Arachidonic acid increases in a rapid and dramatic manner the production of cyclic AMP and in parallel the late expression of GPDH activity and triacylglycerol accumulation; it is also able to amplify the terminal differentiation promoted by other cyclic AMP-elevating agents and to induce polyphosphoinositide breakdown. The triggering of cyclic AMP and inositol phospholipid pathways is accompanied by at least one round of cell division and within a few days all the cells become differentiated. Since these effects of arachidonic acid are prevented by indomethacin or aspirin, it has been postulated that one or more of the various prostaglandins produced by Ob17 cells as well as by human adipose cells, i.e. PGE_2, PGI_2 and $PGF_{2\alpha}$, could actually be involved[20]. We have thus proposed that a combination of signals – each present above a threshold level – is required for terminal differentiation of cells having expressed early markers. This combination involves prostacyclin (acting via the cyclic AMP pathway) and IGF-I as key hormones and $PGF_{2\alpha}$ and insulin as modulating hormones. According to this model, it has been predicted (and actually shown) that (i) antibodies able to neutralize PGI_2 and $PGF_{2\alpha}$ are able to block the terminal differentiation induced by arachidonic acid, (ii) any hormone active on the release of arachidonic acid and/or on the production of prostaglandins should behave as a mitogenic-adipogenic stimulus; this is indeed the case with glucocorticoids which are able to trigger terminal differentiation of Ob1771 cells by means of an increased production of PGI_2,[13] and (iii) a critical "window" of hormone action should be expected; this is the case since prostacyclin becomes unable to stimulate cAMP production once the cells become differentiated.

Another important prediction can be made since stromal-vascular cells have already expressed early markers (as shown for mouse and rat, with respect to pOb24 mRNA and IGF-I mRNA) and thus have been possibly "primed" by various hormones *in vivo*. It is assumed that the hormonal requirements for terminal differentiation of preadipocytes may well be rather limited. This is indeed the case for rat[9], mouse (D. Gaillard *et al.*, unpublished results), rabbit[26] and human preadipocytes[14] that require *in vitro* IGF-I, insulin and glucocorticoids for terminal differentiation (see Fig. 1). Last but not least, since these stimuli have to be present at the same time above threshold levels, it is assumed that the hormonal signals have to be in phase with each other. Since dormant, early marker-expressing cells are present *in vivo*, we postulate that frequent ill-timed hormone secretion, induced by diets or other means, increases the probability of such events to take place and therefore may lead to hyperplasia of adipose tissue.

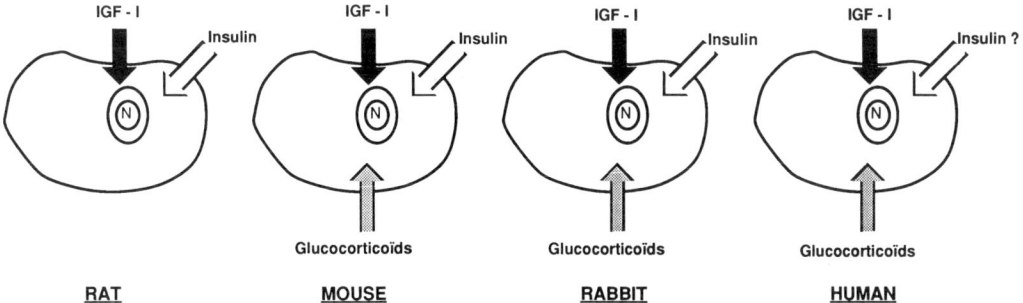

Fig. 1. *Minimal hormonal requirements in serum-free medium for terminal differentiation of preadipocytes isolated from adipose tissue.*

Relationships between brown and white adipose cells

Studies on the development of WAT and to a lesser extent on BAT have led to much controversy regarding the existence of distinct precursor cells and the interchangeability between both tissues.

The recent data favour the existence of distinct adipose precursor cells. First, it is clear that the lipolytic response of differentiated Ob17 cells (clonal line established from WAT) and BFC-1 cells (clonal line established from BAT), i.e. their sensitivity toward various β-agonists, is different. Indeed, the higher sensitivity of mouse cells originating from BAT is also observed in differentiated stromal-vascular cells in primary culture[2]. Thus, in the absence of any trophic innervation, a difference between cells originating from mouse BAT and WAT persists. Second, recent and important observations indicate that differentiated cells from BAT precursor cells express UCP in culture, in contrast to differentiated cells from WAT precursor cells[18,24,25]. Regarding the possible transformation of BAT into WAT, it is known that UCP is present in the newborn, in the human infant and in adult patients suffering from pheochromocytoma; its presence has also been recently reported in 22 subjects ranging in age from 3 to 51 years, who were not affected by this disease[8,19,27]. Among domestic species, postnatal changes have been examined with respect to the content of mitochondrial UCP of ovine adipose tissues. The uncoupling protein has been assayed by GDP-binding, photoaffinity labelling with azido-ATP and immunoblots using specific antibodies directed against rat UCP. A protein of 33 kDa has been characterized with properties similar to those of rodent UCP. All adipose tissues examined (perirenal, subscapular, pericardiac and retroperitoneal), except the subcutaneous adipose tissue, contain UCP at birth indicating that these various adipose tissues of newborn lamb can be considered as BAT.[5] It is noticeable that UCP mRNA disappears within 24 h from the peritoneal site and within 6 days from the various sites[6]. Thus the extinction of UCP gene is very rapid and suggests strongly the direct conversion of BAT adipocytes into WAT adipocytes, without excluding in addition the *de novo* formation of mature white adipocytes.

This conversion process has been shown directly by comparing the expression of UCP mRNA in stromal-vascular cells isolated from the perirenal adipose tissue of newborn and 21-day-old lambs, which are able to undergo differentiation in serum-free, chemically-defined medium. Despite the fact that terminal differentiation takes place *in vitro* in both cases (defined by the emergence of GPDH activity and the accumulation of triacylglycerol), differentiated cells from 21-day-old lambs become unable to express UCP mRNA, in contrast to differentiated cells of newborn lambs. Thus, with respect to UCP expression, precursor cells from 3-week-old animals can be considered as white adipocytes[7].

Clearly, studies focused on the "extinction" of the UCP gene, and its "reactivation" in adult animals, should shed some light on its potential role in controlling adipose tissue mass. Among possible strategies to obtain functional brown fat cells the re-expression of UCP gene, accompanied or not by cell hyperplasia, is a stimulating approach. Last but not the least, introduction of a functional UCP gene in nonexpressing UCP somatic cells represents an exciting and future aim.

Acknowledgements

The author is very grateful to the various investigators involved in these studies over the years, particularly Drs. R. Négrel and P. Grimaldi. The efficient secretarial assistance of Mrs. G. Oillaux is gratefully acknowledged.

Abbreviations

BAT, brown adipose tissue; WAT, white adipose tissue; GH, growth hormone; GPDH, glycerol-3-phosphate dehydrogenase; IGF-I, insulin-like growth factor-I; LPL, lipoprotein lipase; UCP, uncoupling protein.

References

1. Ailhaud, G. (1982): Adipose cell differentiation in culture. *Mol. Cell. Biochem.* **49**, 17-31.

2. Ailhaud, G., Amri, E., Barbaras, R., Casteilla, L., Catalioto, R.M., Dani, C., Deslex, S., Doglio, A., Forest, C., Gaillard, D., Grimaldi, P., Négrel, R., Ricquier, D. & Vannier, C. (1987): Adipose cell differentiation: differential expression of specific mRNAs and protein markers in cells from white and brown adipose tissues. In *Recent advances in obesity research: V*, eds. E.M. Berry, S.H. Blondheim, H.E. Eliahou & E. Shafrir, pp. 174-180. London: John Libbey.

3. Ailhaud, G., Amri, E.Z., Bertrand, B., Barcellini-Couget, S., Bardon, S., Catalioto, R.M., Dani, C., Deslex, S., Djian, P., Doglio, A., Figueres-Pradines, A., Forest, C., Gaillard, D., Grimaldi, P., Negrel, R. & Vannier, C. (1990): Cellular and molecular aspects of adipose tissue growth. In *Obesity: towards a molecular approach*, eds. G. Bray, D. Ricquier & B.M. Spiegelman, pp. 219-236. New York: Alan R Liss.

4. Burdi, A.R., Poissonnet, C.M., Garn, S.M., Lavelle, M., Sabet, M.D. & Bridges, P. (1985): Adipose tissue growth patterns during human gestation: a histometric comparison of buccal and gluteal fat depots. *Int. J. Obes.* **9**, 247-256.

5. Casteilla, L., Forest, C., Robelin, J., Ricquier, D., Lombet, A. & Ailhaud, G. (1987): Characterization of the mitochondrial uncoupling protein in bovine foetus and new-born calf. Disappearance in lamb during ageing. *Am. J. Physiol.* **252**, E627-E636.

6. Casteilla, L., Champigny, O., Bouillaud, F., Robelin, F. & Ricquier, D. (1989): Sequential changes in the expression of mitochondrial protein mRNA during the development of BAT in bovine and ovine species. Sudden occurence of uncoupling protein mRNA during embryogenesis and its disappearance after birth. *Biochem. J.* **257**, 665-671.

7. Casteilla, L., Nougues, J., Reyne, Y. & Ricquier, D. (1991): Differentiation of ovine brown adipocyte precursor cells in a chemically defined serum-free medium. Importance of glucocorticoids and age of animals. *Eur. J. Biochem.* 198, 195-199.

8. Cunningham, S., Leslie, P. & Hopwood, D. (1985): The characterization and energetic potential of brown adipose tissue in man. *Clin. Sci.* **69**, 343-348.

9. Deslex, S., Negrel, R. & Ailhaud, G. (1987): Development of a chemically defined serum-free medium for complete differentiation of rat adipose precursor cells. *Exp. Cell. Res.* **168**, 15-30.

10. Djian, P., Roncari, D.A.K. & Hollenberg, C.H. (1985): Adipocyte precursor clones vary in capacity for differentiation. *Metabolism* **34**, 880-883.

11. Djian, P., Roncari, D.A.K. & Hollenberg, C.H. (1983): Influence of anatomic site and age on the replication and differentiation of rat adipocyte precursors in culture. *J. Clin. Invest.* **72**, 1200-1208.

12. Gaillard, D., Négrel, R., Lagarde, M. & Ailhaud, G. (1989): Requirement and role of arachidonic acid in the differentiation of preadipose cells. *Biochem. J.* **257**, 389-397.

13. Gaillard, D., Wabtisch, M., Pipy, B. & Négrel, R. (1991): Control of terminal differentiation of adipose precursor cells by glucocorticoids. *J. Lipid Res.* **32**, 569-579.

14. Hauner, H., Entenmann, G., Wabitsch, M., Gaillard, D., Ailhaud, G., Négrel, R. & Pfeiffer, E. (1989): Promoting effect of glucocorticoids on the differentiation of human adipocyte precursor cells cultured in a chemically defined serum. *J. Clin. Invest.* **84**, 1663-1670.

15. Hausman, G.J. (1987): Identification of adipose tissue primordia in perirenal tissues of pig fetuses: utility of phosphatase histochemistry. *Acta Anat.* **128**, 236-242.

16. Ibrahimi, A., Bardon, S., Bertrand, B., Ailhaud, G. & Dani, C. (1991): Identification of a marker of the preadipose state as a protein of the extracellular matrix. In *Obesity in Europe 91*, eds. G. Ailhaud, B. Guy-Grand, M. Lafontan & D. Ricquier, pp. 347-354. London: John Libbey.

17. Kirkland, J.L., Hollenberg, C.H. & Gillon, W.S. (1990): Age, anatomic site, and the replication and differentiation of adipocyte precursors. *Am. J. Physiol.* **258**, C206-C210.

18. Kopecky, J., Baudysova, M., Zanotti, F., Dagmar, J., Pavelka, 5. & Houstek, J. (1990): Synthesis of mitochondrial uncoupling protein in brown adipocytes differentiated in cell culture. *J. Biol. Chem.* **265**, 22204-22209.

19. Lean, M.J. & James, W.P.T. (1983): Uncoupling protein in human brown adipose tissue mitochondria. *FEBS Lett.* **163**, 235-240.

20. Négrel, R., Gaillard, D. & Ailhaud, G. (1989): Prostacyclin as a potent effector of adipose cell differentiation. *Biochem. J.* **257**, 399-405.

21. Poissonnet, C.M., Burdi, A.R. & Bookstein, F.L. (1984): Critical periods of human adipogenesis: the buccal fat pad model. In *Human growth development*, eds. J. Borms, R. Hauspie, A. Sands, C. Suzanne & M. Hebbelinck, pp. 243-252. New York: Plenum Publishing Corporation.

22. Poissonnet, C.M., Burdi, A.R. & Garn, S.M. (1984): The chronology of adipose tissue appearance and distribution in the human fetus. *Early Hum. Dev.* **10**, 1-11.

23. Poissonnet, C.M., Lavelle, M. & Burdi, A.R. (1988): Growth and development of adipose tissue. *J. Pediatr.* **113**, 1-9.
24. Rehnmark, S., Kopecky, J., Jacobsson, A., Néchad, M., Herron, D., Nelson, B.D., Obregon, M.J., Nedergaard, J. & Cannon, B. (1989): Brown adipocytes differentiated *in vitro* can express the gene for the uncoupling protein thermogenin: effects of hypothyroidism and norepinephrine. *Exp. Cell. Res.* **182**, 75-83.
25. Rehnmark, S., Néchad, M., Herron, D., Cannon, B. & Nedergaard, J. (1990) α- and β-adrenergic induction of the expression of the uncoupling protein thermogenin in brown adipocytes differentiated in culture. *J. Biol. Chem.* **265**, 16464-16471.
26. Reyne, Y., Nouguès, J. & Dulor, J.P. (1989): Differentiation of rabbit adipocyte precursor cells in a serum-free medium. *In Vitro Cell. & Dev. Biol.* **25**, 747-752.
27. Ricquier, D., Nechad, M. & Mory, G. (1982): Ultrastructural and biochemical characterization of human brown adipose tissue in pheochromocytoma. *J. Clin. Endocrinol.* **54**, 803-807.
28. Rosen, B.S., Cook, K.S., Yaglom, J., Groves, D.L., Volanakis, J.E., Damm, D., White, T. & Spiegelman, B.P. (1989): Adipsin and complement factor D activity: an immune-related defect in obesity. *Science* **244**, 1483-1486.
29. Waggoner, D.W. & Bernlohr, D.A. (1990): *In situ* labelling of the adipocyte lipid binding protein with 3-[^{125}I]Iodo-4-azido-N-hexadecylsalicylamide. *J. Biol. Chem.* **265**, 11417-11420.
30. Wang, H., Kirkland, J.L. & Hollenberg, C.H. (1989): Varying capacities for replication of rat adipocyte precursor clones and adipose tissue growth. *J. Clin. Invest.* **83**, 1741-1746.

Chapter 2

Human Obesities: Chaos or Determinism?

Claude BOUCHARD
Physical Activity Sciences Laboratory, Laval University, Québec, Canada

Introduction

How important are the concepts of chaos and determinism in obesity research for the 1990s? It is the view of this author that it is absolutely essential to incorporate both, not only in the efforts to define the causes and consequences of human obesities but also in designing new and better paradigms for the treatment of the various obese conditions.

As obesity scientists and clinicians, we need all the relevant data that experimental reductionism can generate[14]. Having recognized the significance of the data generating process of modern-day science and its immense power, we must also appreciate that the reductionist approach works best with simple systems or simplified models of more complex realities. Unfortunately, human obesities are not simple systems. They are, as is recognized by most, complex phenotypes evolving under the interactive influences of dozens of affectors rooted in the social, behavioural, physiological, metabolic, cellular and molecular domains. As a result, the reductionist approach in the narrow sense has limitations despite its considerable strengths. It is essential to move some distance away from simple empirical and reductionist evidence from time to time and attempt to understand the usefulness of the data accumulated. We need to appreciate what the data are truly telling us when seen in the context of the holistic phenomenon of human obesities. Then, chaos and determinism become crucial notions that have not been considered to any extent in the past but should become regular agenda topics in the future.

Defining chaos and determinism

Before attempting to illustrate the implications of the concepts for obesity research, it is probably not superfluous to describe briefly what they mean in concrete and obesity-oriented terms. From the history of science perspective, determinism is the oldest of both concepts. Chaos, on the other hand, is the new kid on the block.

In general terms, determinism can be defined as the view or doctrine that events, facts or states reflect nature and are caused by natural laws[11,20,21]. In a strict sense, determinism implies that all phenomena, including human behaviour, have sufficient causes and can be predicted from natural laws. Thus, physics, chemistry and biology provide the set of facts and laws to understand man as an individual and social being. Determinism has been the most wonderful and fertile ideological milieu for science, reductionist science, to emerge and thrive. As scientists, we marvel at the numerous accomplishments that became possible because of reductionist science and are firm believers in the bounties it can bestow upon mankind in the immediate and more remote future.

In the context of obesity research and the human obese conditions, determinism is the precept that individual differences or fluctuations with time in body mass or body energy content have sufficient causes and can be predicted from natural laws. Here, molecular and cellular mechanisms, metabolism, organ physiology, behaviour and a variety of social conditions impact on the phenotype and exemplify nature. It should be apparent that determinism of the human obese conditions must be put in a broad conceptual framework and cannot be reduced to the so-called *gene machine*[11]. It has nonetheless both genetic and nongenetic connotations.

Chaos is a relatively newcomer in the showcase of science. It is almost the equivalent of a midlife crisis[13] for modern science and a deterministic view of nature and the world. The concept evolved from the seminal observations of Edward Lorenz, a meteorologist at MIT, around 1961, and has rapidly attracted the attention of a small group of non-conventional scientists who were fascinated by the observations that systems are never in a perfect steady state, that they are constantly influenced by small local perturbations, and that they exhibit a sensitive dependence on initial conditions[13]. Fundamentally, chaos is a state of disorder. Its presence implies that the predictive process of today's science can only be performed successfully at a distance from the actual phenomenon, where chaos is too faint to be detected and appreciated. In other words, if it was not for the naivety of our approach, or relative ignorance, or the crudeness of our observational tools, we would come to realize that predictability can be achieved only when blinded to the fine local details of the phenomenon. Biological or behavioural systems are constantly in a state of instability and we would come to realize that they are characterized by much intrinsic chaos if we could observe and scrutinize them closely. The dissipative structure described by Prigogine bears considerable resemblance to this concept[18].

One manifestation of chaos, the *butterfly effect*, initially described by Lorenz as a slight perturbation in a large system that may have considerable effects later, after passage through a number of bifurcations[13], is of relevance to obesity research. An apparently slight local perturbation affecting perhaps energy intake or food preference or level of physical activity or sensitivity to norepinephrine or one's body image may have serious implications for energy balance over months and years. Intrinsic chaos and the butterfly effect are rich notions that should be integrated in our research paradigms on both the causal chain of events of the various obesity phenotypes and their metabolic consequences. Let us examine briefly some of the evidence for the presence of chaos and determinism in the human obese condition, assuming that, like in other physical or biological realities, it is never exclusively a case of either chaos or determinism but rather an interactive network of random and predictable conditions.

Chaos or determinism or both?

We believe that the evidence for a role of chaos and *butterfly effect* in human obesities is strong. Let us retain the excess body mass or body energy content adjusted for height phenotypes[10] as the focus of the argument. The case could also be made for the phenotypes of regional fat distribution but space does not permit us to elaborate on them here.

One example of a large random component relevant to our topic can be seen in the day to day fluctuations of energy intake, macronutrient intake and alcohol intake. Thus, the within-person coefficient of variation of intake over 7 days amounts to about 25 per cent for energy and macronutrient intake and is more that 100 per cent for alcohol intake[15]. Day to day variation in level of physical activity may also be quite large[1,2,16] and this could constitute a critical factor for the lack of a tight coupling between energy intake and energy expenditure on a day to day basis. Moreover, resting metabolic rate is characterized by intraindividual variation that may amount to about 4 to 6 per cent[2,6,19]. We must also remember that the thermic response to food, even to a standardized meal test, exhibits considerable intraindividual variation when the challenge is repeated on different days. In other words, the day to day fluctuations in the various components of energy balance are quantitatively important.

It should not be surprising, therefore, that the coupling between instantaneous or daily energy intake with metabolic rate or daily energy expenditure is rather loose[10]. This has been suggested by a score of experiments but perhaps most notably by the classic observations made more than 35 years ago by Edholm and colleagues on 12 cadets followed for 14 days[12]. On the other hand, if chaos is a major actor in the short term, some kind of determinism must also be operating as suggested by the approximate convergence of the energy balance components over long periods of time in the majority of individuals.

Another facet of the chaos and determinism dyad may be reflected in the large number of low correlations that are recovered almost universally in epidemiological and experimental obesity research. Indeed, one of the major challenges of the obesity scientist remains to uncover specificity, to detect the valid signals in a situation where the noise to signal ratio appears to be particularly high. We believe that the low level of heritability (about 15 per cent) for total body energy content adjusted for stature[10] or total body fat (25 per cent)[3] provides further support for the presence and the interactive effects of both chaos and determinism in the coupling between energy intake, energy expenditure and energy storage mechanisms over time. The relative importance of whatever determinism there is in energy balance and energy storage mechanisms does not appear to be overwhelming. As a matter of fact, the heritability data suggest that if determinism is defined in terms of DNA sequence variations that impact on the outcome phenotype, its relative importance is quite low among the other sources of variation from a population point of view. Of course, the corollary of the population data is that DNA sequence variation determinism is of trivial importance for a large number of individuals. It seems as if whatever genetic determinism there is for the energy balance components and energy storage mechanisms, it is easily overridden by food preferences, social factors and a variety of behavioural adjustments. However, one cannot yet rule out the possibility that some forms of DNA sequence variation determinism may define the high-risk persons. I believe that we have come to recognize that being at risk for the development of an excessive body energy content is not equivalent to being a case because of the large behavioural component of obesity but also perhaps because of chaos.

Response to overfeeding: chaos or determinism?

One may learn much from cross sectional correlations or group comparisons and, needless to say, these study designs dominate in the field of obesity research. However, cross-sectional data may, at times, be misleading and, in fact, support conclusions opposite to those reached from longitudinal observations or experimental interventions. This was recently illustrated by Zurlo et al.[22] who reported that, while a low respiratory quotient is generally observed in obese subjects studied cross-sectionally, a low respiratory quotient was protective from weight gain over a mean of 25 months in 111 Pima Indians ($r = 0.24; P = 0.01$). It seems reasonable to assume that one can potentially learn more about chaos and determinism on body mass fluctuations from longitudinal data, particularly from intervention studies with controls over the energy balance components. Our recently completed long term experimental overfeeding study with 12 pairs of identical twins would seem to provide this type data.

Twelve pairs of male identical twins ate a 4.2 MJ (1000 kcal) per day caloric surplus, 6 days a week, during a period of 100 days for a total overfeeding stimulus of 353 MJ (84,000 kcal)[8]. Significant increases in body weight, fat mass, fat-free mass, and body energy content were observed after the period of overfeeding. Data showed that there were considerable interindividual differences in the adaptation to excess calories and that the variation observed was not randomly distributed, as indicated by the significant within-pair resemblance in response. There was at least 3 times more variance in response between pairs than within pairs for the gains in body mass, fat mass, fat-free mass, and body energy content. This is illustrated in Fig. 1 which describes the mean change, the individual response and the twin resemblance in the response to overfeeding for body weight. These data, and those that we have reported earlier for the response to short-term overfeeding[4,17], demonstrate that some individuals are more at risk than others of gaining weight when energy intake surplus is clamped at the same level for everyone and when all subjects are confined to a sedentary lifestyle. The within-identical-twin pair response to the standardized caloric surplus suggests that the amount of body mass gained is likely influenced by the genotype. The genetic effect is, however, moderate and can only account at most for about 50 per cent of the variation in the response to the overfeeding protocol as suggested by the intraclass coefficient computed with the changes in weight gain (Fig. 1). This value is likely to represent the maximal estimate for the genetic effect. In reality the value is probably less as the within-pair similarity in behaviour as well as in physiology and metabolism, resulting from past similar experiences, may have also contributed in an unknown manner to the within-pair resemblance in weight gain.

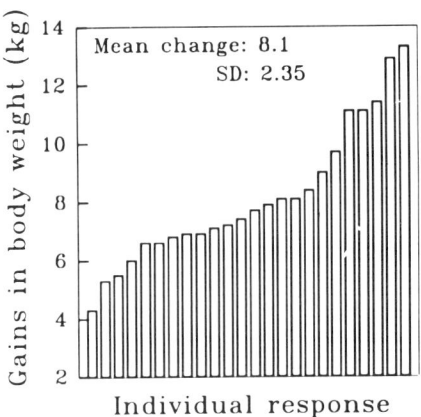
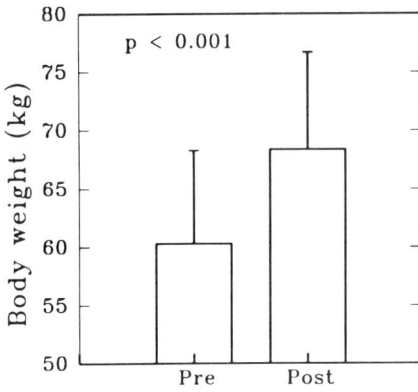

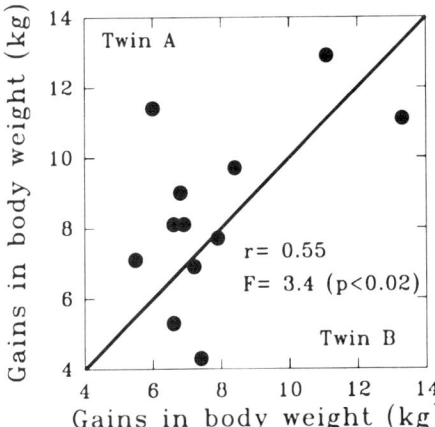

Fig. 1. The response of body weight to a standardized 100-day overfeeding protocol in 12 pairs of identical twins. Adapted from Bouchard et al. (1990): N. Engl. J. Med. **322**, 1477-1482, by permission from the Massachusetts Medical Society.

The mean body-mass gain for the 24 subjects of the 100-day overfeeding experiment was 8.1 kg, of which 5.4 kg were fat mass and 2.7 kg were fat-free mass increases. Thus, a total of 222 MJ were recovered on the average as body-mass changes. This represents about 63 per cent of the excess energy intake. While the mean gain of fat mass to fat-free mass ratio was 2 to 1, there were individual differences in response among the 24 subjects. The variations in the fat mass to fat-free mass ratio (as an indicator of nutrient partitioning) changes in response to overfeeding were correlated with the changes in body mass, and the coefficient reached 0.61 ($P < 0.01$)[8]. In other words, about 37 per cent of the variation in weight gain as a result of exposure to long term overfeeding was associated with nutrient partitioning. Those who gained more fat relative to fat-free tissues were the high gainers for body mass while those who gained relatively more lean tissues were the low gainers. Again, however, there was about 3 times more variance between pairs than within pairs (intraclass coefficient of 0.53) for the changes in fat mass to fat-free mass, hardly an indication of a very strong genetic determinism for this indicator of nutrient partitioning.

The data therefore suggest that when energy intake with a relatively constant macronutrient composition is clamped at the same level above baseline, two main classes of factors are involved in determining the changes in body mass. These are schematically illustrated in Fig.2[7,10]. It would seem from the long term overfeeding study summarized here that nutrient partitioning is the single most important factor to explain the individuality in body mass changes under these experimental conditions. Thus, nutrient partitioning, which reflects current local status of energy storage mechanisms, carries considerable implications for the risk of becoming obese or the protection from obesity. The chances are that a substantial proportion of those prone or resistant to obesity find themselves in this vulnerable or desirable position because of inherited or acquired differences in nutrient-partitioning mechanisms. The other class of factors is one which includes the various components of energy expenditure, i.e. basal and resting metabolic rates, thermic response to food, temperature-induced thermogenesis, energy expenditure of physical activity and fidgeting, and perhaps others. Here, low level relationships with body mass fluctuations are universally reported. This is undoubtedly a class of determinants in which the signal to noise ratio is high as a result of several factors including frequent local perturbations. In addition, let us keep in mind that energy intake and macronutrient composition of the diet are never kept constant and that they fluctuate over a wide range of values for the same individual.

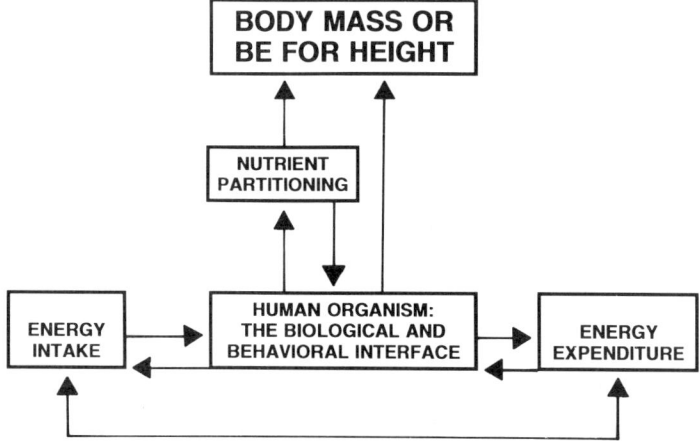

Fig. 2. A paradigm of the major affectors of body mass or body energy content adjusted for height. Modified from Bouchard, C. (1990): Revue du Praticien **40**, 1773-1776.

In my judgement, the main message of this experimental overfeeding study with twins is that it provides support for a role of both chaos and genetic and nongenetic determinism. No long term experimental intervention study with human subjects can be perfect even when full compliance with the treatment can be achieved. Recognizing this fact, the individual differences in response are too large and the twin resemblance is so moderate in this experiment to conclude that genetic variations (between pairs) determine the whole response to overfeeding or that it is even the major determinant. It is unfortunate that a similar experiment but with a clamp over energy expenditure is not feasible, as it could provide information on the extent of energy intake and nutrient composition fluctuations when metabolic rates and activity levels are standardized.

The challenge of uncovering genetic determinism

Our current body of knowledge on the genetic basis of body energy content, overweight or obesity is quite limited and of generally poor quality. There are several reasons for this situation but two are particularly damaging. The first problem lies with the fact that most studies have been conducted with a poorly measured phenotype. A properly assessed phenotype is a sine qua non condition for a valid genetic study. Thus we have not learned much by relying on the body mass index, specially when neither body weight and stature were measured or when recall body weight was used, as the phenotype for genetic investigation and the yield will likely not improve with time. Why the body mass index is a poor phenotype is shown in Table 1. It does not constitute an acceptable proxy variable for the fat content, the fat-free mass, the amount of subcutaneous fat or for the regional distribution of subcutaneous fat in men or in women.

Table 1. Common variance ($r^2 \times 100$) between BMI and body composition in adults[*]

	BMI in 342 males	BMI in 356 females
Per cent fat	41	40
Fat-free mass	37	25
Sum 6 skinfolds	58	67
Trunk/limb skinfolds	10	8

[*]35 to 54 years of age

The second reason is that too few investigators are designing genetic studies or experiments to address specific genetic issues. Scientists were originally justified in massaging existing data bases to ascertain whether there was familial resemblance for the body mass index and to compute heritability estimates. We have long passed this stage now and we need properly designed genetic studies with adequate phenotype assessment and measurements of the physiological, metabolic and behavioural affectors, allowing for testing hypotheses about relevant candidate causes and candidate genes. The task is very complex if the view presented in this paper about the role of chaos and determinism is realistic, which we believe it is. Based on the above and our recent reviews of the available data[5,9,10], we propose that the scenario summarized in Table 2 is one that obesity scientists must come to terms with. It specifies that the current evidence is to the effect that variation in body energy content adjusted for stature has a low heritability level, with no detectable single gene effect, no clear maternal or paternal effect, no X or Y chromosome specific effect and no sex-specific effect. It is, however, characterized by a large number of biological affectors, a large number of behavioural and social correlates and a large number of potential candidate genes. This is clearly the least desirable scenario if one is interested in the genetic basis of a complex quantitative phenotype. The noise to signal ratio in the relationship between a candidate gene and a relevant obesity phenotype is likely to be quite high, particularly in cross-sectional observations. Defining the haplotypes at risk will therefore be a complex undertaking requiring innovative approaches and solid data bases.

Table 2. A summary of the current status of our knowledge about the genetic basis of body fat or body energy content phenotypes

Low level of heritability
No major gene effect
No maternal or paternal effect
No sex-specific effect
No X or Y effect
Large number of biological affectors
Large number of non-biological correlates
Large number of potential candidate genes

We need all the power that experimental reductionism can contribute to improve our understanding of human obesities This is particularly true in light of the perceived urgency and necessity to define the genetic basis of excessive body energy content. Of course, it applies also to the regional fat distribution profile, especially to the size of the atherogenic abdominal visceral fat depot. Until the role of DNA sequence variation at relevant genes is properly understood, it will be impossible to be precise about individual differences in susceptibility to develop excessive body energy content, about risk levels and about the importance of chaos and of genetic and nongenetic determinism. The optimism of this author is dampened by the fact that the currently available data imply that the worst possible scenario for the study of a quantitative multifactorial phenotype is one which seems most likely to apply to the obesity phenotypes. We therefore believe that an understanding of genetic versus nongenetic determinism of obesities is a long way off. In addition, because predictability is generally low in human obesity research paradigms, even under the best of circumstances, the task of defining the true contribution of chaos in the energy balance equation and body energy storage mechanisms will probably have to await further development.

Acknowledgements

The research of the author on the genetics of obesity is supported by the Medical Research Council of Canada (MA-10499) and the National Institutes of Health of the USA (DK-34624).

References

1. Bouchard, C., Tremblay, A., Leblanc, C., Lortie, G., Savard, R. & Thériault G. (1983): A method to assess energy expenditure in children and adults. *Am. J. Clin. Nutr.* **37**, 461-467.
2. Bouchard, C. (1985): Reproducibility of body composition and adipose-tissue measurements in humans. In *Body composition assessments in youth and adults*. Report of the 6th Ross conference on medical research, ed. A.F. Roche, pp.9-14. Columbus, Ohio: Ross Laboratories.
3. Bouchard, C., Pérusse, L., Leblanc, C., Tremblay, A. & Thériault, G. (1988): Inheritance of the amount and distribution of human body fat. *Int. J. Obes.* **12**, 205-215.
4. Bouchard, C., Tremblay, A., Despres, J.P., Poehlman, E.T., Theriault, G., Nadeau, A., Lupien, P., Moorjani, S. & Dussault, J. (1988): Sensitivity to overfeeding: the Quebec experiment with identical twins. *Prog. Food Nutr. Sci.* **12**, 45-72.
5. Bouchard, C. (1989): Genetic factors in obesity. *Med. Clin. North Am.* **73**, 67-81.
6. Bouchard, C., Tremblay, A., Nadeau, A., Després, J.P., Thériault, G., Boulay, M.R., Lortie, G., Leblanc, C. & Fournier, G. (1989): Genetic effect in resting and exercise metabolic rates. *Metabolism* **38**, 364-370.
7. Bouchard, C. (1990): L'obésité est-elle héréditaire? *Rev. Prat.* **40**, 1773-1776.
8. Bouchard, C., Tremblay, A., Després, J.P., Nadeau, A., Lupien, P.J., Thériault, G., Dussault, J., Moorjani, S., Pinault, S. & Fournier, G. (1990): The response to longterm overfeeding in identical twins. *N. Engl. J. Med.* **322**, 1477-1482.

9. Bouchard, C. (1991): Heredity and the path to overweight and obesity. *Med. Sci. Sports Exerc.* **23**, 285-291.
10. Bouchard, C., Tremblay, A., Després, J.P., Deriaz, O. & Dionne, F.T. : The genetics of body content and energy balance: an overview. In *The science of food regulation*, ed. G.A. Bray, New Orleans: Louisiana University Press. (in press).
11. Dawkins, F. (1978): *The selfish gene*, pp. 224. Oxford: Oxford University Press.
12. Edholm, O.G., Fletcher, J.G., Widdowson, E.M. & McCance, F.A. (1955): The energy expenditure and food intake of individual men. *Br. J. Nutr.* **9**, 286-300.
13. Gleick, J. (1988): *Chaos: making a new science*, pp. 352. New York: Penguin Books.
14. Hirsch, J. (1987): Willendorf Lecture: The judgment of Solomon (I Kings 3, 16-28). In *Recent advances in obesity research: V*, ed. E.M. Berry, S.H. Blondheim, H.E. Eliahou & E. Shafrir, pp. 1-4. London: John Libbey.
15. McGee, D., Rhoads, G., Hankin, J., Yano, K. & Tillotson, J. (1982): Within-person variability of nutrient intake in a group of Hawaiian men of Japanese ancestry. *Am. J. Clin. Nutr.* **36**, 657-663.
16. Pérusse, L., Tremblay, A., Leblanc, C. & Bouchard, C. (1989): Genetic and environmental influences on level of habitual physical activity and exercise participation. *Am. J. Epidemiol.* **129**, 1012-1022.
17. Poehlman, E.T., Tremblay, A., Després, J.P., Fontaine, E., Pérusse, L., Thériault, G. & Bouchard, C. (1986): Genotype-controlled changes in body composition and fat morphology following overfeeding in twins. *Am. J. Clin. Nutr.* **43**, 723-731.
18. Prigogine, I. & Goldbeter, A. (1979): Nonequilibrium self-organization in biochemical systems. In *Biochemistry of exercise IV-A*, eds. J. Poortmans & G. Niset, pp. 3-12. Baltimore: University Park Press.
19. Ravussin, E. & Bogardus, C. (1989): Relationship of genetics, age, and physical fitness to daily energy expenditure and fuel utilization. *Am. J. Clin. Nutr.* **49**, 968-975.
20. Thuillier, P. (1981): *Les biologistes vont-ils prendre le pouvoir?*, pp. 327. Bruxelles: Editions Complexe.
21. Wilson, E.O. (1978): *On human nature*, pp. 260. Cambridge, Massachusetts: Harvard University Press.
22. Zurlo, F., Lillioja, S., Esposito-Del Puente, A., Nyomba, B.L., Raz, I., Saad, M.F., Swinburn, B.A., Knowler, W.C., Bogardus, C. & Ravussin, E. (1990): Low ratio of fat to carbohydrate oxidation as predictor of weight gain: study of 24-h RQ. *Am. J. Physiol.* **259** (*Endocrinol. Metab.* **22**), E650-E657.

Section I
Multifaceted aspects of human obesity

Chapter 3

Self-reported Intake as a Measure for Energy Intake
A Validation Against Doubly Labelled Water

K.R. WESTERTERP, W.P.H.G. VERBOEKET-VAN de VENNE, G.A.L. MEIJER
and F. ten HOOR
Department of Human Biology, University of Limburg, 6200 MD Maastricht, The Netherlands

Introduction

In nutrition research, data on energy intake (EI) are used for comparison of energy balance between subjects, to detect changes in energy balance within subjects or as a basis for nutrition intervention. Recently, there has been discussion on the reliability of the results of self-reported intake as a measure for EI with the introduction of doubly labelled water as a method to measure energy expenditure (EE)[7]. The doubly labelled water method allows validation of data on EI in situations where subjects are in energy balance.

There are several methods for measuring dietary intake. Commonly used are dietary recall, including dietary history, and dietary records. We chose dietary records to measure EI. The dietary record is supposed to be superior to the dietary recall with regard to actual consumption, not relying on the memory of the subject. The disadvantage is that subjects, having to record all they eat, may change their feeding habits.

Data on EI were compared with EE measured with doubly labelled water. The doubly labelled water method measures EE under normal living conditions with an accuracy of 1–3 per cent and a precision of 2–8 per cent[6]. When subjects are in energy balance EI equals EE. Thus, doubly labelled water is the ideal method to validate measurements of EI. The present study compares data on EI and EE in three different settings:

(a) A comparison between obese and lean subjects[3]
(b) The change of energy metabolism in subjects after an activity intervention[9]
(c) Subjects fed according to their reported dietary intake.

Methods

Subject characteristics are presented in Table 1, grouped according to the three studies: comparison between lean and obese (A), activity intervention (B), and feeding intervention study (C), respectively. Study A and B included females and males, study C was in males only. All subjects were adults covering the age range between 22 and 62. Most of them had regular jobs or were engaged in house-work. The mean body mass index (BMI) in the lean groups in study A was slightly but not significantly lower than the mean BMI of subjects of the same gender in study B and C. Obese subjects in study A had significantly higher BMI values than subjects of the same gender in study B and C.

Table 1. Subject characteristics in three studies, A: Comparison of lean and obese, B: Activity intervention, C: Feeding intervention

Study	Subject		n	Age (y)	Height (m)	Body mass (kg)	BMI (kg/m^2)
A	Women	lean	5	28 ± 7	1.66 ± 0.04	53.8 ± 2.1	19.7 ± 1.3
		obese	6	34 ± 7	1.73 ± 0.11	94.5 ± 19.9	31.3 ± 3.3
	Men	lean	6	37 ± 3	1.75 ± 0.05	74.0 ± 8.4	24.0 ± 1.5
		obese	4	37 ± 4	1.83 ± 0.06	109.2 ± 20.1	32.3 ± 4.2
B	Women		8	36 ± 4	1.68 ± 0.07	67.0 ± 6.9	23.7 ± 2.0
	Men		8	37 ± 3	1.78 ± 0.06	71.0 ± 5.4	22.4 ± 2.0
C	Men		9	41 ± 11	1.77 ± 0.06	77.0 ± 12.9	24.5 ± 3.5

Study A was designed to compare energy metabolism of obese men and women under free-living conditions. There was no interference with either EI or EE. In study B, the effect of an increase in physical activity on energy balance was investigated, not interfering with energy intake. Initially sedentary subjects were trained during 40 weeks to run a 1/2 marathon. In study C, the effect of the pattern of energy intake on energy expenditure was investigated. Subjects were fed over two weeks with a fixed amount of energy, based on their recorded intake. For one week the food provided had to be consumed in two big meals per day and for the other week in seven small meals.

Energy intake was measured with a 7-day dietary record. Subjects recorded all foods consumed in a diary, including brand names and cooking recipes where applicable. The diary was divided into 7 periods a day, 3 meals and 4 inter-meal periods. The foods were weighed or quantified in household measures. Volumes of repeatedly used utensils were measured with a 400 ml cup with 10 ml scaling. A dietician instructed the subjects before the observation period started. The diary included a written out example of a full day's intake and subjects were contacted by telephone in the middle of the week to solve any problems. During a short session with the subject at the end of the week the diary was examined to eliminate inconsistencies etc. The energy content of the foods was calculated using the Dutch food composition table[2].

Energy expenditure was measured over two weeks with doubly labelled water. In study A and B, the first week of the two-week interval coincided with the measurement of EI. In study C, subjects were fed over the two-week interval according to their reported intake as recorded over a week preceding the interval. Subjects drank a weighed amount of an isotope mixture of 10APE ^{18}O and 5APE ^{2}H. The dose was calculated to create an excess of 300 ppm ^{18}O and 150 ppm ^{2}H. The isotope mixture was administered in the evening between 22.00 and 23.00 h, just before subjects went to sleep, after collecting a background sample. Isotopes were measured in urine using an Aqua Sira® Isotope Ratio Mass spectrometer from VG-Isogas Ltd, Middlewich, Cheshire, England. Further urine samples were collected on days 1, 8, and 15 after dosing from the second voiding in the morning. Carbon dioxide production was calculated from isotope ratios in baseline, and 1-day, 8-day, and 15-day samples with the equation from Schoeller as described by Westerterp et al.[10]. Carbon dioxide production was converted to EE by using a respiratory quotient of 0.85, the average food quotient of the subjects as calculated from the 7-day dietary records.

Energy balance over the two week observation interval with doubly labelled water was measured by weighing subjects (study A and C). Subjects stayed the night before the start of the interval and the last night of the interval in a respiration chamber. Here, body mass was measured upon rising, after emptying the bladder and without clothes, on the same balance ±0.1 kg. The energy balance of the subjects in study B was calculated from changes in body mass and body composition over the full 40 week intervention period. Here, EI, EE, and body composition were measured before and at the end of the training period.

Results

Subjects in study A were in energy balance over the two-week observation interval with doubly labelled water. Body mass changes were nonsignificantly different from zero in all groups, i.e. 0.1 ± 1.3, -0.2 ± 1.2, 0.0 ± 1.3, and -1.1 ± 0.9 kg (mean $\pm$ SD), for lean and obese females and for lean and obese males, respectively. Combining females and males the body mass changes were nonsignificant as well, i.e. -0.1 ± 0.6 and -0.5 ± 1.1 kg, for the lean and the obese, respectively. Thus, there was a tendency for a slight but nonsignificant weight loss. Differences between reported EI and measured EE were -11 ± 15 and -30 ± 18 per cent of EE, for the lean and the obese, respectively. Thus, there was no significant difference between EI and EE in the lean group but EI in the obese group was systematically lower than EE (Wilcoxon signed rank, $P < 0.01$). The difference between EI and EE was not related to body mass changes, neither in the lean group and the obese group separately, nor in the group as a whole. The difference between EI and EE was related to the degree of overweight as expressed in the value of the BMI (Fig. 1A, Pearson $r = 0.56$, $P < 0.01$).

Subjects in study B were weight stable before the start of the training period (B_0). Over the 40 week training interval EE increased 30 per cent (B_{40}). Females did not show a significant

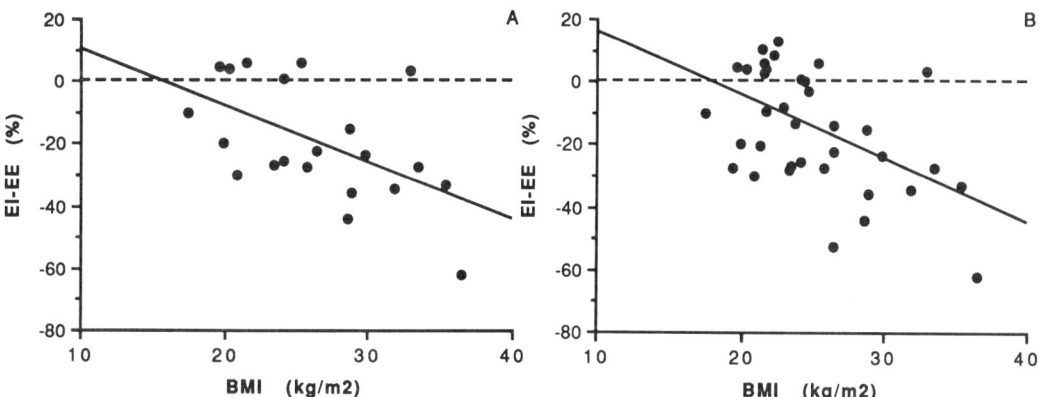

Fig. 1. Reported energy intake (EI) minus measured energy expenditure (EE), expressed as a percentage of EE and plotted as a function of the body mass index (BMI) with the calculated linear regression line. A: results from study A, n = 21; B: results from study A and B_0, n = 37.

change in body mass, losing on average 2.8 kg fat mass (FM) and gaining 2.1 kg fat-free mass (FFM). Males showed an average body mass change of -1.3 kg, losing 4.5 kg FM and gaining 3.2 kg FFM. Before the start of the training intervention, the difference between EI and EE was -5 ± 28 per cent, a result comparable to the observation in the lean subjects of study A. Average EI was not different from average EE though on the individual level discrepancies ranged between +22 and -52 per cent. In Fig. 1B the results from study A and study B_0 are plotted together, strenghtening the result already shown in Fig. 1A. Out of the original 16 subjects, 13 completed the training and were observed again after 40 weeks. At that time, there was a significant difference between intake and expenditure, EI−EE= -19 ± 17 per cent ($P < 0.01$). Figure 2 shows EI plotted as a function of EE, before and at the end of the training in the 13 subjects. Before the training EI was higher than EE in 6 out of 13 and at the end of the training in only 1 out of 13 subjects.

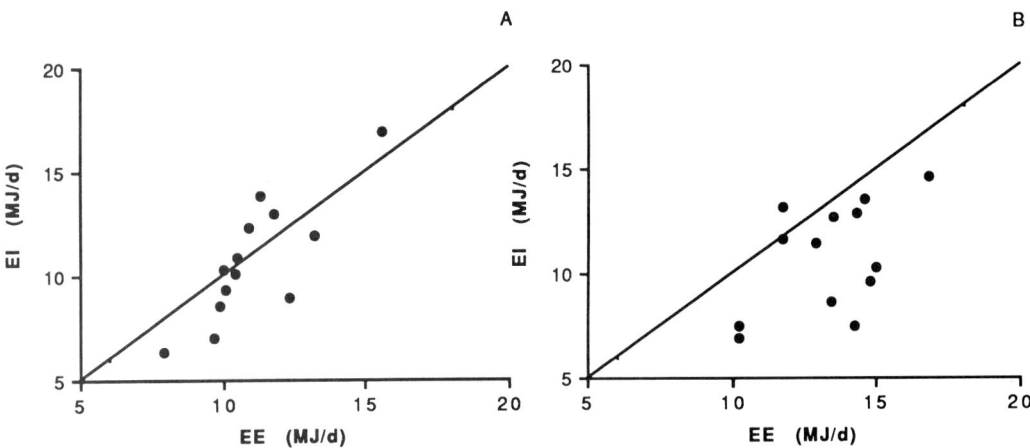

Fig. 2. Reported energy intake (EI) plotted as a function of measured energy expenditure (EE) with the line of identity. A: results from 13 subjects before the start of a training programme; B: results from the same 13 subjects at the end of a 40 week training programme.

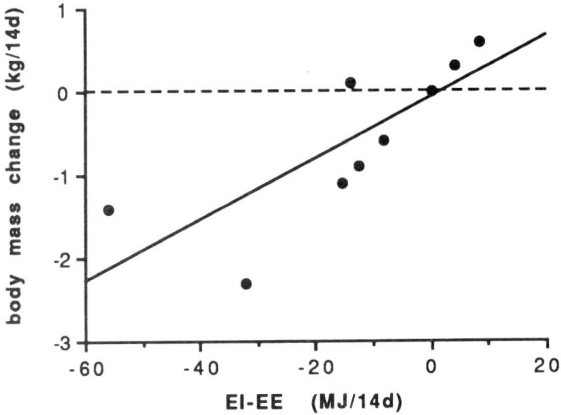

Fig. 3. Body mass change over a 14 day interval plotted as a function of energy intake (EI) minus energy expenditure (EE) over the same interval with the calculated linear regression line. EI is the energy content of the food as supplied according to reported intake, and EE is then measured (see text for further details).

Subjects in study C were fed for two weeks according to their reported EI. The average body mass change was −0.6 ± 0.9 kg over the two week interval. Individual body mass changes ranged between +0.6 and −2.3 kg. There was a significant relationship between the discrepancy between EI and EE and the body mass change over the observation interval (Pearson r = 0.80, $P < 0.01$), subjects with the highest energy deficit losing most weight (Fig. 3).

Discussion

In all three studies reported EI tended to be lower or was significantly lower than measured EE. There are two possible reasons for this discrepancy: subjects were not in energy balance or underreported their intake, assuming the procedure used to calculate EI from the 7-day diary was accurate as well as the calculated EE from the doubly labelled water method. The two reasons mentioned above will be discussed after discussion of the two assumptions.

Subjects reported their intake mainly in household measures instead of weighing every item to facilitate the procedure. This might introduce bias and therefore the measured volumes of the utensils of their own household were used to calculate the quantities. Using the national food composition table with added information on local foods guaranteed the most accurate procedure to convert the quantities to energy.

The measurement of EE with doubly labelled water has proved to be accurate and precise. Differences between simultaneous measurement of carbon dioxide production with doubly labelled water and respirometry have shown the validity of the method[6]. There is consensus regarding the calculation procedure of carbon dioxide production from the isotope elimination rates[5]. In the present study, the conversion of carbon dioxide production to energy expenditure needs further discussion. The energy equivalent of carbon dioxide depends on the energy substrate used, i.e. carbohydrate, protein, or fat. For pure carbohydrate oxidation the value is 21.1 kJ/l, at pure fat oxidation 27.5 kJ/l, and for pure alcohol it goes up to 30.5 kJ/l. In practice the body uses a fuel mixture which can be assessed from the nutrient composition of the diet, correcting for changes in body composition. This procedure reduces the potential error from this source to less than 2 per cent[1]. Even in the situation of imbalance between EI and EE like the situation in study C and during the activity intervention in study B, the potential error from this source is below 2 per cent. In any case the calculated value of EE increases when body fat contributes to oxidation at a negative energy balance as can be seen from the energy equivalents referred above. Thus, the discrepancy between EI and EE seen in all studies is not overestimated, because subjects were in energy balance or tended to be in a negative energy balance.

In conclusion, self reported dietary intake underestimates energy needs, even when a reliable method is used to measure intake. We can only speculate about the reasons for underreporting. Obese people often suggest that their intake is normal or even lower than normal and consequently suggest a low level of EE as the reason for overweight. Prentice et al.[4] showed that EE in obese people is significantly higher than in lean controls. They observed a mean difference between reported EI and measured EE of 33 per cent while the corresponding difference in the lean group was only 2 per cent, which is in line with the present study. The reason for underreporting in the obese might be the wish to eat less and consequently underestimate real intake. Lean people are not expected to have any reason for underreporting on purpose. We only measured significant underreporting in lean subjects in study B, when EE was increased by 30 per cent with a training programme and they had to report their intake again. Both factors are probably important. Subjects may have reported with a bias to their usual, lower, intake. The fact that they had to keep a 7-day dietary record for the fourth time appeared to be a real burden according to their reactions. Results from the second and third dietary record, 8 and 20 weeks after the start of the training period are not reported here as EE was only measured in a subselection of subjects. Finally, keeping a dietary record possibly influences habitual intake in a negative sense. It is impossible to discern whether the small differences between EI and EE in the lean subjects are due to underreporting or dieting. Whatever the reason might be, data on self reported intake have to be interpreted with great care, particularly in the obese.

Summary

In nutrition research, a 7-day dietary record is often used as a measure for energy intake (EI). The doubly labelled water method allows us to validate this method in situations where subjects are in energy balance. Here three such studies are presented:

(a) 11 Obese and 11 lean subjects kept a 7-day dietary record.

(b) 13 Lean subjects kept a 7-day dietary record before and 40 weeks after the start of an activity intervention.

(c) 9 Subjects were fed for two weeks according to their 7-day reported dietary intake.

In all three studies energy expenditure (EE) was measured simultaneously with doubly labelled water. Subjects in study A and B were weight stable, indicating energy balance (EI = EE). Reported EI was not different from measured EE in the lean subjects of study A and the subjects, first observed, in study B (EI – EE = –12 ± 17% of EE, mean ± SD). Overweight subjects underreported (EI – EE = –26 ± 18% of EE) and underreporting was closely related to the degree of overweight (BMI, $P < 0.01$). Lean subjects also significantly underreported when observed for a second time (study B, $P < 0.01$). Subjects fed according to their first recorded EI (study C) were in negative energy balance (EI – EE = –17 ± 9% of EE). EI – EE was related to the change in body mass over the two week observation period ($P < 0.05$). In conclusion, self reported dietary intake underestimates energy needs, even when the most reliable method is used: the 7-day record.

References

1. Black, A.E., Prentice, A.M. & Coward, W.A. (1986): Use of food quotients to predict respiratory quotients for the doubly labelled water method for measuring energy expenditure. *Hum. Nutr. Clin. Nutr.* **40C**, 381-391.
2. Hautvast, J.G.A.J. (1975): Ontwikkeling van een systeem om gegevens van voedings-enquetes met behulp van een computer te verwerken. *Voeding* **36**, 356-361.
3. Meijer, G.A.L. (1990): Physical activity: implications for human energy metabolism. Thesis Rijksuniversiteit Limburg, Maastricht: Datawyse.
4. Prentice, A.M., Black, A.E., Coward, W.A., Davies, H.L., Goldberg, G.R., Murgatroyd, P.R., Ashford, J., Sawyer, M. & Whitehead, R.G. (1986): High levels of energy expenditure in obese women. *B. M. J.* **292**, 983-987.
5. Prentice, A. M. (1990): The doubly-labelled water method for measuring energy expenditure, technical recommendations for use in humans. Nahres-4, International Atomic Energy Agency, Vienna.
6. Schoeller, D.A. (1988): Measurement of energy expenditure in free-living humans by using doubly labelled water. *J. Nutr.* **118**, 1278-1289.
7. Schoeller, D.A. (1990): How accurate is self-reported dietary energy intake. *Nutr. Rev.* **48**, 373-379.
8. Schultz, S., Westerterp, K.R. & Brück, K. (1989): Comparison of energy expenditure by the doubly labelled water technique with energy intake, heart rate, and activity recording in man. *Am. J. Clin. Nutr.* **49**, 1146-1154.
9. Westerterp, K.R., Meijer, G.A.L., Janssen, E.M.E., Saris, W.H.M. & ten Hoor, F.: Long term effect of physical activity on energy balance. *Br. J. Nutr.* (in press).
10. Westerterp, K.R. & Saris, W.H.M. (1991): Limits of energy turnover in relation to physical performance, achievement of energy balance on a daily basis. *J. Sports Sci.* **9**, 1-15

Chapter 4

Effect of a Very Low Calorie Diet on Muscle Bioenergetics at Rest and During Exercise: 31-P Nuclear Magnetic Resonance Study

V. ŠTICH, M. HÁJEK, A. HORSKÁ, V. HAINER, J. VĚTVICKA, J. HRDINA, and M. KUNEŠOVÁ

Obesity Unit, 4th Department of Internal Medicine, Charles University, U nemocnice 2, 128 08 Prague 2; Institute of Clinical and Experimental Medicine, Videnska 800, Prague 4; Institute of Sports Medicine, Prague, Czechoslovakia

Summary

The effect of a 28 days' very low calorie diet (1600 kJ/day) on bioenergetics in the calf muscle at rest and during moderate aerobic exercise was studied in six obese patients (BMI 40.1 ± 2.1 kg/m^2; weight 112.3 ± 8.2 kg) using 31-P NMR *in vivo* spectroscopy. The mean weight loss was 11.2 ± 0.70 kg. The phosphocreatine to inorganic phosphate ratio (PCr/P$_i$) declined after the diet ($P < 0.05$) at rest and showed a tendency towards decreased values after the diet at exercise. Other indices of the metabolic cost of the work were not changed in the course of the diet. The mean PCr/P$_i$ value at rest prior to diet in the obese group did not differ from that of normal-weight subjects. The phosphocreatine to phosphodiester ratio at rest in obese subjects was lower compared to normals and further decreased significantly ($P < 0.05$) after the diet. The results suggest that severe caloric restriction in obese patients may affect bioenergetics of the skeletal muscle.

Introduction

Previous studies have shown that hypocaloric diet or fasting alter skeletal muscle function in humans[5,6,7] and experimental animals[5,11] and modify skeletal muscle bioenergetics at rest[10,11]. Very low calorie diets (VLCD) are used in the treatment of obesity in conjunction with exercise. It is essential, for the safe prescription of exercise during the course of the diet, to be aware of the effects of VLCD on muscle energy metabolism. NMR 31-P spectroscopy appears to be an ideal tool for the longitudinal follow-up of intramuscular changes during the diet. To our knowledge up to today no study has paid attention to the changes in phosphagen concentration in the muscles of patients treated by VLCD.

Subjects and methods

Six obese patients, 5 females and 1 male without a concurrent disease participated in the study. Their mean age was 41 ± 2.7 years, weight 112 ± 8.2 kg, BMI 40.1 ± 2.1 kg/m^2. The patients received a VLCD diet of 1600 kJ/day (33 g protein, 50 g carbohydrate, 6 g fat) for 28 days[4]. Before starting the VLCD the subjects were on their normal diet. During the week prior to VLCD treatment and during the last week of the diet, NMR spectroscopy measurements were carried out as well as submaximal tests on a bicycle ergometer, routine hormonal tests (using commercially available kits) and anthropometric measurements. Body fat was determined using the 10 skinfold method[9].

NMR measurements

NMR spectroscopy was performed in the 1.5 T magnet of a Magnetom (Siemens) clinical whole body system operating at 25.7 MHz for 31-P nuclei. An 8 cm surface coil was used to acquire spectra from the calf muscle as a whole. Spectra were acquired with a repetition time of 1.9 s with 128 and 32 acquisitions during rest and exercise respectively, resulting in measurement duration of 4.3 and 1 min respectively. No correction for saturation was applied.

Exercise protocol

The subjects were asked to flex the ankle (plantar flexion) with a frequency of 1/per 2 s against a load of 20 kg for 4 min. Total work was calculated by multiplying the load by the height of a lift of the load multiplied by the number of lifts. A submaximal test was performed at 80 W.

Data treatment

Base line correction and peak integration were made with a standard software routine of Magnetom. The ratios of phosphocreatine (PCr) to inorganic phosphate (P_i) concentrations, PCr to adenosintriphosphate (ATP) and PCr to phosphodiester (PDE) concentrations were determined. pH was calculated according to the Henderson–Hasselbach formula using the chemical shift difference between P_i and PCr. V_{max} was calculated according to Chance[3], being introduced as an expression of maximal oxidative metabolism of a working muscle in steady state conditions:

$$V_{max} = V*(1 + 0.6/[P_i/PCr])$$

where V is the work performed during the exercise (J/min).

Results

The evolution of anthropometric data during the course of the VLCD are presented in Table 1. The mean weight reduction was 11.2 ± 0.7 kg, the mean lean body mass (LBM) decrease was 4.6 kg. Table 2 presents some of spiroergometric data of the submaximal test before and after the diet. The reduction of the steady-state oxygen consumption, being significant for the absolute values, is not significant anymore when related to LBM. No change in heart rate during the submaximal test due to diet was found. T_3 plasma levels before and after the diet (2.13 ± 0.23 and 1.97 ± 0.18 nmol/l respectively) were not significantly different.

Table 1. Effect of VLCD on anthropometric data of the subjects

	Weight (kg)	BMI (kg/m^2)	Waist/hip	% fat	LBM (kg)
Before	112.3	40.1	0.932	31.5	77.1
SE	8.2	2.1	0.031	0.9	6.4
After	101.1*	36.4*	0.921	28.1*	72.5*
SE	8.4	2.3	0.04	0.8	6.4

Values are means (n=6) ± SE.
*Significant difference ($P < 0.001$) between the values before and after the diet by paired t-test.

Table 2. Effect of VLCD on oxygen consumption and heart rate during submaximal ergometry test

	VO_2 (l/min)	VO_2/LBM (ml/min.kg)	Heart rate (beats/min)
Before VLCD	1.687	21.9	134.8
SE	0.120	0.23	8.2
After VLCD	1.451*	19.8	131.7
SE	0.181	1.1	7.8

Values are means ± SE (n = 6).
* Significant difference ($P < 0.05$) between the values before and after the diet. VO_2/LBM is the value of VO_2 divided by lean body mass in kg.

The concentration ratios for PCr/P_i, PCr/ATP and PCr/PDE at rest, the intramuscular pH and the value of recovery time of PCr/P_i were compared with normal values previously determined in a group of 30 healthy volunteers (normal values: PCr/P_i = 6.7 ± 1.1, PCr/ATP = 1.1 ± 0.1, PCr/PDE = 8.4. ± 2.4, pH = 7.1 ± 0.1 recovery time = 2 min). The only variable exhibiting a difference between our group of obese patients and the normals was PCr/PDE ratio: it was significantly lower in obese (i.e. the relative concentration of PDE is higher).

After the VLCD, the PCr/P_i ratio was significantly ($P < 0.05$) lower compared with pre-diet values (Table 3). The PCr/P_i value during the exercise declined after VLCD, but the fall was not significant. Nevertheless the exercise values were lower after VLCD for all but one subject, thus the tendency towards a decline caused by the diet seems to be obvious. No differences between the pre-diet and post-diet values were found for V_{max} and for recovery time of PCr/P_i (Table 3).

Table 3. Effect of VLCD on PCr/P_i at rest and exercise and on related parameters

	PCr/P_i rest	PCr/P_i exercise	Recovery time (min)	V_{max} (J/min)
Before VLCD	5.78	2.41	2	560
SE	0.45	0.19	0.1	36.4
After VLCD	4.78*	2.09	2	550.5
SE	0.31	0.26	0.1	49.6

Values are means ± SE (n = 6).
*Significant difference ($P < 0.05$) between the values before and after VLCD. V_{max} value is calculated according to Chance[3]: $V_{max} = V(1 + 0.6/[PCr/P_i])$, V is work per min (J/min) performed during the steady-state exercise.

Table 4. Effect of VLCD on ATP, phosphodiesters (PDE) at rest and pH at rest and exercise

	PCr/ATP	PCr/PDE	pH rest	pH exercise
Before VLCD	1.082	5.49	7.1	7.0
SE	0.04	0.49	0.1	0.1
After VLCD	1.158	3.58*	7.1	7.0
SE	0.05	0.33	0.1	0.1

Values are means ± SE (n = 6).
*Significant difference ($P < 0.05$) between the values before and after VLCD.

No change induced by the VLCD was observed either for the PCr/ATP ratio at rest or for intramuscular pH at rest and during the exercise (Table 4). No difference was observed between the rest and exercise values of pH, which proves that the exercise remained in the aerobic state. The PCr/PDE ratio at rest decreased significantly ($P < 0.05$) after the diet (Table 4).

Discussion

VLCD resulted in a significant weight loss, of which 41 per cent accounted for LBM reduction. VLCD induced a decrease in the oxygen cost of the submaximal exercise which accounted mostly for the LBM reduction as it is expressed by only a non-significant change of oxygen consumption when it is related to LBM.

We did not observe any major differences in the bioenergetics of the muscle between our obese group and normals at rest. The higher relative content of phosphodiesters in the muscle is difficult to explain. According to Burt[2] the peak in PDE area corresponds (among the compounds we can expect in the muscle) to glycerol-3-phosphorylcholin (GPC) and he describes the specific occurrence of GPC in slow-twitch muscles. Thus the higher occurrence of the PDE peak could correspond to the higher proportion of slow-twitch fibres in the calf muscles in obese subjects compared to normals, however, we cannot find any previous studies supporting this statement. On the contrary our obese subjects having rather high waist/hip ratio would be expected to have a higher proportion of type II fibres.

VLCD resulted in a decrease of PCr/P_i ratio which was obvious at rest and a clear tendency was observed in exercise, exercise values being, of course, significantly lower compared with the rest. PCr/P_i is considered to be a reflection of the cellular bioenergetic state[3] and was reported to be lower in hypocalorically fed rats[10]. The cause could be a state of energy deficiency of the muscle under the hypocaloric diet, in agreement with some previous reports[5,7,10,11].

Nevertheless this should be also reflected in an alteration of maximal oxidative capacity of the muscle expressed by the V_{max} value and this is not the case. Moreover, if we calculate a relative decrease of PCr/P_i induced by exercise we do not find differences before and after the diet, which reflects again the same metabolic cost of the work performed. The inhibition of the exercise-induced P_i/PCr increase (= decrease of PCr/P_i) reported by Lunt[7] was observed in starving subjects and for the anaerobic exercise, hence in conditions non-comparable with our protocol.

Another reason for the diet-induced decline of PCr/P_i could be a change in the proportion of the mass of the slow-twitch and fast-twitch fibres contributing to NMR spectra of the calf muscles. In animals, slow-twitch muscles have significantly lower PCr/P_i values at rest when compared to fast-twitch muscles[8]. A few studies report an atrophy of type II fibres during dieting (for review see[5,11]) or a tendency towards a decrease in cross-sectional area of these fibres during VLCD[6]. Even the tendency to the decreased cross-sectional area would result in a smaller mass of the type II fibres in a given volume of the calf muscles contributing to the NMR spectra and consequently in a lower PCr/P_i value.

Based on one study on a decline of the rest PCr/P_i value in hypothyroid patients[1], we could speculate about a possible effect of a low-T_3-syndrome induced by VLCD on the decrease of PCr/P_i in our group. However, the decrease of T_3 after the VLCD was not significant in our group and plasma T_3 levels were not in the hypothyroid range.

No changes induced by the diet were observed for intramuscular pH, neither at rest nor at exercise. No change of pH in the course of exercise confirms it remained aerobic.

The relative amount of phosphodiester in the muscle, already higher in the obese group compared to normals before the diet, further increased in the course of the diet. The finding of increased occurrence of phosphodiesters during hypocaloric diet is in agreement with the animal model[10]. As mentioned above, the PDE-like substances could be identified with GPC, occurring in slow-twitch muscles. The increased proportion of GPC after the diet could reflect the higher contribution of the slow-twitch fibres to NMR spectra after the diet and thus could support, together with the decrease of PCr/P$_i$ value, the suggestion about a tendency to an atrophy of type II fibres due to the diet.

In conclusion, the results of our preliminary NMR spectroscopy study suggest that in obese patients VLCD induces mild alterations in the intracellular state of the muscle which can correspond either to structural or purely bioenergetic changes. Further studies on this subject are to be encouraged, as the bioenergetics of the muscle may be crucial for understanding the overall energy metabolism of obesity.

References

1. Argov, Z., Renshaw, P.F., Boden, B., Winokur, A. & Bank, W.J. (1988): Effects of thyroid hormones on skeletal muscle bioenergetics. *J. Clin. Invest.* **81**, 1695-1701.
2. Burt, C.T., Glonek, T. & Barany, M. (1976): Phosphorus-31 nuclear magnetic resonance detection of unexpected phosphodiesters in muscle. *Biochemistry* **15**, 4850-4853.
3. Chance, B., Leigh, J.S, Clark, B.J., Maris, J., Kent, J., Nioka, S. & Smith, D. (1985): Control of oxidative metabolism and oxygen delivery in human skeletal muscle: a steady-state analysis of the work/energy cost transfer function. *Proc. Natl. Acad. Sci. USA* **82**, 8384-8388.
4. Hainer, V., Kunesova, M., Stich, V. & Parizkova, J. (1989): Very low energy formula diet in the treatment of obesity. *Int. J. Obes.* **13** (suppl.1), 185-188.
5. Jeejeebhoy, K.N. (1986): Muscle function and nutrition. *Gut.* **27**, 25-39.
6. Krotkiewski, M., Grimby, G., Holm, G. & Szczepanik, J. (1990): Increased muscle dynamic endurance associated with weight reduction on a very-low-calorie-diet. *Am. J. Clin. Nutr.* **51**, 321-330.
7. Lunt, I.A., Allen, P.S., Brainer, M., Swinamer, D., Treimer, F.O. & King, E.G. (1986): An evaluation of the effect of fasting on the exercise induced changes in pH and P$_i$/PCr from skeletal muscle. *Mag. Res. Med.* **3**, 946-952.
8. Meyer, R.A., Brown, T.R. & Kushmerick, M.J. (1985): Phosphorus nuclear magnetic resonance of fast- and slow-twitch muscle. *Am. J. Physiol.* **248** (*Cell Physiol.* **17**), C279-C287.
9. Parizkova, J. (1977): *Body fat and physical fitness*, pp. 1-30. The Hague: Martinas Nijhoff.
10. Pichard, C., Vaughan, C., Struk, R., Armstrong, R.L. & Jeejeebhoy, K.N. (1988): Effect of dietary manipulations (fasting, hypocaloric feeding and subsequent refeeding) on rat muscle energetics as assessed by nuclear magnetic resonance spectroscopy. *J. Clin. Invest.* **82**, 895-901.
11. Russel, D.M., Atwood, H.L., Whittaker, J.S., Itakure, T., Walker, P.M., Mickle, D.A.G. & Jeejeebhoy, K.N. (1984): The effect of fasting and hypocaloric diets on the functional and metabolic characteristics of rat gastrocnemius muscle. *Clin. Sci.* **67**, 185-194.

Chapter 5

Increased Metabolic Efficiency in a Subset of Obese Patients

M. WECK[1], S. FISCHER[1], H. KARST[2], R. NOACK[2], W. LEONHARDT[1], K. FÜCKER[1], and M. HANEFELD[1]

[1]*Lipid Research Unit, Clinic of Internal Medicine, Medical Academy "Carl Gustav Carus" Dresden, Fetscherstr. 74, D(0)-8019 Dresden and* [2]*Central Institute of Nutrition, D(0)-1510 Potsdam*

Summary

We investigated the interrelationships between resting energy expenditure (REE), postprandial thermogenesis after protein application (PPT), adipose tissue lipolysis and Na^+/K^+-ATPase activity in 40 normotensive obese subjects (18 men, 22 women, BMI 27–45). On average we observed no significant differences between lean and obese subjects with respect to REE % (100.5 ± 1.9 vs. 96.6 ± 1.3%) and PPT (261.2 ± 21.3 vs. 235.1 ± 114.9 kJ/6 hours). In a small subset of the obese group we registered very low metabolic rates at rest and after protein application. This subset (n=7) was characterized by low NE (norepinephrine) stimulated adipose tissue lipolysis and reduced ATPase-activity. Highly significant interrelationships between PPT, Na^+/K^+-ATPase-activity and glycerol release of adipose tissue were found.

Introduction

Differences in the efficiency of energy utilization have been postulated to be a pathogenetic factor in the development and maintenance of obesity [3]. Reduced substrate cycling including the TG/FFA cycle and decreased activity of the Na^+/K^+-ATPase are considered to contribute to diminish energy expenditure and increasing fat mass[1,3,29].

Subjects and methods

Subjects: selection criteria

(1) An energy intake below predicted values, (2) indicators of a genetic background that means onset of obesity in childhood and at least one obese relative, (3) stable weight during the year before the investigations, (4) no other metabolic or endocrine disorders, and normal blood pressure according to WHO criteria, and (5) the age range between 20 and 40 years.

40 obese patients (18 men, 22 women) with a body mass index (BMI) between 27 and 45 took part in the study. As control group for investigation of REE and PPT we determined these parameters in 11 non-obese, healthy volunteers and as the control for Na-pump activity we examined 16 normal weight, normotensive volunteers without metabolic disorders (BMI 20–25, seven men and nine women) (Table 1).

The habitual daily food intake before the investigations was calculated by 7-day dietary records[5]. The individual total energy requirement of the subjects was calculated from the predicted metabolic rate (BMR) according to Kleiber[1]. The patients were all informed about the procedures and gave their written consent.

Table 1. Physical characteristics of the obese subjects and controls (mean ± SEM)

	Obese n = 40	Control group 1 n = 11	Control group 2 n = 16
Sex (men/women)	18/22	7/4	7/9
Age (years)	31.9 ± 0.9	33.9 ± 2.2	34.8 ± 2.2
BMI			
weight (kg)/height (m^2)	35.6 ± 0.7	21.4 ± 0.7[#]	21.7 ± 0.6[#]
Body fat (%)	39.7 ± 1.1	19.7 ± 1.8[#]	–
LBM (kg)	60.3 ± 1.5	54.4 ± 2.8	–
Energy intake			
MJ/die	9.65 ± 0.62	11.29 ± 0.44	–
(%)[†]	76.3 ± 4.1	104.1 ± 5.0*	–
Blood pressure (mmHg)			
systolic	128 ± 2	121 ± 2	125 ± 3
diastolic	84 ± 1	79 ± 1	82 ± 2

[†]Intake in per cent of the total energy requirements calculated from the predicted basal metabolic rate according to Kleiber.
Obese vs. Control group 1 and 2 respectively: *$P < 0.001$, [#] $P < 0.0001$.

Measurements of energy metabolism

1. Resting energy expenditure

REE was determined by indirect calorimetry using an open circuit system (Beckman MMC equipment). The total energy expenditure (E) was calculated according to Scheunert and Trautmann[4]: E (kJ) = 16.18 litres $\dot{V}O_2$ + 5.02 litres $\dot{V}CO_2$ – 5.99 g N. REE was measured during 8 hours (7.30 a.m. to 3.30 p.m.). The measured REE was expressed as a percentage of the theoretically predicted BMR[1].

2. Postprandial thermogenesis

PPT was determined by the same procedure as for REE. After measuring the premeal metabolic rate (PMR, 7.30–9.30 a.m.) the test meal (1MJ casein) was eaten and then the postprandial metabolic rate (PPMR) was recorded for 6 h. PPT was calculated using the following equation: PPT (kJ) = PPMR (kJ) – PMR (kJ).

Adipose tissue lipolysis

Subcutaneous adipose tissue was obtained from the abdominal and femoral region. The fat cells were isolated by the method of Rodbell. Aliquots of the cell suspension were incubated at 37°C for 60 min without and with added norepinephrine (NE) 0.9 and 2.25 µg/ml. Glycerol release was determined in the infranatant.

Sodium/potassium ATPase of erythrocytes

The activity of the Na$^+$/K$^+$-ATPase was determined by ^{86}Rb influx. The cellular uptake of ^{86}Rb that was specifically mediated by the Na$^+$/K$^+$-ATPase was calculated as the difference between the total radioactivity taken up by the cells and that taken up in the presence of excess ouabain.

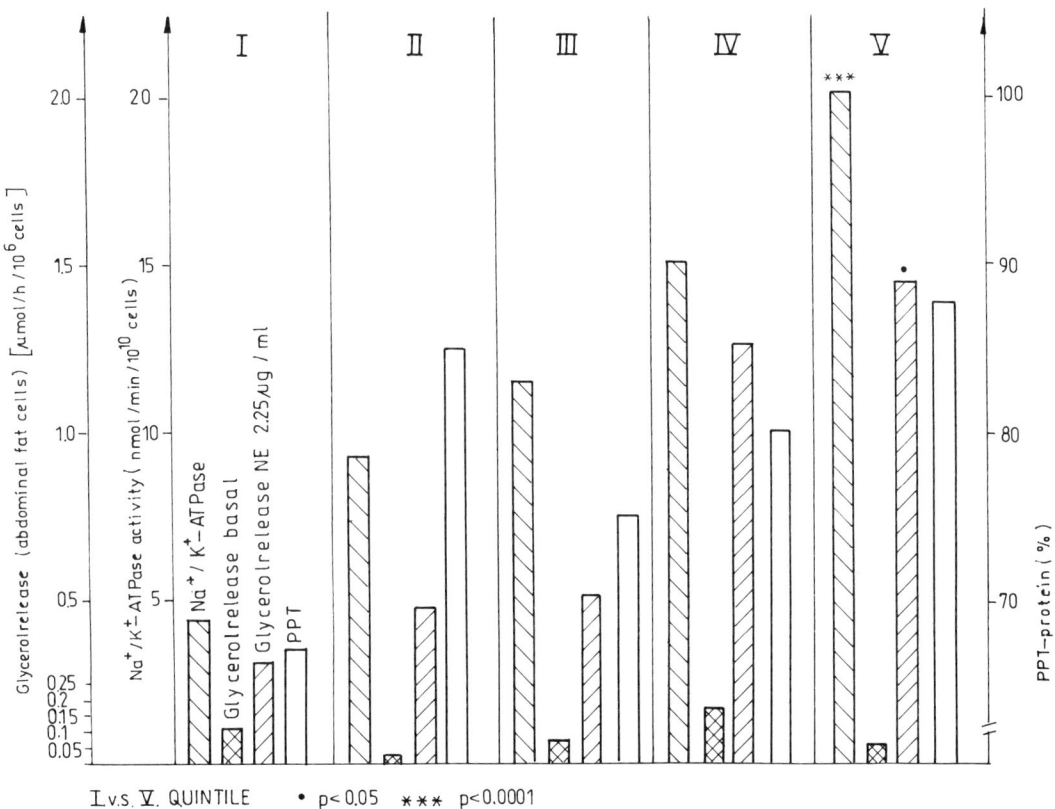

Fig. 1. Interrelations of Na⁺/K⁺-ATPase activity of erythrocytes with adipose tissue lipolysis and PPT in obese subjects (n = 40). Quintiles of the Na⁺/K⁺-ATPase.

Results

Because of their greater metabolic active mass the REE of obese patients was found significantly higher. However, with respect to REE% (measured REE/predicted BMR according to Kleiber x 100), PTT and Na⁺/K⁺-ATPase activity, we observed on average no significant differences between lean and obese subjects but marked inter-individual variation (Table 2). Figure 1 illustrates the interrelationships between thermogenesis, adipose tissue lipolysis and Na⁺ pump within quintiles of the Na⁺/K⁺-ATPase in the obese group. At the bottom quintile of this enzyme we found significantly lower glycerol release after NE-stimulation of abdominal adipocytes, whereas basal lipolysis was quite similar (Fig. 1). There is a tendency to increasing PPT with higher Na⁺/K⁺-ATPase activity (Fig. 1). Table 3 summarizes the Pearson correlations between the parameters investigated with a significance level of more than 0.05.

From the entire obese population we selected patients with "low" metabolic rates and compared them with their counterparts with "normal" metabolic rates in order to differentiate an obese subgroup with high efficiency of energy utilization. The following cut-off limits were defined: (1) for subjects with low metabolic rates, that means "high" efficiency of energy metabolism: REE (%) < 95 and casein-induced PPT (%) < 70; (2) for patients with normal metabolic rates: REE (%) > 100 and casein-induced PPT (%) > 80. Within these criteria about 20% of the highly selected obese "small eaters" demonstrate a high efficiency of energy utilization (Table 4). In obese patients with high efficiency of energy metabolism the NE-stimulated glycerol release of abdominal adipose tissue was significantly lower compared to the counterparts with "normal" metabolic rates ($P < 0.05$) and the lipolytic responsiveness of abdominal adipocytes was found to be significantly higher ($P < 0.05$) than that of femoral fat cells in subjects with normal efficiency of energy metabolism. This difference was equalized at the "high" efficiency group (Table 4). The activity of the Na^+/K^+-ATPase of red cells was nearly 50% lower in subjects with low metabolic rates compared to patients with normal rates (Table 4) but without statistical significance.

Table 2. Body fat content, parameters of energy metabolism and Na^+/K^+ATPase activity of obese subjects compared to normal-weight controls (mean ± SEM)

	Obese, n = 40	Controls, n = 11	P
Body fat (%)	39.7 ± 1.2	19.8 ± 2.2	< 0.0001*
REE (MJ/die)	7.85 ± 18	6.84 ± 0.26	< 0.05
Predicted REE (MJ/die)[1]	8.16 ± 0.19	6.81 ± 0.26	< 0.01
REE (%)[2]	96.6 ± 1.3	100.5 ± 1.9	ns
REE/LBM (kJ/kg/die)	131.6 ± 1.7	125.8 ± 1.8	ns
PPT-protein (kJ/6 h)	235.1 ± 14.9	261.2 ± 21.3	ns
PPT-protein (%)[3]	79.2 ± 5.0	87.9 ± 7.2	ns
Na^+/K^+ATPase (n = 16) (nmol/min/10^{10} cells)	12.2 ± 0.9	9.6 ± 0.7	ns

[1]predicted REE was calculated according to Kleiber.
[2]REE (%) = measured REE (kJ) / predicted REE (kJ) x 100.
[3]PPT-protein (%) = measured PPT (kJ) / mean PPT (kJ) of a reference group x 100.
*Mann–Whitney U-test.

Table 3. Pearson correlations between Na^+/K^+ATPase activity of red blood cells, PPT and adipose tissue lipolysis in obese subjects (n = 40)

	Na-K-ATPase
Postprandial thermogenesis	0.33*
Glycerol release	
Abdominal AT:	
Basal	0.04
NE 2.25 µg/ml	0.39#
Gluteal-femoral AT	
Basal	0.41#
NE 2.25 µg/ml	0.38*

*$P < 0.05$, #$P < 0.01$.

Discussion

Different results with respect to REE and PPT in obesity may partly be due to the heterogeneity of the study populations. Therefore, we have chosen the initially described strict selection criteria. Despite this we observed, on average, only graded differences between lean and obese subjects with respect to REE% and PTT.

Only about 20% of all obese patients seem to have a particularly effective energy utilization. Corresponding with these reports we have illustrated that only in a small subset of highly selected fat people does obesity seem to be associated with increased efficiency of energy utilization, as is evident by the simultaneous reduction of REE% and PPT. Trayhurn and James[5] subdivide postprandial thermogenesis into an obligatory and facultative form. The facultative component has been attributed to sympathetic nervous stimulation of obese tissue after food intake, increased substrate cycling and elevated activity of the Na^+/K^+-ATPase.

Table 4. REE, PPT, Na^+/K^+-ATPase of red cells and adipose tissue lipolysis in obese subjects with different efficiency of energy utilization (mean ± SEM)

	Obese Efficiency of energy utilization	
	"high" (n = 7)	"normal" (n = 7)
Body fat (%)	41.6 ± 2.9	37.4 ± 1.4
REE (%)	91.1 ± 0.9	106.6 ± 2.1*
PPT-protein (%)	52.7 ± 5.0	109.4 ± 2.1*
Na^+/K^+-ATPase (nmol/min/10^{10} cells)	8.7 ± 2.7	15.3 ± 2.8
Adipose tissue lipolysis (glycerol release) µmol/h/10^6 cells		
Abdominal		
basal	0.08 ± 0.06	0.06 ± 0.04
NE 2.25 µg/ml	0.39 ± 0.21	1.32 ± 0.37**
Femoral		
basal	0.07 ± 0.22	0.16 ± 0.10
NE 2.25 µg/ml	0.31 ± 0.09	0.62 ± 0.29**

*$P < 0.05$, **$P < 0.001$.
(Mann–Whitney U-test).

Our investigations provide evidence that NE-stimulated glycerol release of abdominal fat cells is markedly reduced under conditions of impaired metabolic rates (basal, postprandial). Recently most authors failed to observe any difference between lean and obese subjects with respect to the red cell Na^+/K^+-ATPase[6]. We have found a correlation between Na^+/K^+-ATPase activity of erythrocytes and the efficiency of energy utilization (PPT corresponds to lower values of the enzyme activity), and a direct relationship between red cell Na^+/K^+-ATPase and norepinephrine-stimulated lipolysis of abdominal adipose tissue. Thus, low metabolic rates appear to correspond to reduced activity of the Na^+/K^+-ATPase of erythrocytes and to low values of NE-stimulated adipose tissue lipolysis.

References

1. Kleiber, M. (1967): *Der Energiehaushalt von Mensch und Haus tier*. Hamburg: Parey.
2. McNeill, B., McBride, A., Smith, J.S. & James, W.P.T. (1989): Energy expenditure in large and small eaters. *Nutr. Res.* **9**, 363-372.
3. Ravussin, E., Lillioja, S., Knowler, W.C., Christins, L., Freymond, D., Abbott, W.G.H., Boyce, V., Howard, B.Y. & Bogardus, G. (1988): Reduced rate of energy expenditure as a factor for bodyweight gain. *N. Engl. J. Med.* **318**, 467-472.
4. Scheunert, A. & Trautmann, A. (1976): *Lehrbuch der Veterinar-Physiologie*. pp. 331-332. Berlin: Parey.
5. Trayhurn, P., James, W.P.T. (1981): Thermogenesis: dietary and non-shivering aspects. In *The body weight regulatory system: normal and disturbed mechanisms,* eds. L.A. Cioffi, W.P.T. James & T.B. van Italie, pp. 97-105. New York: Raven Press.
6. Pasquali, R., Strocchi, G., Malini, P., Casimirri, P., Melchionda, N., Ambosioni, E. & Lobo, G. (1985): Heterogeneity of the erythrocyte Na-K pump status in human obesity. *Metabolism* **34,** 802-807.

Chapter 6

The Effect of Weight Loss on Erythrocyte Membrane Function in Patients with Morbid Obesity

Yishai LEVY, Nizar ELIAS, Uri COGAN and Daniel YESHURUN

Lipid Research Unit, Rambam Medical Center, Department of Medicine A, Bnai Zion Medical Center, and Faculty of Medicine and Department of Food Engineering and Biotechnology, Technion-Israel Institute of Technology, Haifa 31096, Israel

Summary

Morbid obesity is one of the commonest metabolic disorders. There is no agreement about the mechanisms leading to the derangement in energy balance and fat accumulation. Alterations in membrane composition and function may serve as biological markers of the disorders. Ten patients with morbid obesity were investigated while fasting, maintained on a zero calorie diet for 10 days. Erythrocyte ghosts were separated and membrane function was quantitated by steady state fluorescent polarization using 1,6-diphenyl-1,3,5-hexatriene (DPH) as a fluorescent probe. The patients with morbid obesity showed a significant decrease in erythrocyte membrane lipid fluidity compared to a normal weight group. Upon significant weight loss of 8%, the anisotropy parameter at 37°C was not changed. Thus, morbid obesity is followed by alterations in erythrocyte membrane function. The inability to reverse these alterations upon weight loss is suggestive of a membrane disorder which may play a role in the metabolic processes leading to obesity.

Introduction

The fluid mosaic model proposed by Singer and Nicholson[17] suggests that proteins move within the lipid matrix and that their structural and functional properties are affected by the physical state of the lipid microenvironment[7]. Abnormalities in membrane function have been described in experimental and human obesity; there is reduced Na^+/K^+-ATPase[6,9,12], reduced adenylate cyclase[5], a decrease in insulin receptors[2], and a decrease in glucose transport[3]. Alterations in erythrocyte membrane lipid fluidity have also been demonstrated[1,4,19]. There is no evidence yet that the alterations in membrane function have a primary role in the pathogenesis of obesity.

We have undertaken the present study in order to investigate the membrane lipid fluidity of erythrocyte ghosts from patients with morbid obesity. The relationship between being overweight and membrane function was investigated by repeating fluidity studies after fasting for 10 days with zero calorie diet which resulted in a significant weight loss. Steady state fluorescent polarization with 1,6-diphenyl-1,3,5 hextriene (DPH), as a fluorescent probe, was used to determine membrane fluidity.

Patients and methods

Patients

Ten otherwise healthy patients were recruited from those attending the obesity clinic at the Bnai Zion Medical Center. All the patients were above 150% of their ideal body weight, with a BMI of more than 35 kg/m^2. There were 10 females with an age range of 19–58, mean 43 ± 9 yr. The patients were admitted to the department of medicine and maintained on a zero calorie diet with *ad libitum* drinking water. Allopurinal at a dose of 300 mg daily was administered. Safety tests included routine biochemical blood and urine tests and ECG monitoring throughout the study.

Fluidity measurements were done on the first day and on the eleventh day, at the end of the fasting. The results were compared to a normal weight group of eight patients with a mean age of 36 ± 10 years and a BMI of 23 ± 1 kg/m^2.

Ghost preparation

Morning fasting blood samples were collected using EDTA as an anticoagulant. After removal from plasma the erythrocytes were dispersed in 0.2 M isotonic phosphate buffer, pH = 7.4, and washed repeatedly by centrifugation at 1075 **g** with Sorwall RC-5B centrifuge. Ghosts were prepared by hypotonic lysis in phosphate buffer 5 mM, pH = 8, according to the procedure of Dodge *et al.*[8] Ghosts were washed repeatedly in hypotonic buffer until the haemoglobin was removed.

Fluidity measurements

Fluidity was measured by determining the fluorescent depolarization using 1,6-diphenyl-1,3,5 hexatriene (DPH) as a fluorescent probe, according to the method of Shinitzky and Barenholz[16]. This method has been extensively utilized in our laboratory[11]. Erythrocyte ghosts' protein was analysed according to the method of Lowry *et al.*[13] and was standardized to a concentration of 50 µg/ml.

The polarization of fluorescence, expressed as the fluorescence anisotropy r, and the anisotropy parameter $[r_0/r^{-1}]^{-1}$ is calculated with the limiting anisotropy of DPH value of r_0 = 0.362[16]. The anisotropy parameter is directly related to the microviscosity and inversely related to the lipid fluidity. Comparisons between the groups were made using a Student t-test.

Results

The ten patients finished the study without any side effects. Figure 1 summarizes the effect of the 10 day zero calorie diet on BMI. There was a significant ($P < 0.05$) 7% drop in BMI from 39 ± 5 to 36 ± 5 kg/m^2.

Figure 2 depicts the fluidity measurements at 37°C in the obese patients as compared to the normal controls. There was a significant decrease in ghost fluidity at 37°C with an anisotropy parameter of 1.417 ± 0.093 compared to an anisotropy parameter of 1.279 ± 0.043 in the normal controls ($P < 0.01$). Upon significant weight loss there was no change in the fluidity; the anisotropy parameter at 37°C was 1.401 ± 0.110 after ten days zero calorie diet (Fig. 2).

Discussion

In the erythrocyte membranes of obese patients we observed a decrease in fluidity by means of the fluorescent polarization method using DPH as a fluorescent probe. Alterations in membrane fluidity have been correlated with changes in many membrane functions, including enzyme activity, ligand receptor interaction and transport[18]. The relationship between membrane fluidity and obesity has been addressed by very few studies in the past.

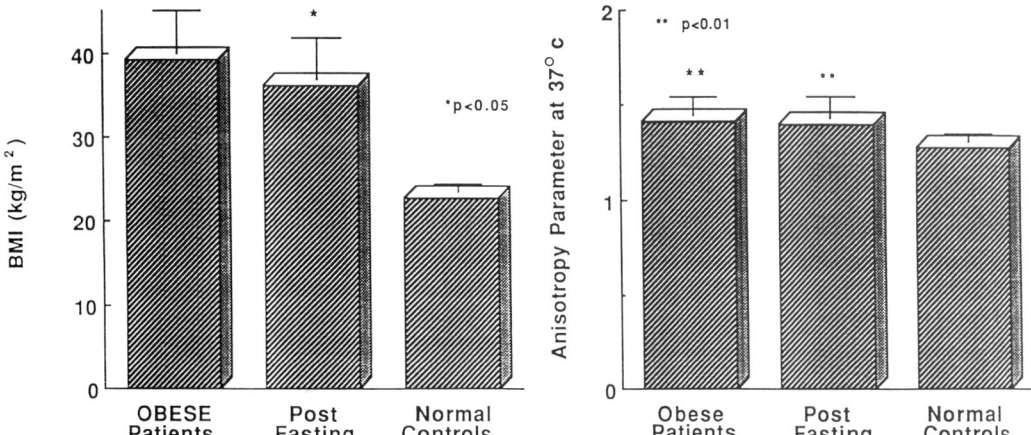

Fig. 1 (left). The effect of fasting, 10 days zero calorie diet, on body mass index (BMI) of ten patients with morbid obesity. *P < 0.05 compares post-fasting BMI to baseline BMI.
Fig. 2 (right). The effect of fasting, 10 days zero calorie diet on erythrocyte membrane fluidity, presented as the diphenyl hexatriene fluorescent anisotropy parameter at 37°C. **P < 0.01 compares ten patients with morbid obesity at baseline and post-fasting to eight normal controls.

In an experimental model using the same technique, York et al.[19] have shown a decrease in polarization value in a wide range of membranes. It is interesting to note that the erythrocyte membrane behaved in an opposite direction to the other membranes examined. The fluidity changes were accompanied by changes in the fatty acid composition of membrane phospholipids. In a human study, Beguinot et al.[1] demonstrated an alteration in erythrocyte membrane fluidity which was correlated with an increased cholesterol-to-phospholipid ratio. A recent study, using an electron spin resonance technique[4], showed a decrease in fluidity at the surface and in the hydrophobic core of erythrocyte membranes from obese subjects. All these studies found a good correlation between the degree of obesity and erythrocyte membrane fluidity.

We have followed, for the first time, the effect of significant weight loss on membrane lipid fluidity in obesity. The inability to reverse the altered membrane fluidity in our patients raises some suggestions which are speculative at this time. As membrane fluidity is dependent on cholesterol content and fatty acid composition, we should make better definitions of erythrocyte membrane composition before and after significant weight loss.

Studies in siblings clearly indicate the contribution of genes that influence metabolic regulation in obesity[15]. It is assumed that processes which lead to an increased metabolic efficiency, decreased thermogenesis and decreased basal metabolic rate, cause fat accumulation[10]. Other receptor mediated and enzymatic reactions which have been described in obesity[14], are potentially involved in the pathogenesis of the disorder. Thus, the alterations in erythrocyte membrane fluidity in obesity which are resistant to weight loss suggest a membrane disorder which may be a marker or a cause of processes mediating metabolic pathways, leading to fat accumulation and to obesity.

Acknowledgements

This work was supported by the Technion V.P.R. Fund for Laboratory Research (Haifa, Israel). The excellent secretarial work of Mrs. Ruth Rose is gratefully acknowledged.

References

1. Beguinot, F., Tranontano, D., Duileo, C., Formisano, S., Beguinot, L., Mattioli, P., Mancini, M. & Alog, S. (1985): Alteration of erythrocyte membrane lipid fluidity in human obesity. *J. Clin. Endocrinol. Metab.* **60**, 1226-1230.
2. Chang, K., Huang, D. & Cuatrecasas, P. (1975): The defect in insulin receptors in obese-hyperglycemic mice: a probable accompaniment of more generalized alterations in membrane glycoproteins. *Biochem. Biophys. Res. Commun.* **64**, 566-573.
3. Cuendet, G.S., Loten, E.G., Jeanrenaud, B. & Renold, A.E. (1976): Decreased basal, noninsulin-stimulated glucose uptake and metabolism by skeletal soleus muscle isolated from obese-hyperglycemic (ob/ob) mice. *J. Clin. Invest.* **58**, 1078-1088.
4. Curatola, G., Ferretti, G., Bertoli, E., Dott, M., Bartolotta, E. & Giorgi, P. (1987): Changes in membrane fluidity in erythrocytes of obese children. A spin label study. *Ped. Res.* **22**, 141-144.
5. Deahaye, J.P., Winand, J. & Christophe, J. (1978): Adenylate cyclase activity in the epididymal adipose tissue from obese-hyperglycemic mice. *Diabetologia* **15**, 45-51.
6. De Luise, M., Blackburn, G.L. & Flier, J.S. (1980): Reduced activity of the red-cell sodium-potassium pump in human obesity. *N. Engl. J. Med.* **303**, 1017-1022.
7. Dipple, I. & Houslay, M.S. (1978): The activity of glucagon stimulated adenylated cyclase from rat liver plasma membranes is modulated by the fluidity of its lipid environment. *Biochem. J.* **174**, 179-190.
8. Dodge, J.T., Mitchell, C. & Hanahan, D.J. (1963): The preparation and chemical characteristics of hemoglobin-free ghosts of human erythrocytes. *Arch. Biochem. Biophys.* **100**, 119-130.
9. Klines, I., Magulesparan, M., Unger, R.H., Aronoff, S.L. & Mott, D.M. (1982): Reduced Na^+,K^+-ATPase activity in intact red cells and isolated membranes from obese man. *J. Clin. Endocrin. Metab.* **54**, 721-724.
10. Lardy, H. & Shargo, E. (1990): Biochemical aspects of obesity. *Ann. Rev. Biochem.* **59**, 689-710.
11. Levin, G., Cogan, U., Levy, Y. & Mokady, S. (1990): Riboflavin deficiency and the function and fluidity of rat erythrocyte membranes. *J. Nutr.* **120**, 857-861.
12. Lin, M.H., Romos, D.R., Akera, T. & Leveille, G.A. (1978): Na^+,K^+-ATPase enzyme units in skeletal muscle from lean and obese mice. *Biochem. Biophys. Res. Commun.* **80**, 398-404.
13. Lowry, O.H., Rosebrough, N.J., Farr, A.L. & Randall, R.J. (1951): Protein measurement with the folin phenol reagent. *J. Biol. Chem.* **193**, 265-275.
14. Neufeld, N.D., Ezrin, C., Corbo, L., Long, D. & Bush, M.A. (1986): Effect of caloric restriction and exercise on insulin receptors in obesity: association with changes in membrane lipids. *Metabolism* **35**, 580-587.
15. Roberts, S.E., Savage, J., Coward, W.A., Chew, B. & Lucas, A. (1988): Energy expenditure and intake in infants born to lean and overweight mothers. *N. Engl. J. Med.* **318**, 461-466.
16. Shinitzky, M. & Barenholz, Y. (1978): Fluidity parameters of lipid regions determined by fluorescence. *Biochim. Biophys. Acta* **515**, 367-394.
17. Singer, S.J. & Nicholson, G.L. (1972): The fluid mosaic model of the structure of cell membranes. *Science* **175**, 720-731.
18. Spector, A.A. & Yorek, M.A. (1985): Membrane lipid composition and cellular function. *J. Lipid Res.* **26**, 1015-1025.
19. York, D.A., Hyslop, P.A. & French, R. (1982): Fluorescence polarization and composition of membranes in genetic obesity. *Biochem. Biophys. Res. Commun.* **106**, 1478-1483.

Section II
Neuro-endocrine regulation of food intake

Chapter 7

Fat Intake, Fat Digestion and the Satiety Signal for Fat Intake

Charlotte ERLANSON-ALBERTSSON and Jie MEI
Department of Medical and Physiological Chemistry, University of Lund, P.O. Box 94, S-221 00 Lund, Sweden

Evolution does not produce novelties from scratch. It works on what already exists, either transforming a system to give it new functions or combining several systems to produce a more elaborate one.
(François Jacob, *Evolution and Tinkering*)

Summary

Enterostatin, a pentapeptide derived from pancreatic procolipase, was demonstrated to suppress high-fat food intake in rats as opposed to low-fat food after central administration, in agreement with earlier findings, as well as after intraduodenal administration. Endogeneous enterostatin was also measured for the first time by an ELISA method. It was found that enterostatin was present in the intestinal contents of rat and man during feeding and that the concentration of the peptide was increased after high-fat feeding 1.2-fold after 4 h and threefold after 24 h. The peptide in the intestinal contents was partially associated with the lipid particles. A close association between intestinal fat digestion and regulation of fat intake by enterostatin is suggested.

Introduction

The diet in Western industrial nations is characterized by a high amount of fat. The proportion of calories derived from fat in this diet is around 40% as opposed to 11%, for instance, in the traditional Japanese diet[13]. Since a high fat intake is a characteristic feature of overweight people[1,7], it is of a great importance to know if there are signals that specifically regulate fat intake and the identity of these. The existence of signals associated with fat intake seems to be without any doubt[2], the satiety after fat intake being characterized as a long-term highly efficient satiety[16]. The identity of these signals has hitherto been unknown.

We have found that a peptide[9,10] named *enterostatin*[17], derived from pancreatic procolipase, specifically inhibits fat intake[11,14], when injected into rats either peripherally or centrally or when given orally as the parent molecule procolipase[9]. Pancreatic colipase is a protein cofactor for pancreatic lipase and necessary for optimal fat digestion in the intestine[4,12].

In the following, the properties of enterostatin in reducing fat intake will be described, as well as the measurements of endogenous enterostatin in man and rat and its relationship to high-fat feeding.

Methods

Female Sprague-Dawley rats (200 g) (ALAB, Sollentuna, Sweden) were used throughout the study. Prior to experiments the rats were housed in individual cages with free access to water and standard pellets. In the short-term feeding experiments the rats were fasted for 17 h. Thereafter the rats (five in each group) were fed either a low-fat diet (standard pellets, containing 5.2% fat by weight) or a high-fat diet (containing 17.8% by weight). After 4 h of feeding the rats were killed. Ten cm of the intestine starting from pylorus was excised. The intestinal contents were emptied into a test tube and rinsed with 5 ml 0.15 M NaCl. The samples were immediately frozen at –20°C until further analysed.

In the long-term experiments the rats in groups of five were fed with low-fat food (standard pellets) or high-fat food for 24 h, 48 h and 72 h. Intestinal contents were collected during 20 minutes through a catheter (Silastic tubing 0.030 in ID; 0.065 in OD), that was inserted under anaesthesia into the duodenum through incision in the intestinal wall.

The intestinal contents of man were collected from the first part of the jejunum after intubation with a polyethylene cannula according to standard procedures[5]. A standard fluid test meal of 300 ml (16% protein, 31% fat and 53% carbohydrate by energy) was given after overnight fasting of the patient. Intestinal content was collected over ice by siphonage in six 10-min and two 30-min fractions following the test meal and kept frozen at –20°C until analysed.

Analysis of enterostatin was carried out by an ELISA-based method using antibodies specific for enterostatin developed in rabbits[6].

Lipase and colipase activity measurements were carried out using tributyrin dispersed in bile salt as substrate with a titrimetric method[3]. For lipase determinations an excess of pure colipase was added[8], while for colipase determinations an excess of pure lipase was added[15].

Results

Properties of enterostatin during feeding

In Fig. 1 is shown the food intake pattern of rats after injection i.c.v. with enterostatin during low-fat feeding (5.2% fat) compared to high-fat feeding (17.8% fat). As can be seen, the suppressive effect of enterostatin on food intake is *longlasting*, i.e. over the whole experimental period and significant only during *high-fat feeding*.

Enterostatin during a single meal with low-fat feeding and high-fat feeding

Immunreactive enterostatin was found to be present in the intestinal contents of rats following a 4 h meal. Interestingly enough, enterostatin was found to be present at a higher concentration during high-fat feeding compared to low-fat feeding (Fig. 2). Lipase and colipase activities were in the same order of magnitude in these two different situations (Fig. 2).

Effect of prolonged high-fat feeding on enterostatin

Immunreactive enterostatin was found to be increased two- to threefold already after 24 h of high-fat feeding compared to low-fat feeding. The high level of enterostatin persisted during the 72 h investigated. In this situation there was a parallel increase of lipase and colipase activities in the intestinal content starting also after 24 h of high-fat feeding.

Enterostatin in intestinal contents of man

Enterostatin, when measured in the intestinal contents of man was found to be present in micromolar concentration. Filtration of intestinal contents through a Sephadex G-25 Superfine column showed the enterostatin to be eluted in two different peaks, one corresponding to a molecular size of 600 Da and the other appearing in the void volume together with the lipid particles of the intestinal contents (Fig. 3).

Chapter 7 – Fat Intake, Fat Digestion and the Satiety Signal for Fat Intake

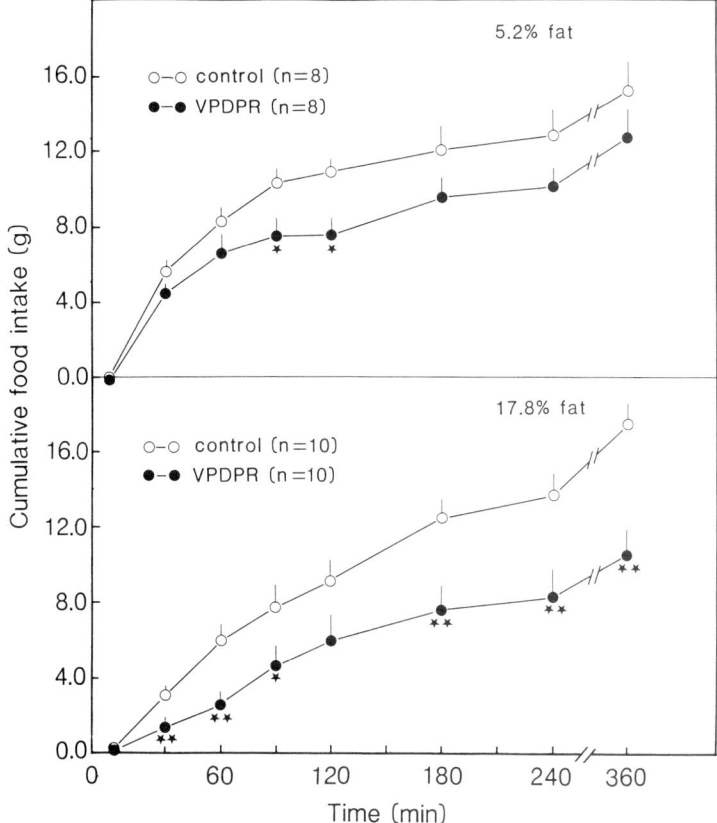

Fig. 1. Effect of i.c.v. injection of enterostatin 333 pmol (VPDPR) on low-fat feeding compared to high-fat feeding on 18 h fasted female Sprague-Dawley rats, adapted to a 6 h feeding period and provided with a permanent cannula into the lateral ventricle. Student's t-test was used for comparison of control injected with peptide injected animals. $*P < 0.05$, $**P < 0.001$.

Discussion

In these studies exogenous enterostatin when given to Sprague-Dawley rats was found to specifically reduce high-fat feeding, in agreement with previous observations[11,14]. A suppressive effect on food intake was also observed after intraduodenal administration of the peptide. The long-term action of this peptide is to be noted since this is in agreement with the high satiating power of dietary fat described recently[2].

In these studies endogenous enterostatin was also measured in intestinal contents from rats and man. Immunoreactive enterostatin was definitely present in intestinal contents and after a single meal (in man) found to be present for several hours after feeding.

One important observation was that enterostatin was present at an apparently higher concentration during high-fat feeding compared to low-fat feeding, already after a single meal, but definitely and two- to threefold higher during prolonged high-fat feeding. In the latter case the increase of enterostatin occurred parallel with an increased synthesis of pancreatic lipase and colipase, in agreement with earlier reports[18].

Enterostatin in intestinal contents partially associated with the lipid particles and proteins into a macromolecular form as demonstrated by gel filtration. Such an interaction could be

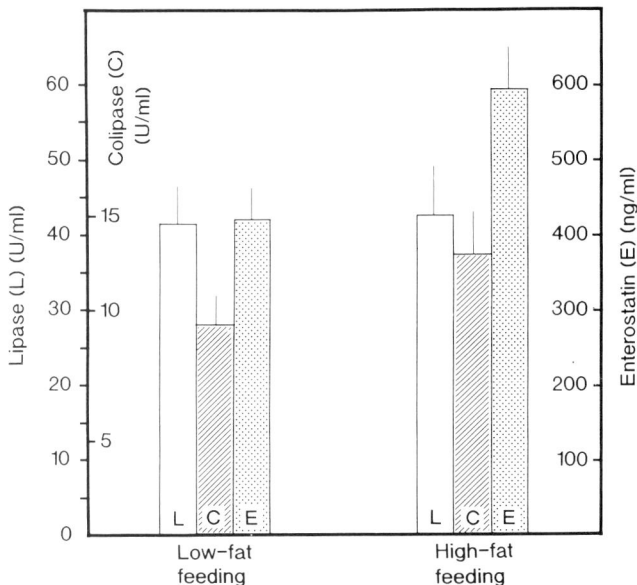

Fig. 2. Immunreactive enterostatin (E), pancreatic lipase (L) and pancreatic colipase (C) in intestinal washings after 4 h of feeding with low-fat food (5.2% fat) or high-fat food (17.8% fat). Enterostatin is expressed as ng/ml and lipase and colipase activities in units/ml.

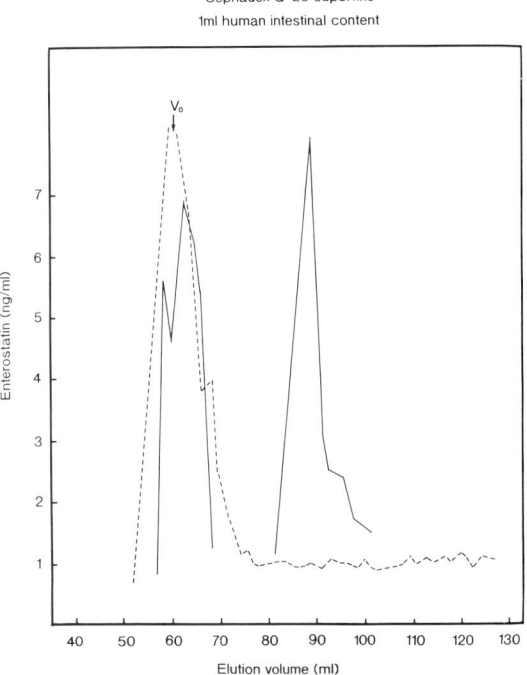

Fig. 3. Gel filtration of 1 ml human intestinal content aspirated 2 h after a single fluid meal of 300 ml containing 31% fat, 16% protein and 53% carbohydrate by energy. Immunoreactive enterostatin was measured in each fraction and expressed in ng/ml. The void volume, indicated by V_0, was measured by absorbance at 280 nm.

responsible for a greater stability of the peptide against proteolysis and thereby a higher concentration during high-fat feeding. Whether this is the explanation for the selective fat-reducing effect of enterostatin is not known, but may be one important factor.

In conclusion, fat intake, fat digestion and regulation of fat intake may be very closely associated through enterostatin and its parent molecule pancreatic procolipase.

Acknowledgements

This research was supported by grants from the Swedish Medical Research Council (B91-03X-07904-05C). Ms Ulla Johannesson and Ms Yajun Cheng are thanked for skilful technical assistance and Ms Ruth Lovén for secretarial assistance.

References

1. Berry, E.M., Hisch, J., Most, J. & Thornton, J. (1986): The role of dietary fat in human obesity. *Int. J. Obes.* **10**, 123-131.
2. Blundell, J.E. & Burley, V.J. (1990): Evaluation of the satiating power of dietary fat in man. Abstr. *Int. J. Obes.* **14**, suppl. 2.
3. Borgström, B. & Erlanson, C. (1973): Pancreatic lipase and colipase. Interactions and effects of bile salts and other detergents. *Eur. J. Biochem.* **37**, 60-68.
4. Borgström, B. & Erlanson-Albertsson, C. (1984): Pancreatic colipase. In *Lipases*, eds. B. Borgström & H.L. Brockman, pp. 151-184. Amsterdam: Elsevier North-Holland.
5. Borgström, B. & Hildebrand, H. (1975): Lipase and colipase activities of human small intestinal contents after a liquid test meal. *Scand. J. Gastroent.* **10**, 585-591.
6. Bowyer, R.C., Jehanli, A.M.T., Patel, G. & Herman-Taylor, J. (1991): Development of enzyme-linked immunosorbent assay for free human procolipase activation peptide. *Clin. Chim. Acta* (in press).
7. Dreon, D.M., Hewitt, B., Ellsworth, N., Williams, P.T., Terry, R.B. & Wood, P.D. (1988): Dietary fat: carbohydrate ratio and obesity in middle-aged men. *Am. J. Clin. Nutr.* **47**, 995-1000.
8. Erlanson, C., Fernlund, P. & Borgström, B. (1973): Purification and characterization of two proteins with colipase activity from porcine pancreas. *Biochim. Biophys. Acta* **310**, 437-445.
9. Erlanson-Albertsson, C. & Larsson, A. (1988): A possible physiological function of procolipase activation peptide in appetite regulation. *Biochimie* **70**, 1245-1250.
10. Erlanson-Albertsson, C. & Larsson, A. (1988): The activation peptide of pancreatic procolipase decreases food intake in rats. *Regul. Pept.* **22**, 325-331.
11. Erlanson-Albertsson, C., Jie, M., Okada, S., York, D. & Bray, G.A. (1991): Pancreatic procolipase activation peptide – enterostatin – specifically inhibits fat intake. *Phys. Behav.* **49**, 1191-1194.
12. Hildebrand, H., Borgström, B., Békássy, A., Erlanson-Albertsson, C. & Helin, I. (1982): Isolated colipase deficiency in two brothers. *Gut* **23**, 243-246.
13. Kromhout, D., Keys, A., Aravanis, C., Buzina, R., Fidanza, F., Giamaoli, S., Jensen, A., Menotti, A., Nedeljovic, S., Pekkarinen, M. *et al.* (1989): Food consumption patterns in the 1960s in seven countries. *Am. J. Clin. Nutr.* **49**, 889-894.
14. Okada, S., York, D.A., Bray, G.A. & Erlanson-Albertsson, C. (1991): Enterostatin (Val-Pro-Asp-Pro-Arg) the activation peptide of procolipase selectively reduces fat intake. *Phys. Behav.* **49**, 1185-1189.
15. Rovery, M., Boudouard, M. & Bianchetta, J. (1978): An improved large scale procedure for the purification of porcine pancreatic lipase. *Biochim. Biophys. Acta* **575**, 373-379.
16. Sepple, C.P. & Read, N.W. (1990): Effect of prefeeding lipid on food intake and satiety in man. *Gut* **31**, 158-161.
17. Shargill, N.S., Tsujii, S., Bray, G.A. & Erlanson-Albertsson, C. (1991): Enterostatin suppresses food intake following injection into the third ventricle of rats. *Brain Research* **544**, 137-140.
18. Wicker, C. & Puigserver, A. (1987): Effects of inverse changes in dietary lipid and carbohydrate on the synthesis of some pancreatic secretory proteins. *Eur. J. Biochem.* **162**, 25-30.

Chapter 8

Absence of Complete Caloric Compensation Following Mild Deprivation at the End of the Dark Phase in Lean Female Rats

Mary Lisa SASSANO, Francoise J. SMITH and L. Arthur CAMPFIELD
Neurobiology and Obesity Research, Hoffmann-La Roche Inc., Nutley, NJ 07110, USA

The effects of food deprivation at the end of the dark cycle on the meal pattern of female intact rats were studied. Following stable recordings of 24 h food intake and meal pattern, 14 animals were subdivided into two groups: control (n = 4) and experimental (n = 10). The experimental group was food deprived for the last 2 h of the 12 h dark cycle on four occasions that were randomly chosen to be 1 to 4 days apart over a 2 week period in two separate studies. The control animals always had free access to food. Daily food intake was significantly reduced on food deprived days compared to *ad libitum* days (14.2 ± 0.4 g versus 18.1 ± 0.4 g, respectively). On the days following food deprivation, daily food intake was 19.8 ± 0.8 g. Thus, a 24 ± 3% reduction in daily food intake was observed on food deprivation days while an increase of only 12 ± 2% was observed the day after food deprivation. Compensation, on the day following food deprivation, was only partial (56–78%) when calculated over the 24 and 6 h intervals following food deprivation or the 12 h interval across the dark/light transition. These studies demonstrate that daily food intake can be reduced without total compensation during the following day when food deprivation is imposed at the *end* of the dark cycle.

Introduction

The purpose of this study was to assess the consequences of mild food deprivation at the *end* of the dark phase of the light/dark cycle on the meal pattern of intact female Sprague-Dawley rats. An important issue in the control of food intake and the effect of drugs reducing food intake is the optimal timing for the most robust suppression. Many other investigators have shown that periods of food deprivation at the *beginning* of the dark cycle are compensated completely by the end of the dark phase (e.g. Kersten et al.[2]; Strubbe et al.[3]; Tempel et al.[4]). This study was designed to determine if the dark/light phase transition was fundamentally different from the light/dark transition with respect to caloric compensation.

Methods

Female Sprague-Dawley (Charles-River) intact rats (230-260 g) were maintained on a 12/12 light/dark cycle and housed in individual cylindrical plastic cages in a temperature-controlled room with constant access to powdered rat chow (except during food deprivation) and tap water. The meal pattern of the individual rats was measured using a special food cup fitted with strain gauge weighing apparatus (microbalance) set in a metal alcove. The analogue outputs of the strain gauge food cup weighing apparatus were sampled four times a minute, amplified, digitized and interfaced to an IBM computer (Campfield et al.[1]).

Twenty-four hour food intake and body weight were monitored throughout the experiment. A total of 14 animals were used in the two separate replications (2-week duration) of the study and subdivided into two groups, control (n = 4) and experimental (n = 10). The animals in the control and experimental groups were selected on the following criteria:

1. A stable baseline daily food intake and meal pattern maintained for 4 days (CV < 10%).
2. Insignificant amounts of food spillage from the instrumented cup (equipped with an anti-spillage cover).

The experimental group was food deprived for the last 2 h of the dark cycle: food in the instrumented cup was replaced at lights "on". Four periods of food deprivation were applied in a randomized order, separated by 1 to 4 days of free-feeding. The control group had free access to food throughout the study. In addition, all rats were subjected to a sham experiment on non-experimental days in which food cups were removed and then replaced to eliminate the possibility of the rats becoming entrained to the food deprivation paradigm.

In order to evaluate the degree of compensation in food intake, analysis of food intake was subdivided into four 6 h intervals: the first and last 6 h of the light and dark cycles. Analyses were made comparing the intake between *ad libitum* days and food deprivation days as well as the days after food deprivation. All data were first averaged across individual rats, then averaged across all animals within the study.

Calculations

Two different methods of assessing the percentage compensation in food intake were used as shown in the following equations.

Equation I (over 12 h interval across dark/light transition):

$$\% \text{ compensation} = \frac{\text{last 6 h dark (fd)} + \text{first 6 h light (dafd)}}{\text{first 6 h light (nfd)} + \text{last 6 h dark (nfd)}} \times 100$$

Equation II (over the next 6 h of access to food):

$$\% \text{ compensation} = \frac{\text{first 6 h light (dafd)}}{\text{last 6 h dark (nfd)} - \text{last 6 h dark (fd)}} \times 100$$

dafd = day after food deprivation; fd = food deprivation day; nfd = non food deprived day

Results

The animals in the control group (n = 4) maintained a stable 24 h food intake over the 2 week period. Mean daily food intake of the experimental animals is shown in Fig. 1 (Study 1) and Fig. 2 (Study 2). When the data were combined over all trials of both studies, daily food intake was significantly reduced on food deprivation days compared to non-food deprivation days (14.2 ± 0.4 g versus 18.1 ± 0.4 g, respectively; $P < 0.05$). On the day following food deprivation, daily food intake was 19.8 ± 0.8 g. Therefore, a $24 \pm 3\%$ reduction in daily food intake occurred on food deprivation days. During the 24 h following food deprivation, food intake was increased by $12 \pm 2\%$. As a result, compensation in daily food intake on the day after food deprivation was only partial, ranging from 50 to 60%.

The percentage compensation during the 12 h interval across the dark/light transition was calculated using Equation I. The mean percentage compensations for the individual rats over the four trials in each study are shown in Fig. 3. Compensation for all the rats in Study 1 (n = 6) was $77 \pm 11\%$ and in Study 2 (n = 4) was $80 \pm 5\%$. When averaged across all the rats in both studies, compensation was only partial on the day after food deprivation trials compared to non-food deprivation trials in nine out of ten animals, ranging from 50 to 125% with a mean of $78 \pm 6\%$.

The percentage compensation during the first 6 h of the light phase following food deprivation

Chapter 8 – Absence of Complete Caloric Compensation Following Mild Deprivation

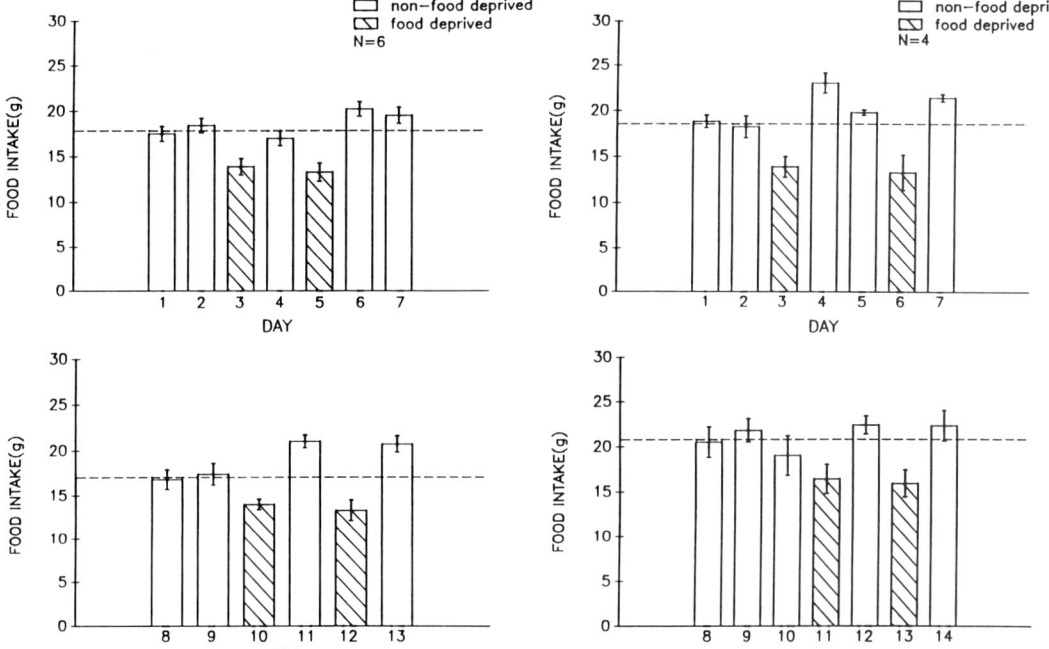

Fig. 1. Study 1: Averaged mean 24 h food intake of six experimental animals over 13 days. The open bars represent non-food deprived days while the hatched bars represent the days of food deprivation. Each bar represents the mean ± SEM. Twenty-four hour food intake on days 3, 5, 10 and 12 was significantly reduced compared to the other days (P < 0.05).

Fig. 2. Study 2: Averaged 24 h food intake of four experimental animals over 14 days. The open bars represent non-food deprived days while the hatched bars represent the days of food deprivation. Each bar represents the mean ± SEM. Twenty-four hour food intake on days 3, 6, 11 and 13 was significantly reduced compared to the other days (P < 0.05).

was calculated using Equation II. The percentage compensation on the day after each trial of food deprivation for the rats in Study 1 (n = 6) and Study 2 (n = 4) is shown in Fig. 4. The averaged percentage compensation the day after food deprivation over the four trials for Study 1 was 52 ± 5% and for Study 2 was 61 ± 8%. When the data from the two studies were combined, compensation for the "blocked meals" was only partial in 28 out of 36 trials (nine out of ten rats), ranging from 0 to 174% with a mean of 56 ± 5%.

Discussion

These studies demonstrate that daily food intake can be reduced without complete compensation the following day, when food deprivation was imposed at the end of the dark cycle. In sharp contrast with our results, similar studies utilizing equivalent periods of food deprivation imposed at the *beginning* of the dark phase resulted in complete compensation by the end of the dark phase (e.g. Kersten et al.[2]; Strubbe et al.[3]; Tempel et al.[4]). These findings are in agreement with those of Kersten et al.[2] obtained in animals maintained on mixed diets and deprived of food for 3 h across the dark/light transition and those of Tempel et al.[4] obtained in animals maintained on pure macronutrient diets and deprived of food for hours 10 and 11 of the dark cycle. In this study, a meal was observed in the light phase immediately following the restriction of food access. However, the size of the meal was insufficient to compensate for the blocked intake during the end of the dark. Thus, these rats could adjust

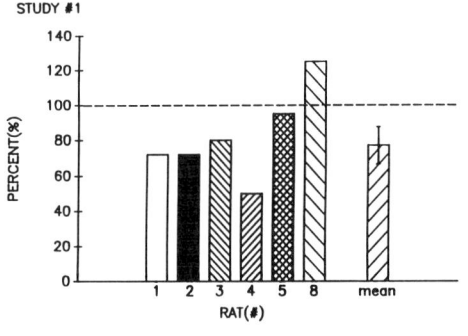
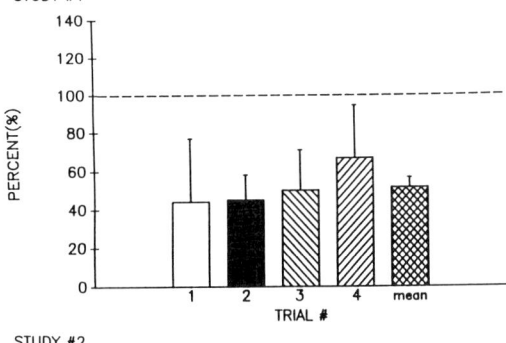
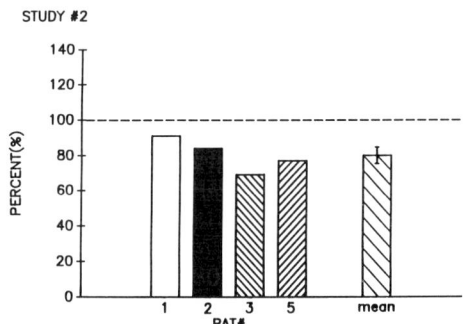
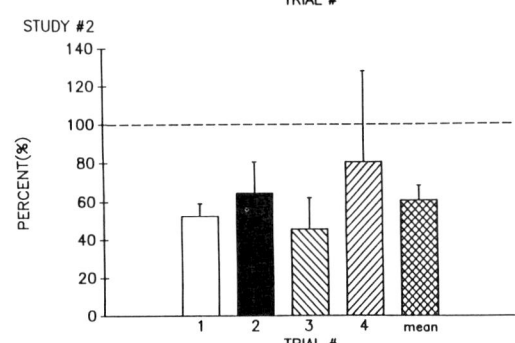

Fig. 3. Averaged compensation during the 12 h interval across the dark/light transition (Equation I). The mean percentage compensation for the individual rats over the four trials and the cumulative mean percentage compensation across rats ($X \pm SEM$) for Study 1 ($n = 6$) and Study 2 ($n = 4$) are represented.

Fig. 4. Averaged percentage compensation during the first 6 h of the light phase following food deprivation (Equation II). Mean percentage compensation ($X \pm SEM$) for the day after each trial of food deprivation and the cumulative mean of the four trials in Study 1 ($n = 6$) and Study 2 ($n = 4$) are represented.

the distribution of meals in response to this mild food deprivation but the mechanisms controlling meal size were insufficiently plastic to allow complete compensation. These experiments suggest that the mechanisms underlying caloric compensation are distinctly different in the light/dark compared to the dark/light phase transitions and they imply an inherent plasticity of these regulatory mechanisms. Therefore, agents that suppress food intake may be more effective across the dark/light than the light/dark transition in rats.

Acknowledgements: We would like to acknowledge the technical assistance of Debra Howell, Constantino Michailidis, Kimberly Moore and Joseph Sia.

References

1. Campfield, L.A., Brandon, P. & Smith, F.J. (1985): On-line continuous measurement of blood glucose and meal pattern in free-feeding rats: the role of glucose in meal initiation. *Brain Res. Bull.* **14**, 605-616.
2. Kersten, A., Strubbe, J.H. & Spiteri, N.J. (1980): Meal patterning of rats with changes in day length and food availability. *Physiol. Behav.* **25**, 953-958.
3. Strubbe, J.H., Keyser, J., Dijkstra, T. & Prins, J.A. (1986): Interaction between circadian and caloric control of feeding behavior in the rat. *Physiol. Behav.* **36**, 489-493.
4. Tempel, D.L., Shor-Posner, G., Dwyer, D. & Leibowitz, S.F. (1989): Nocturnal patterns of macronutrient intake in freely feeding and food-deprived rats. *Am. J. Physiol.* **256**, R541-R548.

Chapter 9

Intracerebroventricular Injection of Monosodium Glutamate (MSG) Stimulates Food Intake in Long-Evans Rats

A. STRICKER-KRONGRAD, B. BECK, J.P. MAX, J.P. NICOLAS and C. BURLET

INSERM U.308, Mécanismes de Régulation du Comportement Alimentaire, 38, rue Lionnois, 54000 Nancy, France

Systemic injection of monosodium glutamate (MSG) promotes hyperphagia in the adult rats. To test the hypothesis of a possible role of brain glutamate in feeding behaviour regulation, Long-Evans adult rats were centrally injected with MSG and feeding behaviour was analysed. Results showed that central MSG strongly stimulated food intake with marked effects on the first meal after injection. These effects were obtained with a dose of MSG several thousand-fold smaller than those used in systemic injection. The peripheral effect of MSG on food intake might therefore be partly related to the passage of MSG in the central compartment and its action on central circumventricular areas.

Introduction

Monosodium glutamate (MSG) is a well-known food additive. When injected subcutaneously in neonatal rats and mice, it produces a marked decrease in food intake and an increase in adipose tissue mass[3,4]. These effects are related to its neurotoxic properties[2,5]. On the other hand, in the adult rat, systemic injections of MSG produce a dose-dependent increase in food intake[6]. The exact mechanism of this effect of MSG is not known but we supposed that it could be partly related to the passage of MSG in the central compartment. To test this hypothesis, we determined the effects of intracerebroventricular injection of MSG on the feeding pattern of adult Long-Evans rats. If our hypothesis is true, central injection of MSG might reproduce the effects of systemic injection with a higher potency.

Material and methods

Fifteen male Long-Evans rats (Centre d'Elevage R. Janvier. Le Genest-Saint Isle, France) weighing 290 ± 2.7 g were housed in individual wire cages in an air-conditioned room with an automatic light-dark cycle (dark between 19.00 and 7.00). The animals were fed on a well-balanced diet. 54 per cent, 30 per cent and 16 per cent of energy were provided by carbohydrate, fat and protein respectively. Its exact composition has been previously described[1]. Diet and tap water were available *ad libitum*. After 7 days of habituation to these conditions, the rats were implanted with a stainless steel guide cannula (27 gauge, Terumo Corporation, Leuven, Belgium) aimed in the right lateral brain ventricle. To avoid its occlusion, a stylet was inserted into the cannula. After 7 days of recovery, the rats were injected either with vehicle (artificial cerebrospinal fluid; CSF) or with MSG (3 mg/brain

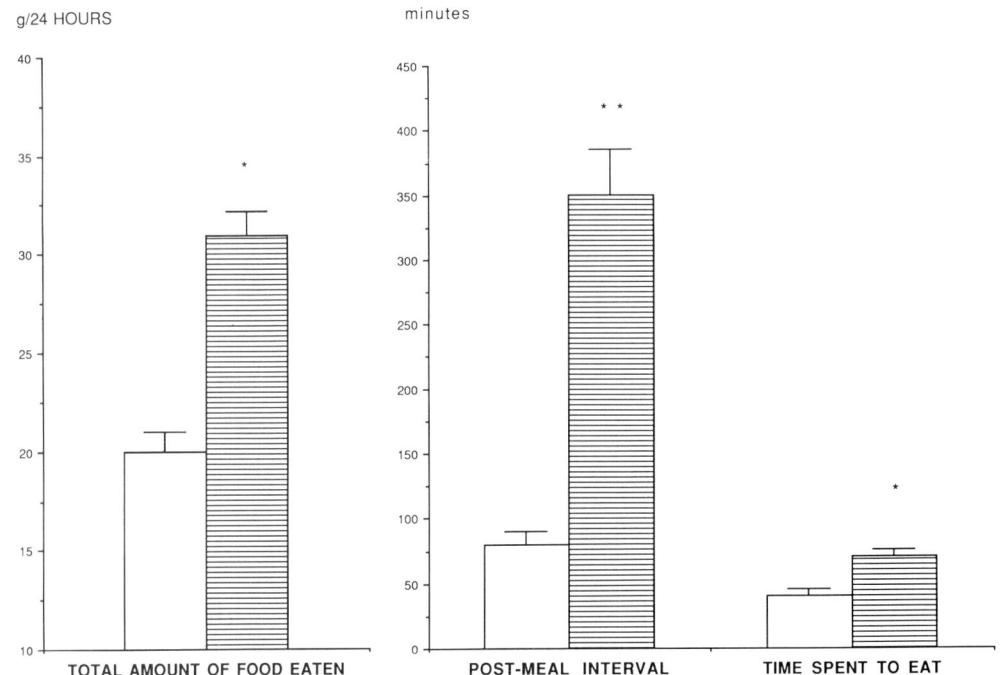

Fig. 1. Total amount of food eaten, time spent to eat during 24 h post-injection and post-meal interval of the first meal of the same rats (n = 15) injected either with CSF (open bars) or with MSG (stripped bars). *$P < 0.01$ and **$P < 0.001$ between CSF and MSG injections. Values represent mean $\pm$ SEM.

diluted in 5 µl of CSF) under light ether anaesthesia. The feeding pattern of the rats was recorded during 24 h through a complete automatic system driven by a computer.

Effects of injection were compared with those of the cerebrospinal fluid only, for the same animals. All values were compared with Student's paired t-test (two-tailed) with a 5 per cent upper level of significance.

Results and discussion

Total amount of food eaten, time spent to eat during the 24 h that followed injection of CSF or MSG and the post-meal interval after the first meal are shown in Fig. 1. During the 24 h that followed the injection, rats injected with MSG ate significantly more food (+21 per cent; $P < 0.01$) and spent much more time to eat (+40 per cent; $P < 0.01$) than when injected with vehicle only. These effects were present in spite of the augmentation of the post-meal interval that followed the first meal (x4; $P < 0.001$). Central MSG injection induced therefore the same effects as systemic injections during these 24 h[6]. During this period, the structure and pattern of feeding behaviour were strongly modified (cf. Fig. 2). The size of the first meal after MSG injection was greatly increased (+285 per cent; $P < 0.001$). This augmentation of meal size was accompanied by a subsequent augmentation of meal duration (x10; $P < 0.001$). These increases were observed for all meals of this 24 h period. They reached +44 per cent ($P < 0.01$) for meal size and +53 per cent ($P < 0.01$) for meal duration. However they were smaller than the effects on the first meal ($P < 0.01$ and $P < 0.01$ for size and duration respectively).

MSG injection produced very strong and rapid, as well as relatively long lasting, modifications of feeding behaviour. This study showed that monosodium glutamate must be considered as a potent stimulant of food intake when administered by a central route. This effect

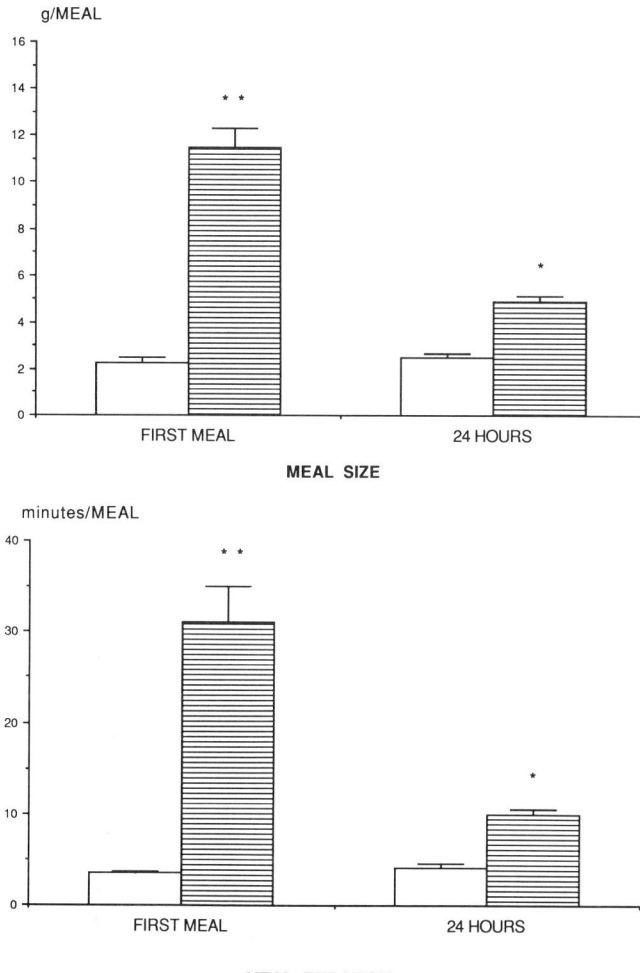

*Fig. 2. Meal size (top panel) and meal duration (bottom) of the first meal and of the all other meals of the 24 h period of the same rats (n = 15) injected either with artificial CSF (open bars) or with MSG (stripped bars). *P < 0.01 and **P < 0.001 between CSF and MSG injections. Values represent mean ± SEM.*

was more powerful than that observed when systemically injected[6], even if we used a several thousand-fold smaller dose. It is therefore possible that central glutamate might be implicated in hyperphagia observed after peripheral injection. The importance of the passage of MSG from peripheral to central compartment and the eventual circumventricular areas involved in this action remains to be determined.

References

1. Beck, B., Stricker-Krongrad, A., Burlet, A., Nicolas, J.P. & Burlet, C. (1990): Influence of diet composition on food intake and hypothalamic neuropeptide Y (NPY) in the rat. *Neuropeptides* 17, 197-203.
2. Dawson, R. & Annau, Z. (1983): A behavioral assessment of arcuate nucleus damage after a single injection of monosodium glutamate to mice. *Neurobehav. Toxicol. Teratol.* 5, 399-406.

3. Kanarek, R.B., Meyers, J., Made, R. & Mayer, J. (1979): Juvenile onset obesity and deficits in caloric regulation in MSG-treated rats. *Pharmacol. Biochem. Behav.* **10**, 717-721.
4. Olney, J.W. (1969): Brain lesions, obesity and other disturbances in mice treated with monosodium glutamate. *Science* **164**, 719-721.
5. Olney, J.W., Rhee, V. & DeGubareff, T. (1977): Neurotoxic effects of glutamate on mouse area postrema. *Brain Res.* **120**, 151-157.
6. Reddy, V.M., Meharg, S.S. & Ritter, S. (1986): Dose-related stimulation of feeding by systemic injection of monosodium-glutamate. *Physiol. Behav.* **38**, 465-470.

Chapter 10

Stress Related Overeating, d-Fenfluramine and Neuroendocrine Responses in the Ageing Rat

Francoise LACOUR, Denis RAVEL, Bernard KERDELHUÉ*, Joseph ESPINAL and Jacques DUHAULT

Institut de Recherches SERVIER, 11 rue des Moulineaux, 92150 Suresnes, France; *Laboratory for Reproductive Neurobiology, CNRS, 78360 Jouy en Josas, France

The 12-month-old rat (SD) presents some of the characteristics of the overweight population: hyperinsulinaemia, hypertriglyceridaemia and a decrease in glucose tolerance. The purpose of this study was to observe the effects of an i.p. administration of 1 mg/kg of d-fenfluramine on the neuroendocrine responses to a tail pinch (TP) session (a stress-related overeating) in young (3 months of age) and aged (12 months of age) male Sprague-Dawley rats.

Blood samples were collected for plasmatic determinations (glucose, insulin, ACTH, β-endorphin and corticosterone) prior to and after TP and at the end of a recovery period (2 h). During the 120 s of TP trial, the 12-month-old rat ate significantly more than the 3-month-old rat (105 s *versus* 91 s, respectively $P = 0.019$). d-Fenfluramine induced the same significant reduction in the duration of eating in the two groups of treated rats (–20%). All animals responded to the tail pinch by increasing plasma insulin. However, the corticosterone, ACTH and β-endorphin responses were decreased in the 12-month-old group when compared to the 3-month-old rats. d-Fenfluramine administration significantly reduced these responses in the 3-month-old rats but was without significant effect in the aged rat. The reduction in the stress-related overeating in response to d-fenfluramine, could be related to the reduction of stress, independently of its own anorectic effect.

Introduction

In experimental pharmacology unstressed animals are generally used to study the mechanism of action of drugs. However, in humans and animals, mildly stressful daily events occur which can induce behavioural, neuroendocrine and metabolic responses.

Ageing has been associated with a deterioration in glucose tolerance, insulin resistance[16], hypertriglyceridaemia and a consequent increase in adipose tissue deposits[12,7]. Ageing is also characterized by a systemic loss of adaptation to neuroendocrine responses. Glucocorticoids released in stress conditions could contribute to the ageing process and to neuronal loss[13,19]. The 12-month-old male SpragueDawley rat parallels the profile of human non-insulin dependent diabetes mellitus. This elderly rat presents some of the characteristics of the overweight population[15]: hyperinsulinaemia, hypertriglyceridaemia and a decrease in glucose tolerance[8].

It has been shown that stress-related overeating in humans and a stress such as TP eating in rats show similar responses to certain anorectic agents[3]. A mild stress such as tail pinch

(TP)[2,17] which induces eating in fed rats, may thus produce different responses in the ageing insulin-resistant rat.

The serotoninergic antiobesity agent d-fenfluramine (dF) is known to decrease food intake by acting through an enhancement of brain serotonin tone *via* an inhibition of reuptake and an increase of serotonin release from presynaptic neurons[4]. When given acutely, dF is a potent inhibitor of stress-related eating[17]. The purpose of this study was to observe the effects of an intraperitoneal administration of 1 mg/kg of dF on the neuroendocrine responses to a tail pinch session in young (3 months of age) and aged (12 months of age) male Sprague-Dawley rats.

Methods

Tail pinch was performed as in published procedures[21]. Blood samples were collected, through an indwelling catheter in the jugular vein, for determination of blood glucose (glucose oxidase method), plasma insulin (Phadeseph, Pharmacia), corticosterone, ACTH and β-endorphin, which were determined using specific RIA's. All parameters were determined before and after the tail pinch (TP) session and 30 and 120 min later.

Results

Stress overeating

The mean duration of tail pinch induced eating in fed rats was significantly different in the 12-month- and 3-month-old rats (105 s and 91 s respectively, $P = 0.019$) (Fig. 1). d-Fenfluramine induced a similar reduction (20%) in the duration of eating in the two groups of rats.

Blood glucose

TP induced a small increase in blood glucose but it was not significant in both groups. dF significantly reduced blood glucose by 16% only in the 3-month-old group 30 min after the stress ($P = 0.036$) (Fig. 2 a,b).

Plasma insulin

Higher insulin values were observed in the 12-month-old rat (Fig. 3b) when compared to the 3-month-old rat throughout the test but the difference was not significant. dF reduced

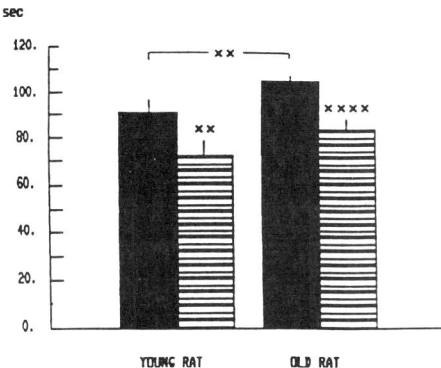

Fig. 1. Duration of eating during 120 s of tail pinch. Rats received an IP administration of saline or d-fenfluramine (1 mg/kg) 30 min prior to the TP.
■ NaCl treated rats; ≡ d-fenfluramine treated rats; n = 15 in each group.
Values were expressed as means ± SE and compared using Student's t-test
** $P \leq 0.025$, **** $P \leq 0.005$

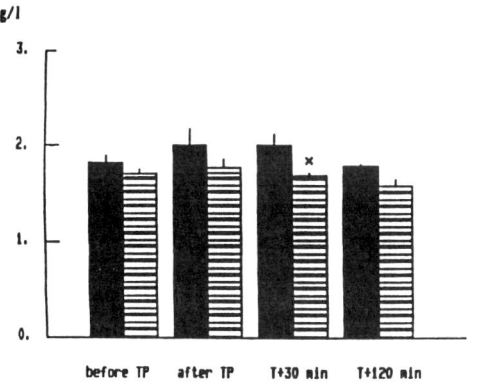
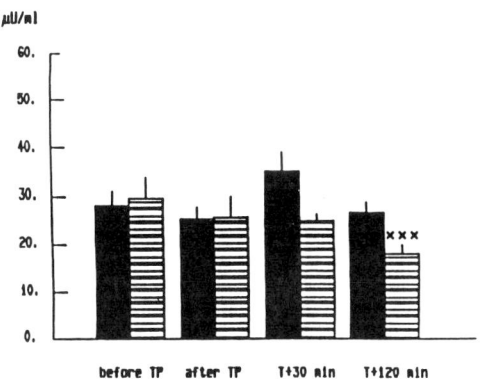
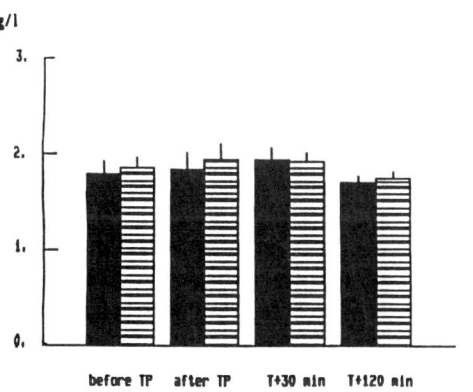
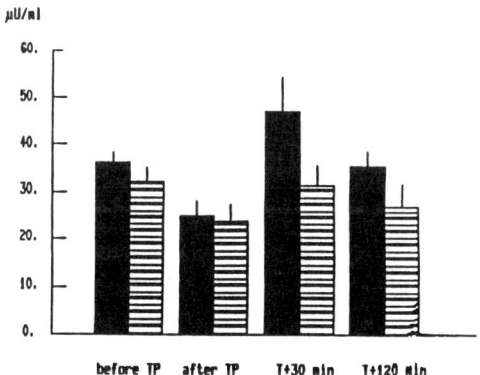

Fig. 2 (left). Blood glucose and d-fenfluramine in the young rat (a) and in the old rat (b).
n = 5 in the young groups; n = 6 in the old groups.
■ *NaCl treated rats;* ≡ *d-fenfluramine (1 mg/kg, IP) treated rats.*
Results are expressed as means ± SE and were compared using a 2-way analysis of variance
* $P \leq 0.05$, *** $P \leq 0.01$.
Blood samples were taken before and after the TP and during the post-stress period (T + 30 min and T + 120 min) via a jugular catheter.

Fig. 3 (right). Plasma insulin and d-fenfluramine in the young rat (a) and in the old rat (b).
n = 5 in the young groups; n = 6 in the old groups.
■ *NaCl treated rats;* ≡ *d-fenfluramine (1 mg/kg, IP) treated rats.*
Results are expressed as means ± SE and were compared using a 2-way analysis of variance
* $P \leq 0.05$, ***$P \leq 0.01$
Blood samples were taken before and after the TP and during the post-stress period (T + 30 min and T + 120 min) via a jugular catheter.

significantly the insulin response to the TP throughout the 2 h after stress in the 3 month group only (Fig. 3a).

Plasma corticosterone

Whereas the corticosterone response to tail pinch was similar in the two groups of rats, the post-stress recovery was impaired with sustained higher corticosterone values in the 12-

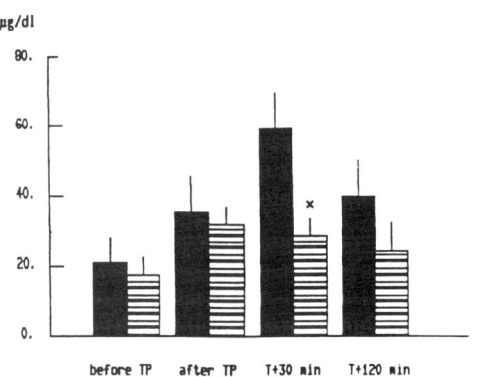
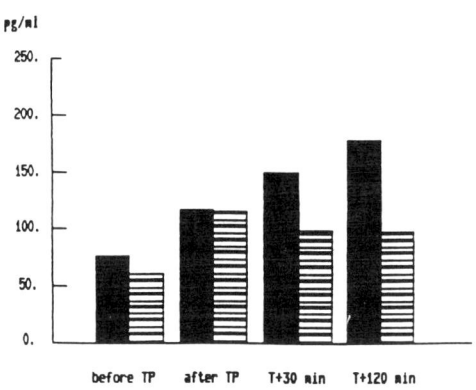
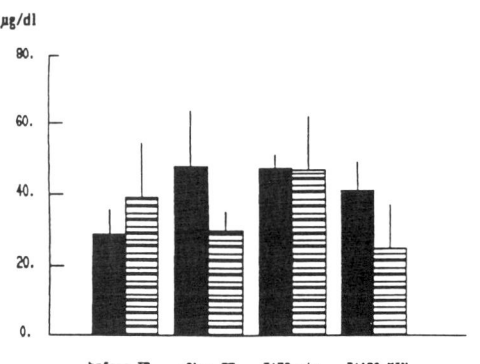
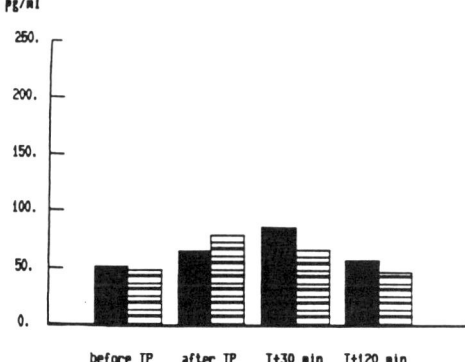

Fig. 4 (left). Plasma corticosterone and d-fenfluramine in the young rat (a) and in the old rat (b).
n = 6 in the young groups; n = 5 in the old groups.
■ *NaCl treated rats;* ≡ *d-fenfluramine (1 mg/kg, IP) treated rats.*
Results are expressed as means ± SE and were compared using a 2-way analysis of variance
* $P \leq 0.05$
Blood samples were taken before and after the TP and during the post-stress period (T + 30 min and T + 120 min) via a jugular catheter.

Fig. 5 (right). Plasma ACTH d-fenfluramine in the young rat (a) and in the old rat (b).
Each bar represents a pool of six rats.
■ *NaCl treated rats;* ≡ *d-fenfluramine treated groups*
Blood samples were taken before and after the TP and during the post-stress period (T + 30 min and T + 120 min) via a jugular catheter.

month-old group (Fig. 4b). dF induced a significant decrease only in the 3-month-old group (–51%, 30 min after the stress, $P = 0.03$) (Fig. 4a).

Plasma ACTH

Old rats responded to stress with a decreased ACTH secretion when compared to young rats (Fig. 5a). In young rats, dF caused a fast return to baseline levels, whereas it was without effect in old rats (Fig. 5b). Thus, a decreased sensitivity to stress in the liberation of ACTH is observed in old rats.

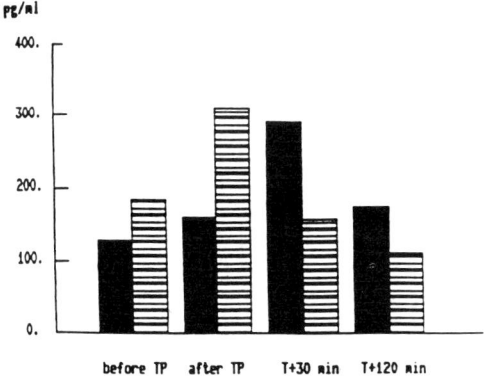
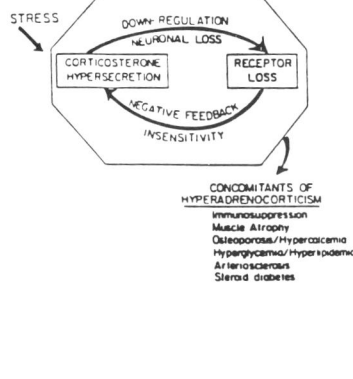
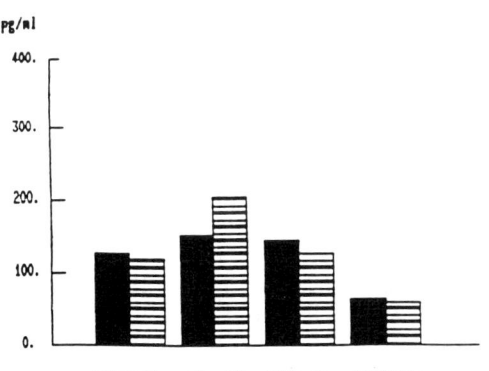

Fig. 6 (left). Plasma β-endorphin and d-fenfluramine in the young rat (a) and in the old rat (b).
Each bar represents a pool of six rats.
■ NaCl treated rats; ≡ d-fenfluramine treated groups.
Blood samples were taken before and after the TP and during the post-stress period (T + 30 min and T + 120 min) via a jugular catheter.

Fig. 7 (right). Sapolsky's model of glucocorticoid cascade hypothesis, 1986.

Plasma β-endorphin

β-endorphin secretion in response to stress was dramatically decreased in the 12-month-old rats. Pretreatment with dF increased the initial secretion of β-endorphin and caused a faster return to baseline levels in both groups (Fig. 6a, b).

Discussion

The present results show that ageing rats are more responsive to tail pinch than the young rats in terms of the duration of eating. There is no concomitant significant alteration in the circulating levels of glucose and insulin. The aged male rat showed no impairment in its early ACTH, β-endorphin and corticosterone responses to stress immediately after the tail pinch session. Nevertheless, the neuroendocrine system can be considered impaired, as suggested by the sustained secretion of corticosterone (Fig. 4).

Previous studies have reported that in the rat, the ageing process decreases the capacity to elicit an adequate adrenocortical response to stress[10]. Sapolsky et al.[18] have also observed an elevation of basal corticosterone which could explain the decline in sensitivity to negative-feedback control.

Our results are in agreement with those of Erisman et al.[10] despite the use of different stress conditions. The same results in plasma corticosterone levels have been observed also in young and old Fisher rats after 60 min of immobilization[20]. It was hypothesized that the hippocampus is a mediating locus of glucocorticoid feedback inhibition at the end of stress and that in the aged rats, the observed hippocampal degeneration is responsible for the loss of sensitivity to feedback inhibition (see Sapolky's model in Fig. 7). Thus, rat hypothalamus CRF released after perception of a stressor stimulates the release of ACTH from the pituitary which in turn stimulates release of glucocorticoids from the adrenal gland[11]. The degenerative loss of neurons and receptor depletion (B and GC, corticosterone and glucocorticoid receptors, respectively) desensitizes the structure to the presence of circulating corticosterone and causes circulating concentrations of the steroids to be underestimated[20]. Odio et al.[14] observed that the ability of the pituitary adrenal system to show adaptation of the early response to stress declines with advancing age and with chronic exposure to stress.

In our study, d-fenfluramine reduced the duration of tail pinch-induced eating to the same extent in both 3 month- and 12 month-old rats. The effects observed in young rats are in agreement with previously published results[17,21]. Fenfluramine failed to decrease significantly blood glucose and plasma insulin levels in the old rat. However, a significant reduction in these two parameters occurred after the stress in the 3-month-old rat. The effect of d-fenfluramine on insulin levels has been described previously by ourselves and others[9,4].

Following df administration, the pattern of corticosterone ACTH and β-endorphin was the same for both young and old rats. Thus, d-fenfluramine administration tended to result in a faster return to baseline levels of all three hormones. d-Fenfluramine also induced a greater secretion of β-endorphin in both groups.

We can therefore conclude that the effects of df on stress-induced eating may in part be related to alterations in the patterns and levels of secretion of neuroendocrine mediators, such as glucocorticoids and endorphins. Interestingly, we found that following TP, the plasma concentration of β-endorphin was greater than that of ACTH in df-treated animals. Since both of these peptides derive from the same gene (proopiomelanocortin), it is tempting, if not necessarily justified, to speculate on a possible selective effect of d-fenfluramine on post translational processing of these peptides. The molecular mechanisms controlling these processes are unclear at present[6].

Acknowledgements

The authors are grateful to S. Laurin for statistical treatment of this study.

References

1. Amir, S. (1979): The role of endorphins in stress: evidence and speculations. *Neurosci. Biobehav. Rev.* **4**, 77-86.
2. Antelman, S.M. (1975): Tail pinch-induced eating, gnawing and licking behavior in rats: dependence on the nigrostriatal dopamine system. *Brain Res.* **99**, 319-337.
3. Antelman, S.M. (1978): Tails of stress-related behavior: a neuropharmacological model. In *Animal models in psychiatry and neurology*, eds. I. Hanin & E. Usdin, pp. 227-245. Oxford: Pergamon Press.
4. Arnaud, O. (1990): Antiobesity and lipid-lowering agents with antidiabetic activity. In *New antidiabetic drugs*, eds. C.J. Bailey & P.R. Flatt, pp. 133-142. London: Smith-Gordon.
5. Asny, G.M. (1988): The neuroendocrine response to fenfluramine in depressives and normal controls. *Biol. Psychiatry* **24**, 117-120.
6. Boscaro, M. (1990): Inhibition of pituitary β-endorphin by ACTH and glucocorticoids. *Neuroendocrinology* **61**, 561-664.

7. Brindley, D.N. (1989): Possible connections between stress, diabetes, obesity, hypertension and altered lipoprotein metabolism that may result in atherosclerosis. *Clin. Sci.* **77**, 463-461.
8. Duhault, J. (1987): Animal models of pancreatic and peripheral decrease in glucose tolerance. *Lessons from animal diabetes*. London: John Libbey.
9. Duhault, J. (1989): Relationship between fenfluramine effects and adiposity status. Abs. No. 23. New York: New York Academy of Sciences.
10. Erisman, S.(l990): The effects of stress on plasma ACTH and corticosterone in young and aging pregnant rats and their fetuses. *Life Sci.* **47**, 1527-1533.
11. Keller-Wood, M. (1984): Corticosteroid inhibition of ACTH secretion. *Endocr. Rev.* **5**, 1.
12. Kirkland, J.L. (1984): Adipocyte hormone responsiveness and aging in the rat: problems in the interpretation of aging research. *J. Am. Geriatr. Soc.* **32**, 219-228.
13. Lorens, S.A. (1990): Neurochemical, endocrine and immunological responses to stress in young and old Fisher 344 male rats. *Neurobiol. Aging* **11**, 139-150.
14. Odio, M. (1989): Age-related adaptation of pituitary-adrenocortical responses to stress. *Neuroendocrinology* **49**, 382-388.
15. Porte, D. (1991): β-cells in type II diabetes mellitus. *Diabetes* **40**, 166-179
16. Reaven, G.M. (1988): Role of insulin resistance in human disease. *Diabetes* **37**, 1595-1607.
17. Rowland, N.E. (1988): Dexfenfluramine: effects on food intake in various animal models. *Clin. Neuropharmacol.* **11**, 33-50.
18. Sapolsky, R.M. (1983): The adrenocortical stress-response in the aged male rat: impairment of recovery from stress. *Exp. Gerontol.* **18**, 55-64.
19. Sapolsky, R.M. (1984): Do vasopressin-related peptides induce hippocampal corticosterone receptors? Implications for aging. *J. Neurosci.* **4**, 1479-1485.
20. Sapolsky, R.M. (1986): The neuroendocrinology of stress and aging: the glucocorticoid cascade hypothesis. *Endocr. Rev.* **7**, 284-301.
21. Souquet, A.M. (1989): Effect of chronic administration of dexfenfluramine on stress- and palatability-induced food intake in rats. *Physiol. Behav.* **46**, 145-149.

Chapter 11

Evaluation of the Action of a Non-absorbable Fat on Appetite and Energy Intake in Lean, Healthy Males

Victoria J. BURLEY and John E. BLUNDELL

BioPsychology Group, Psychology Department, University of Leeds, Leeds, LS2 9JT, UK

Introduction

Recent evidence suggests that the incidence of obesity is increasing in Britain. The proportion of the population classified as overweight or obese has increased by 15% in men and 12% in women between 1980 and 1986[2]. It is generally recognized that the intake of dietary fat in the developed world is excessive. In the United Kingdom fat intake continues to provide in the region of 40% of our energy intake. An estimated one-third of Britons manage to limit their energy intake from fat to 35 per cent, a figure which is recommended in the reports of a number of advisory bodies in the UK[1,4]. For the remaining 65% of the population their excessive dietary fat intake may predispose them to the development of obesity since it is known that a dietary intake high in fat is strongly correlated with weight gain[5]. Furthermore, evidence from studies such as that conducted by Lissner *et al.*[3] suggests that the provision of high-fat food facilitates passive overconsumption.

One apparently easy way of reducing dietary fat and/or energy intake whilst maintaining the palatability of the diet is to use a non-absorbable fat substitute, such as the sucrose polyester, olestra. Little is known, however about the consequences of a reduction in dietary fat (or its replacement by a fat substitute) on satiety and energy intake.

Methods

In order to investigate the action of dietary fat on the expression of appetite we have conducted a study to compare the satiating effect of breakfasts containing differing amounts of fat. A proportion of the fat was replaced in two of the breakfasts by substituting olestra, a sucrose polyester that mimics fat but is not digested by lipases and thus has no energy value. The nutritional composition of the test breakfasts is shown in Table 1.

Twenty four lean (BMI 19–25), healthy, well-regulating males were selected for this study. Using a within-subject, double-blind design each subject consumed a test breakfast after an overnight fast. The breakfast meals (scone, spread, jam and a hot drink) were similar in every respect except for their fat and energy content. For 24 h after consumption, energy and nutrient intakes, and motivational states including hunger were monitored by a combination of measured test meals (at lunch and dinner), food diaries, checklists and visual analogue ratings. *Ad libitum* test meals (lunch and dinner) were carefully constructed from a range of low, medium and high fat foods in order to permit selection of a high or low fat intake. An outline of the experimental schedule is illustrated in Fig. 1.

Table 1. Nutritional composition of experimental breakfasts in the olestra study

Nutrient	Treatment		
	0 g olestra	20 g olestra	36 g olestra
Energy, kcal	761	587	440
Carbohydrate, g	74	74	74
Protein, g	10	10	10
Fat, g	48	28	12

Table 2. 24 hour intake of energy (kcal) and macronutrients (gram and percentage energy), including the test breakfasts in the olestra study

Nutrient	Treatment					
	0 g olestra		20 g olestra		36 g olestra	
	Mean	SE	Mean	SE	Mean	SE
Energy, kcal	3480	89.8	3353	103	3476	103
Carbohydrate, g	343	12	345	12	378	12
Protein, g	156	5	158	5	163	5
Fat, g	161	5	146*	5	140*	6
% Carbohydrate	39	0.8	41*	0.7	44*	0.9
% Protein	18	0.3	19	0.4	19	0.5
% Fat	42	0.8	39*	0.7	36*	0.8

*Mean value significantly different from 0 g olestra breakfast.

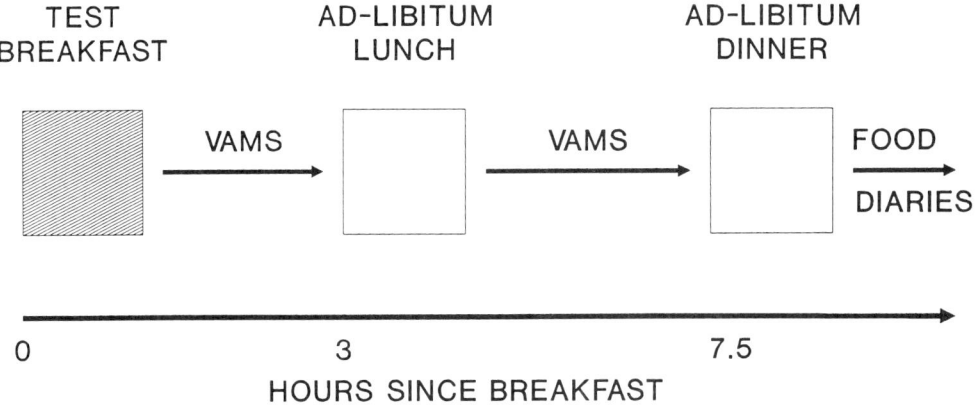

Fig. 1. Experimental schedule of the olestra study (VAMS = Visual Analogue Mood Scales).

Results

The major outcome of the study is shown in Table 2. Caloric intakes for the full 24 h period (including the test breakfast) were not statistically different. Consequently the withdrawal of fat from this meal (fat minus manipulation) and its substitution by olestra lead to almost complete caloric compensation for the caloric deficit sustained. However, two further features should be noted. Firstly, caloric intakes at the test lunch taken 3 h after the breakfast were not statistically different. Subjects compensated for the lower energy intake at breakfast partly by consuming more at the second test meal (dinner), but primarily by snacks during the evening. In these subjects almost complete energy compensation occurred in the 24 h following consumption of the fat-substituted meals. The second important outcome was that since fat compensation did not occur, the percentage of energy derived from fat over the whole 24 h period was reduced by the use of olestra in a single breakfast meal.

Discussion

Taken in isolation thus study suggests that dietary fat does exert some control over appetite and has the capacity to suppress food intake later on in the day.

Using this experimental strategy to remove fat from a breakfast, subjects made up for the energy deficit by consuming more later on in the day. The mechanism responsible for this late action has yet to be defined. This study implies that the substitution of fat in the diet (by a non-absorbable fat such as olestra) may be a useful strategy for the reduction of total fat intake, even when energy balance is maintained. However, certain factors should be mentioned in interpreting the data presented here. Other studies, using a different type of manipulation, have suggested that fat has a lower satiating power than protein or carbohydrate[6]. Secondly, these conclusions may only strictly apply to the type of subjects used in this study, i.e. lean individuals who exhibit good day-to-day energy intake regulation. There is a clear need for further studies to be conducted on other types of subject who may not show such precise energy intake regulation. It appears that dietary fat may exert differing effects on appetite in different types of human subjects.

References

1. Committee on Medical Aspects of Food Policy (1983). Department of Health and Social Security. *Report on health and social subjects, No. 28*. London: HMSO.
2. Gregory, J., Foster, K., Tyler, H. & Wiseman, M. (1990). Office of Population Censuses and Surveys. *The dietary and nutritional survey of British adults*. London: HMSO.
3. Lissner, L., Levitsky, D.A., Strupp, B.J., Kalkwarf, H.J. & Roe, D.A. (1987): Dietary fat and the regulation of energy intake in human subjects. *Am. J. Clin. Nutr.* **46**, 886-892.
4. National Advisory Committee for Nutrition Education (1983). *Proposals for nutritional guidelines for nutrition education*. London: Health Education Council.
5. Tremblay, A., Plourde, G., Despres, J.P. & Bouchard, C. (1989): Impact of dietary fat content and fat oxidation on energy intake and oxidation in humans. *Am. J. Clin. Nutr.* **49**, 799-805.
6. Van Amelsvoort, J.M.M., Van Stratum, P., Kraal, J.H., Lussenburg, R.N. & Houtsmuller, U.M.T. (1989): Effects of varying the carbohydrate-fat ratio in a hot lunch on post-prandial variables in male volunteers. *Br. J. Nutr.* **61**, 267-283.

Chapter 12

The Effect of Myco-protein on Hunger, Satiety and Subsequent Food Consumption

W.H. TURNBULL, D. BESSEY, J. WALTON and A.R. LEEDS
Department of Nutrition and Dietetics, King's College London, University of London, Campden Hill Road, London W8 7AH, UK

Introduction

Myco-protein is a food produced by continuous fermentation of *Fusarium graminearum* (Schwabe) on a carbohydrate substrate. The development of myco-protein began in the mid 1960s (Owen et al.[5], Edelman et al.[2], Udall et al.[8]) and after 20 years of extensive research UK authorities approved it for sale to the general public in 1985. The raw product and a large number of prepared dishes are now available through major food retailers. The product is sold under the trade name of Quorn (reg. trade mark of Marlow Foods, UK).

Previous studies on myco-protein (Turnbull et al.[7], Udall et al.[8]) to investigate its effects on blood variables in man demonstrated that subjects felt quite full after consuming a meal containing myco-protein. It was postulated that the effects seen on appetite may have been due to the fact that myco-protein contains a considerable dietary fibre component. For this reason it was decided to design the described study to investigate the effects of myco-protein on appetite and energy consumption in man.

The terms hunger, appetite, and satiety are commonly used, although they are not always clearly defined. Appetite might be regarded as a process which comes into operation once eating has begun and guides the selection of foods (Blundell et al.[1]). Hunger is a motivational construct with the logical status of an intervening variable (McQuorquodale et al.[4], Udall et al.[8]). The layman recognizes hunger in terms of the conscious sensations linked to a desire to obtain and eat food. Satiety can be defined as the "state of inhibition over further eating", whereas satiation is the process which brings eating to a close (Blundell et al.[1]).

Methods

Materials

The nutrient content of myco-protein is shown in Table 1. The myco-protein meal and the control meal (containing chicken) were nutrient balanced (Table 2) except for the dietary fibre found in myco-protein (6.7 g/meal). The fibre content of myco-protein (25% of dry matter) is attributable to its cell wall components, approximately 1/3 chitin (poly n-acetyl glucosamine) and 2/3 insoluble beta glucan.

Table 1. Nutrient content of myco-protein per 100 g

Protein, g	11.8
Dietary fibre, g	4.8
Total fat, g	3.5
Saturated fat, g	0.6
Monounsaturated fat, g	0.7
Polyunsaturated fat, g	1.3
Other lipids, g	0.9
Carbohydrate, g	2.0
Energy, kcal	86
MJ	0.36

Table 2. Nutrient content of meals

	Chicken	Myco-protein
Energy, kcal	579	561
MJ	2.43	2.36
Protein, g	44.5	44.2
Fat, g	10.9	10.2
Carbohydrate, g	80.8	76.8
Dietary fibre, g	10.1	16.8

Subjects

Thirteen female subjects (BMI < 25.0 kg/m^2) were found suitable to participate in the study after screening using an eating habits questionnaire in order to eliminate subjects who were restrained eaters. Subjects were not aware of the nature of the study.

Study procedure

Subjects were randomly allocated to attend the metabolic unit, after fasting from midnight, to consume a set meal. 100 mm visual analogue scales (VAS) were completed before the meal asking questions about desire to eat, hunger, fullness and prospective consumption. The meal was then presented and subjects were asked to consume everything. Immediately after the meal subjects were given another VAS which in addition to the pre-meal questions requested information on the pleasantness of the meal. Further VAS were give at 1, 2 and 3 h post meal. Subjects had no verbal or visual contact with each other during the meal. Weighed dietary records were kept on the day before the study, on the day of the study and the following day. This procedure was repeated the following week until all subjects had consumed both meals.

Results

There was a decrease in desire to eat after eating myco-protein compared with chicken (Fig. 1). There was a decrease in hunger after eating myco-protein compared with chicken (Fig. 2). Fullness increased after eating myco-protein compared with chicken (Fig. 3). Prospective consumption decreased after the myco-protein meal compared with chicken (Fig. 4). There was a decrease in energy intake of 263 kcal/d after consuming the myco-protein meal compared with the chicken (Fig. 5).

Chapter 12 – The Effect of Myco-protein on Hunger, Satiety and Subsequent Food Consumption

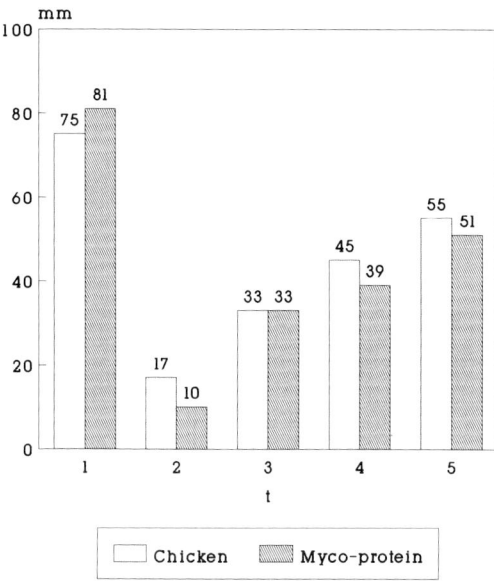

Fig. 1. Desire to eat
1 = immediately pre-meal; 2 = immediately post-meal; 3–5 = 1, 2 & 3 h post-meal.

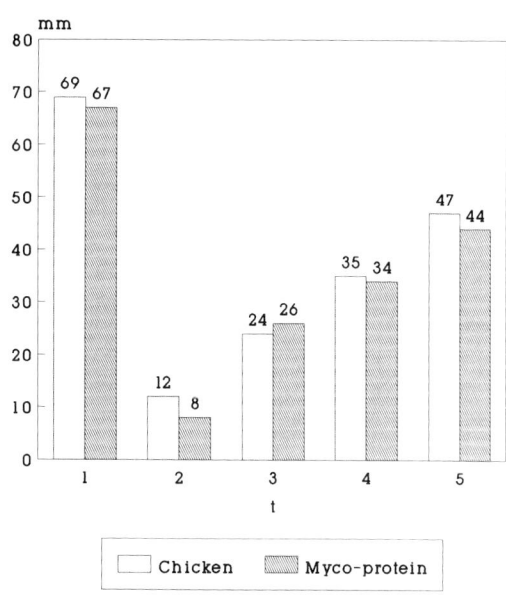

Fig. 2. Hunger
1 = immediately pre-meal; 2 = immediately post-meal; 3–5 = 1, 2 & 3 h post-meal.

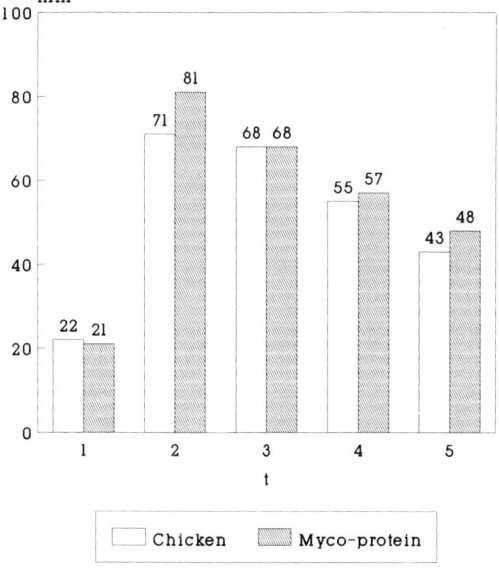

Fig. 3. Fullness
1 = immediately pre-meal; 2 = immediately post-meal; 3–5 = 1, 2 & 3 h post-meal.

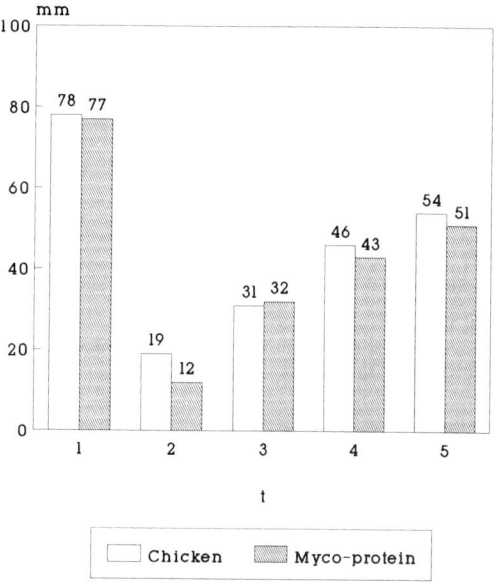

Fig. 4. Prospective consumption
1 = immediately pre-meal; 2 = immediately post-meal; 3–5 = 1, 2 & 3 h post-meal.

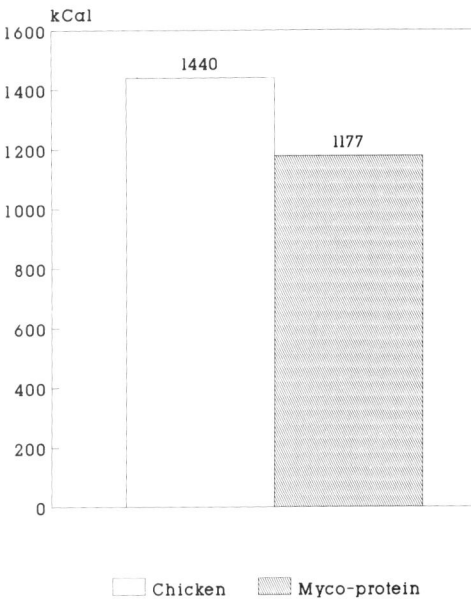

Fig. 5. Energy intake for rest of test day.

Discussion

It seems from this first study investigating the effect of myco-protein on appetite variables that food intake can be reduced without the perception of feeling hungry. Because both meals were macro-nutrient balanced the effects may be due to the difference in the dietary fibre composition of the meals. Other studies have shown similar effects of dietary fibre (Levine et al.[3]).

Much of the effect on appetite variables is seen 2 to 3 h after the meal or even later when energy intake was considerably reduced. The larger physical volume of the myco-protein meal could have caused greater gastric distension, which could initiate satiety at an earlier stage than the chicken meal, thus reducing the desire to eat and prospective consumption. Myco-protein may have delayed gastric emptying (possibly by increasing stomach content viscosity) and may also have decelerated intestinal transit thus extending the state of satiety.

Conclusion

It seems that there is an effect of myco-protein on energy intake and appetite variables and it may be of some use in the treatment of obesity although we can not be over-confident at this early stage in this research. Further studies are underway using more complex methods of study design.

References

1. Blundell, J.E. & Burley, V.J. (1987): Satiation, satiety and the action of fibre on food intake. *Int. J. Obes.* **11**, (supp. 1), 9-25.
2. Edelman, J., Fewell, A. & Solomons, G.L. (1983): Mycoprotein – a new food. *Nutr. Abstr. Rev.* **53**, 472-479.
3. Levine, A.S., Tallman, J.R., Grace, M.K., Parker, S.A., Billington, C.J. & Levitt, M.D. (1989): Effect of breakfast cereals on short term food intake. *Am. J. Clin. Nutr.* **50**, 1303-1307.
4. McQuorquodale, K. & Meehl, P.E. (1948): The distinction between hypothetical constructs and intervening variables. *Psychol. Rev.* **55**, 95-109.
5. Owen, D.E., Munday, K.A., Taylor, T.G. & Turner, M.R. (1975): Hypocholesterolaemic action of wheat bran and a mould (*Fusarium*) in rats. *Proc. Nutr. Soc.* **34**, 16A-17A (abstr.).
6. Royce, J.R. (1963): Factors as theoretical constructs. *Am. J. Psychol.* **18**, 522-528.
7. Turnbull, W.H., Leeds, A.R. & Edwards, G.D. (1990): Effect of myco-protein on blood lipids. *Am. J. Clin. Nutr.* **52**, 646-650.
8. Udall, J.N., Lo, C.W., Young, V.R. & Scrimshaw, N.S. (1984): The tolerance and nutritional value of two microfungal foods in human subjects. *Am. J. Clin. Nutr.* **40**, 258-292.

Chapter 13

Buspirone and Food Intake in Women Volunteers in Relation to the Menstrual Cycle

Elizabeth GOODALL, Mary WHITTLE, John COOKSON and Trevor SILVERSTONE

Academic Unit of Human Psychopharmacology, Medical Colleges of St. Bartholomew's and the Royal London Hospitals, London E9 6SR, UK

The effect of menstrual phase and buspirone on food intake was examined in 10 healthy women not on a contraceptive pill in a double-blind placebo-controlled study using 10 mg and 20 mg buspirone. Following placebo, protein intake was higher in the follicular phase compared to the luteal phase, an observation not previously recorded. No increase in carbohydrate/fat was seen in the luteal phase although subjects experienced other premenstrual symptoms. The response to buspirone was varied.

Introduction

Increased consumption of food has been reported during the premenstrual luteal phase in healthy women[6,14,19,20]. The increase is largely of carbohydrate and/or fat[1,8,18]. The relationship between changes in food intake and other premenstrual symptoms is not clear. Appetite ratings increased premenstrually in control subjects and in women with Premenstrual Syndrome (PMS) but were correlated with depression, anxiety and irritability ratings only in PMS subjects[5], although others have failed to find such a relationship[3,7].

Drugs such as fenfluramine, which enhance levels of 5-HT, reduce food intake in human subjects[15] although women are less responsive in the luteal phase[17,18].

Chronic treatment with buspirone (a 5-HT 1A agonist) in women with PMS significantly improved their symptoms including food craving[21]. Single doses of 8-OH-DPAT, buspirone, and gepirone increase food intake in rats[9,12,13], possibly *via* 5-HT 1A auto-receptor stimulation which leads to increased feeding by reducing output of 5-HT[4,10]. If 5-HT receptor sensitivity is enhanced by sex hormones[23], it could be that the hyperphagia seen in women in the luteal phase is due to an increase in the sensitivity of 5-HT 1A autoreceptors, induced by such changes. This would reduce 5-HT release, resulting in an increase in food intake.

We predicted that (1) buspirone would increase food intake in women, and (2) that this increase would be greater in the luteal phase than in the follicular phase.

Method

Design. Double blind placebo-controlled dose response study over three menstrual cycles using 10 mg and 20 mg buspirone. Subjects received one treatment per cycle in random order. Within each cycle the subject received the treatment condition twice, once in the follicular phase (one day in the week after her period ceased, median day 10) and once the luteal phase (one day in the week before menses was expected, median day −4). Half the subjects entered the study in each phase.

Subjects. Twelve women aged 22–41 years (mean BMI = 22.7 (17.6–29.8)) with regular menstrual cycles (26–32 days), not taking any contraceptive pill. No subject was being treated for PMS or had abnormal eating (as determined by scores on the EAT[11] and BITE[16] rating scales).

The subjective feelings of hunger, desire to eat, arousal, contentment and of five premenstrual symptoms (breast tenderness, bloatedness, depressed mood, irritability, anxiety) were rated using visual analogue scales (VAS).

Food was provided in a 10-channel automated food dispenser containing bread, lean meat, cheese and fruit so that subjects could make a lunch time meal which could vary in nutrient content; and also high carbohydrate/fat snacks, such as crisps and chocolate, which women reported that they consumed more of premenstrually.

Subjects attended the unit in the morning at approximately the same time on each occasion having eaten their usual breakfast. 5 ml blood samples were taken for progesterone assay[22]. The nine VAS were completed before drug, 1 h later and after lunch. Oral temperature was recorded before and 1 h after drug. Subjects received either 10 mg or 20 mg buspirone or matching placebo. After 1 h 15 min subjects ate their lunch.

Results were analysed by ANOVA and ANCOVA with *post hoc* group comparisons by the least significant difference (lsd) test.

Results

Two subjects had anovulatory cycles or deficient luteal responses and their results were excluded. No differences in total energy intake were seen, the mean overall intake being 2253 kJ (538 kcal). Significant drug condition/phase interactions were found for protein intake ($F = 5.096$, df 2,18, $P < 0.018$). Energy intake derived from total protein was significantly greater after placebo in the follicular phase than in the luteal, and also compared to 20 mg buspirone in the follicular phase (Fig. 1). This held true for protein energy derived from nonsweet foods ($F = 4.076$, $P < 0.035$; lsd test $P < 0.05$). Significant interaction effects were also seen for sweet protein and fat intakes. A dose difference was found, with intake of these nutrients being significantly higher in the 20 mg luteal phase compared to 10 mg luteal.

Hunger and desire-to-eat ratings were not affected by buspirone or by menstrual phase. Food intake correlated highly with hunger and appetite. When differences in appetite had been adjusted for, the significant phase/condition effect for total and nonsweet protein remained ($F = 4.91$, $P < 0.021$). Response to buspirone varied widely, some experiencing an adverse dizzy response. There was some indication that intake was greater after 20 mg buspirone in the luteal phase (Fig. 2). Breast tenderness, bloatedness, temperature, irritability, anxiety and discontent, but not depression, all increased in the luteal phase.

Discussion

The main findings of this study are (1) an increased consumption of protein in the placebo follicular phase and (2) no increased intake of carbohydrate/fat in the mid/late luteal phase, a time in which premenstrual symptoms were clearly being experienced. Preferential selection of protein has not been recorded before. It is clearly of potential physiological importance at a time when the follicle and endometrium of the uterus are proliferating. By day 10 of the cycle oestrogen is rising and this might be responsible for the increased protein intake. Modulation of neurotransmitter control of food intake by ovarian steroids has received little attention, although the human menstrual cycle is a natural experimental model for the study of such effects. The results show there to be endogenous modulation of nutrient selection of likely biological significance within the menstrual cycle in healthy women. This finding corroborates the suggestion[2] that women may be more susceptible than men to abnormalities in neurotransmitter function brought about by exogenous factors such

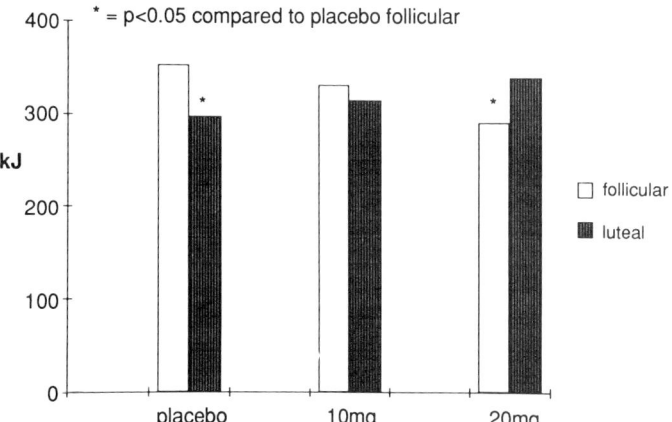

Fig. 1. Effect of menstrual cycle phase on energy intake (kJ) derived from total protein following placebo, 10 mg and 20 mg buspirone in 10 healthy women.

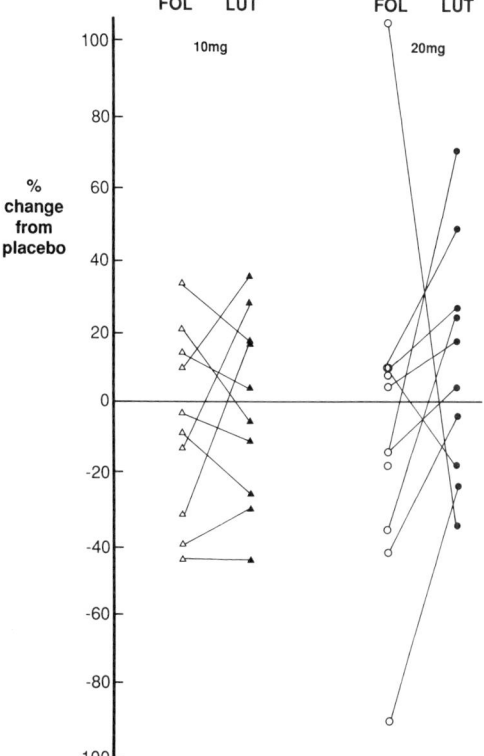

Fig. 2. Effect of menstrual cycle phase on total energy intake following 10 mg and 20 mg buspirone expressed as the percentage change from the intake following placebo for each phase. Individual values are shown.

as dieting and that this may lead to women developing eating disorders such as bulimia nervosa or anorexia nervosa.

Acknowledgements: The authors thank Mr. Brian Miller, Chief Pharmacist, for his contribution; Mr. L. Perry, Dept. of Reproductive Physiology, for the progesterone assay and Bristol Myers Co. Ltd. for supplying the buspirone and placebo and for their donation towards expenses.

References

1. Anantharaman-Barr, H.G., Clavien, H., Gmunder, B. & Pollet, P.E. (1988): Nutrient intake and the menstrual cycle. Abstract – 1st European Congress on Obesity, Stockholm, June 1988.
2. Anderson, I.M., Parry-Billings, M., Newsholme, E.A., Fairburn, C.G. & Cowen, P.J. (1990): Dieting reduces plasma tryptophan and alters brain 5-HT function in women. *Psychol. Med.* **20**, 785-791.
3. Bancroft, J., Cook, A. & Williamson, L. (1988): Food craving, mood and the menstrual cycle. *Psychol. Med.* **18**, 855-860.
4. Bendotti, C. & Samanin, R. (1986): 8-Hydroxy-2 (di-n-propylamino)tetralin (8-OH-DPAT) elicits eating in free-feeding rats by acting on central serotonin neurones. *Eur. J. Pharmacol.* **121**, 147-150.
5. Both-Orthman, B., Rubinow, D.R., Hoban, M.C., Malley, J. & Grover, G.N. (1988): Menstrual cycle phase-related changes in appetite in patients with Premenstrual Syndrome and in control subjects. *Am. J. Psychiatry* **145**, 628-631.
6. Bowen, D.J. & Grunberg, N.E. (1990): Variations in food preference and consumption across the menstrual cycle. *Physiol. Behav.* **45**, 287-291.
7. Cohen, I.T., Sherwin, B.B. & Fleming, A.S. (1987): Food cravings, mood and the menstrual cycle. *Horm. Behav.* **21**, 457-470.
8. Dalvit-McPhillips, S.P. (1983): The effect of the human menstrual cycle on food intake. *Physiol. Behav.* **31**, 209-212.
9. Dourish, C.T., Hutson, P.H., Kennett, G.A. & Curson, G. (1986a): 8-OH-DPAT-Induced hyperphagia: Its neural basis and possible therapeutic relevance. *Appetite* **7**, (suppl.), 127-140.
10. Dourish, C.T., Hutson, P.H. & Curzon, G. (1986b): Para-chloro-phenylalanine prevents feeding induced by the serotonin agonist 8-hydroxy-2-(di-n-propylamino)tetralin (8-OH-DPAT). *Psychopharmacology* **89**, 467-471.
11. Garner, D.M. & Garfinkel, P.E. (1979): The eating attitudes test: an index of the symptoms of anorexia nervosa. *Psychol. Med.* **9**, 273-279.
12. Gilbert, F. & Dourish, C.T. (1987): Effects of the novel anxiolytics gepirone, buspirone and ipsapirone on free feeding and on feeding induced by 8-OH-DPAT. *Psychopharmacology* **93**, 349-352.
13. Gilbert, F., Dourish, C.T., Brazell, S., McClue, S. & Stahl, S.M. (1988): Relationship of increased food intake and plasma ACTH levels to 5-HT1A receptor activation in rats. *Psychoneuroendocrinology* **13**, 471-478.
14. Gong, E.J., Garrel, D. & Calloway, D.H. (1989): Menstrual cycle and voluntary food intake. *Am. J. Clin. Nutr.* **49**, 252-258.
15. Goodall, E. & Silverstone, T. (1988): Differential effect of d-fenfluramine and metergoline on food intake in human subjects. *Appetite* **11**, 215-227.
16. Henderson, M. & Freeman, C.P.L. (1987): A self-rating scale for Bulimia, the BITE. *B. J. Psychiat.* **150**, 18-24.
17. Hill, A.J. & Blundell, J.E. (1989): Food selection, body weight and the Premenstrual Syndrome (PMS)-effect of d-fenfluramine. Abstract from Physiology of Food and Fluid Intake Conference, Paris. *Appetite* **12**, 215.
18. Leiter, L.A., Hrboticky, N. & Anderson, G.H. (1987): Effects of L-tryptophan on food intake and selection in lean men and women. *Ann. N.Y. Acad. Sci.* **499**, 327-328.
19. Lissner, L., Stevens, J., Levitsky, D.A., Rassmussen, K.M. & Strupp, B.J. (1988): Variations in energy intake during the menstrual cycle: implications for food intake research. *Am. J. Clin. Nutr.* **48**, 956-962.
20. Manocha, S., Choudhuri, G. & Tandon, B.N. (1986): A study of dietary intake in pre- and post-menstrual period. *Hum. Nutr. Appl. Nutr.* **40A**, 213-216.
21. Rickels, K., Freeman, E. & Sondheimer, S. (1989): Buspirone in the treatment of Premenstrual Syndrome. *Lancet*, **i,** 777.
22. Wathen, N.C., Perry, L., Lilford, R.J. & Chard, T. (1984): Interpretation of single progesterone measurement in diagnosis of anovulation and defective luteal phase: observations on analysis of the normal range. *B.M.J.* **288**, 7-9.
23. Yatham, L.N. Barry, S. & Dinan, E.G. (1989): Serotonin receptors, buspirone and premenstrual syndrome. *Lancet*, **i,** 1447-1448.

Section III
Genetics of obesity in animal models and humans

Chapter 14

Genetics of Obesity in Animal Models and in Humans

Paul TRAYHURN
Division of Biochemical Sciences, Rowett Research Institute, Bucksburn, Aberdeen AB2 9SB, Scotland, UK

Introduction

It is axiomatic that for obesity to develop, energy intake must be in excess of energy expenditure. From this it follows that those individuals who become obese do so as a consequence of either a higher than normal food intake, or an abnormally low rate of energy expenditure. Obesity is clearly dependent on environmental factors in that it requires a sufficient level of energy intake; equally, the disorder cannot be initiated on unusually low levels of intake. Environmental factors interact, however, with the genetic endowment of an individual in the development of obesity. It is emphasized that any genetic tendency to fatness – or leanness – may in principle operate on either, or both, of the central components of energy balance, i.e. appetite control, or the constituent parts of energy expenditure (e.g. basal metabolic rate).

This article provides a brief, general, overview of the genetic basis of obesity in both animals and in man.

Genetics of obesity in animals

Wild animals

It is generally considered that wild animals are lean[8], at least compared with man and laboratory animals. Several wild species that are 'lean' in their natural habitat have, however, been shown to become obese when maintained under laboratory conditions (e.g. spiny mouse, sand rat)[12]. Seasonal changes in body fat are well-recognized in certain species in the wild, and although this can be subject to environmental cues it has a genetic basis. Hibernating animals such as Richardson's ground squirrel may double their body weight between March, when they emerge from hibernation, and July/August when the period of winter hibernation recommences; all, or almost all, of this endogenously-driven weight change is due to body fat. The fat provides an energy store for the period of hibernation itself and for the regular phases of arousal that take place.

In a similar manner, birds that undergo seasonal migration generally deposit large amounts of fat in summer and during the pre-migration period. The fat provides the substrate required to fuel the substantial energy costs of long-distance flight.

Agricultural species

Major differences in body fat and the tendency to fatness are apparent between different strains of agricultural animal. This is particularly well illustrated in the case of pigs. Modern breeds such as the Pietrain and the Landrace, for example, are lean, while at the other extreme the Chinese Meishan has a high body fat content. Amongst European breeds, the current reduction in the tendency to fatness is the result of intensive genetic selection. Historically, fatness in pigs has been prized, but more recently selection has been directed towards leanness in response to consumer and health preferences.

Genetics of obesity in laboratory animals

Variations between inbred strains of laboratory rodent in the tendency to fatness, particularly in response to specific dietary regimens such as high fat diets, are well-recognized. The Osborne-Mendel rat, for example, becomes considerably obese when fed a high fat diet, while the S5B/Pl strain remains essentially lean[9].

In addition to strain differences in the susceptibility to fattening in normal animals, there are a number of laboratory rodents in which frank obesity is genetically transmitted. They range from the mild obesity of the KK mouse to the extreme obesity of animals such as the obese *(ob/ob)* mouse and the Zucker, or fatty, *(fa/fa)* rat[12]. In some types of genetic obesity a polygenic inheritance is involved, with a number of interacting genes, while in others there is a mutation in a single (recessive) gene[12].

The single gene mutants – particularly the *ob/ob* mouse and the *fa/fa* rat – have been extensively studied as animal models in obesity research. These mutants exhibit a constellation of problems, in addition to extreme obesity, including hyperinsulinaemia, insulin resistance, reduced sympathetic activity, hyperphagia and reduced skeletal muscle mass[3,12]. A major attraction of the single gene mutants as experimental subjects in obesity research is that the disorder can, in principle, be localized to a change in a *single* protein – be it enzyme, receptor, carrier, etc. Identification of the altered protein will enable the metabolic sequalae which result in obesity to be unravelled, and fresh insight into general metabolic control systems is likely to be obtained.

In terms of the fundamental energetics of obesity, the major obese mutants exhibit a low rate of energy expenditure, leading to a high efficiency of energy utilization, together with hyperphagia (see[12,13]). The hyperphagia appears, however, to be a secondary event, occurring only *after* the obese syndrome has been initiated. Such studies provide convincing evidence that obesity is not necessarily a simple problem of overeating.

Genetics of obesity in man

Certain genetic disorders in man are associated with obesity, as well as with other abnormalities. Perhaps the best known is the Prader–Willi syndrome, which occurs at an incidence of approximately 1 in 20,000. The syndrome is characterized by hyperphagia, hypogonadism, and short stature[4]. Other genetic disorders which are linked with obesity include the Bardet–Biedl syndrome, Cohen's syndrome, and Carpenter's syndrome[4]. The genes that produce these disorders have not been identified.

Within populations, family studies, twin studies, and adoption studies have increasingly indicated that there is a genetic basis to general obesity in man[1,2,4,11]. Interaction with environmental factors (food) is again important, and the situation is most appropriately described in terms of there being a *genetic predisposition to obesity*. Not only is there a genetic basis to human obesity, but fat distribution also appears to have an hereditable component[2].

It has been emphasized that obesity in human populations is unlikely to result from a simple Mendelian inheritance[1]; a polygenic inheritance with a large number of interacting genes would be anticipated. However, the possibility that obesity is associated with the transmission of a major recessive gene is raised elsewhere in this symposium[10]. As noted above, genetic influences may operate at a number of the loci involved in energy balance.

It has been argued that there is a "thrifty genotype" associated with diabetes and obesity[5,7].

This hypothesis suggests that in evolutionary terms a genetic predisposition to these disorders would be advantageous in that a high efficiency of energy utilization, resulting from a low level of energy expenditure, in man, would increase survival in the face of severe, or intermittent, food deprivation. Thus selective pressures would clearly favour those individuals with a thrifty genotype. However, once food supply is no longer limiting then the genotype would become disadvantageous with an ensuing high incidence of diabetes and obesity.

Examples which are consistent with this view include the situation appertaining with Australian aborigines[7]. A low incidence of diabetes and obesity is evident in aborigines in the bush, but following acculturation into urban Australia both disorders become widespread.

Molecular biological approaches

Molecular biological techniques enable specific genes which may be involved in the development of particular diseases to be identified. Such approaches are now being applied to obesity. In principle, the defective gene involved in the single gene obese mutants, such as the fa/fa rat and the ob/ob mouse, should be particularly amenable to identification. Several candidate genes have been explored in initial studies, based on metabolic systems that are recognized to be altered. In the fa/fa rat these have included the genes for growth hormone, neuropeptide Y, adipsin and lipoprotein lipase[6]. None, however, appears to be the site of the primary mutation for obesity, but rapid progress in this area is to be expected in the near future.

In the case of human obesity, candidate genes are also being examined, as presented elsewhere in this symposium[14]. Neither the insulin receptor gene, nor the genes for the glucose transporters (GLUT 1) appear to be involved.

Summary

A genetic basis to differences in fatness between different breeds of agricultural animal is well-recognized. Mutants in which obesity is inherited as a result of a change in a single gene are well-documented in laboratory rodents. It is increasingly evident that obesity in humans has a genetic component, and specific genetically transmitted disorders, such as the Prader–Willi syndrome, are found in which obesity occurs. Expression of a genetic predisposition to obesity requires the appropriate environmental conditions (food). Molecular biological techniques should enable the genes responsible for obesity and leanness to be identified, in both mutant animals and in man.

References

1. Bouchard, C. (1987): Genetics of body fat, energy expenditure and adipose tissue metabolism. In *Recent advances in obesity research: V*, eds. E.M. Berry, S.H. Blondheim, H.E. Eliahou & E. Shafrir, pp. 16-25. London: John Libbey.
2. Bouchard, C., Pérusse, L., Leblanc, C., Tremblay, A. & Thériault, G. (1988): Inheritance of the amount and distribution of body fat. *Int. J. Obes.* **12**, 205-215.
3. Bray, G.A. (1984): Integration of energy intake and expenditure in animals and man: the autonomic and adrenal hypothesis. *Clin. Endocrinol. Metab.* **13**, 521-546.
4. Bray, G.A. (1991): Weight homeostasis. *Ann. Rev. Med.* **42**, 205-216.
5. Coleman, D.L. (1978): Diabetes and obesity: thrifty mutants? *Nutr. Rev.* **36**, 129-132.
6. Greenwood, M.R.C. & Johnson, P.R. (1991): Mollecular and cellular aspects of fa/fa obesity. In *Progress in obesity research 1990*, eds. Y. Oomura, S. Tarui, S. Inoue & T. Shimazu, pp. 423-429. London: John Libbey.

7. James, W.P.T. & Trayhurn, P. (1977): An integrated view of the metabolic and genetic basis for obesity. *Lancet* **ii**, 770-773.
8. Rothwell, N.J. & Stock, M.J. (1981): Thermogenesis: comparative and evolutionary considerations. In *The body weight regulatory system: normal and disturbed mechanisms*, eds. L.A. Cioffi, W.P.T. James & T.B. Van Itallie, pp. 335-343. New York: Raven Press.
9. Schemmel, R., Mickelsen, O. & Gill, J.L. (1970): Dietary obesity in rats: body weight and body fat accretion in seven strains of rats. *J. Nutr.* **100**, 1041-1048.
10. Sørensen, T.I.A., Holst, C. & Stunkard, A.J. (1991): Recessive inheritance of a major gene for human obesity? Analysis of the Danish adoption study. In *Obesity in Europe 91*, eds. G. Ailhaud, B. Guy-Grand, M. Lafontan & D. Ricquier, pp. 85-88. London: John Libbey.
11. Stunkard, A.J., Sørensen, T.I.A., Hanis, C., Teasdale, T.W., Chakraborty, R., Schull, W.J. & Schulsinger, F. (1986): An adoption study of human obesity. *N. Engl. J. Med.* **314**, 193-198.
12. Trayhurn, P. (1984): The development of obesity in animals: the role of genetic susceptibility. *Clin. Endocrinol. Metab.* **13**, 451-474.
13. Trayhurn, P. (1986): Brown adipose tissue and energy balance. In *Brown adipose tissue*, eds. P. Trayhurn & D.G. Nicholls, pp. 299-338. London: Edward Arnold.
14. Weaver, J.U., Kopelman, P.G. & Hitman, G.A. (1991): Glucose transporter (GLUT 1) as a possible candidate gene for obesity. In *Obesity in Europe 91*, eds. G. Ailhaud, B. Guy-Grand, M. Lafontan & D. Ricquier, pp. 000-000. London: John Libbey.

Chapter 15

Losses of Total Body Fat and of Abdominal Adipose Tissue and the Response of Plasma Lipoproteins to Aerobic Exercise Training in Identical Twins

Jean-Pierre DESPRÉS, Sital MOORJANI, Paul J. LUPIEN, Angelo TREMBLAY, André NADEAU, Germain THÉRIAULT and Claude BOUCHARD

Physical Activity Sciences Laboratory, PEPS, Laval University, Ste-Foy, Quebec, Canada, G1K 7P4

Plasma lipoprotein levels show marked individual variation in their response to aerobic exercise training. The origin of such variation is partly unknown. In an attempt to quantify the role of heredity in determining the sensibility of plasma lipid transport to aerobic exercise training, we have used the identical twin design in short term (22 days) and long term (100 days) exercise training experiments. Results obtained in both protocols clearly suggest that there is a marked heterogeneity in the response of plasma lipoproteins to standardized exercise training. However, the variance observed in the response of plasma lipoproteins within MZ twin pairs was consistently smaller than the variance measured among twin pairs, suggesting that the response of plasma lipoproteins is significantly influenced by genetic variation. In other words, some individuals are more susceptible than others to favourable environmental changes aiming at reducing the risk of CHD, whereas others show some resistance to exercise training. The mechanisms involved in determining the genetic susceptibility of lipoprotein metabolism to exercise training clearly warrant further studies.

Introduction

The marked heterogeneity in the individual response of plasma lipoproteins to aerobic exercise training is a well-known phenomenon. The reasons for such heterogeneous responses are partly unknown. Several factors have been suggested as being involved such as subjects' age, sex, the initial level of body fatness, as well as the weight loss produced by exercise training[10]. In addition, we have suggested that genetic variation is also an important correlate for the metabolic response to exercise training[6-8]. In order to study the role of heredity in determining the sensibility of plasma lipid transport to aerobic exercise training, we have used the identical twin design to investigate the effect of prolonged exercise training on plasma lipoprotein levels in two different protocols.

Effects of short term (22 days) aerobic exercise training

In the first experiment, six pairs of male monozygotic (MZ) twins exercised 2 h per days for 22 consecutive days at 58% of their $\dot{V}O_2$ max[1]. At the end of the training protocol, subjects showed a significant increase in $\dot{V}O_2$ max, and a reduction in body fat mass. The exercise programme also induced metabolic improvements that included reductions in plasma insulin and triglyceride levels and an increase in the HDL-CHOL/CHOL ratio ($P < 0.05$)[1]. In addition, substantial individual variation was noted in the response of plasma lipoproteins to the training protocol. In other words, some individuals were resistant to exercise-training-induced changes in body composition and metabolism, whereas others showed marked improvements in plasma lipid transport. However, significant within MZ pair resemblance in the response of plasma cholesterol (CHOL)($r_i = 0.92$, $P < 0.01$), apoprotein B ($r_i = 0.88$, $P < 0.01$), LDL-CHOL ($r_i = 0.90$, $P < 0.01$), HDL-CHOL ($r_i = 67$, $P < 0.05$) and HDL-CHOL/CHOL ($r_i = 0.83$, $P < 0.01$) was observed[1]. Furthermore, the loss of trunk fat measured by changes in subcutaneous skinfolds was significantly correlated with the response of plasma CHOL, apo B, LDL-CHOL and plasma insulin levels to exercise training[1]. These results suggested that part of the genetic effect on the response of plasma lipoproteins to exercise training was mediated by the twin resemblance for changes in regional fat deposition.

Effects of long term (100 days) aerobic exercise training

To study further the interrelations between the genotype, body fatness, adipose tissue distribution and plasma lipoprotein responses, we have, in another experiment, exercise trained seven pairs of male monozygotic twins for a period of 100 days (Després et al., unpublished observations). Subjects exercised about 2 h/day on bicycle ergometers in order to induce a net 4.2 MJ daily energy deficit, six days/week, for a period of 100 days. After training, a significant reduction in body weight (5 kg, $P < 0.001$) was observed, that was entirely explained by the reduction in body fat mass ($P < 0.005$), as fat-free mass was preserved. A significant increase in maximal aerobic power was also noted ($P < 0.001$). As in the short-term exercise training experiment, substantial variation in plasma lipoprotein responses to the exercise training programme was observed among twin pairs, some individuals showing marked improvements whereas other twins showed little change. However, significant within twin pair resemblance was observed for changes in plasma triglyceride (TG), VLDL-TG, VLDL-cholesterol (CHOL), LDL apoprotein (apo) B, HDL_2-CHOL, and for changes in the HDL-CHOL/LDL-CHOL and HDL-apo A-I/LDL-apo B ratios (results not shown). Finally, individual changes in plasma HDL-CHOL and HDL_2-CHOL levels were equally well correlated with reductions in total body fatness, and in CT-measured abdominal and mid-thigh adipose tissue areas (results not shown). Therefore, results from this long term exercise training study have confirmed our previous observations[1] that the response of plasma lipoproteins to prolonged aerobic exercise training is, to a significant extent, determined by the genotype. Furthermore, as previously suggested[2-5,9-11], the magnitude of total and abdominal adipose tissue loss is a significant correlate of the change in plasma HDL-CHOL levels observed in response to endurance exercise training.

Acknowledgement

Supported by the National Institutes of Health, the Natural Sciences and Engineering Research Council of Canada, and by the Fonds de la recherche en santé du Québec (FRSQ). J.P. Després is a FRSQ scholar.

References

1. Després, J.P., Moorjani, S., Tremblay, A., Poehlman, E.T., Lupien, P.J., Nadeau, A. & Bouchard, C. (1988): Heredity and changes in plasma lipids and lipoproteins following short-term exercise training in men. *Arteriosclerosis* **8**, 402-409.
2. Després, J.P., Tremblay, A., Moorjani, S., Lupien, P.J., Thériault, G., Nadeau, A. & Bouchard, C. (1989): Long-term exercise training with constant energy intake. 3: effects on plasma lipoprotein levels. *Int. J. Obes.* **14**, 85-94.
3. Després, J.P., Pouliot, M.C., Moorjani, S., Nadeau, A., Tremblay, A., Lupien, P.J., Thériault, G. & Bouchard, C. (1991): Loss of abdominal fat and metabolic response to exercise training in obese women. *Am. J. Physiol. (Endocrinol. Metab.)*, **261** E159-E167.

4. Haskell, W.L. (1984): Exercise-induced changes in plasma lipids and lipoproteins. *Prev Med.* **13**, 23-26.
5. Leon, A.S., Conrad, J., Hunninghake, D.B. & Serfass, R. (1979): Effects of a vigorous walking program on body composition, and carbohydrate and lipid metabolism of obese young men. *Am. J. Clin. Nutr.* **3**, 1776-1787.
6. Poehlman, E.T., Tremblay, A., Marcotte, M., Pérusse, L., Thériault, G. & Bouchard, C. (1987): Heredity and changes in body composition and adipose tissue metabolism after short-term exercise training. *Eur. J. Appl. Physiol.* **56**, 398-402.
7. Poehlman, E.T., Tremblay, A., Nadeau, A., Dussault, J. Thériault, G. & Bouchard, C. (1986): Heredity and changes in hormones and metabolic rates with short-term training. *Am. J. Physiol. (Endocrinol. Metab.)* **250**, E711-E717.
8. Tremblay, A., Poehlman, E.T., Nadeau, A., Pérusse, L. & Bouchard, C. (1987): Is the response of plasma glucose and insulin to short-term exercise training genetically determined? *Horm. Metab. Res.* **19**, 65-67.
9. Williams, P.T., Krauss, R.M., Vranizan, K.M., Albers, J.J., Terry, R.B. & Wood, P.D. (1989): Effects of exercise-induced weight loss on low density lipoprotein subfractions in healthy men. *Arteriosclerosis* **9**, 623-632.
10. Wood, P.D. & Stefanick, M.L. (1990): Exercise, fitness, and atherosclerosis. In *Exercise, fitness, and health. A consensus of current knowledge*, eds. C. Bouchard, R.J. Shephard, T. Stephens, J.R. Sutton & B.D. McPherson, pp. 409-427. Champaign (IL): Human Kinetics Publishers.
11. Wood, P.D., Stefanick, M.L., Dreon, D.M., Frey-Hewitt, B., Garay, S.C., Williams, P.T., Superko, H.R., Fortmann, S.P., Albers, J.J., Vranizan, K.M., Ellsworth, N.M., Terry, R.B. & Haskell, W.L. (1988): Changes in plasma lipids and lipoproteins in overweight men during weight loss through dieting as compared with exercise. *N. Engl. J. Med.* **319**, 1173-1179.

Chapter 16

Recessive Inheritance of a Major Gene for Human Obesity? Analysis of the Danish Adoption Study

Thorkild I.A. SØRENSEN, Claus HOLST and Albert J. STUNKARD

Institute of Preventive Medicine, Copenhagen Health Services, Copenhagen Municipality Hospital, Copenhagen, Denmark, DK-1399; Statistical Research Unit, University of Copenhagen, Blegdamsvej 3, Copenhagen, Denmark, DK-2100; and Department of Psychiatry, University of Pennsylvania, Philadelphia, Pennsylvania, 19104-3246, USA

We assessed whether the mode of inheritance of adult obesity in adoptees and their biological relatives is compatible with recessive or dominant transmission of a single major fully penetrant gene. Analysis of the prevalence of obesity, defined by either the 92nd or 96th percentile of BMI, in adoptees and in their biological mothers (344), fathers (269), full (57) and half siblings (341) strongly rejected dominant transmission. Recessive transmission of 92nd percentile obesity was also rejected, but less strongly. For obesity defined by the 96th percentile, recessive transmission was similarly rejected for the parents, but not for the siblings. The estimated frequencies of the recessive gene for obesity ranged from 0.11 to 0.18. The observed prevalence of obesity was less than expected under the recessive model, perhaps for methodological reasons. We conclude that our results are incompatible with a major dominant gene for obesity, but they may be compatible with a fairly common major recessive gene.

Introduction

Recent studies of genetically related individuals separated early in life – parents and offspring[5,13,14], siblings[14,15], and twins[3,12] – have established that the BMI across its entire range is under strong genetic control. Recent segregation analyses of the distribution of BMI in intact families indicate the presence of a major recessive gene for obesity with a frequency of 0.21–0.24[4,6,8]. In such studies, however, the genetic effects may be confounded by effects of the shared environment. We have earlier reported a distribution of the mean values of the BMI that was suggestive of recessive inheritance of elevated BMI in a large sample of the biological parents and siblings of adult adoptees separated from their relatives very early in life[13,15]. We now report a further analysis addressing the mode of transmission of obesity defined by the extreme of the BMI distribution.

Methods

The 5455 non-familial adoptions granted in the Copenhagen area between 1924 and 1947 form the basis for the study population[1]. Adoptees were usually separated from their biological mothers immediately after birth and either transferred directly to the adoptive parents or reared in foster homes until adoption. Ninety per cent of the adoptees were transferred to the adoptive parents within the first year of life.

A questionnaire asking for height and weight was mailed to 4643 still living in Denmark, of whom 3580 replied. Mean (SD) age of the adoptees was 42.2 (8.1) years, and 56 per cent were women. For the family study, four groups including total 548 adoptees were selected within gender and five age strata on the basis of their BMI – thin, medium weight, overweight, and obese – each comprising 4 per cent of the population. Information on height and weight of the adult members of the biological families was sought by mailed questionnaires. For the parents we asked about the weight at the age when the adoptees went to school. When we had no self-reported weight from the parent, we used offspring's report on the parent.

Two series of analyses were performed using different definitions of obesity. In the adoptees, obesity was defined by either the 92nd or the 96th percentile according to the sampling scheme. The BMI values of these percentiles for each gender and age stratum were used to identify the obese among the siblings. For the parents we used definitions corresponding to the approximate 92nd (mothers: 30.5 kg/m^2; fathers: 30.0 kg/m^2) and 96th percentiles (mothers: 33.0 kg/m^2; fathers 31.5 kg/m^2) of their own BMI distribution.

The statistical analysis attempted to assess the extent to which the distribution of obesity in these families were compatible with the simplest case of Mendelian inheritance – either an autosomal dominant or an autosomal recessive single gene[17]. The analysis assumes full penetrance of the gene, no assortative mating, no polygenic inheritance, and no cases of obesity that were not caused by the gene (no sporadic phenocopies).

For each of the biological relatives of the adoptees – the fathers, the mothers, the full siblings, and the half siblings – the expected frequency of obesity when the adoptee was either obese or non-obese were based on Li and Sacks' ITO-matrix method[2,17]. The frequency of the disease related gene under either the dominant or recessive model was estimated by an iterative maximum likelihood procedure for each pair of relatives. This resulted in likelihood ratio tests (which follows a χ^2 distribution with one degree of freedom) for the fit of the observed to the expected frequencies under each model.

Since several adoptees had more than one sibling, random selection of one sibling within the sibships was performed 1000 times, and the estimation procedure was carried out for each of these 1000 samples. We present the median results of the estimated observed and expected prevalence rates, gene frequencies and likelihood ratio tests among the 1000 analyses.

Results

The observed prevalence of obesity among the biological relatives of the obese adoptees were lower than the expected prevalence rates under both the recessive and dominant transmission models (Table 1). As judged from the likelihood ratio test the differences between the observed and expected values were highly significant for the dominant model, irrespective of definition of obesity. For obesity defined by the 92nd percentile BMI, the recessive model was also rejected, but less strongly. When the 96th percentile definition was used, the recessive model was similarly rejected for the parents, but accepted for the siblings.

The gene frequencies estimated for each model are shown in Table 1. The recessive model for 96th percentile obesity resulted in frequencies of the assumed obesity gene between 0.11 and 0.18, implying that between 1.2 and 3.2 per cent of the population are homozygous obese.

Discussion

This study indicates that the familial occurrence of obesity is incompatible with dominant inheritance. The pattern fits better to recessive inheritance, but with prevalence rates possibly too low even for this mode of transmission.

Segregation analysis of two large populations of families (Lipid Research Clinic[4,6] and Community Health Study of Tecumseh[8]) showed a distribution of BMI that indicated a combination of a polygenic and major recessive inheritance for obesity. In the Lipid Research Clinic study, the frequency of the obesity gene was estimated at 0.21, and in the Tecumseh study at 0.24 (approximate value). These frequencies correspond to a prevalence of homozygous obesity of 4 and 6 per cent, respectively.

Table 1. Analysis of occurrence of obesity, defined by either the 92nd or the 96th percentile level of the body mass index distribution*, among biological relatives of adult adoptees under an autosomal recessive or dominant single gene model of inheritance

Biological relative	Percentiles defining obesity	Pairs N	Prevalence of obesity among relatives of obese adoptees			Recessive model		Dominant model	
			Observed	Expected recessive	Expected dominant	Gene frequency	LR test†	Gene frequency	LR test
Mother		344							
	92nd		0.12	0.17	0.52	0.17	7.01	0.024	123.5
	96th		0.07	0.15	0.52	0.15	6.98	0.024	76.9
Father		269							
	92nd		0.10	0.16	0.52	0.16	9.80	0.027	111.5
	96th		0.06	0.16	0.52	0.16	9.98	0.031	69.3
Full siblings‡		57							
	92nd		0.10	0.30	0.51	0.11	5.05	0.015	15.9
	96th		0.09	0.31	0.51	0.11	1.33	0.015	5.8
Half siblings‡		341							
	92nd		0.08	0.13	0.28	0.21	7.95	0.025	49.5
	96th		0.08	0.11	0.27	0.18	1.02	0.018	20.8

*For the parents, the percentile levels were estimated from the observed distribution of each of the parents. For the siblings, the limits were those defining the 92nd and 96th percentile levels among the adoptees within each gender and age stratum.
†Likelihood ratio test, which follows a χ^2 distribution with one degree of freedom.
‡The results for the siblings are the median result of 1000 analyses with random sampling of one among multiple siblings of the adoptee. No distinction was made between maternal and paternal half-siblings.

A strength of the present study is the separation of genetic from possible shared family environment effects. However, some limitation may weaken the possibility of our detecting specific genetic effects on obesity. First, the prevalence of obesity may have been underestimated among both adoptees and biological family members: non-response rates is increased in obesity[9], and weights reported by obese people are lower than their true weights[10,11]. The latter problem is particularly relevant for the biological parents whose weights several years earlier were reported, either by themselves or by their offspring[11,16]. Second, effects of gender and age on BMI among the parents were only indirectly adjusted for, via the gender and age balanced sampling design of the adoptees. The crude definition of obesity by a cut-off point in the BMI distribution rather than by an underlying component BMI distribution may result in misclassification of obese and non-obese[7]. It is possible that a more stable result might have been obtained if the family members had been analysed together rather than pairwise. Finally, the assumptions of the analysis[17], as mentioned under *Methods*, may not have been met. With these reservations in mind, we conclude that our results are incompatible with a major dominant gene for obesity, and possibly compatible with a relatively common major recessive gene.

References

1. Kety, S.S., Rosenthal, D., Wender, P.H. & Schulsinger, F. (1967 & 1968): The types and prevalence of mental illness in the biological and adoptive families of adopted schizophrenics. *J. Psychiatr. Res.* **6** (Suppl 1), 345-362.
2. Li, C. & Sacks, L. (1954): The derivation of joint distribution and correlation between relatives by the use of stochastic matrices. *Biometrics* **10**, 347-360.
3. MacDonald, A. & Stunkard, A.J. (1990): Body-mass indexes of British separated twins [Letter]. *N. Engl. J. Med.* **322**, 1530.
4. Ness, R., Laskarzewski, P. & Price, R.A. (1990): Inheritance of extreme overweight in black families. *Hum. Biol.* **63**, 39-52.
5. Price, R.A., Cadoret, R.J., Stunkard, A.J. & Troughton, E. (1987): Genetic contributions to human fatness: an adoption study. *Am. J. Psychiatry.* **144**, 1003-1008.
6. Price, R.A., Ness, R. & Laskarzewski, P. (1990): Common recessive inheritance of extreme overweight. *Hum. Biol.* **62**, 747-765.
7. Price, R.A., Sørensen, T.I.A. & Stunkard, A.J. (1989): Component distributions of body mass index defining moderate and extreme overweight in Danish women and men. *Am. J. Epidemiol.* **130**, 193-201.
8. Province, M.A., Arnqvist, P., Keller, J., Higgins, M. & Rao, D.C. (1990): Strong evidence for a major gene for obesity in the large unselected total Community Health Study of Tecumseh (Abstract). *Am. J. Hum. Genet.* **47** (Suppl), A143.
9. Sonne-Holm, S., Sørensen, T.I.A., Jensen, G. & Schnohr, P. (1989): Influence of fatness, intelligence, education and sociodemographic factors on response rate in a health survey. *J. Epidemiol. Comm. Health* **43**, 369-374.
10. Stevens, J., Keil, J.E., Waid, L.R. & Gazes, P.C.(1990): Accuracy of current, 4-year, and 28-year selfreported body weight in an elderly population. *Am. J. Epidemiol.* **132**, 1156-1163.
11. Stunkard, A.J. & Albaum, J.M. (1981): The accuracy of self-reported weights. *Am. J. Clin. Nutr.* **34**, 1593-1599.
12. Stunkard, A.J., Harris, J.R., Pedersen, N.L. & McClearn, G.E. (1990): The body-mass index of twins who have been reared apart. *N. Engl. J. Med.* **322**, 1483-1487.
13. Stunkard, A.J., Sørensen, T.I.A., Hanis, C., Teasdale, T.W., Chakraborty, R., Schull, W.J. & Schulsinger, F. (1986): An adoption study of human obesity. *N. Engl. J. Med.* **314**, 193-198.
14. Sørensen, T.I.A., Holst, C., Stunkard, A.J. & Skovgaard, L.T. (1991): Correlations of body mass index of adult adoptees and their biological and adoptive relatives. *Int. J. Obes.*, in press.
15. Sørensen, T.I.A., Price, R.A., Stunkard, A.J. & Schulsinger, F. (1989): Genetics of obesity in adult adoptees and their biological siblings. *B. M. J.* **298**, 87-90.
16. Sørensen, T.I.A., Stunkard, A.J., Teasdale, T.W. & Higgins, M.W. (1983): The accuracy of reports of weight: children's recall of parents' weights 15 years earlier. *Int. J. Obes.* **7**, 115-122.
17. Weiss, K.M., Chakraborty, R. & Majumder, P.P. (1982): Problems in the assessment of relative risk of chronic disease among biological relatives of affected individuals. *J. Chron. Dis.* **35**, 539-551.

Chapter 17

Glucose Transporter (Glut 1) as a Possible Candidate Gene for Obesity

Jolanta U. WEAVER, Peter G. KOPELMAN and Graham A. HITMAN
Medical Unit, The Royal London Hospital, Whitechapel, London E1 1BB, UK

In rodents the hypothalamus appears to play an important role in the maintenance of normoglycaemia by integrating the afferent signals at the level of glucosensors and subsequent central regulation of the autonomic stimulation to the pancreas and insulin secretion. Glucose uptake by mammalian cells is mediated by a family of structurally related integral membrane proteins (the glucose transporters) that have tissue specific pattern of expression. Glut 1 is mainly expressed in the brain. We have therefore investigated Glut 1 as a candidate gene for obesity in 56 obese (mean ± SEM, 40 ± 1), premenopausal, nondiabetic women and 31 normal weight, female controls. The obese subjects were characterized by parameters of insulin secretion and insulin resistance – fasting insulin, insulin resistance as determined by homeostatic model of assessment (HOMA), stimulated insulin secretion during an oral glucose tolerance test and insulin-induced glucose disposal (SSPG). DNA was extracted from the whole blood samples, digested with Xba I restriction enzyme and studied by Southern blot hybridization method using a ^{32}P-labelled Glut 1 probe. Two alleles were detected, size 5.8 and 6.2 kb. The genotype distribution for 5.8 homozygous, 5.8/6.2 heterozygous and 6.2 homozygous in obese subjects were 49%, 47%, 4% respectively; corresponding figures in normal weight subjects were 61%, 35%, and 3%; (P = NS). No association within obese subjects was found between parameters of body weight, insulin resistance, insulin secretion or fat distribution. Those findings suggests that Xba I polymorphism of Glut 1 is not a useful genetic marker for obesity.

Introduction

Obesity is likely to be a multifactorial disease being determined by both environmental and genetic factors. The evidence for significant genetic component comes from animal models and, in man from family, twin and adoption studies. The primary metabolic defect in obesity remains uncertain but there is evidence to suggests that a hypothalamic dysfunction leads to altered autonomic function with an imbalance between the parasympathetic and the sympathetic system. Increased parasympathetic stimulation of the pancreas appears to result in excessive insulin secretion, increased food intake and fat deposition. Reduced sympathetic stimulation leads to lower energy dissipation. An association between abnormalities of the hypothalamic-pituitary axis and peripheral endocrine function has been found in genetically obese animals[13], and has been recently reported in man[15]. It has been proposed that the glucose-sensitive neurones (GSN) in the lateral hypothalamus (LH, hunger centre) and glucoreceptor neurones (GRN) in the ventromedial nucleus of the hypothalamus (VMH, satiety centre) play an important role in the maintenance of normoglycaemia by integrating the afferent signals at the hypothalamic level[12]; the importance of the satiety centre is demonstrated by the induction of obesity in rats with VMH lesions. Glucose uptake by mammalian cells is mediated by a family of structurally related integral membrane proteins (the glucose transporters) which have tissue specific pattern of expression[2,10]. One of these transporters, Glut 1, is predominantly expressed in brain tissue and, although termed insulin sensitive, mainly facilitates basal glucose transport in adipocytes and muscle. Abnormal Glut 1 expression has been found in adipocytes of aged rats which results in alterations of Glut 1 distribution between the plasma membrane and cytoplasm which is thought to be due to increased glucose transporter intrinsic activity.[5] The Glut 1, glucose transporter is a plausible candidate gene in obesity as it may contribute to the abnormality of the "glucosensor system" within the central nervous system leading to hypothalamic dysfunction and may also play an additional role in developing and maintaining obesity by translocating glucose into cells regardless of the insulin concentration.

Subjects studied

The control group consisted of 31 normal weight, British, unrelated Caucasoids, healthy, female volunteers, nondiabetic, body mass index expressed as weight in kg/height in metres^2 (BMI), mean 22.5 (range 20–25), age 31 years (range 23–50) who were drawn from the hospital staff. They had no family history of obesity or diabetes. The obese group consisted of 56 severely obese, unrelated, premenopausal British Caucasoids, who were recruited from the Obesity Clinic at the Royal London Hospital. The obese subjects were nondiabetic as documented by a normal oral glucose tolerance test (WHO criteria) and had mean BMI of 40 (range 31–59) and mean age of 32 years (range 18–54). The majority of women included in the study had a family history of obesity but this was not confirmed by photographs. They had previously been studied for various parameters of insulin resistance and secretion as described below. All subjects gave their informed written consent for the study.

Methods

Different methods for assessment of insulin sensitivity were used within a period of 10 days in the same patients whose weight had remained unchanged for at least 6 weeks. Not all the patients were studied by each of the methods.

1. Fasting insulin (FI) was measured at 9.00 a.m. after an overnight fast.

2. Relative insulin resistance was calculated using ambulatory fasting plasma insulin and glucose levels after an overnight fast by the homeostatic model of assessment (HOMA) method[9].

3. Insulin-induced glucose disposal was measured after a 16 h fast by determining the steady state plasma glucose (SSPG) during simultaneous intravenous infusion of dextrose (420 mg/min) and insulin (0.77 U/kg body weight/min) using somatostatin (500 µg/h) to suppress endogenous insulin secretion. Measurements of plasma insulin and glucose were performed at the beginning of the infusion and then every 30 min for a further 150 min. Steady state plasma insulin and glucose were achieved after 90 min infusion. The arithmetical mean of the measurements at 90, 120 and 150 min gave a qualitative index of insulin resistance, SSPG[11].

4. The insulin secretion in response to a 75 g oral glucose tolerance test was measured by calculating the area under the curve (AUC) using the trapezoid method.

Insulin assay

Serum immunoreactive insulin was determined by a double antibody RIA, using Guildhay antisera. The inter- and intra-assay CVs were 10 and 7 per cent respectively, with a minimal detectable limit of 3 mU/l.

Fat distribution

Fat distribution was assessed by single observer using a flexible tape measure with the subject standing and breathing shallowly. The standardized measurements (in centimetres) were taken at the level half-way between the lower rib margin and the iliac crest for the waist and widest hip circumference for the hip, and expressed as a waist to hip ratio[16]. Reproducibility for the measurements was confirmed by the observer repeating the measurement on a separate occasion for each subject.

Restriction fragment length polymorphism (RFLP) studies of erythrocyte/HepG2-type glucose transporter (Glut 1) locus

DNA was extracted from the whole blood samples and studied by Southern blot hybridization methods as previously described.[6] We used Xba I restriction enzyme and phGT2-2 (vector pBR327) probe[14,17].

Statistics

To assess differences between genotypic or allelic frequencies in the obese and normal weight groups the chi square test was used with the Yates correction when applicable. FI, HOMA, SSPG, W/H, AUC, variables which describe the phenotype of the obese subjects, were logarithmically transformed prior to analysis. Associations with genotypes were assessed by one way analysis of variance. The significance levels between the difference of the mean values of parameters measured, correcting for multiple comparisons, were determined by Tukey's alternative tests, (SSPC/PC+). If significant inhomogeneity of variance was detected (Cochran's C), then an independent t-test using separate rather than pooled variances was employed.

Results

The following RFLPs were identified sized 5.8 and 6.2 kb as illustrated in Fig. 1.

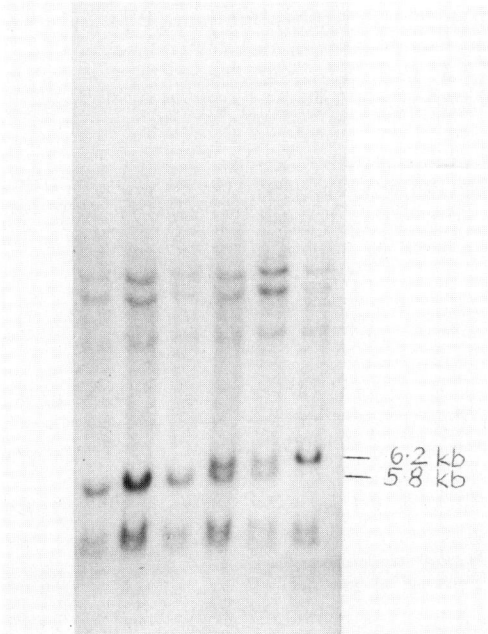

Fig. 1. Autoradiograph showing hybridization of glucose transporter, Glut 1, Xba I restriction fragment length polymorphism with phGT2-2 ^{32}P-labelled probe.

The genotype distribution for 5.8 homozygous, 5.8/6.2 heterozygous and 6.2 homozygous in obese subjects were 49, 47 and 4 per cent respectively; corresponding figures in slim subjects were 61, 35 and 3 per cent; (P = NS, chi square test).

The obese subjects showed marked fasting hyperinsulinaemia (mean value ± SEM), 26 ± 1 mU/l, range 4.2–76.1 (reference mean 7 ± 0.04 mU/L). with significant relative insulin resistance as calculated by HOMA model 6.6, range 1–20; (reference mean 1 ± 0.3). Their mean insulin under curve area during oral GTT (AUC) was 11.02 U/l x min, mean reference 4.4 ± 0.6 U/l x min, W/H ratio 0.86 and varied between 0.73 and 1.06. Mean SSPG was 8.0 ± 0.4 mmol/l. It was not possible to obtain a SSPG value for the control subjects, because the degree of insulinaemia achieved (mean 35.0 ± 1.0 mU/l) during the infusion was considered insufficient to suppress hepatic glucose production[4]. There was no association of Glut 1 polymorphism with any variables studied (Table 1).

Discussion

This is the first study to examine the potential role of the Glut 1 glucose transporter gene locus as a candidate gene for human obesity and its relationship to insulin resistance, hyperinsulinaemia and topographical distribution of body fat in severe obesity. Interestingly Glut 1 gene locus is localized on chromosome 1, which is the same chromosome in which mutation was recently found in an animal model of obesity, the db/db mouse[1]. We used the population approach study as obesity is a very heterogeneous disease and likely to be caused by several susceptibility genes. No association was found of Xba I Glut 1 RFLPs and obesity or various parameters of insulin resistance and insulin secretion. Before an association of the locus with obesity can be confidently excluded at the population level further RFLPs of Glut 1 locus need to be studied. Previous studies of the Xba I RFLPs have been focused on NIDDM. In the original report by Li and colleagues, an association was found between these RFLPs and NIDDM in Italians and Japanese but not in British Caucasoids[8]. Further studies however failed to confirm these observations in a variety of ethnic groups[3], as well as using different restriction enzymes. Taking all data together it seems unlikely that a primary abnormality of Glut 1 accounts for obesity although this may only be confidently ruled out by sequencing studies.

Table 1. Variation of anthropometric measurements and indices of insulin secretion and insulin resistance with polymorphism of the Glut 1 gene locus

	5.8/5.8 genotype	6.2 +ve genotype [5.8/6.2; 6.2/6.2]	F ratio	P value
BMI	41.6 (n=25) (39.3–44.0)	39.1 (n=27) (41.1–37.2)	2.7	0.1
W/H	0.87 (n=25) (0.84–0.91)	0.84 (n=27) (0.81–0.86)	2.7	0.1
FI	23.9 (n=25) (19.8–28.7)	20.3 (n=23) (15.2–27.0)	1.2	0.3
HOMA	5.9 (n=25) (4.76–7.2)	5.2 (n=23) (3.9–7.1)	0.42	0.5
AUC	10230 (n=18) (7891–13262)	8957 (n=15) (6358–12622)	0.4	0.5
SSPG	7.7 (n=15) (6.6–9.1)	7.2 (n=13) (5.9–8.8)	0.4	0.5

Acknowledgements

We would like to thank G.I. Bell (Howard Hughes Medical Institute, Chicago, Illinois, USA) for release of the glucose transporter clones, K. Noonan (The Royal London Hospital Medical College, London, UK) for insulin assay and R.D. Cohen for helpful discussion.

References

1. Bahary, N., Leibel, R.L., Joseph, L. & Friedman, J.M. (1990): Molecular mapping of the mouse db mutation. *Proc. Natl. Acad. Sci., USA* **87**, 8642-8646.
2. Bell, G.I., Kayano, T., Buse, J.B. *et al.* (1990): Molecular biology of mammalian glucose transporters. *Diabetes* **13**, 198-208.
3. Cox, N.J., Xiang, K-S., Bell, G.I. & Karam, J.H. (1988): Glucose transporter gene and non-insulin-dependent diabetes (letter). *Lancet* **ii**, 793-794.
4. De Fronzo, R.A. (1987): Use of the splanchnic/hepatic balance technique in the study of glucose metabolism. In *Clinical endocrinology and metabolism*, Vol. 1, eds. K.G.M. Alberti, P.D. Home & R. Taylor, pp. 837-862. London: Bailliere.
5. Ezaki, O., Fukuda, N. & Itakura, H. (1990): Role of two types of glucose transporters in enlarged adipocytes from aged obese rats. *Diabetes* **39**, 1543-1549.
6. Hitman, G.A., Jowett, N.I., Williams, L.G, Humphries, S., Winter, R.M. & Galton, D.J. (1984): Polymorphisms in the 5′ flanking region of the insulin gene and non-insulin dependent diabetes. *Clin. Sci.* **66**, 383-388.
7. Jeanrenaud, B. (1985): A hypothesis on the aetiology of obesity: dysfunction of the central nervous system as a primary cause. *Diabetologia* **28**, 502-513.
8. Li, S.R., Oelbaum, R.S., Baroni, M.G., Stock, J. & Galton, D.J. (1988): Association of genetic variant of the glucose transporter with non-insulin-dependent diabetes mellitus. *Lancet* **ii**, 368-370.
9. Matthews, D.R., Hosker, J.P., Rudenski, A.S., Naylor, B.A., Tracher, D.F. & Turner, R.C. (1985): Homeostasis model assessment: insulin resistance and b cell function from plasma glucose and insulin concentrations in man. *Diabetologia* **28**, 412-419.
10. Mueckler, M. (1990): Family of glucose-transporter genes. Implications for glucose homeostatis and diabetes. *Diabetes* **39**, 6-11.
11. Nagulesparan, M., Savage, P.J., Unger, R.H. & Bennett, P.H. (1979): A simplified method using somatostatin to assess *in vivo* insulin resistance over a range of obesity. *Diabetes* **28**, 980-983.
12. Oomura, Y. (1988): Contributions of endogenous substances to control of feeding. *Obesity in Europe 88*, eds. P. Björntorp & S. Rossner, pp. 101-107. London: John Libbey.
13. Sinha, Y.N., Salocks, C.B. & Vanderlaan, W.P. (1976): Control of prolactin and growth hormone secretion in mice by obesity. *Endocrinology* **99**, 881-886.
14. Shows, T.B., Eddy, R.L. & Byers, M.G. *et al.* (1987): Polymorphic human glucose transporter gene (Glut) is on chromosome 1p31.3-p35. *Diabetes* **36**, 546-549.
15. Weaver, J.U., Noonan, K. & Kopelman, P.G. (1991): Association between central and peripheral endocrine function in obesity. *Clin. Endocrinol.* **35**, 97-102.
16. WHO (1988): Measuring obesity-classification and description of anthropometric data. WHO document. Geneva: World Health Organization.
17. Xiang, K., Cox, N.J., Karam, J.H. & Bell, G.I. (1987): Bgl II RFLP at the human erythrocyte/HepG-type glucose transporter (Glut 1) locus on chromosome I. *Nucl. Acid Res.* **15**, 9101.

Chapter 18

White Adipocytes from Young Obese Zucker Rats Maintain Excessive Lipogenic Enzyme Activity in Long Term Culture

Véronique BRIQUET-LAUGIER, Annie QUIGNARD-BOULANGE, Isabelle DUGAIL, Bernadette ARDOUIN, Xavier LE LIEPVRE and Marcelle LAVAU
Physiopathologie de la Nutrition, INSERM U177, Institut Biomédical des Cordeliers, 15 rue de l'Ecole de Médecine, 75006 Paris, France

We used a system of long-term culture to examine whether isolated adipocytes from genetically obese Zucker rats were able to maintain excessive fat storage capacity when withdrawn from their *in vivo* environment. During culture in the absence of insulin, glucose consumption (GC) of cells from obese rats was twofold higher than that of cells from lean rats. Chronic treatment of adipocytes with insulin (10 nM) elicited an increment of glucose consumption which was more pronounced in obese (180 per cent) than in lean cells (50 per cent). After 9-day culture, cells from obese rats displayed a very sharp increase in specific activity of malic enzyme, glycero-3P-dehydrogenase, fatty acid synthetase and lipoprotein lipase: this genotype-mediated increase was amplified twofold after chronic treatment with insulin.

We concluded that adipocytes from genetically obese Zucker rats were able to maintain their hyperactive glucose metabolism, and therefore their excessive lipid storage capacity, even after long-term culture. This suggests the presence of intrinsic alterations in adipocytes from mutant rats.

Introduction

Over the past several years, we have been actively investigating the mechanism responsible for increased fat storage capacity in the genetically obese Zucker rat. Previous findings demonstrated that, at the onset of obesity, adipocytes from obese displayed a several-fold increase in lipid storage-related enzyme activities together with an increase in glucose transport and metabolism[1,3,7,8]. Although the reason why dietary substrates were preferentially channelled into body fat has not yet been elucidated, several hypotheses, including hyperphagia[2] and hyperinsulinaemia[1], which are characteristic features of this obesity syndrome, have been ruled out as aetiological factors.

The present study was undertaken to examine whether adipocytes from genetically fa/fa Zucker rats were able to maintain their characteristic increased fat storage capacity when withdrawn from their *in vivo* neuro-hormonal environment. For this purpose, we used long-term primary cultures of mature adipocytes, ensuring the maintenance of the metabolic activity of these cells.

Experimental procedures

Thirty-day old obese (fa/fa) and lean (Fa/fa) Zucker rats were killed by decapitation, and the subcutaneous inguinal fat pads were removed under sterile conditions. Tissues were pooled according to the genotype and subjected to collagenase treatment as previously described[7]. Isolated fat cells were filtered through sterile nylon mesh (190 µm), washed twice with Hank's solution and once with insulin-free DMEM containing 20 mM Hepes, 1% BSA, penicillin (62.5 U/ml) and streptomycin (62.5 µg/ml), pH 7.4 according to Marschall et al.[12] and supplemented or not by 1% FCS. Cells were then diluted with the cultured medium and the adipocyte number was determined by dividing the lipid content of an aliquot of cell suspension by the fat cell weight. Freshly prepared adipocytes (1–2 x 10^6) were incubated at 37°C in 35 mm dishes (multiwell Falcon) for various times in a humidified atmosphere (CO_2/air; 7.5%/92.5%) and the medium was changed every day. After 48 h of culture, cells were treated with or without 10 nM insulin.

Glucose consumption (GC) by cells was determined in each well by measuring glucose concentration in the medium using an industrial analyser (YSI 27).

After 9 days in culture, cells from 3–6 dishes were pooled, rinsed twice with Hank's buffer and homogenized in appropriate buffer. Lipoprotein lipase (LPL) activity was determined using acetone powder extract of cells, as described by Dugail et al.[4]. Malic enzyme (ME), fatty acid synthetase (FAS) and glycerol-3-phosphate dehydrogenase (GPDH) activities were measured in the cytosolic fraction. as previously described by Bazin et al.[1,10]. All enzyme activities were expressed per 10^6 cells.

Results

In a first set of experiments, we attempted to use a well-defined medium (FCS-free) for mature adipocyte cultures. Glucose consumption (GC) was measured daily during 1 week of culture in obese rat adipocytes maintained in either FCS-supplemented or FCS-free medium; in this experiment, insulin, when added, was present from day 0. Figure 1 shows that, when the cells were maintained in a basal medium (no insulin, panel A), the absence of FCS provoked a twofold decrease in GC throughout the culture time. In insulin-treated cells, there was a rapid twofold increase in GC which persisted until day 7, when FCS-supplemented medium was used. In the absence of FCS, the high level of GC exhibited by insulin-treated cells could not be sustained after 2 days of culture (panel B). Thus, the presence of FCS allowed the adipose cells to keep their relative insulin-stimulated glucose consumption. In all further experiments undertaken to examine the genotype effect, cells were maintained in DME supplemented with 1% FCS. Glucose consumption of adipocytes from either obese or non-obese rats was assessed during the 9-day culture. In cells from lean rats, GC did not change throughout the experimental period. The continual addition of insulin to culture medium increased GC by 50 per cent (1.6 ± 0.3 and 2.5 ± 0.4 µmol/24 h/10^6 cells in basal and insulin-stimulated conditions, respectively). Similarly, in obese cells, GC remained constant until day 9 and insulin triggered a more pronounced effect (190 per cent), as shown by the following data: 2.9 ± 0.5 versus 5.6 ± 1.0 µmol/24 h/10^6 cells under basal and insulin-stimulated conditions, respectively. Regardless of the presence of insulin, cells from obese rats displayed a twofold increase in GC when compared to cells from lean rats.

Figure 2 shows the effect of genotype on several enzyme activities in fat cells maintained for 9 days in culture. Under basal conditions, and for all enzymes studied, cells from obese rats exhibited levels of enzyme activities four- to fivefold higher than those from non-obese rats. In insulin-treated cells, the genotype effect was stronger, such that there was an eight- to 10-fold increase in enzyme activities in obese cells compared to lean cells.

Taken together, these results show that, regardless of the presence of insulin, we observed a genotype effect upon GC and lipogenic enzyme activities in cells, which was maintained

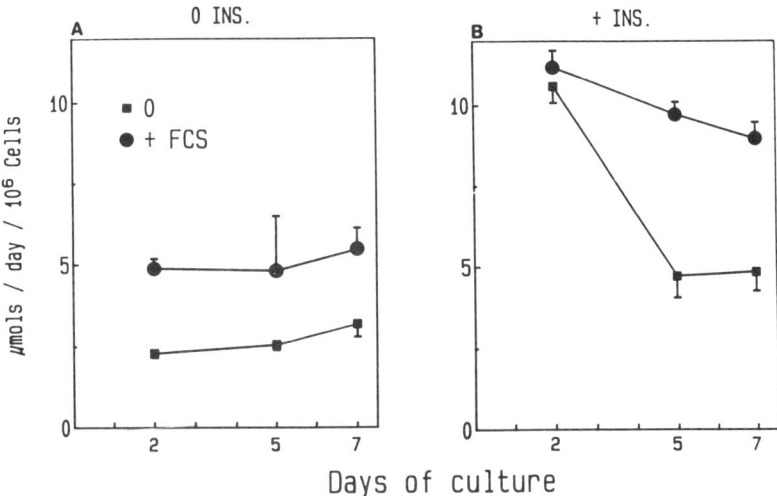

Fig. 1. Effect of FCS addition on the ability of obese adipocytes to consume glucose. Obese rats' adipocytes were maintained in either FCS-supplemented (●) or FCS-free (■) medium. At the indicated time, we measured glucose consumption of adipose cells maintained in the absence (panel A) or in the presence (panel B) of 10 nM insulin. Each point represents the mean ± SEM of three culture dishes.

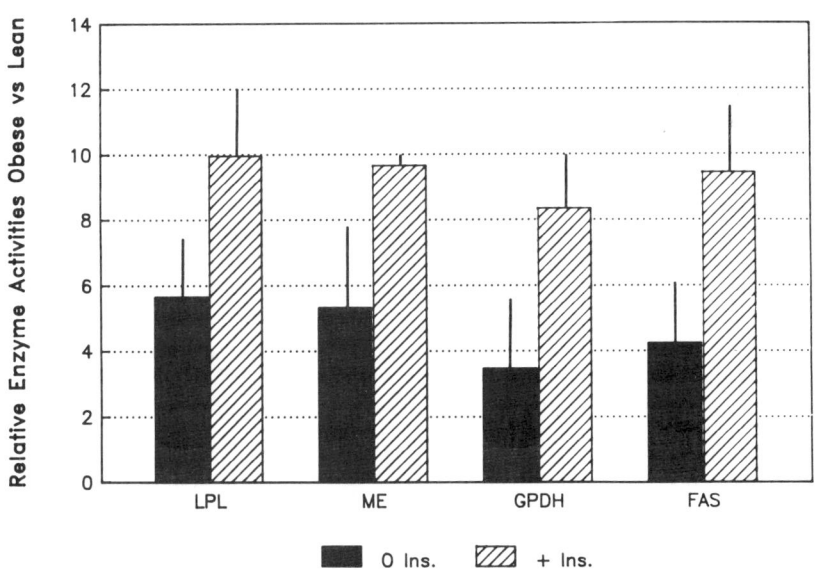

Fig. 2. Genotype effect on enzyme activities in cells maintained for 9 days in culture. After a 9-day culture, with or without insulin (10 nM), malic enzyme, fatty acid synthetase, glycerol-3-phosphate dehydrogenase and lipoprotein lipase activities were measured in adipocytes. Each bar represents mean value ± SEM for the increase factor in enzyme activities of obese versus lean cells.

even after a long-term culture. Moreover, this genotype effect was amplified when cells were submitted to chronic treatment with insulin.

Discussion

In this study, we used a model of long-term primary culture of mature adipocytes to compare the ability of cells from either genetically obese or lean Zucker rats to uptake glucose from the medium and to maintain a lipid storage capacity. In an attempt to eliminate all factors that condition the *in vivo* environment and modulate the metabolic activity of these cells, we modified the system described by Marschall *et al.*[12] by extending the time of culture over 9 days. We also used an FCS-free medium, but demonstrated that the presence of FCS even at a very low concentration (1 per cent) was necessary to maintain stable glucose consumption by cells. It is very likely that different components of FCS enabled the cells to maintain an active metabolic state.

Among different characteristic abnormalities of adipose tissue in genetically obese rats, adipocytes from young obese rats, under physiological concentrations of insulin, exhibit a several-fold increase in glucose transport activity both *in vivo* and *in vitro*, as compared to fat cells from their lean littermates[7,11]. The present data show that the genotype-linked increase in basal and insulin-stimulated glucose consumption is maintained after 1 week of culture, whereas lactate production by cells does not differ between obese and lean cells throughout the duration of culture (data not shown). In agreement, a similar twofold higher glucose uptake by freshly isolated adipocytes of obese rats compared to lean rats has been recently reported[9].

After 9 days in culture, adipocytes from obese rats, when deprived of their *in vivo* environment, exhibit a several-fold increase in lipogenic enzyme activities. These results reflect an intrinsic overcapacity of these cells for lipid storage, independently of the presence of any *in vivo* stimulating factors. Given the half-lives of these different enzymes, ranging from 60 min for LPL[13] to 45 h for FAS[15], these results, obtained after 9 days in culture, strongly suggest that the genotype effect is mediated by intrinsic factor(s). Insulin-mediated stimulation was observed for all enzymes regardless of the genotype, but this effect was more pronounced in obese cells compared to lean cells, in such a manner that the differences between obese and lean cells were amplified in chronically insulin-supplemented medium. In such insulin-treated cells, the differences in enzyme activity between the two genotypes were very similar to those previously reported *in vivo*[1,3,4].

Our present data indicate that the fatty genotype increases the fat storage capacity independently of a neuro-hormonal environment, suggesting that it acts through intrinsic factor(s). Recently, we demonstrated that there is transcriptional overexpression of genes encoding for these lipid storage-related enzymes in adipose tissue of genetically obese rats[5,6]. These results, obtained in our *in vitro* model, suggest the presence in the obese rat of factors triggering overtranscription of these genes and intrinsically expressed in the adipocytes. This model could be suitable for studying the hormonal regulation of gene transcription.

References

1. Bazin, R. & Lavau, M. (1982): Development of hepatic and adipose tissue lipogenic enzymes and insulinemia during suckling and weaning on to a high-fat diet in Zucker rats. *J. Lipid Res.* **23**, 839-849.
2. Boulangé, A., Planche, E. & de Gasquet, P. (1979): Onset of genetic obesity in the absence of hyperphagia during the first week of life in the Zucker rat (fa/fa). *J. Lipid Res.* **20**, 857-864.
3. Boulangé, A., Planche E. & de Gasquet P. (1981): Onset and development of hypertriglyceridemia in the Zucker rat fa/fa. *Metabolism* **30**, 1045-1052.
4. Dugail, I., Quignard-Boulangé, A., Brigant, L., Etienne, J., Noe, L. &. Lavau, M. (1988): Increased lipoprotein lipase content in the adipose tissue of suckling and weaning obese Zucker rats. *Biochem. J.* **249**, 45-49.

5. Dugail, I., Quignard-Boulangé, A., Bazin, R., Le Liepvre, X. & Lavau, M. (1988): Adipose tissue specific increase in glyceraldehyde 3-phosphate dehydrogenase activity and mRNA amounts in suckling pre-obese Zucker rats. *Biochem. J.* **254**, 483-487.
6. Dugail, I., Le Liepvre, X., Guichard, C., Quignard-Boulangé, A. & Lavau, M. (1990): Increased transcription of genes encoding for lipid storage-related enzymes in adipose tissue of young obese Zucker rats. *Int. J. Obesity* **14**, (suppl.2) 151A.
7. Guerre-Millo, M., Lavau, M., Horne, J.S. & Wardzala, L.J. (1985): Proposed mechanism for increased insulin-mediated glucose transport in adipose cells from young obese Zucker rats. Large intracellular pool of glucose transporters. *J. Biol. Chem.* **260** (4), 2197-2201.
8. Gruen, R., Hietanen, R. & Greenwood, M.R. (1978): Increased adipose tissue lipoprotein lipase activity during the development of the genetically obese rat (fa/fa). *Metabolism* **27**, 1955-1966.
9. Hainault, I., Guerre-Millo, M., Guichard, C. & Lavau, M. (1991): Differential regulation of adipose tissue glucose transporters in genetic obesity (fatty rats). Selective increase in the adipose cell/muscle glucose transporter (Glut4) expression. *J. Clin. Invest.* **87**, 1127-1131.
10. Kozak, L.P. & Jansen, J.T. (1974): Genetic and developmental control of multiple forms of L-glycerol-3-phosphate dehydrogenase. *J. Biol. Chem.* **249**, 7775-7781.
11. Krief, S., Bazin, R., Dupuy, F. & Lavau, M. (1988): Increased *in vivo* glucose utilization in 30-day-old obese Zucker rats: role of white adipose tissue. *Am. J. Physiol.* **254**, E342-E348.
12. Marshall, S., Garvey, W.T. & Geller, M. (1984): Primary culture of isolated adipocytes a new model to study insulin receptor regulation and insulin action. *J. Biol. Chem.* **259**, 6376-6384.
13. Ong, J.M., Kirchgessner, T.G., Schotz, M.C., & Kern, P.A. (1988): Insulin increases the synthetic rate and messenger RNA level of lipoprotein lipase in isolated rat adipocytes. *J. Biol. Chem.* **263**, 12933-12938.
14. Spydevold, S.O. & Greenbaum, A.L. (1978): Adaptive responses of enzymes of carbohydrate and lipid metabolism to dietary alteration in genetically obese Zucker rats (fa/fa). *Eur. J. Biochem.* **89**, 329-339.
15. Weiss, G.H., Rosen, O.M. & Rubin, C.S. (1980): Regulation of fatty acid synthetase concentration and activity during adipocyte differentiation. Studies on 3T3-L1 cells. *J. Biol. Chem.* **255**, 4751-4757.

Chapter 19

Development of Thyroxine 5′ Monodeiodinase Activity in Brown Adipose Tissue of Young Zucker Rats

V. MARIE, F. DUPUY and R. BAZIN
INSERM U. 177, 15 rue de l'Ecole de Médecine, 75006 Paris, France

This study was undertaken to determine whether the capacity of triiodothyronine production was altered in brown adipose tissue of Zucker *fa/fa* rats. Thyroxine 5′-deiodinase activity was measured in *Fa/fa* and *fa/fa* littermates from day 2 to day 30 after birth. In the early suckling period (from day 2 to day 16) the enzyme activity was significantly reduced in BAT of pre-obese compared to lean pups. In *fa/fa* pups, a moderate cold stress or an acute injection of β-agonist drug (BRL 35135) were able to restore the enzyme activity to the level of their lean *Fa/fa* counterparts. On the contrary, deiodinase activity was more elevated in *fa/fa* than in *Fa/fa* during the suckling to weaning transition.

These results confirm that BAT is a very early site of *fa/fa* genotype expression and are consistent with the hypothesis that a defect in the autonomic nervous system may be a primary cause of this genetic obesity.

Introduction

Genetic obesity in Zucker *fa/fa* rats is characterized early in life by decreased energy expenditure[17] which precedes the increased growth of white adipose tissue[18]. In newborn or young rats, brown adipose tissue (BAT) represents the most important site of facultative thermogenesis. In Zucker rats, BAT thermogenic capacity is lower in *fa/fa* than in their lean littermates at as early as 2 days of age[1], consistent with a decrease in the uncoupling protein message level[19]. Thermic activity of BAT is controlled chiefly by norepinephrine released through sympathetic innervation of the tissue[16]; moreover, Silva and Larsen have demonstrated that thyroid hormones and the sympathetic nervous system act synergistically in the regulation of the thermogenic activity of BAT[20] and that the local production of T_3 plays an important role in modulating thermogenesis[3]. The present study was undertaken to determine whether the reduced capacity of pre-obese Zucker pups for BAT thermogenesis could be related to a reduced capacity to convert T_4 to T_3 in this tissue.

Methods

Zucker rats are bred in our laboratory from obese *(fa/fa)* males and lean *(Fa/fa)* females. Pups and their mother were housed in a temperature-controlled (22–23°C) room at a fixed 12 h-light (07:00-19:00 h)/12 h-dark cycle. The dams were fed stock diet (M25, Pietrement, France) *ad libitum*. The rats were used at 2, 7, 14, 16, 18 and 21 days of age during suckling, and after weaning at 30 days of age. In 2- and 7-day old pups, interscapular BAT samples (20–30 mg) were surgically removed under light diethyl ether anaesthesia, so that the pups could be kept alive for later genotype identification. Rats used after 2 weeks of age were killed and genotype identification was made by plotting inguinal fat pad weight *versus* body weight as previously described[13].

Frozen tissue samples were homogenized in a glass-glass-potter in ice-cold 0.25 M sucrose, 0.2 mM EDTA, 1 mM HEPES buffer, pH 7.2 (in 20 vol, w/v). Protein content was measured by the method of Bradford[4].

Thyroxine 5′-deiodinase (T 5′-D) was assayed in infranatants (below the fat layer) of 600 **g** centrifuging for 10 min of tissue homogenates according to Visser *et al.*[23]. The reaction was carried out with 100,000 cpm of [^{125}I-]T$_4$ (Amersham, France) plus 2 nM unlabelled T$_4$ in 200 mM potassium phosphate, 1 mM EDTA, 20 mM DTT, pH 7.0 medium. Serum insulin was measured by a radioimmunoassay (CIS, France) with a rat insulin standard (Novo, Denmark). BRL 35135 (Dr M.A. Cawthorne, Beecham Pharmaceuticals) was injected intraperitoneally (10 µg/g body wt) 2 h before sacrifice of the pups.

Results are expressed as mean ± SEM. The level of significance in the difference between groups was calculated either by Student's *t*-test or by a two-way analysis of variance.

Results

During the first week of life, the *fa/fa* genotype had no detectable effect on body weight (Table 1). From 14 days of age, *fa/fa* pups were heavier than their lean *Fa/fa* littermates. In the third week of life, the genotype of the pups was easily detectable and whole interscapular BAT was totally dissected out and weighed after sacrifice of the pups. In *fa/fa* as compared with *Fa/fa* pups, BAT weight increased by 20–30 and 75 per cent in the suckling period and after weaning, respectively (Table 1). This increased tissue weight observed in *fa/fa* rats was totally accounted for by lipid content, so that fat-free masses of tissues were not significantly different between the two genotypes (data not shown).

Table 1. Body weight, interscapular BAT weight, T 5′-D specific activity and insulinaemia in lean (*Fa/fa*) and obese (*fa/fa*) Zucker rats

Age (days)		Body weight (g)	IBAT weight (mg)	Deiodinase (U/mg prot)	Insulin (µU/ml)
2	Fa/fa	7.2 ± 0.12 (22)	nd	77.5 ± 7.92 (22)	nd
	fa/fa	7.1 ± 0.12 (20)	nd	54.4 ± 5.85 (20)**	nd
7	Fa/fa	12.5 ± 0.15 (25)	nd	79 ± 19.9 (11)	27.1 ± 4.39 (5)
	fa/fa	12.7 ± 0.28 (14)	nd	38.6 ± 7.85 (8)*	45.8 ± 5.50 (6)*
14	Fa/fa	21.6 ± 0.37 (27)	86 ± 3.9 (27)	56.2 ± 5.72 (15)	57.4 ± 4.61 (23)
	fa/fa	24.6 ± 0.79 (16)**	115 ± 7.6 (16)**	31.8 ± 5.61 (11)**	92.7 ± 11.78 (15)**
16	Fa/fa	25.6 ± 0.50 (15)	94 ± 3.5 (15)	29.5 ± 2.58 (22)	nd
	fa/fa	27.7 ± 0.58 (19)**	117 ± 3.6 (16)**	15.8 ± 0.77 (26)**	nd
18	Fa/fa	27.2 ± 0.31 (7)	105 ± 5.0 (7)	24.8 ± 4.03 (7)	nd
	fa/fa	28.9 ± 0.38 (10)**	133 ± 5.3 (10)**	26.8 ± 1.97 (10)	nd
21	Fa/fa	37.5 ± 0.58 (15)	167 ± 1.2 (15)	25.1 ± 2.14 (15)	53.5 ± 6.48 (8)
	fa/fa	37.7 ± 0.67 (12)	199 ± 7.3 (12)**	45.8 ± 4.94 (12)**	87.6 ± 10.19 (11)**
30	Fa/fa	71.5 ± 1.72 (9)	146 ± 5.8 (19)	37.1 ± 2.82 (19)	57.7 ± 3.06 (8)
	fa/fa	79.6 ± 1.31 (10)**	255 ± 10.6 (20)**	65.0 ± 7.78 (20)**	244 ± 34.5 (8)**

Values are mean ± SEM; number of rats is in parentheses. Statistically significant at *$P < 0.05$ or **$P < 0.01$; *fa/fa versus Fa/fa*. nd, value not determined. One Unit of enzyme is defined as the amount that will catalyse the formation of one femtomole of product/h at 37°C.

Table 2. Effect of cold exposure on specific activity of BAT T 5′-D in 7-day-old Zucker pups

	28°C	15°C
Lean (Fa/fa)	42.8 ± 7.86 (8)	85.6 ± 11.82 (12)[a]
Obese (fa/fa)	21.8 ± 1.43 (9)*	39.5 ± 6.27 (6)**,[b]

Values are mean ± SEM; number of rats is in parentheses. Statistically significant at * $P < 0.05$ or ** $P < 0.01$, fa/fa versus Fa/fa; a $P < 0.05$ or b $P < 0.01$, 15°C versus 28°C within the same genotype. Enzyme activity is expressed as femtomole/h/mg protein.

Table 3. Effect of BRL injection on BAT T 5′-D specific activity in 14-day-old Zucker pups.

(Fa/fa)	(fa/fa)	Treated (fa/fa)
56.2 ± 5.72 (15)	31.8 ± 5.61 (11)**	64.6 ± 10.96 (8)[a]

Values are mean ± SEM; number of rats is in parentheses. Statistically significant at ** $P < 0.01$ fa/fa versus Fa/fa, or a $P < 0.05$ treated fa/fa versus fa/fa. Enzyme activity is expressed as femtomole/h/mg protein at 37°C.

Table 1 also shows the developmental pattern of thyroxine 5′-deiodinase in BAT of lean and pre-obese rats.

In lean pups, the high level of enzyme activity observed during the first week of life fell significantly during the second week and remained at a low level during the suckling period. Weaning was accompanied by a significant 50% increase in enzyme activity, but at 30 days of age, it was only half of the value observed in the first days of life.

From 2 to 16 days of age, the pattern of development of T 5′-D activity in the pre-obese pups was similar to that observed in tissues of lean pups in terms of developmental changes. However, the enzyme activity was significantly lower in pre-obese than in lean rats at as early as two days of age. In BAT of fa/fa rats from 16 to 30 days of age, the enzyme activity rose to reach the value observed at two days of age. After weaning, BAT deiodinase activity was twofold higher in obese than in lean rats.

During the suckling period, insulinaemia was significantly increased, by 60–70%, in pre-obese pups compared with their lean counterparts (Table 1). After weaning, the difference between the two genotypes was much more pronounced (x4). Exposure of 7-day old Zucker pups to a cold environment (15°C, 30 min) resulted in similar increased enzyme activity (x2) in both lean and obese pups (Table 2).

In 14-day old pre-obese pups, an acute injection of β-agonist, BRL 35135, was able to restore the enzyme activity to the level observed in their lean littermates (Table 3).

Discussion

In lean Zucker pups, the developmental pattern of BAT T 5′-D was very close to that observed in the Wistar rat by Iglesias et al.[8]. The high level of enzyme activity during the first week of life correlates with the known increase in tissue thermogenic activity occurring after birth[5], thus reinforcing the suggestion that local 3′,3,5-triodothyronine generation could be an important event related to thermogenesis in BAT[3].

The present study clearly demonstrates that a reduced capacity for T_3 production characterizes BAT of pre-obese pups at as early as two days of age. This result is in good agreement with the decreased thermogenic capacity previously reported in this tissue[1]. Thus, the low activity of T 5′D in BAT of pre-obese pups might induce limited local production of T_3 and contribute to the reduced thermic activity of this tissue. However, in suckling pups, no change was detectable in circulating T_3 (data not shown), reinforcing the hypothesis that under basal conditions, BAT does not contribute in any major way to circulating T_3.[6,21]

In pre-obese rats, the impaired capacity of T_3 production by BAT was totally restored during the suckling to weaning transition. Moreover, after weaning, BAT T 5'-D activity was higher in obese than in lean rats. Since insulin and meal-feeding are potent activators of BAT T 5'-D[6,22], this change in enzyme activity could be explained by dramatic hyperinsulinaemia and/or hyperphagia[2] which characterized weaned fa/fa rats.

The present developmental study points out that an alteration in T_4 to T_3 conversion of very early emergence in fa/fa rats could be totally masked or reversed after weaning, as we previously reported for glucose uptake[11,12]. In adult rats, the report of an unchanged T_4 to T_3 conversion in BAT of obese compared with lean rats[7,24] suggests that deiodinase activity continues to evolve with ageing.

A subnormal response of BAT T 5'-D to cold has been widely demonstrated in animal models of obesity, such as db/db, ob/ob mice and fa/fa rats[9,10,24]. At variance with results reported in adult Zucker rats[24], our data clearly show that 7-day old fa/fa pups exposed to physiological cold stress normally respond by increasing BAT T 5'-D activity.

In BAT, T 5'-D is well known to be activated by noradrenaline[20]. In Zucker fa/fa pups, as was demonstrated for thermogenic activity[19], an acute injection of a β-agonist drug totally restored the capacity for T_4 to T_3 conversion in BAT.

These results strongly suggest that reduced sympathoadrenal activity which characterizes adult Zucker fa/fa rats[14,15] is present very early in life and plays a key role in the onset of this genetic obesity.

In conclusion, this study confirms that BAT is a very early site of fa/fa genotype expression. In pre-obese pups, the capacity for T_4 to T_3 conversion is totally restored by sympathetic activation, consistent with the hypothesis that a defect in the autonomic nervous system may be a primary cause of this genetic obesity.

References

1. Bazin, R., Etève, D. & Lavau, M. (1984): Evidence for decreased GDP binding to brown-adipose-tissue mitochondria of obese Zucker (fa/fa) rats in the very first days of life. *Biochem. J.* **221**, 241-245.
2. Bell, G.E. & Stern, J.S. (1977): Evaluation of body composition of young obese and lean Zucker rats. *Growth* **41**, 63-80.
3. Bianco, A.C. & Silva, J.E. (1987): Optimal response of key enzymes and uncoupling protein to cold in BAT depends on local T_3 generation. *Am. J. Physiol.* **253**, E255-E263.
4. Bradford, M.M. (1976): A rapid and sensitive method for the quantitation of microgram quantities of protein utilizing the principle of protein-dye binding. *Anal. Biochem.* **72**, 248-254.
5. Giralt, M., Martin, I., Iglesias, R., Vinas, O., Villaroya, F. & Mampel, T. (1990): Ontogeny and perinatal nodulation of gene expression in rat brown adipose tissue. Unaltered iodothyronine 5'-deiodinase activity is necessary for the response to environmental temperature at birth. *Eur. J. Biochem.* **193**, 297-302.
6. Glick, Z., Wu, S.Y., Lupien, J., Reggio, R., Bray, G.A. & Fisher, D.A. (1985): Meal-induced brown fat thermogenesis and thyroid hormone metabolism in rats. *Am. J. Physiol.* **249**, E519-E524.
7. Goldberg, J.R., Ehrmann, B. & Katzeff, H.L. (1988): Altered triiodothyronine metabolism in Zucker fatty rats. *Endocrinology* **122**, 689-693.
8. Iglesias, R., Fernandez, J.A., Mampel, T., Obregon, M.J. & Villaroya, F. (1987): Iodothyronine 5'-deiodinase activity in rat brown adipose tissue during development. *Biochim. Biophys. Acta* **923**, 233-240.
9. Kaplan, M.M. & Young, J.B. (1987): Abnormal thyroid hormone deiodination in tissues of ob/ob and db/db obese mice. *Endocrinology* **120**, 886-893.
10. Kates, A-L. & Himms-Hagen, J. (1985): Defective cold-induced stimulation of thyroxine 5'-deiodinase in brown adipose tissue of genetically obese (ob/ob) mouse. *Biochem. Biophys. Res. Commun.* **130**, 188-193.

11. Krief, S., Bazin, R., Dupuy, F. & Lavau, M. (1988): Increased *in vivo* glucose utilization in 30-day-old obese Zucker rat: role of white adipose tissue. *Am. J. Physiol.* **254**, E342-E348.
12. Krief, S., Bazin, R., Dupuy, F. & Lavau, M. (1989): Role of brown adipose tissue in glucose utilization in conscious pre-obese Zucker rats. *Biochem. J.* **263**, 305-308.
13. Lavau, M. & Bazin, R. (1982): Inguinal fat pad weight plotted versus body weight as a method of genotype identification in 16-day-old Zucker rats. *J. Lipid Res.* **23**, 941-943.
14. Levin, B.E., Triscari, J. & Sullivan, A.C. (1980): Abnormal sympathoadrenal function and plasma catecholamines in obese Zucker rats. *Pharmacol. Biochem. Behav.* **13**, 107-113.
15. Levin, B.E., Triscari, J. & Sullivan, A.C. (1981): Defective catecholamine metabolism in peripheral organs of genetically obese Zucker rats. *Brain Res.* **224**, 353-356.
16. Nicholls, D.G. & Locke, R.M. (1984): Thermogenic mechanisms in brown fat. *Physiol. Rev.* **64**, 1-64.
17. Planche, E., Joliff, M., de Gasquet, P. & Le Liepvre, X. (1983): Evidence of a defect in energy expenditure in 7-day-old Zucker rat *(fa/fa)*. *Am. J. Physiol.* **245**, E107-E113.
18. Planche, E., Joliff, M. & Bazin, R. (1988): Energy expenditure and adipose tissue development in 2- to 8-day-old Zucker rats. *Int. J. Obesity* **12**, 352-360.
19. Ricquier, D., Bouillaud, F., Toumelin, P., Mory, G., Bazin, R., Arch, J. & Penicaud, L. (1986): Expression of uncoupling protein mRNA in thermogenic or weakly thermogenic brown adipose tissue. Evidence for a rapid β-adrenoreceptor-mediated and transcriptionally regulated step during activation of thermogenesis. *J. Biol. Chem.* **261**, 13905-13910.
20. Silva, J.E. & Larsen, P.R. (1983): Adrenergic activation of triiodothyronine production in brown adipose tissue. *Nature* **305**, 712-713.
21. Silva, J.E. & Larsen, P.R. (1985): Potential of brown adipose tissue type II thyroxine 5′-deiodinase as a local and systemic source of triiodothyronine in rats. *J. Clin. Invest.* **76**, 2296-2305.
22. Silva, J.E. & Larsen, P.R. (1986): Hormonal regulation of iodothyronine 5′-deiodinase in rat brown adipose tissue. *Am. J. Physiol.* **251**, E639-E643.
23. Visser, T.J., Leonard, J.L., Kaplan, M.M. & Larsen, P.R. (1982): Kinetic evidence suggesting two mechanisms for iodothyronine 5′-deiodination in rat cerebral cortex. *Proc. Natl. Acad. Sci. USA.* **79**, 5080-5084.
24. Wu, S.Y., Stern, J.S., Fisher, D.A. & Glick, Z. (1987): Cold-induced increase in brown fat thyroxine 5′-monodeiodinase is attenuated in Zucker obese rat. *Am. J. Physiol.* **252**, E63-E67.

Section IV
Epidemiological aspects of obesity

Chapter 20

Obesity in Europe – Some Epidemiological Observations

J.C. SEIDELL
Department of Human Nutrition, Wageningen University, P.O. Box 8129, 6700 EV Wageningen, The Netherlands

The heavy burden of obesity in Europe

Obesity is a common problem, especially in middle-aged Europeans. A recent compilation of data that will be published by the WHO Regional Office for Europe gives some astonishing figures[3]. Table 1 gives a preliminary impression of some of the data that were compiled. The figures do not reflect the large intra-country variability of the prevalence of obesity in some countries but, rather, gives a weighed average of different studies available for the age-group 40–60 years of age. Within columns, the data are not ranked according to obesity prevalence. It is clear that obesity is generally more common in women than in men and that a very high prevalence (from 20 up to 45 per cent) is present in Mediterranean countries as well as countries from Eastern Europe.

Table 1. Preliminary classification of countries according to the estimated prevalance of obesity (BMI > 30 kg/m^2) in 40–60 year old Europeans

Women		Men	
Prevalence 10–20%	Prevalence 20–45%	Prevalence 5–15%	Prevalence 15–25%
Iceland	Portugal	Iceland	Finland
Denmark	Italy	Denmark	Belgium
Sweden	Spain	Sweden	Germany
Norway	Yugoslavia	Norway	Switzerland
Finland	Poland	Scotland	France
Scotland	Hungary	United Kingdom	Italy
United Kingdom	Czechoslovakia	Netherlands	Yugoslavia
Netherlands	USSR	Portugal	Poland
Belgium		Spain	Hungary
Germany			Czechoslovakia
Switzerland			USSR
France			

The prevalence of obesity in men does not follow exactly the geographic distribution of women. This is illustrated in Figs. 1–3 that show plots of age-adjusted 10th, 50th and 90th percentiles of BMI in 43 centres that participated in the WHO MONICA study in men *versus* women. China is excluded from the plot. The correlation between men and women becomes stronger towards the right side of the distribution of BMI suggesting that obesity but not

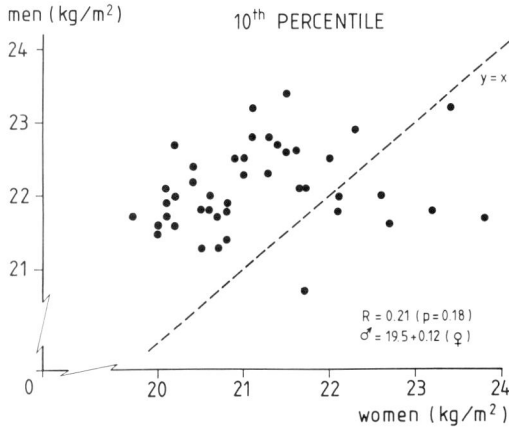

Fig. 1. Plot of age-standardized 10th percentiles of BMI in MONICA populations. Men and women aged 35–64 years.

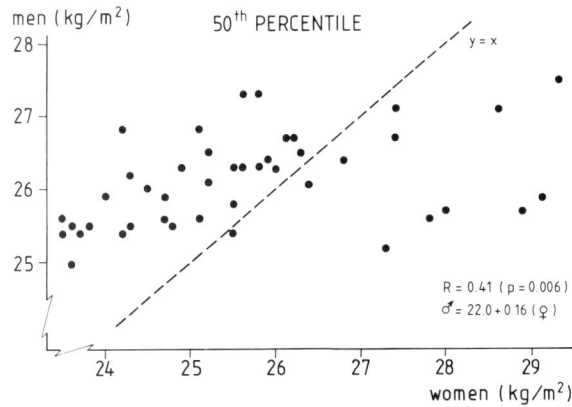

Fig. 2. Plot of age-standardized 50th percentiles of BMI in MONICA populations. Men and women aged 35–64 years.

leanness is shared by men and women in the same communities. In most centres women have a higher 90th but a lower 10th percentile value of BMI. The plots indicate that the variation in BMI in women between centres and within centres is much larger than in men.

Is it always bad to be obese?

One may wonder, in communities where obesity seems to be the norm rather than the exception, if the prevalence of cardiovascular risk factors and cardiovascular events is also very high. Within countries BMI and waist/hip ratio are associated with unfavourable risk profiles in selections of men and women in very different European communities[4,5]. Table 2 shows the correlations between BMI and cardiovascular risk factors in different European population samples. Although the correlation-coefficients differ somewhat there is no clear emerging suggestion of some populations being protected for a rise in serum triglycerides or blood pressure with increasing BMI. Also in other European countries, significant associations between BMI and waist/hip on the one hand and blood pressure, serum triglycerides,

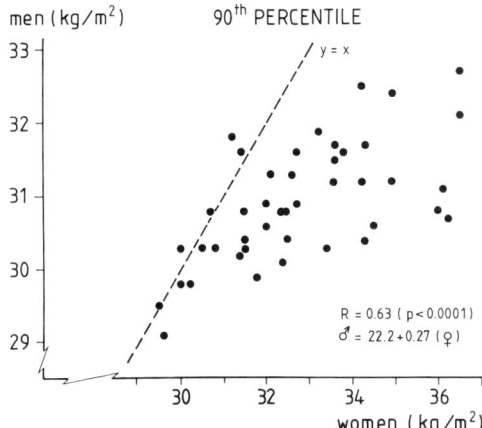

Fig. 3. Plot of age-standardized 90th percentiles of BMI in MONICA populations. Men and women aged 35–64 years.

serum insulin (all positive) and HDL-cholesterol (negative) on the other hand have been observed[2,8]. It is important to note, however, that differences in BMI and waist/hip could not explain the differences in risk factors between populations[4,5].

Moreover, the median and 90th percentile of BMI in centres participating in the WHO MONICA study were weakly correlated with mortality of ischaemic heart disease in women (which became stronger after adjustment for smoking and disappeared after adjustment for hypertension) but not in men (Table 3). Quite consistently, however, the proportion of hypertensives was increased in the heavier populations.

Table 2. Correlations between BMI and risk factors in 38-year old men randomly selected from six European populations[5]

	Netherlands	Sweden	Italy	Poland	Belgium	Portugal
Systolic bp	0.14	0.40**	0.27**	0.28**	0.32**	0.30**
Diastolic bp	0.31**	0.41**	0.18	0.23*	0.44**	0.32**
Serum triglycerides	0.40**	0.44**	0.32**	0.36**	0.49**	0.37**
Serum HDL-cholesterol	−0.13	−0.32**	−0.04	−0.41**	−0.33**	−0.48**
Serum LDL-cholesterol	0.18	0.28*	0.07	0.12	0.16	0.001

Table 3. Correlations between age--standardized 50th and 90th percentiles of BMI with the percentages of hyperytensives and smokers, and the age standardized average annual mortality from ischaemic heart disease in 38 centres participating in the WHO MONICA study (recalculated from[9,10])

	Men BMI 50th%	Men BMI 90th%	Women BMI 50th%	Women BMI 90th%
% actual hypertensives	0.19	0.41*	0.59**	0.65**
% regular smokers	−0.17	0.02	−0.57**	−0.56**
IHD mortality	−0.15	0.08	0.36*	0.29

Although these ecological comparisons must be viewed with caution because they are cross-sectional and do not take other risk factors and life-styles into account, these observations suggest that within population increasing obesity is associated with increased risk for cardiovascular disease but that differences between populations are determined by many factors other than obesity (especially in men where the variation in obesity prevalence is much smaller than in women). With respect to other chronic diseases (such as diabetes mellitus) similar disease patterns have been associated with increasing obesity in, for example, Italian and Dutch populations[1,6]. This suggest that, even in populations where obesity is very common it constitutes a significant health risk.

Conclusion

Obesity is a widespread problem in Europe. This seems to be especially the case in women from southern and eastern parts of Europe. Obesity is within populations quite consistently related to increased blood pressure and unfavourable serum lipid profiles and glucose metabolism. In men, differences in obesity prevalence do not seem to explain mortality rates of ischaemic heart disease in European centres, while in women there is a modest positive association between the level of fatness in populations and mortality of ischaemic heart disease. At this moment there are no clear initiatives for public health policies that make it possible to deal effectively with the treatment of the vast number of obese individuals in Europe. No strategies to prevent individuals from developing obesity nor strategies to prevent an increase in prevalence of obesity in populations have been formulated. In this context it may be appropriate to cite Peter Skrabanek's view on preventive medicine[7]: "The issues of preventive medicine have little to do with science, relative risks, and risk factors. They could be more profitably debated within the framework to which they belong – ethics, politics, and vested interest". Let us hope that politicians responsible for public health will take an interest in obesity in Europe.

References

1. Negri, E., Pagano, R., Decarli, A. *et al.* (1988): Body weight and the prevalence of chronic diseases. *J. Epidemiol. Community Health* **42**, 24-29.
2. Raison, J., Bonithon-Kopp, C., Eglof, M. *et al.* (1990): Hormonal influences on the relationships between body fatness, body fat distribution, lipids, lipoproteins, glucose and blood pressure in French working women. *Atherosclerosis* **85**, 185-192.
3. Seidell, J.C. Obesity in Europe: prevalence and public health implications. WHO Regional Series of Europe (in preparation).
4. Seidell, J.C., Cigolini, M., Charzewska, J. *et al.* (1989): Indicators of fat distribution, serum lipids, and blood pressure in European women born in 1948 – the European fat distribution study. *Am. J. Epidemiol.* **130**, 53-65.
5. Seidell, J.C., Cigolini, M., Deslypere, J.-P *et al.* (1991): Body fat distribution in relation to serum lipids and blood pressure in 38-year old European men: the European fat distribution study. *Atherosclerosis* **86**, 251-160.
6. Seidell, J.C., De Groot, C.P.G.M., van Sonsbeek, J.L.A. *et al.* (1986): Associations of moderate and severe overweight with self-reported illness and medical care in Dutch adults. *Am. J. Public Health* **76**, 264-269.
7. Skrabanek, P. (1986): Preventive medicine. *Lancet* **i**, 143-144.
8. Tuomilehto, J., Marti, B., Kartovaara, L. *et al.* (1990): Body fat distribution, serum lipoproteins and blood pressure in middle aged Finnish men and women. *Epidemiol. Public Health* **38**, 507-516.
9. WHO MONICA project (1989): Assessing CHD mortality and morbidity. *Int. J. Epidemiol.* **18** (Suppl.1), S38-S45.
10. WHO MONICA project (1989): Risk factors. *Int J. Epidemiol.* **18** (Suppl. 1) S46-S55.

Chapter 21

Variations of the Body Mass Index in the French Population from 0 to 87 years

M.F. ROLLAND-CACHERA[1], T.J. COLE[2], M. SEMPÉ[3], J. TICHET[4], C. ROSSIGNOL[5] and A. CHARRAUD[6]

[1]*INSERM, ISTNA, CNAM, 2 rue Conté, 75003 Paris, France;* [2]*MRC Dunn Nutrition Unit, Downhams Lane, Milton Road, Cambridge CB4 1XJ, England;* [3]*INSERM, Groupe d'Auxologie Médico-Sociale, Hôpital Debrousse, rue Soeurs Bouvier, 69005 Lyon, France;* [4]*IRSA, Institut Régional pour la Santé, 37521 La Riche, France;* [5]*Centres de Bilans de Santé de l'Enfant CPAM, Caisse Primaire d'Assurance Maladie Paris, 14 rue Baudelique, 75018 Paris, France;* [6]*INSEE, Institut National de la Statistique et des Etudes Economiques, 18 Bd Adolphe Pinard, 75014, Paris, France*

Body mass index (weight/height^2) values for the French population are given from birth to the age of 87 years. Like direct measurements of fat, the BMI increases during the first year of life, decreases until the age of 6 years, increases again up to 65 years and decreases thereafter. The 50th centile values of wt/ht^2 at the ages of 20, 65 and 85 years are 21.5, 25.5 and 23.6 kg/m^2 for men and 20.6, 24.3 and 22.8 kg/m^2 for women. The values for the 3rd, 50th and 97th centiles in adults are approximately 18, 24 and 32 kg/m^2. The prevalence of obesity when defined by a BMI higher than 25 kg/m^2 is 36% in men and 26% in women and when defined by a BMI higher than 30 is 6% in both sexes.

Introduction

Simple measurements for assessing the level of fatness in populations are necessary in order to pick up variations over time and to compare different groups or countries. The BMI is a reasonable index of adiposity to be used both in children[14] and adults[9]. It has been shown to be correlated with many related health indices[12]. In particular, it is linked with the mortality ratio[1,21]. Cut off points for defining malnutrition[11] or obesity[8], have been proposed for adults. These limits plotted against curves presenting the distribution of the BMI in a representative sample of a population show to which percentiles they correspond.

The present report gives wt/ht^2 values for the French population, from birth to age 87 years. Details of this study have been reported earlier[17]. The wt/ht^2 curves give a general indication of how the index changes with age in males and females. Prevalence of different grades of nutritional status are given by age and sex.

Subjects and method

The data used to construct the curves were derived from four samples. During growth, most of the data were longitudinally recorded. The study started between 1953 and 1960 and finished at adult age in 1979. Data at birth were derived from the files of the Centre de Bilans de Santé de l'enfant de la Région Parisienne of the Caisse Primaire d'Assurance Maladie (CPAM). For adults, two samples were available. One from the IRSA, CNAMTS, included

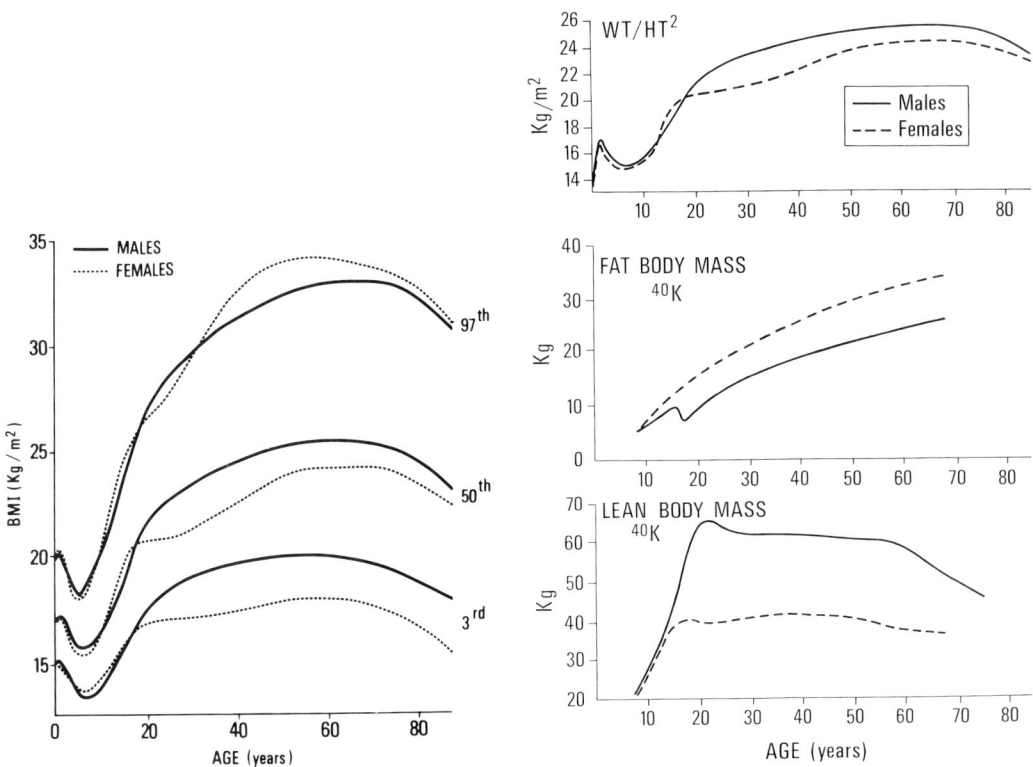

Fig. 1. Weight/height² (kg/m²) 3rd, 50th and 97th centiles by age in both sexes.

Fig. 2. Changes of BMI (present study) and body composition (after[4,5]) by age in both sexes.

21,569 males and 23,284 females. The data were recorded in 1977. The other was from the decennial Health survey 1980 made by the National Institute for Statistics and Economic Studies (INSEE)[10]. The measurements were precisely recorded in the IRSA sample, but the group studied were not representative of the whole French population. Conversely, the INSEE sample was representative, but the measurements used were provided by the subjects themselves. However, the distributions of data in adjacent samples were very similar at the points where they overlapped[17]. The INSEE sample was selected as it covered all adults of all ages up to, and beyond, 85 years. Values corresponding to the 3rd, 10th, 25th, 50th, 75th, 90th and 97th percentiles were obtained for each age and sex group, and these were smoothed using the LMS method[3]. The distribution of wt/ht² is very skew, so that the Z-scores and percentiles cannot be calculated from the mean and standard deviation assuming a normal distribution. In addition, the amount of skewness in the distribution changes with age. The LMS method takes both these features of the data into account in smoothing the percentiles. The method also converts wt/ht² values in individuals to Z-scores and percentiles. Individual charts of the BMI for males and females and detailed tables with 7 percentiles and L, M, and S values are available*.

---

* BMI charts (1 month to 21 years and birth to 87 years) and detailed tables with 7 percentiles and L, M, S values to calculate Z-scores are available from Dr Rolland-Cachera, ISTNA – CNAM, 2 rue Conté 75003 Paris, France.

Results and discussion

BMI changes with age

Figure 1 shows the wt/ht^2 changes from birth to age 87 years. During the first year of life, the BMI increases in both sexes; it decreases until the age of 6 years and increases again until the end of growth. These changes are similar with changes of fatness as assessed by skinfold measurements[22] or radiographs[23]. The decrease in fatness between 1 and 6 years is dramatic. A child situated on the 50th centile at the age of 1 year looks fat. A child on the same centile at the age of 6 years looks thin. From the age of 6 years the BMI curve rises. This increase named adiposity rebound[15] occurs earlier in industrialized than in developing countries. It occurs earlier in obese than in normal weight children. As a rule, we have shown that an individual's age at rebound is correlated with subsequent adiposity: the earlier the rebound, the higher the subsequent adiposity. The age at adiposity rebound can be used as a predictor of adult obesity[16]. During adult life, the BMI continues to increase up to 65 years, after which time it decreases. The data indicate that most of the wt/ht^2 increase in adults occurs by the age of 50 years, it plateaus until the age of 70 and then decreases. The median values of wt/ht^2 at the ages of 20, 65 and 85 years are 21.5, 25.5, 23.6 kg/m^2 in men and 20.6, 24.3, 22.7 kg/m^2 in women. The changes indicate a weight increase of about 11 kg for men and women between the ages of 20 and 65 years, and weight decrease of 5 kg between 65 and 85 years of age. The wt/ht^2 difference between sexes is small during childhood. The 50th centile of wt/ht^2 is always higher in men than in women from the age of 18. The greatest difference occurs in young adults (maximum at age 30 years: 23.4 *vs* 21.2 kg/m^2). The higher value of the BMI in males for the mean curve reflects their higher lean body mass (LBM)[4,5]. The average values of the 3rd, 50th and 97th percentiles in adults are 19, 24.5, 31 kg/m^2 in men and 17, 23, 32 kg/m^2 in women. As LBM decreases during adult life[5], the increase of the index until the age of 65 years corresponds to an increase of fat body mass (FBM) only (Fig. 2). After this age, the decrease of the curve reflects both FBM and LBM changes. BMI changes are similar to total FBM changes assessed by ^{40}K in both sexes. They are similar to skinfolds changes in females but not in males[7,13] (subcutaneous fat hardly increases). This can be explained by the fact that with age, most men accumulate fat at the intra-abdominal level. This fat cannot be picked up by measuring skinfolds.

Cross-sectional and longitudinal changes

The BMI changes observed during growth are actual longitudinal variations. During adulthood, the study is cross-sectional, but the variations mainly reflect longitudinal changes of fatness[5]. Longitudinal studies of changes in BMI[13,19] have shown that weight gain is common in the young even in those with a high initial BMI, and weight loss is associated with old age.

Energy intake variations with age

The IRSA study included dietary records. Description of the method and part of the results of this study on intake and adiposity relationship were published earlier[18]. The BMI changes between 20 and 65 years cannot be explained by an increase of energy intake, as a regular decrease is observed from the age range 30–35 years in both sexes (Fig. 3). The sex and age variations in energy intake (Fig. 3) are similar to LBM variations and opposite to FBM variations (Fig. 2).

Comparison between different countries

Figure 4 compares the BMI percentile curves in different countries: England[20], Finland[13], France[17], The Netherlands[19], USA[6]. It calls for a few comments:

1. The fiftieth centile curves have a similar pattern in all countries, i.e. an increase until the age of 60 years followed by a decrease.

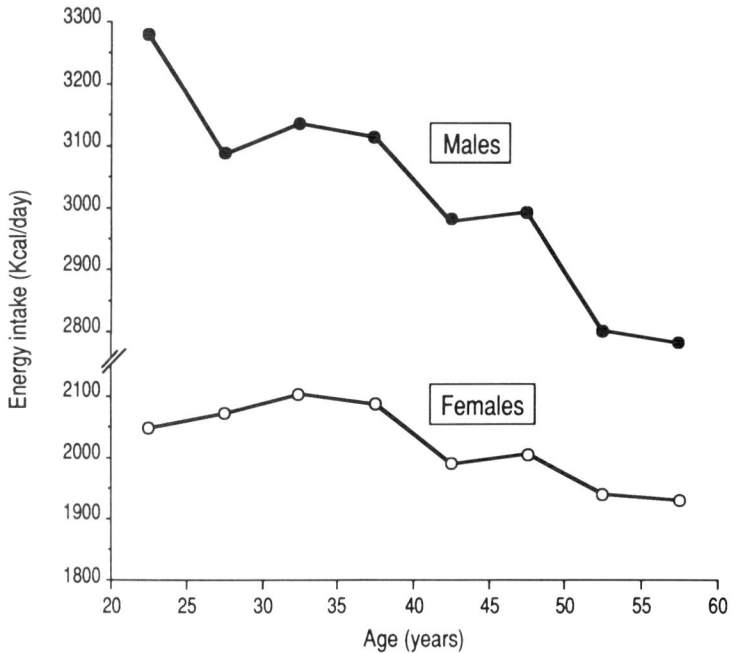

Fig. 3. Energy intake variation with age in both sexes.

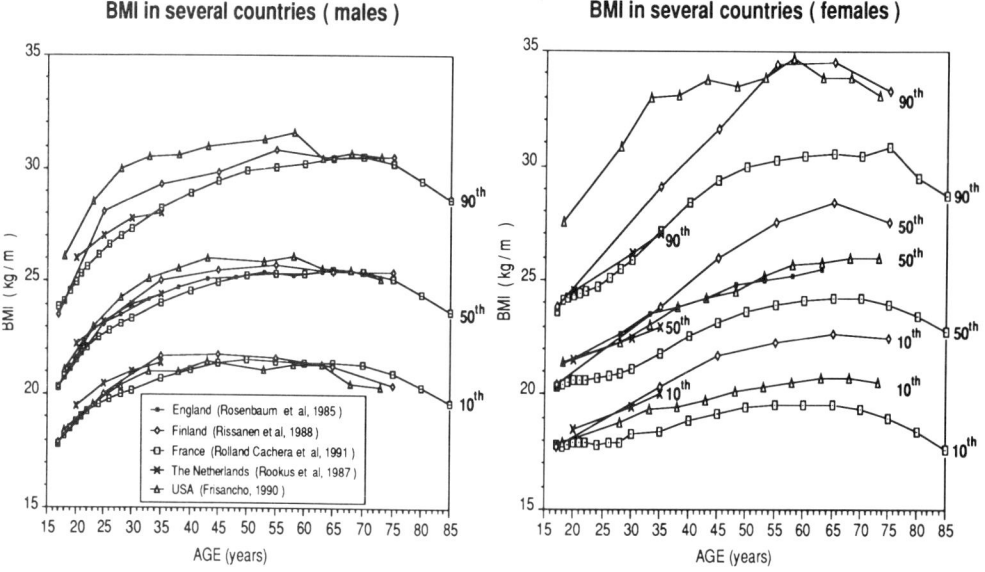

Fig. 4. BMI variations of the 10th, 50th and 90th centiles in four countries and of the mean values for England, by age and sex.

2. Differences between countries are smaller in men than in women.

3. In men, the main differences between countries appear in young adults, especially for the 90th centile. The differences are small after the age of 60 years. In women, differences appear for all centiles and at all ages.

Chapter 21 – Variations of the Body Mass Index in the French Population from 0 to 87 years

Table 1. Percentages of subjects in 8 grades of nutritional status by age and sex

Males								
Age (years) / BMI (Kg/m²)	20-29	30-39	40-49	50-59	60-69	70-79	80 +	Total
> 40	0.2	0.2	0.2	0.1	0.1	0.2	0	0.2
30 - 39.9	1.8	3.6	7	9	10	11.5	5	6
25 - 29.9	15	30.2	39	43.4	44	38	38	33
20 - 24.9	71	61	50.7	44	42	44	59	55
18.5 - 19.9	8.6	3.6	2.4	2.6	3	4.5	4	4.1
17 - 18.4	3	1.1	0.4	0.5	0.8	1.3	3	1.3
16 - 16.9	0.1	0.2	0.1	0.2	0.1	0.2	1	0.2
< 16	0.3	0.1	0.2	0.2	0	0.3	0	0.2
	100 %	100 %	100 %	100 %	100 %	100 %	100 %	100 %
n =	1466	1413	1213	1248	729	578	161	6808

Females								
Age (years) / BMI (Kg/m²)	20-29	30-39	40-49	50-59	60-69	70-79	80 +	Total
> 40	0.1	0.1	0.5	0.5	0.2	0.2	0	0.3
30 - 39.9	1.5	3	7	9	9.5	10	4	6
25 - 29.9	7	12.5	20.5	27.7	32	29.6	29	20
20 - 24.9	51	56	56	51	46	46	43	52
18.5 - 19.9	26	20	11.3	8	8	7	9.5	14
17 - 18.4	12	7	4	3	3.2	4	6.5	6
16 - 16.9	1.9	1.1	0.5	0.4	1	2	4	1.2
< 16	0.5	0.3	0.2	0.4	0.1	1.2	4	0.5
	100 %	100 %	100 %	100 %	100 %	100 %	100 %	100 %
n =	1509	1397	1272	1325	834	797	282	7425

4. The different countries can be listed in descending order: in men, the highest values are observed for the US population, followed by Finland. In women, for most centiles the highest values are observed in Finland. However, the highest 90th centile up to the age of 45 years corresponds to the American women. For men and women, the next orders are for England and The Netherlands. As a rule, the French values are the lowest for all centiles in both sexes. Among other factors, the lowest BMI in the French population can account for the

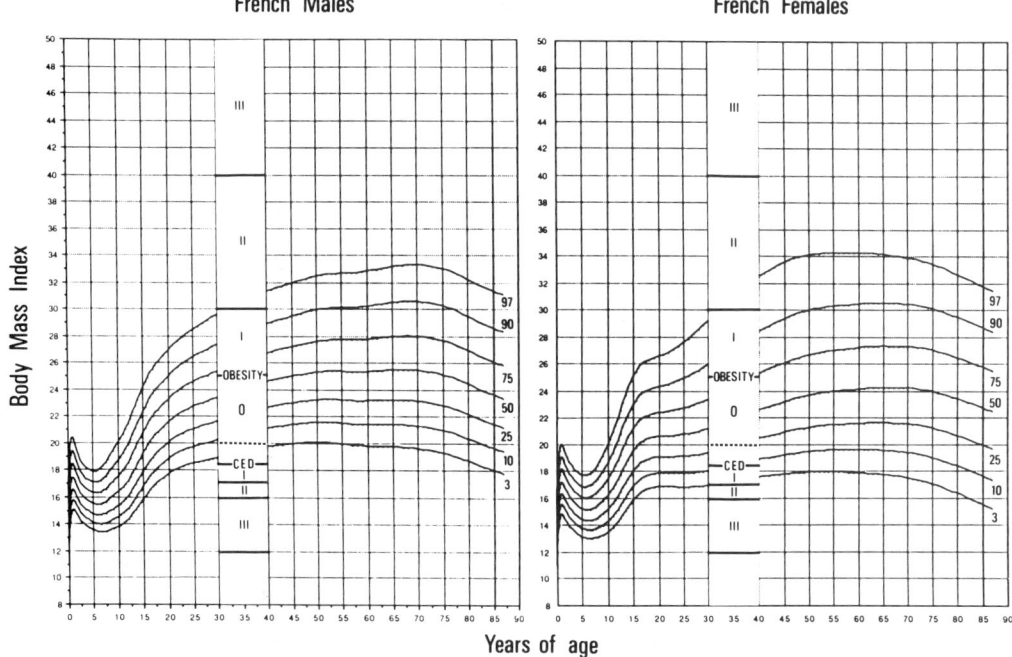

Fig. 5. Grades of nutritional status plotted against the BMI curves in French males and females.

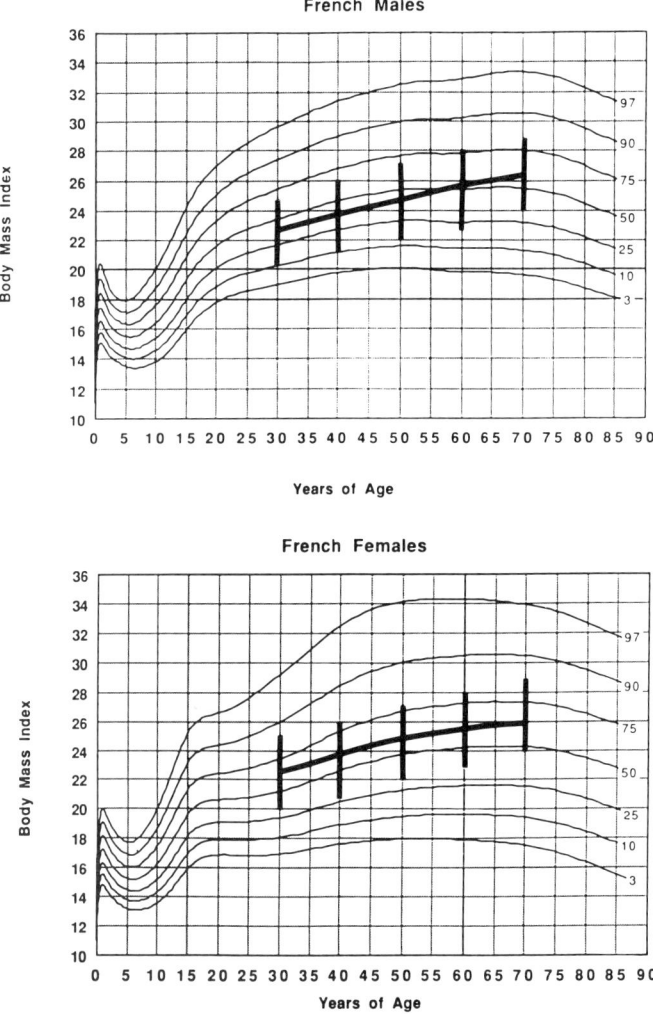

Fig. 6. Recommendations that the normal BMI range 20–25 should change with age increasing by 1 kg/m² for each decade of life between 30 and 70 years (after²) plotted against the French BMI curves.

lowest incidence of coronary, heart diseases[24]. The differences observed between countries reflect different levels of fatness. They can also reflect differences in body frame as suggested by the differences observed even for the lowest percentiles.

Classification of nutritional status

Classifications of nutritional status have been proposed on the basis of the BMI. They consist of three grades of chronic energy deficiency (CED)[11] with cut-off points of: 18.5, 17 and 16; and three grades of obesity[8] with cut-off points of: 25, 30 and 40. The "desirable weight" falls between 20–25. The range 18.5–20 represents mere thinness. At the age of 30 years, the range 20–25 corresponds to the 10th-75th centiles in French men and to the 30–85th centiles in French women (Fig. 5). The limit for Grade I CED (18.5 kg/m²) corresponds to the 3rd centile in men and to the 10th centile in women. The limit for overweight (30 kg/m²) corresponds to the 97th centile in both sexes. Table 1 gives the percentage of subjects in each category of nutritional status. Six per cent have a BMI higher than 30 kg/m^2. Thirty-three per cent of men and 20% of women have a BMI between 25 and 29.9. Most of the population is within the ideal range: 55 per cent men and 52 per cent women. The BMI cut-off point gives preliminary information but this measure must be combined with the assessment of basal metabolic rate (BMR) in order to confirm the diagnosis of CED and with complementary measures of fatness to confirm the diagnosis of obesity in individuals. These grades of nutritional status do not take age into account. Andres[1] observed that the BMI values associated with the lowest mortality rate increased with age. On this basis, G. Bray[2] recommends that the normal range of 20–25 should change with age increasing by 1 kg/m^2 for each decade of life between 30 and 70 years. Figure 6 indicates that the median of the range of these recommendations is close to the 50th centile of the French population, and the limits of the range close to the 25th and 75th centiles, slightly lower in men and slightly higher in women. This recommendation which takes age into account does not mean that individual BMI has to increase with age. However, the curves can be used as a guide indicating that individual weight gain should not exceed the mean weight gain.

Conclusion

In conclusion, the present study describes the changes in BMI over the whole life-span of the French population. While wt/ht^2 is not a measure of Fat Body Mass alone, it does show a pattern of development which resembles that obtained by direct measurement of fat.

As weight and height measurements are widely available subjects at risk of under- or over-nutrition can be identified. Their status should be checked by complementary anthropometric and laboratory examinations.

The French BMI values (mean and distribution) fit well with usual recommendations. These data should be considered as valuable references to assess and monitor the nutritional status. In addition, the BMI curves show how body shape changes during life. The use of the BMI charts can improve body-weight surveillance.

Acknowledgements

The authors are greatly indebted to H. Valdelièvre (INSEE), S. Vol (IRSA), E. Patois, M. Deheeger, F. Péquignot and M. Niravong (INSERM) who assisted in the treatment of the data, to M. Mormiche (INSEE) who provided useful information and to F. Bellisle for her constructive criticisms.

References

1. Andres, R., Elahi, D., Tobin, J.D., Muller, D.C. & Brant, L. (1985): Impact of age on weight goals. *Ann. Intern. Med.* **103**, 1030-1033.
2. Bray, G.A. (1987): Overweight is risking fate: Definition, classification, prevalence, and risks. *Ann NY Acad. Sci.* **499**, 14-28.
3. Cole, T.J. (1990): The LMS method for constructing normalized growth standards. *Eur. J. Clin. Nutr.* **44**, 45-60.
4. Forbes, G.B. (1972): Growth of the Lean Body Mass in man. *Growth* **36**, 325-338.
5. Forbes, G.B. & Reina, J.C. (1970): Adult Lean Body Mass declines with age: some longitudinal observations. *Metabolism* **19**, 653-663.
6. Frisancho, A.R. (1990): *Anthropometric standards for the assessment of growth and nutritional status*, pp. 189. Ann Arbor: The University of Michigan Press.
7. Garn, S.M. & Clark, D.L. (1976): Trends in fatness and the origins of obesity. *Pediatrics.* **57**, 443-456.
8. Garrow, J.S. (1981): *Treat obesity seriously. A clinical manual.* pp. 246. London: Churchill Livingstone.
9. Garrow, J.S. & Webster, J. (1985): Quetelet's index (W/H^2) as a measure of fatness. *Int. J. Obes.* **9**, 147-153.
10. INSEE (1987): La taille et le poids des français. *Données Sociales*: 462-463.

11. James, W.P., Ferro-Luzzi, A. & Waterlow, J. (1988): Definition of chronic energy deficiency in adults. Report of a working party of the International Dietary Energy consultative group. *Eur. J. Clin. Nutr.* **42**, 969-981.
12. Keen H., Thomas, B.J, Jarrett, R.J. & Fuller, J.H. (1979): Nutrient intake, adiposity and diabetes. *Br. Med. J.* **1**, 655-658.
13. Rissanen, A., Heliövaara, M. & Aromaa, A. (1988): Overweight and anthropometric changes in adulthood: a prospective study of 17 000 Finns. *Int. J. Obes.* **12**, 391-401.
14. Rolland-Cachera, M.F., Sempé, M., Guilloud-Bataille, M., Patois, E., Péquignot-Guggenbuhl, F. & Fautrad, V. (1982): Adiposity indices in children. *Am. J. Clin. Nutr.* **36**, 178-184.
15. Rolland-Cachera, M.F., Deheeger, M., Bellisle, F., Sempé, M., Guilloud-Bataille, M. & Patois, E. (1984): Adiposity rebound in children: a simple indicator for predicting obesity. *Am. J. Clin. Nutr.* **39**, 129-135.
16. Rolland-Cachera, M.F., Deheeger, M., Avons, P., Guilloud- Bataille, M., Patois, E. & Sempé, M. (1987): Tracking adiposity patterns from 1 month to adulthood. *Ann. Hum. Biol.* **14**, 219-222.
17. Rolland-Cachera, M.F., Cole, T.J., Sempé, M., Tichet, J., Rossignol, C. & Charraud, A. (1991): Variation of the Weight/Height^2 index from birth to age 87 years. *Eur. J. Clin. Nutr.* **45**, 13-21.
18. Rolland-Cachera, M.F., Bellisle, F., Tichet, J., Chantrel, A.M., Guilloud-Bataille, M., Vol, S. & Péquignot, G. (1990): Relationship between adiposity and food intake: an example of pseudo-contradictory results obtained in case-control versus between-population studies. *Int. J. Epidem.* **19**, 571-577.
19. Rookus, M.A., Burena, J., Van't Hof, M.A., Deurenberg, P., Van der Wiel-Wetzels, W.A. & Hautvast, J.G. (1987): The development of the Body Mass Index in young adults, 1: Age-reference curves based on a four-years mixed-longitudinal study. *Hum. Biol.* **59**, 599-615.
20. Rosenbaum, S., Skinner, R.K., Knight, I.B. & Garrow (1985): A survey of heights and weights of adults in Great Britain, 1980. *Ann. Hum. Biol.* **12**, 115-127.
21. Seltzer, C.C. (1966). Some re-evaluations of the build and blood pressure study 1959 as related to ponderal index, somatotype and mortality. *N. Engl. J. Med.* **274**, 254-259.
22. Tanner, J.M. & Whitehouse, R.H. (1975): Revised standard for triceps and subscapular skinfolds in British children. *Arch. Dis. Child.* **50**, 142-145.
23. Tanner, J.M., Hughes, P.C.R. & Whitehouse, R.H. (1981): Radiographically determined widths of bone, muscle and fat in the upper arm and calf from age 3–18 years. *Ann. Hum. Biol.* **8**, 495-517.
24. World Health Organisation (1988): Healthy nutrition: preventing nutrition-related disease in Europe (European series 24). Geneva: WHO.

Chapter 22

The Relation of Obesity and Fat Distribution to Blood Lipid Levels

Berit Lilienthal HEITMANN

Research Department of Human Nutrition, Rolighedsvej 25, 1958 Frederiksberg C, Copenhagen, Denmark and The Glostrup Population Studies, Medical Department C, Glostrup Hospital, University of Copenhagen, Denmark

In a population sample (n = 2987) of adult Danish men and women aged 35–65 years the variation in blood lipid levels (HDL-cholesterol, LDL-cholesterol, total cholesterol, VLDL-cholesterol or triglyceride concentrations (mmol/l)) explained by various measures of overall obesity (body fat mass (kg) percentage body fat, body mass index (kg/m^2)) or abdominal obesity (waist/hip ratio, waist/thigh ratio or waist circumference (cm)) was examined.

Only minor differences between the associations of the various indices of obesity/fat-distribution and a given blood lipid were found.

Dependent on the blood lipid up to 11% of the variation was explained, the size of the variation being more dependent on the type of blood lipid than on the measure of obesity.

Introduction

Several prospective studies have shown that both overall and abdominal obesity relates to cardiovascular disease, either through alterations in one or several of the risk factors or directly[2,9,11,12,14]. Thus, in the Framingham study[9] and in the Norwegian study[14], obesity was an independent risk factor for cardiovascular disease. In most studies, however, BMI and not measures of "true" obesity, e.g. body fat mass or body fat percentage, have been used. As BMI has been shown to explain only about 50% of the variation in percentage body fat[6-13], and as it is more plausible that body fat and not body overweight relates to blood lipid levels, stronger associations may be expected between lipids and body fatness than between lipids and BMI.

In the 12 year follow up of Gothenburg men[12] a strong and independent effect of waist/hip-ratio on blood pressure, serum cholesterol, myocardial infarction, angina pectoris and stroke was found, and in the Gothenbourg women[11] an independent effect of waist/hip ratio was found on myocardial infarction, angina pectoris, stroke and death. Thus a stronger association between the lipids and abdominal obesity than between the lipids and overall obesity may be expected.

It is therefore of interest to examine to what extent the contribution to the variation in the blood lipid levels comes from the different measures of overall or abdominal obesity.

Population

A population sample, selected from the Danish personal registry, of 3608 Danish men and women born in 1922, 1932, 1942 or 1952 were invited to participate in the study. The study group has been described elsewhere[8]. Eighty-three per cent (2987) agreed to participate in the study.

The present study (GEN-MONICA) was carried out in 1987/88, in collaboration with the Glostrup Population Studies[10] and was a five year follow-up of the Danish MONICA-I project[5].

Anthropometry

All anthropometric measurements (height, weight and circumference measures) were made in accordance with WHO standards[15].

Height (Ht) was measured without shoes to the nearest 0.5 cm. Body weight (BW) was measured to the nearest 0.1 kg using a SECA scale, subjects wearing only light indoor clothes. Circumference measurements were taken to the nearest 0.5 cm. Waist circumference was measured midway between lower rib margin and the iliac crest in the horizontal plane.

Hip circumference was measured at the point yielding the maximum circumference over the buttocks. Thigh circumference was measured at the point of the maximum circumference.

Measurements of electrical impedance

A BIA-103 RJL-system-analyser (RJL-systems Detroit) was used to measure electrical impedance, following the instructions given by the manufacturer. The measurement was taken using a tetrapolar electrode placement and subjects lying relaxed on a couch.

Measures of overall and abdominal obesity

Body fat (BF) and body fat percentage (BF%) were estimated from measurement of electrical impedance using an algorithm developed on a subgroup of this random sample of Danes[7].

$$BF = 0.819\ BW\ (kg) - 0.279\ Ht^2/R\ (cm^2/ohm) - 0.064\ gender\ {}^*BW\ (kg) + 0.077\ age\ (years) - 0.231\ Ht\ (cm) + 14.941.$$

(gender is coded as 1 for men and 0 for women).

Waist/hip ratio (WH ratio) and waist/thigh ratio (WT ratio) were computed from the circumference measures of waist and hip, and of waist and thigh, respectively. Body mass index (body weight for body height squared) was calculated from measures of body weight (BW) and body height (Ht).

Blood lipids

Blood samples were drawn after a 12 h overnight fast. A commercial enzymatic method was used (Boehringer Mannheim) to measure concentrations of total cholesterol, HDL-cholesterol and triglyceride concentrations (mmol/l) in serum. VLDL-cholesterol and LDL-cholesterol concentrations were calculated using the formula given by Friedewal et al.[4]. This was done only if the triglyceride level was below 4.5 mmol/l. Otherwise no calculation was made and the value is thus missing.

The project was approved by the ethical committee for the Copenhagen County, and is in accordance with the Helsinki II declaration.

Statistical methods

Multiple regression analysis, including different intercepts and slopes for men and women of different ages, and standard F-tests were used to evaluate the effects of gender and age on the associations between obesity and the lipids. The statistical analyses were performed with the SPSS.PC V4.0 and the PC. SAS V6.03 programs.

Results and discussion

Mean body fat (kg) and mean WH ratio by age and gender in 1527 men and 1464 women are

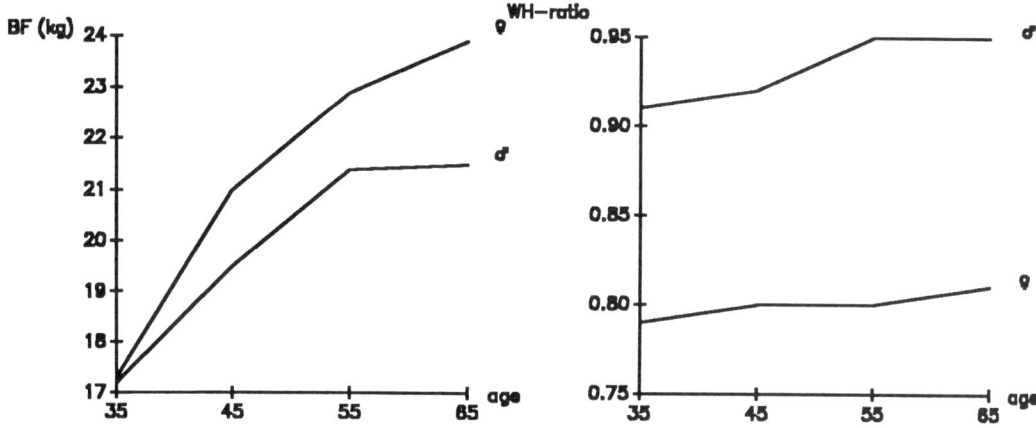

Fig. 1. Mean body fat mass (kg) and WH ratio by age in 1527 men and 1467 women.

shown in Fig. 1. The detailed description of the characteristics of the subjects is given in a previous study[8]. A description of the paricipants and the non-paricipants is also given previously, and it was found that the non-paricipants included slightly more older people than the paricipants, but that within each age/gender group there were no differences in body weight or BMI between paricipants and non-paricipants compared to baseline-data 5 years previously.

Table 1 lists the measures of obesity used to predict HDL, LDL, total cholesterol, VLDL or triglyceride levels. Three measures of overall obesity (BF (kg), BF% and BMI), and three measures of abdominal obesity (WH ratio, WT ratio and waist circumference), were used.

Table 1. Measures of overall and abdominal obesity used in the present study

Measures of overall obesity:
    BF (kg) (impedance)
    BF% (impedance)
    BMI (kg/m^2)

Measures of abdominal obesity:
    WH ratio
    WT ratio
    Waist circumference (cm)

Different prediction of lipid levels has been reported in other literature. Thus, on a sample of 303 men and women aged 18–57 years, Baumgardner et al.[1], report that centripetal fat distribution, percentage body fat and age are responsible for 9–31% of the variance in lipid levels (HDL, LDL, total cholesterol or triglycerides), where the fatness or fat distribution variables are responsible for up to 9%, and age for between 2 and 28%. Similarly, on 368 men and women aged 18–76 years, Foster et al.[3] report that body build, fatness, fat patterning, age and diabetes are responsible for up to 31% of the variation in lipid levels (HDL, LDL or triglycerides), of which the body composition measures are responsible for up to 14%, and age for about 12%.

In the present study 0.5–10% of the variation in HDL, LDL, total cholesterol, VLDL or triglycerides was explained by overall or abdominal obesity. Thus, our data are in agreement with the studies of Baumgardner et al.[1] and Foster et al.[3]. Furthermore, we found only small differences between the predictions from the six different measures of obesity.

Table 2. Range in the variation in lipid levels explained by different obesity measures in different studies

Baumgardner et al.[1]	0–9%
Foster et al.[3]	0–14%
Present study	0–11%

Thus, although we expected to find that more of the variation in the lipid levels could be explained by "true" measures of overall obesity, than by the measure of overweight, only minor differences in the R-squares were found. Nor could the variation in lipid levels be explained any better from measures of abdominal obesity (WH ratio, WT ratio or waist circumference) than from the measures of overall obesity. The explained variation was much more dependent on the type of lipid than on the measure of body fatness.

Acknowledgements: The project was supported by a grant from The Danish Agricultural and Veterinary Research Council, (SJVF 13-4061) and Helsefondet.

References

1. Baumgardner, R.N., Roche, A.F., Chumela, C., Siervogel, R.M. & Glueck, C.J. (1987): Fatness and fat patterns: associations with plasma lipids and blood pressure in adults 18 to 57 years of age. *Am. J. Epidemiol.* **126**, 614-628.
2. Feinleib, M. (1985): Epidemiology of obesity in relation to health hazards. *Ann. Intern. Med.* **103**, (No. 6), 1019-1023.
3. Foster, C.J., Weinsier, R.L., Birch, R., Norris, D.J., Bernstein, R.S., Wang, J., Pierson, R.N. & Van Itallie, T.B. (1987): Obesity and serum lipids: an evaluation of the relative contribution of body fat and fat distribution to lipid levels. *Int. J. Obes.* **11**, 151-161.
4. Friedewald, W.T, Levy, R.I. & Fredrickson, D.S., (1972): Estimation of the concentration of low-density lipoprotein cholesterol in plasma, without use of the preparative ultracantrifuge. *Clin. Chem.* **18**(6), 499-502.
5. Hagerup, L., Eriksen, M., Schroll, M., Hollnagel, H., Agner, E. & Larsen, S. (1981): The Glostrup population studies. Collection of epidemiologic tables. *Scand. J. Soc. Med.* suppl **20**.
6. Heitmann, B.L. (1990): Measurements of body fat in the adult Danish population. A methodological study. *Eur. J. Clin. Nutr.* 831-837.
7. Heitmann, B.L. (1990): Prediction of body water and fat in adult Danes from measurement of electrical impedance. A validation study. *Int. J. Obes.* **14**, 789-802.
8. Heitmann, B.L. (1991): Body fat in the adult danish population aged 35–65 years. An epidemiological study. *Int. J. Obes.* **15**, 535-545.
9. Hubert, H.B., Feinleib, M., McNamara, P.M. & Castelli, W.P. (1983): Obesity as an independent risk factor for cardiovascular disease: A 26-year follow-up of participants in the Framingham heart study. *Circulation* **67**, 968-977.
10. Kirchoff, M., Schroll, M., Kirkby, H., Hansen, B.S., Sanders, S., Sjöl, A., Jørgensen, T. & Hansen, P.F. (1983): Screening I. Danmonica. Part of the MONICA Project (Multinational Monitoring of Trends and Determinants in CVD). *CVD Epidemiology Newsletter* **34**, 32.
11. Lapidus, L., Bengtsson, C., Larsson, B., Pennert, K., Rybo, E. & Sjöström, L. (1984): Distribution of adipose tissue and risk of cardiovascular disease and death. A 12 year follow up of participants in the population study of woman in Gothenburg, Sweden. *Br. Med. J.* **289**, 1257-1261.
12. Larsson, B., Svärdsudd, K., Welin, L., Wilhelmsen, L., Björntorp, P. & Tibblin, G. (1984): Abdominal adipose tissue distribution, obesity, and risk of cardiovascular disease and death: 13 year follow up of participants in the study of men born in 1983. *Br. Med. J.* **288**, 1401-1404.
13. Macdonald, F.C. (1986): Quetelet index as indicator of obesity. *Lancet* **i**, 1043.
14. Waaler, H.T. (1983): The Norwegian study. *Waalers Thesis* 1–56.
15. WHO, Measuring obesity – classification and description of anthropometric data. Report on a WHO Consultation on the Epidemiology of Obesity, Warsaw 21–23 October 1987. Nutrition Unit document, EUR/ICP/NUT 125, WHO Copenhagen, 1989.

Chapter 23

Body Fat Distribution and Breast Cancer Preliminary Results from a Case-control Study in Women from Southern Italy

Renato BORRELLI*, Emilia DE FILIPPO*, Luca SCALFI*, Gelsomina BUGLIONE*, Franco CONTALDO*, Achille MARONE, Valerio PARISI, Franco CREMONA, Francesco SCOGNAMIGLIO, Raffaele PALAIA, Fulvio RUFFOLO and Marco SALVATORE

*Clinical Nutrition, 2nd Medical School, University of Naples and National Cancer Institute (NCI), Naples, Italy

Introduction

It has been largely shown that obesity is characterized by increased risk for breast cancer and cardiovascular disease[6,9,12,14,16,23].

Considerably recent literature suggests that body fat distribution is a better predictor of risk for cardiovascular disease than obesity itself[5,14]. Björntorp[4] has suggested, in particular, that gluteal-femoral obesity could be considered a cosmetic problem rather than a morbid condition, whereas abdominal obesity markedly increases the risk for cardiovascular disease.

The increased risk of abdominal adiposity has been attributed, among others things, to the role of abnormal androgenic/oestrogenic and insulin activity[3,7,10,11,13,15,22]. In fact, abdominal obesity is associated with low serum concentrations of sex hormone binding globulin (SHBG), high levels of free testosterone and hyperinsulinaemia. These hormonal alterations could also be implicated in the development of female carcinomas[17,19].

In this paper the relationship between body fat distribution and breast cancer is evaluated in a case-control study of women from Southern Italy.

Subjects and methods

All women consecutively admitted for suspect primary breast cancer to the National Cancer Institute "Fondazione G. Pascale" in Naples from October 1990 to January 1991 were considered eligible for the study. One hundred and thirty women were contacted. Of these, 15 refused to participate, and the remaining 115 participated in the study. They were submitted to breast biopsy within a few days of the first observation. They were also asked to fill a dietary and a life style questionnaire.

Eighty-two were identified as breast cancer cases and 33 as benign breast disease cases (mastitis, fibrocystic disease, etc.) on the basis of the breast biopsy. No women reported weight loss in the three months preceding the study.

Anthropometry

Anthropometric measurements were taken by a skilled operator. Height was measured with the patients being without shoes with a steel tape attached to the wall. Body weight was measured without any garments or shoes, using a platform scale.

Skinfold thickness (biceps, triceps, suprailiac and subscapular) were measured using the Harpender caliper on the right side of the body.

Chest, waist, hip and arm circumferences were measured by a single examiner with a cloth tape following the standardized procedure[21].

The BMI (body mass index) was calculated as weight in kg divided by height in metres squared. The W/H (waist/hip) ratio and S/T (subscapular/triceps skinfold thickness) ratio were calculated as indices of body fat distribution.

Statistics

The two groups (breast cancer and benign breast disease cases) were compared by the Mann–Whitney U-test[1]. This non-parametric statistical procedure was preferred because it does not need particular assumptions on the distribution of the variables under study.

To measure the risk of incurring breast cancer in the variables categorized into two groups (low and high) by the 50th percentile, the odds ratio (and its 95% confidence limits) was evaluated. The odds ratio is referred to as the approximate relative risk in case-control studies[1].

Table 1. Anthropometric characteristics and age (mean ± SD) odds ratios (its 95% confidence limits) in women with breast cancer and women with benign breast diseases (ben dis)

	ben dis	cancer	P	odds ratio		
				ll	est	ul
n	33	82				
Age (yr)	47 ± 10	56 ± 12	<0.01	1.2	2.7	6.5
Weight (kg)	66.6 ± 10	69.7 ± 13	0.33	0.5	1.2	3.0
Height (cm)	155 ± 6	155 ± 8	0.76	0.3	0.8	2.4
BMI (kg/m^2)	27.2 ± 5	29.3 ± 5	0.06	0.7	2.1	6.2
Skinfold thickness (mm)						
biceps	12 ± 5	14 ± 6	0.21	0.8	2.0	4.5
triceps	24 ± 7	26 ± 7	0.25	0.5	1.2	2.8
suprailiac	22 ± 8	24 ± 10	0.43	0.8	2.1	5.2
subscapular	24 ± 10	29 ± 11	0.02	1.2	2.8	2.5
S/T ratio	1.05 ± 0.33	1.16 ± 0.38	0.11	0.6	1.5	3.5
Circumference (cm)						
arm	30 ± 4	32 ± 4	0.02	1.0	2.6	6.3
chest	95 ± 8	98 ± 8	0.07	1.2	2.9	7.1
waist	93 ± 12	101 ± 13	<0.01	1.3	3.1	7.5
hip	102 ± 11	107 ± 12	0.02	0.9	2.1	5.1
W/H ratio	0.91 ± 0.06	0.94 ± 0.05	0.02	1.2	3.0	7.1

ll = 95% confidence lower limit; est = estimated value; ul = 95% confidence upper limit. P value by Mann–Whitney U-test.

Results

Table 1 reports the mean and standard deviation of the anthropometric variables for the two groups. The women with breast cancer are older and have larger thickness of the subscapular skinfold and larger circumferences (arm, chest, waist and hip). The women with breast cancer are, then, bigger. These findings are confirmed by the greater BMI. More interesting, the W/H ratio is greater in women with breast cancer (0.91 vs 0.94); this difference remained after adjustment for age (0.92 vs 0.94), although the statistical significance was not reached ($P = 0.11$) probably because of the reduction in the test power when doing the covariance analysis.

In Table 1, the odds ratios are also reported. These estimates of the relative risk of having breast cancer in the upper distribution compared to benign breast disease reached statistical significance for age, subscapular skinfold, waist, chest circumferences and waist/hip ratio. These findings, in general, confirm the observations by the Mann–Whitney U-test for the mean differences between the two groups.

Discussion

This study shows that women with breast cancer are bigger (as revealed by the greater circumferences) and have a more pronounced abdominal distribution of fat (as reflected by the higher waist to hip ratio) than women with benign breast disease. Also skinfold thicknesses were different between the two groups although only in the subscapular skinfold was the statistical significance level ($P < 0.05$) reached.

The difference in age between the two groups did not account for the difference in W/H ratio (unadjusted mean 0.911 vs 0.940; adjusted mean 0.917 vs 0.938) although statistical significance level was not reached ($P = 0.11$), probably due to the lesser power of the covariance analysis test.

Increasing evidences in literature relate body fat distribution to breast cancer. Firstly, Lapidus et al.[18], in a longitudinal study on 1462 Swedish women aged 38–60 years, were not able to show a significant relationship between breast cancer incidence and body fat distribution over a 12-year follow up, but their findings were based on only 21 cases. Recently, Schapira et al.[20], in a case-control study with 216 cases aged 25–83 years, reported that breast cancer patients had greater W/H ratio than women randomly selected from a South Florida population register. Ballard-Barbash et al.[2], in the Framingham study on a total of 2201 women aged 30–62 years with a follow up of 28 years for the 106 breast cancer cases, reported that the women in the upper fourth of the distribution of S/T ratio, had an elevated risk for breast cancer over the subsequent 28-year interval (relative risk 1.8). Again, this finding suggests that abdominal adiposity increases the risk of breast cancer. Folsom et al.[8], in a nested case-control study of 41,837 women from Iowa State, aged 55–69 years (229 cases) over 2 years follow up, showed a positive association between abdominal adiposity and breast cancer incidence.

In this study, the control group of women with benign breast disease may be probably not representative of the "normal population". As the women with benign breast disease are likely to be more similar to breast cancer patients than to the "normal" population, any difference between breast cancer cases and "normal population" is probably underestimated. This is also expected on the basis of the quite high W/H ratio in this control group (0.91) if compared to W/H ratio in 38 year-old women (0.82) randomly selected from a population register of the same geographical area[22].

The possible explanations for the association between breast cancer and abdominal distribution of body fat could be the hormonal abnormalities found in abdominal obesity (reduced levels of SHBG, increased levels of free androgens, oestrone, increased levels of insulin, etc.).

In conclusion, body fat distribution could represent a risk factor not only for cardiovascular diseases, but also for some female carcinomas, such as breast cancer.

References

1. Armitage, P. & Berry, G. (1987): *Statistical methods in medical research*. Oxford: Blackwell Scientific Publications.
2. Ballard-Barbash, R., Schatzkin, A., Carter, C.L., Kannel, W.B., Kreger, B.E., D'Agostino, R.B., Splansky, G.L., Anderson, K.M. & Helsen, W.E. (1990): Body fat distribution and breast cancer in the Framingham study. *J. Natl. Cancer Inst.* **82**, 286-290.
3. Barbieri, R.L., Makris, A., Randall, R.W., Daniels, G., Kistner, R.W. & Ryan, K.J. (1986): Insulin stimulates androgen accumulation in incubations of ovarian stroma obtained from women with hyperandrogenism. *J. Clin. Endocrinol. Metab.* **62**, 904-910
4. Björntorp, P. (1990): How should obesity be defined? *J. Intern. Med.* **227**, 147-149.
5. Desprès, J.P. (1991): Obesity and lipid metabolism: relevance of body fat distribution. *Curr. Opin. Lipid* **2**, 5-15.
6. deWaard, F., Poortman, J. & Collette, R.J. (1981): Relationship of weight to the promotion of breast cancer after menopause. *Nutr. Cancer* **2**, 237-240.
7. Evans, D.J., Hoffmann, R.G. & Kalkhoff, R.K. (1983): Relationship of androgenic activity to body fat topography and metabolic profiles in premenopausal women. *J. Clin. Endocrinol. Metab.* **57**, 304-310.
8. Folsom, A.R., Kaye, S.A., Prineas, R.J., Potter, J.D., Gapstur, S.M. & Wallace, R.B. (1990): Increased incidence of carcinoma of the breast associated with abdominal adiposity in postmenopausal women. *Am. J. Epidemiol.* **131**, 794-803.
9. Garfinkel, L. (1985): Overweight and cancer. *Ann Int. Med.* **1030** (6 pt 2), 1034-1036.
10. Glass, A.R., Burnam, K.D. & Dahms, Wt. et al. (1981): Endocrine function in human obesity. *Metabolism* **30**, 89-104.
11. Haffner, S.M., Katz, S.M., Stern, M.P. & Dunn, J.F. (1989): Relationship of sex hormone binding globulin to overall adiposity and body fat distribution in a biethnic population. *Int. J. Obesity* **13**, 1-9.
12. Helmrich, S.P., Shapiro, S. & Rosenberg, L. et al. (1983): Risk factors for breast cancer. *Am. J. Epidemiol.* **117**, 35.
13. Kissebah, A.H., Evans, D.J. & Peiris, A. et al. (1985): Endocrine characteristics in regional obesities: role of sex steroids. In *Metabolic complications of human obesity*. eds. J. Vague, P. Björntorp & B. Guy-Grand et al., pp.115. Amsterdam: Excerpta Medica.
14. Kissebah, A.H., Freedman, D.S. & Peiris, A.N. (1989): Health risks of obesity. *Med. Clin. North Am.* **73**, 111-138.
15. Kopelman, P.G., Pilkington, T.R.E. & White, N. et al. (1980): Abnormal sex steroid secretion and binding in massively obese women. *Clin. Endocrinol.* **12**, 363-369.
16. La Vecchia, C., Franceschi, S. & Gallus, G. (1982): Estrogens and obesity as risk factors for endometrial cancers in Italy. *Int. J. Epidemiol.* **11**, 120-126.
17. Langley, M.S., Hammond, G.L., Bardsley, A., Sellwood, R.A. & Anderson, D.C. (1985): Serum steroid binding proteins and the bioavailability of estradiol in relation to breast diseases. *J. Natl. Cancer Inst.* **75**, 823-829.
18. Lapidus, L., Helgesson, O., Merck, C. & Björntorp, P. (1988): Adipose tissue distribution and female carcinoma, a 12 years follow-up of participants in the population study of women in Gothenburg, Sweden. *Int. J. Obesity* **12**, 361-368.
19. Moore, J.W., Clark, G.M.G., Bulbrook, R.D., Hayward, J.L., Murai, J.T., Hammond, G.L. & Siiteri, P.K. (1982): Serum concentrations of total and non-protein-bound oestradiol in patients with breast cancer and in normal controls. *Int. J. Cancer* **29**, 17-21.
20. Schapira, D.V., Kumar, N.B., Lyman, G.H. & Cox, C.E. (1990): Abdominal obesity and breast cancer risk. *Ann Int. Med.* **112**, 182-186
21. Seidell, J.C., Cigolini, M., Charzewska, J., Contaldo, F., Ellsinger, B. & Björntorp, P. (1988): Measurement of regional distribution of adipose tissue. In *Obesity in Europe 1*. eds. P. Björntorp & S. Rossner, pp. 351-359. London: John Libbey.
22. Seidell, J.C., Cigolini, M., Charzewska, J., Ellsinger, B., Di Biase, G., Björntorp, P., Hautvast, J.G.A.J., Contaldo, F., Szostak, V. & Scuro, L. (1990). Androgenicity in relation to body fat distribution and metabolism in 38-year-old women. The European fat distribution study. *J. Clin. Epidemiol.* **43**, 21-34.
23. Staszewski, J. (1977): Breast cancer and body build. *Prev. Med.* **6**, 410-415.

Chapter 24

Weight Changes Among 13,097 Adult Finns Over Six Years

M. KORKEILA, J. KAPRIO, A. RISSANEN, M. KOSKENVUO[1] and K. HEIKKILÄ

Department of Public Health, University of Helsinki, Haartmaninkatu 3, 00290 Helsinki; [1]Department of Public Health, University of Turku, Lemminkäisenkatu 1, 20520 Turku, Finland

We have studied weight changes in 13,097 subjects aged 18–54 years from The Finnish Twin Cohort. Self-reported weight was obtained by mailed questionnaires in 1975 and 1981. Women being pregnant during and between the two questionnaires (1975 and 1981) were excluded (n = 2361).

Weight changes between the two studies ranged from +45 kg to –38 kg, with a mean gain of 2.5 kg (SD = 5.1) in men and 1.7 kg (SD = 4.4) in women. 23.7% of subjects gained and 5.5% of subjects lost more than 5 kg. Young subjects (18–24 years) gained most with a mean gain of 3.0 kg (SD = 5.6) among men and 1.8 kg (SD = 4.2) among women, and oldest subjects (50–54 years) gained least (0.8 kg, SD = 4.7 men, and 0.6 kg, SD = 4.7 women). Weight gain was inversely related to initial weight, i.e. those with initial weight BMI < 20 kg/m^2 gaining an average of 4.6 kg (SD = 5.1) among men and 2.5 kg (SD = 3.4) among women, while those with BMI > 30 kg/m^2 remained at almost stable weight (–0.7 kg, SD = 8.1 men and 0.2 kg, SD = 7.7 women). Age and initial BMI together explained 8% and 2% of the variance among men and women respectively. Other determinants of weight change need to be further investigated.

Introduction

It is well recognized that body weight is not stable over time, but studies on weight changes among large population samples are few[7]. Most of the studies on weight changes have focused on human metabolism[6], morbidity[1,2,9,11] and fat redistribution[8,10,12]. The aim of this report is to describe the weight changes among 13 097 adult Finns in relation to gender, age and initial weight.

Material and methods

The Finnish Twin Cohort

The present report is based on data from the nationwide Finnish Twin Cohort compiled in 1974, where all Finnish same-sexed twins born before 1957 with both members alive in 1967 are included[3]. Data was obtained by mailed questionnaires in 1975, and again in 1981. The nearly identical questionnaires included questions about health status, physical characteristics, psychosocial and behavioural factors. Response rates were 89% and 84% in respective years. The cohort can be regarded as fairly representative of the entire population[4,5].

Data set

The Twin Cohort includes 22,218 twin individuals, who responded to both questionnaires in 1975 and 1981. The sample for the present study includes all individuals aged 18–54 years with complete data for weight in 1975 and 1981 and for height in either of the questionnaires. Women being pregnant during or between the two questionnaires were identified and excluded (n = 2361). The final study sample consisted of 7072 males and 6025 non-pregnant females (Table 1).

Table 1. Number of twin individuals. Finnish Twin Cohort, 1975 & 1981 questionnaire studies

Age 1975	18–24	25–29	30–34	35–39	40–44	45–49	50–54	TOTAL
Men	2393	1362	1018	798	588	526	388	7072
Women	1645	916	880	756	705	623	500	6025

Determination of body weight change and initial weight

Self-reported weights and heights were used for the present report. Weight (kg) and height (cm) were rounded to the nearest integral number, if necessary. Body weight change in kilograms was determined as the difference between weights given in questionnaires in 1975 and 1981. Body mass index (BMI), [weight(kg)/height(m)^2] was used as a measure of initial relative body weight in 1975.

Results and discussion

Weight change by age

The mean weight gain was 2.5 kg (SD = 5.1) for men and 1.7 kg (SD = 4.4) for women. Maximal weight change was 45 kg among men and 39 kg among women. Maximal weight losses were 24 kg and 38 kg respectively. 5.5 % of subjects lost and 23.7 % gained more than 5 kg. Among men, subjects aged 18–24 years gained most (3.0 kg, SD = 5.6), while among women the maximal weight gain occurred among those aged 30–34 years (2.1 kg, SD = 4.5). Oldest subjects aged 50–54 years gained least among both genders (0.8 kg, SD = 4.7 among men and 0.6 kg, SD = 4.7 among women) (Fig. 1).

Weight change and initial BMI

Weight gain was inversely related to initial BMI (Fig. 2). Those with lowest initial weight (BMI < 20) gained most (4.6 kg, SD = 5.1 men and 2.5 kg, SD = 3.5 women), while those with initial weight BMI > 30 kg/m^2 remained almost at stable weight (–0.7 kg, SD = 8.1 men and 0.2 kg, SD = 7.7 women).

Weight changes by gender, age and initial BMI are shown in Figs. 3 and 4. Among men those with lowest initial weight gained most in all but one age-group (35–39 years), while those with highest initial weight gained least throughout (Fig. 3). Among women weight changes do not follow a linear pattern, either in relation to age nor initial BMI. The clear trend with age among both genders is, however, that losing weight is commonest among those with high initial weight. These results are very similar to previous work on adults in Finland[7].

In linear regression analysis, age alone explained 6.1% of the male and 1.0% of the female variance. Corresponding values for initial BMI alone were 5.8% for men and 1.4% for women. A combined equation (age75 + age75^2 + BMI75) explained the largest proportion of the variance i.e. 8% among males and 2% among females.

Conclusions

1. Weight change is related to age and initial relative weight.
2. 24% of subjects gained and 6% lost more than 5 kg.
3. Losing weight is commonest among those with high initial weight.
4. Age and initial BMI alone both explained 6% of male and 1% of female variance, while together they explained 8% and 2% among men and women respectively.

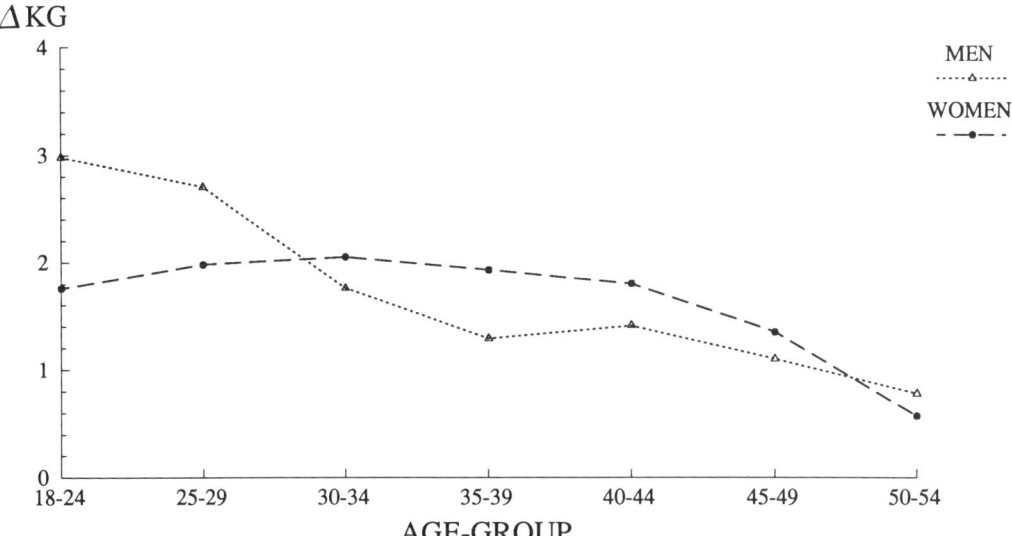

Fig. 1. Six-year weight change by gender and age. Finnish Twin Cohort, 1975 and 1981 questionnaire studies.

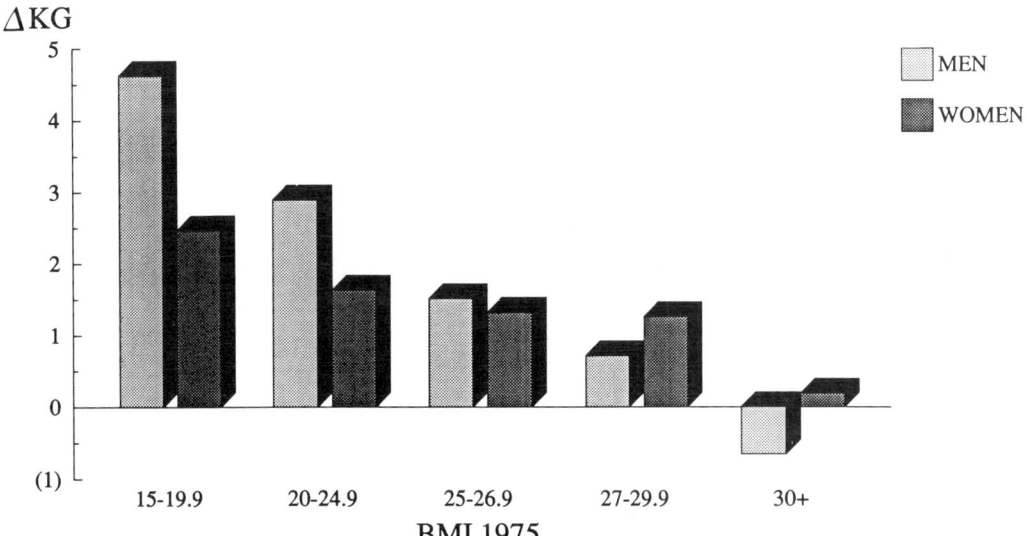

Fig. 2. Six-year weight change by gender and initial BMI. Finnish Twin Cohort, 1975 and 1981 questionnaire studies.

References

1. Borkan, G.A., Sparrow, D., Wisniewski, C. & Vokonas, P.S. (1986): Body weight and coronary disease risk: patterns of risk factor change associated with long-term weight change. *Am. J. Epidemiol.* **124**, 410-419.
2. Hamm, P., Shekelle, B. & Stamler, J. (1989): Large fluctuations in body weight during young adulthood and twenty-five-year risk of coronary death in men. *Am. J. Epidemiol.* **129**, 312-318.

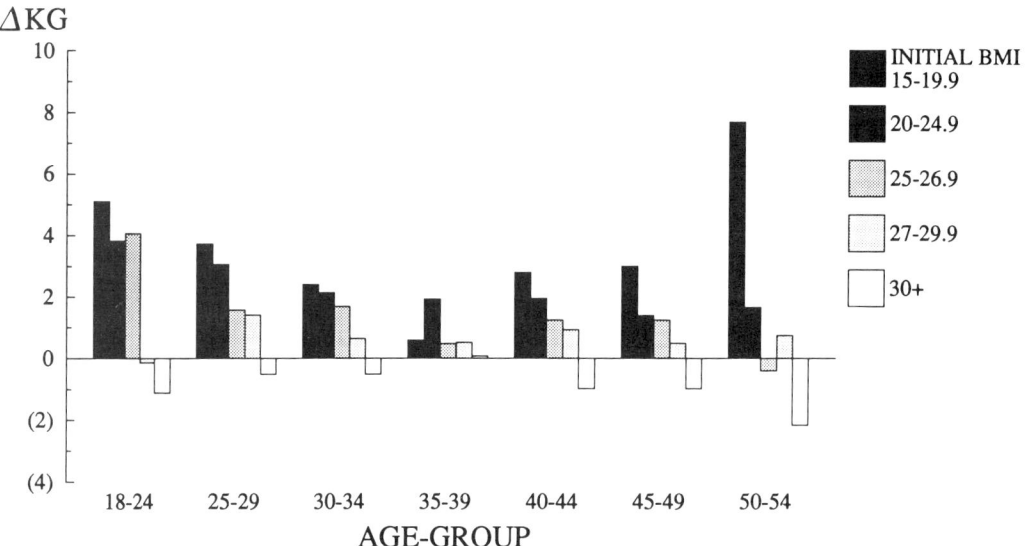

Fig. 3. Six-year weight change by age and initial BMI. Men. Finnish Twin Cohort, 1975 and 1981 questionnaire studies.

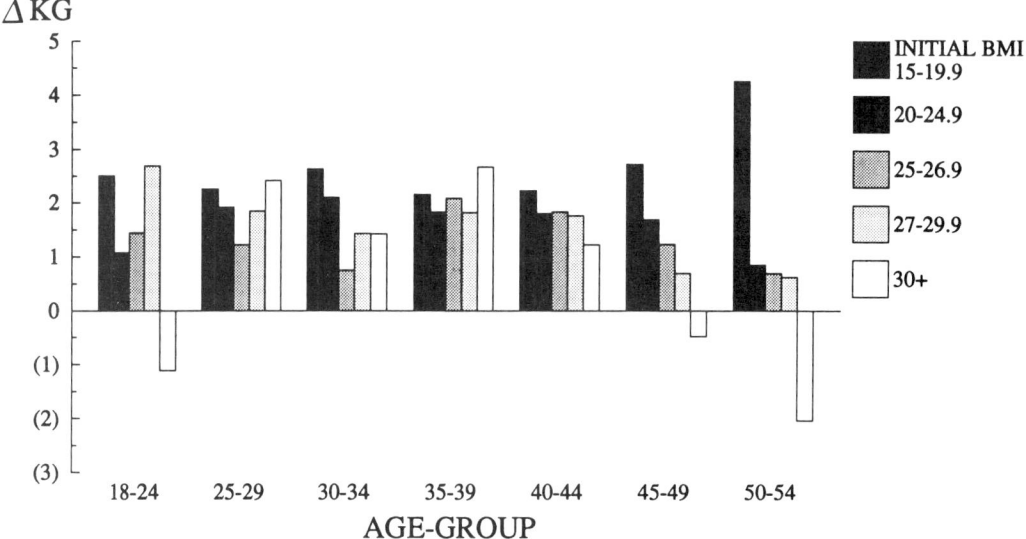

Fig. 4. Six-year weight change by age and initial BMI. Women. Finnish Twin Cohort, 1975 and 1981 questionnaire studies.

3. Kaprio, J., Sarna, S., Koskenvuo, M. & Rantasalo, I. (1978): The Finnish Twin Registry: Formation and compilation, questionnaire study, zygosity determination procedures and research program. *Prog. Clin. Biol. Res.* **24B**, 179-184.
4. Kaprio, J., Rose, R.J., Sama, S., Langinvainio, H., Koskenvuo, M., Rita, H. & Heikkilä, K. (1978): Design and sampling considerations, response rates, and representativeness in a Finnish Twin Family Study. *Acta Gen. Med. Gemellol.* **36**, 79-93.
5. Koskenvuo, M., Langinvainio, H., Kaprio, J., Rantasalo, I. & Sarna, S. (1979): The Finnish Twin Registry: Baseline characteristics. Section III. Occupational and psychosocial factors. Publication of The Department of Public Health Science M49, Helsinki, 1979.
6. Lissner, L., Andres, R., Muller, D.C. & Shimokata, H. (1990): Body weight variability in men: metabolic rate, health and longevity. *Int. J. Obes.* **14**, 373-383.
7. Rissanen, A., Heliövaara, M., Aromaa, A., Reunanen, A., Knekt, P. & Maatela, J. : Determinants of weight gain and overweight in adult Finns. *Eur. J. Clin. Nutr.* (in press).
8. Rodin, J., Radke-Sharpe, N., Rebuffé-Scrive, M. & Greenwood, M.R.C. (1990): Weight cycling and fat distribution. *Int. J. Obes.* **14**, 303-310.
9. Rookus, M.A., Thomas, D.W., Davies, M. & Baghurst, K. (1990): Relationship between weight change and blood lipids in men and women: " The Adelaide 1000". *Int. J. Obes.* **14**, 439-450.
10. Shimokata, H., Anders, R., Coon, P., Elahi, D., Muller, D.C. & Tobin, J.D. (1989): Studies on the distribution of body fat. II. Longitudinal effects of changes in weight. *Int. J. Obes.* **13**, 455-464.
11. Sonne-Holm, S., Sörensen, T.I.A., Jensen, G. & Schnohr, P. (1989): Independent effects of weight change and attained body weight prevalence of arterial hypertension in obese and non-obese men. *Br. Med. J.* **299**, 767-770.
12. Wadden, D.A., Stunkard, A.J., Johnston, F.E., Wanf, J., Pierson, R.N., Van Itallie, T.B., Costello, E. & Pena, M. (1988): Body fat deposition in adult obese women. II. Changes in fat distribution accompanying weight reduction. *Am. J. Clin. Nutr.* **47**, 229-234.

Chapter 25

Relationships of Fasting Plasma Insulin to Anthropometry and Blood Lipids in European Subjects: Influence of Gender

M. CIGOLINI[1], J.C. SEIDELL[2], J.P. DESLYPERE[3], J. CHARZEWSKA[4], B.M. ELLSINGER[5], L. ZAMBELLI[1], M.G. ZENTI[1] and F. CONTALDO[6]

[1]*Metabolic Diseases, University Hospital, I-37134 Verona, ltaly;* [2]*Department of Human Nutrition, Wageningen, The Netherlands;* [3]*Department of Endocrinology, Ghent, Belgium;* [4]*Natl. Inst. Food & Nutrition, Warsaw, Poland;* [5]*Department of Internal Medicine, Göteborg, Sweden;* [6]*Department of Internal Medicine and Metabolic Diseases, Naples, Italy*

A randomized sample of 38-year-old men and women from different European centres was examined in this study in order to verify the influence of gender on the relationships of fasting plasma insulin to anthropometric and lipid variables. Fasting plasma insulin shows the lowest mean value in both Italian men and women. BMI is consistently correlated with fasting plasma insulin in both men and women in all centres. In pooled data, waist girth is better correlated with fasting plasma insulin in both sexes, than any other anthropometric parameter studied including BMI and circumference ratios.

Waist girth is the only parameter in both sexes still significantly correlated with fasting plasma insulin after adjusting for BMI. Therefore waist circumference seems the anthropometric parameter to be preferred in relation to fasting plasma insulin in both sexes.

Simple and BMI adjusted partial correlations between fasting insulin and blood lipids vary widely among the centres and between the sexes. In a multivariate analysis including fat distribution, BMI, and insulin we found that total, LDL, HDL, cholesterol and HDU/total cholesterol ratio are related to fasting plasma insulin only in pooled European women but not in pooled European men. Triglycerides are related to fasting plasma insulin and to fat distribution, independently of each other and of BMI, in both pooled men and pooled women.

Introduction

Body fat distribution is related to insulin resistance and fasting insulin[4,7]. Fasting insulin was more strongly associated with cardiovascular risk factors than insulin during oral glucose load[8]. The relationships of fasting insulin to fat distribution and metabolic risk factors are not yet fully clarified[1]. We demonstrated that waist circumference was the anthropometric parameter showing the highest correlation with fasting serum insulin in European women from different centres[2]; moreover, in those women, fasting insulin was associated with an unfavourable lipid profile[3]. In the present study we aimed at verifying these findings in European men and at emphasizing the influence of gender in these relationships.

Methods

The European Fat Distribution Study has studied randomized groups of 38-year-old subjects from a total population born and living in different European countries. A first study was performed on women from five centres: Göteborg in Sweden, Ede in The Netherlands, Warsaw in Poland, Verona in northern Italy and Naples in southern Italy[5]. The study on men was done two years later and it included also men from Lumiar in Portugal and Deinze in Belgium[6]. We excluded diabetics, subjects with major chronic diseases, patients under drugs known to affect lipid and glucose metabolism or to influence blood pressure. There were only few exclusions among these 38-year-old subjects. Blood pressure and anthropometric parameters were determined by one observer in each centre following an instruction manual. In this work waist girth is the horizontal circumference measured at the midway between the lower rib margin and the iliac crest. Blood parameters were measured in one laboratory for all centres in each study.

Results and discussion

Table 1 shows mean fasting insulin levels in the two studies, respectively on women and on men.

Table 1. Fasting plasma insulin (µU/ml; means ± SE) in women and men from different European centres. The number of subjects is in parentheses; ANOVA F-values of the comparison among centres are also reported

	Study on women	Study on men
Sweden	10.4 ± 0.4 (88)	20.0 ± 0.61 (83)
Poland	16.1 ± 0.7 (92)	18.8 ± 0.63 (94)
Netherlands	15.2 ± 0.7 (85)	19.0 ± 0.62 (72)
Belgium	—	18.6 ± 0.56 (94)
Italy (Verona)	10.1 ± 0.3 (87)	16.0 ± 0.65 (94)
Italy (Naples)	12.7 ± 0.6 (100)	—
Portugal	—	17.1 ± 0.54 (78)
F value	17	5.5
P	<0.001	<0.001

Table 2. Pearson's coefficients of the simple and BMI-adjusted partial correlations between selected anthropometric parameters and fasting insulin

	Women (n=452)		Men (n=515)	
	Simple	BMI adj.	Simple	BMI adj.
BMI	0.30*	—	0.37*	—
Waist	0.35*	0.18*	0.41*	0.15*
Waist/hip	0.20*	0.07	0.21*	−0.01
Waist/thigh	0.21*	0.09	0.21*	0.09

*$P < 0.001$

In men, mean fasting plasma insulin was different between centres. The lowest mean value was shown by the Italian men; it was statistically lower than for any other centre except Portugal. In women the two Italian centres again showed the lowest mean value, together with Sweden in this case. The low mean fasting insulin in Italy is even lower if the values are adjusted for BMI since the Italian women showed the highest values of BMI.

Table 2 shows the coefficients of the correlations, both the simple and the BMI-adjusted partial correlations, between selected anthropometric parameters and fasting plasma insulin in pooled women and pooled men. As expected insulin is correlated with BMI in both sexes (this was the case for all centres). However the anthropometric parameter showing the best simple correlation with fasting insulin was the waist circumference; that correlation was also better than the correlation of insulin with waist to hip ratio or waist to thigh ratio in both women and men.

Furthermore waist circumference was the only anthropometric parameter considered in these studies which still showed a significant correlation with insulin after adjusting for BMI.

Table 3 shows the coefficients of simple correlations of plasma insulin to blood lipids. Insulin is correlated with triglycerides in all centres and in both sexes except in the Italian men. On the contrary cholesterol is much less consistently correlated with fasting insulin.

Table 3. Pearson's r coefficients of the simple correlations between fasting plasma insulin and selected lipid parameters; significant correlations are indicated by asterisks

	Sweden		Netherlands		Poland		Italy	
	Women	Men	Women	Men	Women	Men	Women	Men
Triglycerides	0.33*	0.32**	0.31**	0.41***	0.45***	0.32**	0.38***	0.06
Total cholesterol	−0.17	0.41***	0.15	0.19	0.15	0.25*	0.46***	0.01
HDL/total cholesterol	−0.15	−0.03	−0.17	−0.23*	−0.30***	−0.03	−0.46***	−0.22*

*$P < 0.05$; **$P < 0.01$; ***$P < 0.001$

If we examine the blood lipid parameters by multivariate analysis we can see that insulin and fat distribution are related significantly to total and LDL cholesterol in women[3] but not in men (not shown).

In women insulin contributes to explain the variance of HDL-cholesterol and HDL to total cholesterol ratio, independently of BMI[3]; whilst in men only fat distribution is related to HDL cholesterol.

Both in women and men, fat distribution and fasting insulin are significantly related to triglycerides independently of BMI (not shown).

Acknowledgements

The authors thank Per Björntorp, Joseph G.A.J. Hautvast, Ludovico Scuro (deceased), Victor Szostak, and Albert Vermeulen for their important contributions to the organization of the study. The participation of the Project Management Group of "Euro Nutrition" (EURO-NUT), a concerted action project on Nutrition and Health of the Comac Epidemiology Group within the Medical Research Council of the European Community, is gratefully acknowledged. Dr. M. Cigolini has received grants 86.00040.04, 87.00077.04 and 88.00466.04 from Italian C.N.R.. Dr. Jacob C. Seidell is a research fellow of the Royal Netherlands Academy of Science.

References

1. Cambien, F., Warnet, J.M., Eschwege, E., Jacqueson, A. Richard, J.L. & Rosselin, G. (1987): Body mass, blood pressure, glucose and lipids: does plasma insulin explain their relationships? *Arteriosclerosis* **7**, 197-202.
2. Cigolini, M., Seidell, J.C., Charzewska, J., Ellsinger, B.M., Di Biase, F., Björntorp, P., Hautvast, J.G.A.J., Contaldo, F., Szostak, V. & Scuro, L.A. (1989): Fat distribution, metabolism and plasma insulin in European women. The European Fat Distribution Study. In *Obesity in Europe '88*, eds. P. Björntorp & S. Rossner, pp. 35-42. London: John Libbey.

3. Cigolini, M., Seidell, J.C., Charzewska, J., Ellsinger, B.M., Di Biase, G., Björntorp, P., Hautvast, J.G.A.J., Contaldo, F., Szostak, V. & Scuro, L.A. (1991): Fasting serum insulin in relation to fat distribution, serum lipid profile and blood pressure in European women. The European Fat Distribution Study. *Metabolism* (in press).
4. Evans, D.J., Hoffman, R.G., Kalkhoff, R.K. & Kissebah, A.H. (1984): Relationship of body fat tomography to insulin sensitivity and metabolic profiles in premenopausal women. *Metabolism* **33**, 68-75.
5. Seidell, J.C., Cigolini, M., Charzewska, J., Ellsinger, B.M., Di Biase, G., Björntorp, P., Hautvast, J.G.A.J., Contaldo, F., Szostak, V. & Scuro, L.A. (1989): Indicators of fat distribution in relation to serum lipid and blood pressure in European women born in 1948. The European Fat Distribution Study. *Am. J. Epidemiol.* **130**, 53-65.
6. Seidell, J.C., Cigolini, M., Deslypere, J.P., Charzewska, J., Ellsinger, B.M. & Cruz, A. (1991): Body fat distribution in relation to physical activity and smoking habits in 38 year old European men. The European Fat Distribution Study. *Am. J. Epidemiol.* **133**, 257-265.
7. Soler, J.T., Folsom, A.R., Kaye, S.A. & Prineas, R.J. (1989): Associations of abdominal obesity, fasting insulin, sex hormone binding globulin and estrone with lipids and lipoproteins in post-menopausal women. *Atherosclerosis* **79**, 21-27.
8. Wing, R.R., Bunker, C.H., Kuller, L.H. & Mattews, K.A. (1989): Insulin, body mass index and cardiovascular risk factors in premenopausal women. *Arteriosclerosis* **9**, 479-484.

Section V
Management of obesity

Chapter 26

Fat Cell Adrenergic Receptors: from Molecular Approaches to Therapeutic Strategies

Max LAFONTAN, Jean-Sébastien SAULNIER-BLACHE, Christian CARPENE, Dominique LANGIN, Jean GALITZKY, Maria PORTILLO, Dominique LARROUY and Michel BERLAN

INSERM Unit 317, Institut Louis Bugnard, Université Paul Sabatier, Faculté de Médecine, Bât L3, 31054 Toulouse Cedex, France

This review contains up-to-date results on fat cell adrenoceptors and major perspectives about therapeutic strategies. A summary of the essential features concerning the characterization of β- and α2-adrenoceptors of the human fat cell is given. Moreover, some new perspectives offered by the recent cloning of the genes encoding for various subtypes of adrenergic receptors are considered. For clarity, we give the interest and limits of various animal and cell-line models and a critical appraisal of the limitations of fat cells of animal models and preadipose cell lines for the study of adrenoceptors and their various hormonal regulations. Most of these models possess adrenoceptors having major pharmacological and genetic differences with those of human fat cells, i.e. β3- and/or other "atypical" β-adrenoceptor isotypes and α2-adrenoceptors which are different from the classical α2A-subtype of the human fat cell. Finally, a brief overview of the prospective pharmacological strategies which could be proposed from the knowledge acquired from adrenoceptor studies is also presented.

Introduction and general considerations

The first step of the cellular action of norepinephrine and epinephrine is its binding to adrenoceptors which are located in the plasma membrane of target cells. The old classification of adrenoceptor subtypes, essentially based on functional approaches needs a rather extensive re-evaluation with all the recent data now available. There is now pharmacological, biochemical, molecular and genetic evidence that beta-(β) and alpha2-adrenoceptors (α2) are heterogeneous structures consisting of a single subunit containing seven stretches of 20–28 hydrophobic amino acids that represent potential membrane-spanning α-helices. Many of these receptors share considerable amino-acid sequence homology, particularly in the transmembrane domains[8,14,23,47,50]. The more recent studies have led to the cloning of genes for a large number of subtypes and isotypes of adrenoceptors existing inside the basic β-, α1- and α2-adrenoceptor families. Structural and functional studies are entering a new area. Many features such as pharmacological specificity, interspecies heterogeneity, regulation and coupling are expected to be unique for each individual receptor subgroup and/or subtype. Understanding these unique features should yield important new insights into the role of the receptor proteins.

This review of fat cell adrenoceptors will contain: (i) a brief summary of the essential features concerning the characterization of the adrenoceptors of the human fat cell; (ii) a critical appraisal of the limitations of the animal models and preadipose cell lines which possess adrenoceptors presenting major pharmacological differences with those of human fat cells and (iii) comments on the prospective pharmacological strategies which could be proposed from the knowledge acquired from adrenoceptor studies.

Catecholamines are the most sophisticated regulators of fat cell function since adipocytes express classical and also probably "atypical" adrenoceptor subtypes. The major function of β- and α2-adrenoceptors is to exert a positive and negative control respectively on plasma membrane adenylyl cyclase and cyclic AMP (cAMP) production. Catecholamines are also able to stimulate phosphoinositide hydrolysis through α1-adrenoceptors leading to increment of Ca^{2+} level and protein kinase C activation. This latter aspect has been more deeply investigated in brown fat cells[49] and will not be considered further in the present review of white fat cell adrenoceptors. Basically, in fat cells, β1, β2 and "atypical" β-adrenoceptors are positively coupled with adenylyl cyclase by a Gs protein while, conversely, α2-adrenergic receptors are negatively coupled with the enzyme by Gi proteins. Increments in cellular cAMP levels result in cAMP-dependent phosphorylation/activation of hormone-sensitive lipase (HSL), the enzyme catalysing the rate-limiting steps in the breakdown of stored triglycerides. However, cAMP elevations, besides HSL activation, also promote desensitization of β-adrenoceptors and activation of cGMP-inhibited low-K_m cAMP phosphodiesterase in fat cells[13]. The latter effects, which are a consequence of cAMP increment and cAMP-dependent protein kinase A activation, probably represent some sort of feed back mechanisms whereby cAMP controls its own turnover. Catecholamines also affect the processes of lipid synthesis and have an impact on glucose uptake and metabolism by the fat cells[11].

It is not intended to give here an exhaustive review but to focus attention on the major questions arising from the very recent studies on fat cell adrenoceptors in humans and currently used animal models. Moreover, the advantages and limits of the more recently available pharmacological tools will also be pointed out.

Human fat cell adrenoceptors

Classification of human fat cell adrenergic receptors was, for a long time, based on the order of potency of different agonists and antagonists. Depending on the specificity of the pharmacological agents used for receptor delineation, fat cell adrenoceptors were firstly considered as being of the β1-subtype. Then, the presence of an α-adrenoceptor, suspected during the early seventies, was followed by the functional and pharmacological characterization of an α2-adrenoceptor in fat cells in the early eighties[30]. The coexistence of β1- and β2-adrenoceptors in fat cells was assessed with the utilization of highly selective β1-(CGP 20712A and bisoprolol) and β2-antagonists (ICI 118551)[29,41].

Binding studies began with the utilization of non-selective drugs for β- and α-adrenoceptor subtype delineation such as [^{3}H]dihydroalprenolol ([^{3}H]DHA) and [^{3}H] dihydroergocryptine respectively but rapidly used subtype-specific agents. Concerning β-adrenoceptors, there is no highly subtype-selective radioligand and the commonly used agents: [^{3}H]DHA, [^{125}I]cyanopindolol ([^{125}I]CYP) and [^{3}H](−) CGP 12177, have been considered as being not subtype selective. Nevertheless, the more recent studies indicate that [^{3}H]DHA and [^{125}I]CYP have a twofold selectivity for β2-adrenoceptors while [^{3}H](−)CGP12177 is β1-adrenoceptor selective[45,46,53]. These differences are not important for the accurate determination of the total number of β1/β2-adrenoceptor binding sites in membrane preparations or on intact fat cells since all these agents give linear Scatchard plots derived from the saturation binding curves. However, when a radioligand with low subtype selectivity is falsely presumed to be non-selective, the estimated binding parameters, i.e. the estimated proportion of β1- and β2-adrenoceptors and the inhibitory constants of the competitor suffer considerable distortions in their estimation. This problem has recently been discussed and improvements of the analytical procedures were proposed[53].

One of the consequences of these problems is that data in the literature are, in reality, only accurately comparable for the same kind of ligand. Nevertheless, the higher selectivity of recent β1- and β2-antagonists such as CGP 20712A and ICI 118551 respectively has considerably improved the reliability of the determinations of the proportion of each subtype in a given fat cell preparation. But, it is still very difficult to accurately assess agonist affinity for each kind of β-site due to the existence of two different affinity states for β1- and also for β2-adrenoceptors.

Concerning α2-adrenoceptors, there is now convincing pharmacological evidence for the existence of an α2A-adrenoceptor in human fat cells which exhibits an equivalent and high affinity for [^{3}H]yohimbine and [^{3}H]rauwolscine. These two radioligands are suitable tools to identify human fat cell α2A-adrenoceptors. However, the recently introduced [^{3}H]RX 821002 radioligand which has a high affinity for α2A-adrenoceptors, labels, in human fat cells, some additional binding sites compared with the others; this discrepancy has not been explained for the moment[20]. Among the partial and full α2-agonists, [^{3}H]clonidine and [^{3}H]UK14304 respectively, when used under suitable conditions, label the higher affinity state of the α2A-adrenoceptor but exhibit discrepancies in their binding kinetics which are explainable by their partial and full-agonist properties on the α2A-adrenoceptor.[21]

Although a few studies have been carried out on β- and α2-adrenoceptors on intact cells, the validity of the determinations performed with lipophilic ligands such as [^{3}H]DHA, [^{3}H]yohimbine and [^{125}I]CYP are highly questionable as discussed previously[32]. [^{3}H](−)CGP 12177 and [^{3}H]RX 821002, which are membrane impermeable due to their poor lipophilicity, appeared, in our hands, to be the most valuable tools for the characterization of β- and α2-adrenoceptors on the intact fat cells and largely overcome the problems occurring with more lipophilic radioligands[20,29,32].

Beta1-, β2- and β3-adrenoceptor genes, isolated from genomic libraries have recently been cloned in humans[16,17,19,28] and rat[7,40]. The mRNAs for β1- and β2-adrenoceptors were identified in human fat cells and an increased transcription activity of the genes encoding for β1- and β2-adrenoceptors has recently been described in abdominal as compared to gluteal fat cells[3] while nothing was revealed with the β3-adrenoceptor probe in human subcutaneous fat cells (personal communication from D. Strosberg). The gene coding for the α2A-adrenoceptor is located on chromosome 10 in humans[47]. Using an antisense mRNA probe for the α2-C10 adrenoceptor (α2A), it was possible to identify the α2A-adrenoceptor mRNA in the human fat cell with solution hybridization studies (unpublished results). It should be determined whether the amount of specific mRNA correlates with the expression of the α2-adrenoceptors in various fat deposits as shown for β1- and β2-adrenoceptors to explain the heterogenous distribution of these binding sites[42]. All the adrenoceptor genes have now been identified in humans and exploration of adrenoceptor regulation at the genetic level will be facilitated[12,14].

Fat cell adrenoceptors in animal models and preadipocyte cell lines

β-adrenergic receptors

On application of binding approaches, currently performed for β-site identification on human fat cells, to the adipocytes of various animal models (dog, rat, hamster and rabbit, etc.) and preadipocyte cell lines[18], the coexistence of both adrenoceptor subtypes (β1/β2) was clearly assessed by competition studies with [^{3}H]DHA, [^{3}H](−)CGP 12177 and [^{125}I]CYP. However, the total number of sites as well as the relative proportion of each kind of site greatly varied according to the species and also between experiments reported on the same species by different authors. These results are easily explainable by the technical problems encountered with β-antagonist ligands mentioned in the previous chapter and also by the differences existing between the various strains of mammal species currently used in laboratories.

Indeed, in most of the mammals classically used in labs, a major element should be pointed out for all the studies on fat cell β-adrenoceptors: whatever the reliability of previous binding experiments, it is now clear that, in addition to the well known β1- and β2-adrenoceptors, an atypical β-adrenoceptor (neither β1- nor β2-) exists in the brown and the white fat cells of most of the species investigated. Its presence is highly questionable in human subcutaneous white fat cells although its putative existence in human brown fat cells can reasonably be suspected. For a long time, the evidence for an atypical β-adrenoceptor was exclusively based on functional studies with subtype-selective atypical β-adrenoceptor agonists[1,2,6,25,26,27,37,55]. Recently, the cloning of a β3-adrenoceptor gene and the identification of specific mRNAs for this new β-adrenoceptor, which could correspond to the atypical β-adrenoceptor, has strongly reactivated an old debate[16]. No selective antagonist for this receptor has yet been developed and various attempts at using traditional radioligands such as [^{3}H](–)CGP 12177 and [^{125}I]CYP for its identification were not really convincing in rat, hamster or dog fat cells ([37] and unpublished results).

Whatever the importance of the limitations inherent to the lack of radioligand, in order to gain further insights into the atypical β-adrenoceptor subtype in fat cells of various species and extend the atypical β-adrenoceptor concept, essentially limited for a long time to the rat, several lipolytic assays were carried out on fat cells from various species in the laboratory. Attention was focused upon rather large interspecies discrepancies in the extent of atypical β-adrenoceptor-mediated lipolytic responses. This functional investigation was based on the utilization of BRL 37344, isoproterenol, noradrenaline, (±)CGP 12177 and SR 58611 in lipolysis measurements as previously established[25,37]. Subtype-selective β1- and β2-antagonists were used to verify the atypical nature of the responses which are weakly blocked by such agents. The results are summarized in Fig. 1. From these experiments, it was possible to roughly delineate three major groups of species depicting clear-cut differences in the atypical β-adrenoceptor-mediated responses.

In fat cells of the first group of animals, composed of the rat and hibernators such as the hamster and garden dormouse, BRL 37344 has a potency that is about 10-fold higher than (–)isoproterenol. Non-selective β1/β2-antagonists such as (–)cyanopindolol and (±)CGP 12177 were partial agonists in rat and hamster fat cells and full agonists in dormouse adipocytes which exhibited the strongest responsiveness to the atypical β-adrenoceptor agonists. Classical β1- and β2-adrenoceptors probably play a minor role in these species since the lipolytic effect of 0.1 µM doses of noradrenaline and isoproterenol were not antagonized by higher doses of β1- and β2-selective antagonists (10 µM), a result clearly indicating the importance of the atypical β-adrenoceptor component of the response initiated by these agents. To conclude, in these small mammal species, BRL 37344 acts solely and isoproterenol predominantly through atypical β-adrenoceptors (Fig. 1).

In the adipocytes of the second group of "larger" mammals, such as the rabbit and the dog, isoproterenol had a higher lipolytic potency than BRL 37344 and the lipolytic effect of the partial agonists (–)cyanopindolol and (±)CGP 12177 was very weak. The effect of the lowest lipolytic concentrations of isoproterenol was blocked by β1/β2-antagonists while the highest doses were poorly antagonized by these compounds. It seems that β1-adrenoceptors play a stronger role in the initiation of the noradrenaline- and isoproterenol-induced lipolysis in these species although the atypical β-adrenoceptor exists. Experiments are currently being performed in the lab to explore the question more deeply and to determine the mechanisms explaining its weaker efficacy.

The third heterogeneous group composed of guinea pig and human fat cells exhibited a standard responsiveness to isoproterenol and a response which was very weak or absent to BRL 37344. Moreover, the fat cells are completely unresponsive to partial agonists such as (–)cyanopindolol and (±)CGP 12177. The β1-adrenoceptors play the essential role in the control of noradrenaline and isoproterenol-induced lipolysis although a β2-adrenergic component can easily be revealed with appropriate selective β2-agonists such as procaterol and fenoterol.

This comparative approach reveals important species-specific differences in atypical β-

Chapter 26 – Fat Cell Adrenergic Receptors: from Molecular Approaches to Therapeutic Strategies

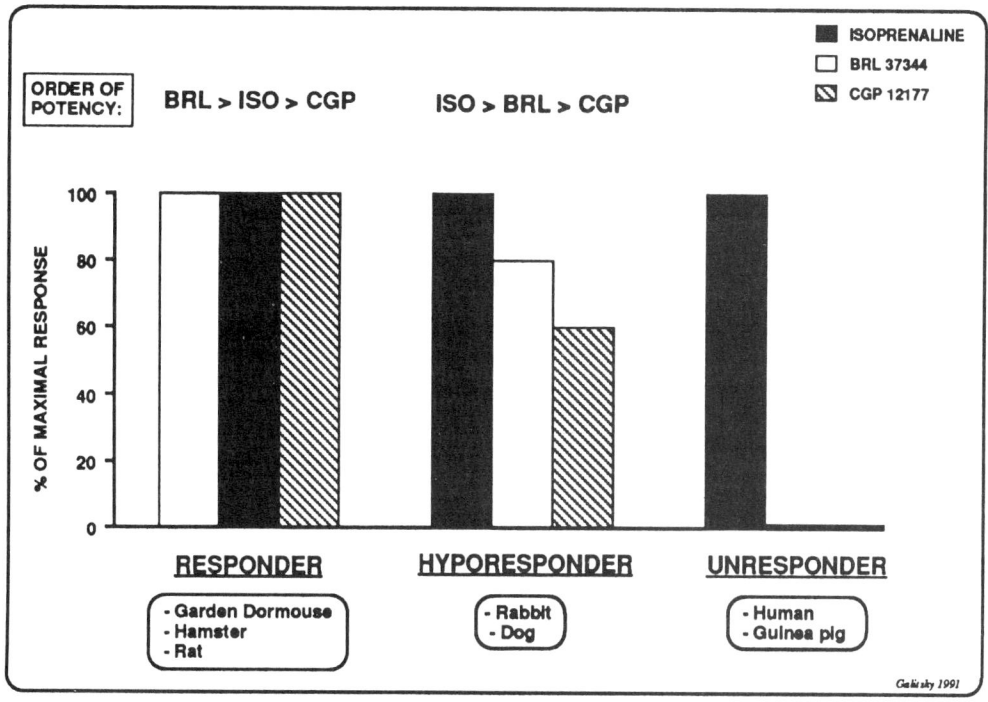

Fig. 1. Diagram delineating the major lipolytic profiles of atypical β-adrenoceptor-mediated responses in fat cells from various mammal species. The delineation was based on the use of BRL 37344 (BRL), isoproterenol (ISO) and (±)CGP 12177 (CGP). Maximal lipolytic effects and the relative order of potency of the various agents were defined. The most responsive fat cells gave similar maximal lipolytic responses with the various agonists while the unresponsive only responded to isoproterenol. The hyporesponsive fat cells exhibited a relative order of sensitivity to the agonists (ISO > BRL > CGP) which was different from that defined in responsive fat cells (BRL > ISO > CGP).

adrenoceptor responsiveness. Several hypotheses could be proposed to explain these differences. The higher lipolytic potency of BRL 37344 observed in rodent fat cells could be linked to the high affinity and selectivity of the drug for the atypical β-adrenoceptor or to an efficient coupling between cAMP generation and lipolysis, e.g. a more efficient activation of protein kinase A and hormone-sensitive lipase. As shown for lipolysis, adenylyl cyclase activation in rat adipocytes by BRL 37344 is obtained solely by an atypical β-adrenoceptor[26], while the effect of isoproterenol will depend on the proportions of β1/β2 and atypical β-adrenoceptor proportions and possibly the relative affinity of the agonist for the various β-adrenoceptor sites. In the absence of any suitable ligand for the atypical β-adrenoceptor, it is difficult to assess the affinity of BRL 37344 and of the other agonists for this receptor. It is not excluded that BRL 37344 is also able to initiate cAMP-dependent as well as cAMP-independent events both leading to lipolysis activation. Nevertheless, the reduction of BRL 37344 efficiency, with preservation of isoproterenol efficiency suggests that the "atypical" β-adrenoceptor-mediated lipolytic component is highly variable between the species. A recent study performed in rabbit fat cells has clearly shown the strong involution of the atypical β-adrenoceptor-mediated lipolytic response with ageing and/or fattening (in preparation). There was similarly a loss of BRL 37344 efficiency in obese rats (500–600 g), a result also suggesting a reduction of the atypical β-adrenergic component in rat fat cells with ageing and/or fattening (unpublished results). More insight should be gained in this

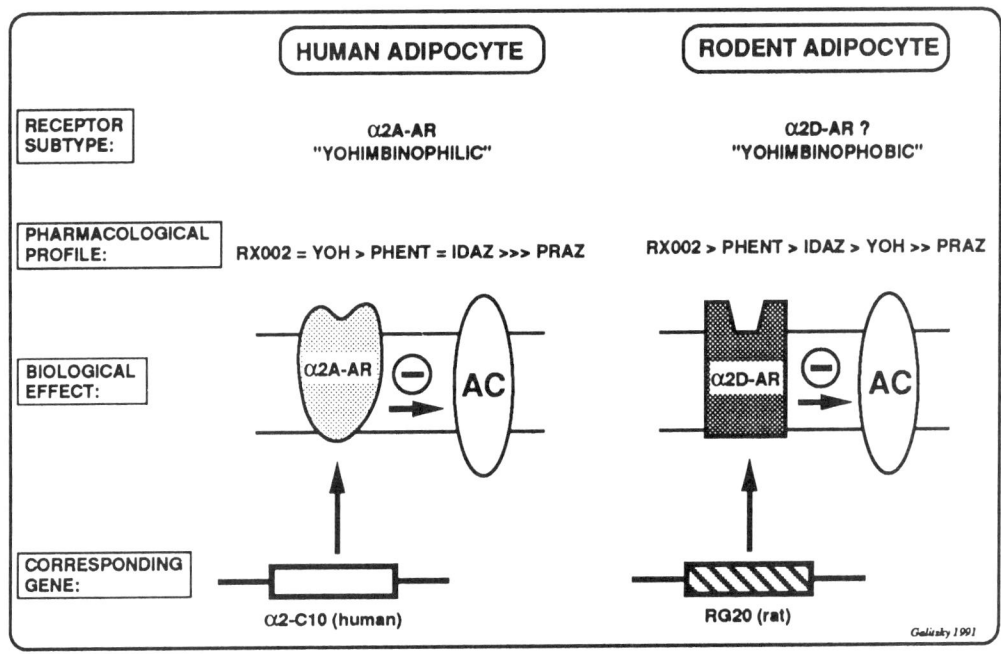

Fig. 2. Diagram showing the essential differences in the α2-adrenoceptor subtype of human and rodent adipocytes. The pharmacological profile, the biological effect and the corresponding gene encoding for the receptor are mentioned on the figure. Abbreviations are the following: adenylate cyclase (AC), RX 821002 (RX002), yohimbine (YOH), phentolamine (PHENT), idazoxan (IDAZ) and prazosin (PRAZ). The stimulation of the α2A- and of the "yohimbinophobic" α2-adrenoceptor promotes inhibition of plasma membrane adenylate cyclase. This effect is blocked by the various α2-antagonists with the order of potency mentioned in the diagram.

matter although the tools usable are rather limited. The lack of a highly specific radioligand having antagonist properties is one of the major limitations for the delineation of the atypical β-adrenoceptor contribution in the control of fat cell function.

The strongest support for the existence of atypical β-adrenoceptors was provided by the recent cloning and sequencing of a human gene encoding for a protein having 50.7 and 45.5% homology with human β1- and β2-adrenoceptors respectively[16]. The pharmacological characterization of this so-called β3-adrenoceptor in CHO cells revealed atypical β-adrenoceptor properties, i.e. high affinity for BRL 37344 and low affinities for ICI 118551 and CGP 20712A. Moreover, it was labelled by [^{125}I]CYP but the K_D for the ligand at this β3-site was at least 10 times higher (i.e. 500 pM) than that defined for classical β1- and β2-adrenoceptors. Apparently, noticeable differences exist between the human β3-receptor and rat atypical β-adrenoceptors which may be due to large phenotypic differences in the CHO cells used for transfection[59]. This aspect still requires further validation. For the moment, it is impossible to assess whether the β3-adrenoceptor gene isolated from human genome, expressed in CHO cells, corresponds to the atypical β-adrenoceptor existing in the fat cell of mammals or is a member of a larger family exhibiting some species-specific differences which still require further genetic characterization[2,36,37]. Recently, two recent reports in mouse and rat have mentioned the cloning of two additional atypical β-adrenoceptor genes which are greatly similar but not identical with the human β3-adrenoceptor[44,51].

Nevertheless the numerous remaining questions, it is clear that three separated β-adrenoceptor subtypes may mediate the same function in fat cells; the respective importance of which has to be determined. For a long time, most of the investigators only focused their interest on β1- and β2-adrenoceptors identified with the classical radioligands for β-adrenoceptors to interpret the lipolytic changes occurring in various physiological and pathological situations in mammal species.

It is essential in the near future: (i) to perform a total reconsideration in terms of the role of efficiency differential recruitment and regulation of the three β-adrenoceptor subtypes coexisting in fat cells of most of the mammals; (ii) to stimulate the involvement of major pharmaceutical groups to find out selective agonists and antagonists for the atypical β-adrenoceptors to improve the amount of available pharmacological tools; the agonists could also have putative interests in animal production if some anabolic actions of β-agonists are associated with atypical β-adrenoceptor stimulation; (iii) to engage a pertinent reflexion about the interest of fat cells of most of the small mammals as models for the understanding of the regulation and dysregulation of human fat cell function since the preponderance of atypical β-adrenoceptor-mediated effects is clearly shown in white fat cells of these species while being very limited or absent in human adipocytes; (iv) to clearly establish if atypical β-adrenoceptors can have physiological relevance in human white or brown fat cells or if some particular fat deposits, still not defined, possess a strong atypical β3-adrenergic control.

α2-adrenoceptors

There is now pharmacological and genetic evidence that α2-adrenoceptors are heterogeneous structures. As is the case with other members of the adrenoceptor family, α2-adrenoceptors exist as subtypes that are encoded by distinct genes and differ in their structural characteristics, ligand recognition properties, tissue distribution, regulation and coupling to transducing systems. Three genes encoding for different α2-adrenoceptor subtypes have been cloned in humans; they are located on separate chromosomes (C2, C4 and C10) and the subtypes are defined by the chromosome location of their genes, i.e. α2-C2, α2-C4 and α2-C10. The latter, α2-C10, corresponds to the α2A-adrenoceptor characterized by classical pharmacological approaches[8,23,47,50]. Concerning fat cells, the α2-adrenoceptor in human as in dog fat cells is of the α2A-subtype[20,21,56] while different α2-subtypes (or isotypes) seem to exist in fat cells of other species (rat, fa/fa rat, hamster, rabbit). The classical α2-antagonist radioligands, [³H]yohimbine and [³H]rauwolscine, have failed to give accurate binding data with adipocyte α2-adrenoceptors in most of the currently used mammal species. Moreover, alpha2-adrenoceptors have never been identified in the various preadipose cell lines (3T3L1, 3T3-F442A and ob17) tested in the laboratory with the radioligands available whatever their differentiation stage. Recently, expression of α2-adrenoceptors has been demonstrated in 25-day post-confluent differentiating cultured hamster preadipocytes while the receptors are not expressed in 8-day post-confluent differentiating cells already having β-adrenergic responses (submitted paper).

The identification of α2-adrenoceptors in fat cells of various species and cultured preadipocytes was recently resolved by our group which optimized the conditions of use of a new α2-antagonist: RX 821002. This compound has a benzodioxan structure and is the 2-methoxy derivative of the α2-antagonist idazoxan[54]. Incidentally, in functional studies on isolated fat cells from various species, it was found that RX 821002 was more potent for the blockade of UK 14304-induced antilipolysis (α2-adrenoceptor-mediated antilipolytic effects) than other commonly used α2-adrenoceptor antagonists such as phentolamine, idazoxan or yohimbine; yohimbine was the weakest antagonist in all the fat cells used[36,52]. It was considered that its labelled form, [³H]RX 821002, could be a valuable tool for the study of fat cell α2-adrenoceptors.

[³H]RX 821002 labelled a homogeneous population of sites, as indicated by the Hill coefficients close to unity, and displayed a high affinity for the sites (equilibrium dissociation constants (K_D) from 0.5–0.6 nM in man, to 0.9-1.5 nM in hamster and rat and 6.0–7.0 nM in rabbit fat cells). The B_{max} values for [^{3}H]RX 821002 binding (expressed in fmol/mg protein) to fat cell membranes were very different according to the species, i.e. from 40–60 in rat fat cells and hamster preadipocytes[9,10] to 100–200 in rabbit adipocytes[36] and from 500–800 in human and hamster fat cells[20,52]. This heterogeneity is amplified by the level of fatness. Indeed, as previously demonstrated by our group in various species, the number of α2-adrenoceptors was directly correlated with the fat cell size (fat cell volume); the larger the fat cells, the higher the number of α2-adrenoceptors in the adipocytes[31].

In order to confirm that [^{3}H]RX 821002 was bound to an α2-adrenoceptor, competition studies were performed. To determine the pharmacological subtype of the α2-adrenoceptor of the adipocyte from the various species used, K_i values obtained for oxymetazoline (an α2A-subtype-selective adrenergic agent) were compared with the K_i values obtained for prazosin and chlorpromazine (two α2B-subtype selective adrenergic agents). K_i values for other compounds such as phentolamine, idazoxan, rauwolscine and yohimbine were also included for a better definition of the binding properties of the α2-adrenoceptors.

The relative order of potency of the reference compounds to inhibit [^{3}H]RX 821002 binding in human fat cell membranes is: RX 821002 > rauwolscine ≥ yohimbine > oxymetazoline > phentolamine > idazoxan > prazosin. This rank order is similar to that obtained in inhibition studies of [^{3}H]yohimbine binding. Thus, the human α2A-adrenoceptor subtype, previously identified with [^{3}H]yohimbine and [^{3}H]rauwolscine in human fat cells[20], brain cortex[57] and adenocarcinoma HT29 cell line[34], is also labelled by [^{3}H]RX 821002[20,35].

In rat, rabbit and hamster fat cell membranes the rank order was clearly different: RX 821002 > phentolamine ≥ idazoxan ≥ oxymetazoline > rauwolscine ≥ yohimbine >> prazosin. The main characteristic of the α2-adrenoceptor of the fat cells from these animal models is its low affinity for yohimbine and its diastereoisomer, rauwolscine (from 30 to 50 nM).

As expected for agonists, competition curves obtained from displacement of [^{3}H]RX 821002 binding by UK 14304, epinephrine, and clonidine exhibited pseudo-Hill coefficients different from unity and allowed the definition of high and low affinity states for the receptor.[21]

To conclude, inhibition studies of [^{3}H]RX 821002 binding by various compounds confirmed the α2A-adrenergic nature of the sites labelled by this new radioligand in human fat cells[21,34,35]. However, it is noticeable that in fat cells of various other species, [^{3}H]RX 821002 labels a "yohimbinophobic" α2-adrenoceptor (having a weaker affinity than expected, for an α2-adrenoceptor, for yohimbine and rauwolscine). However, when referring to the action promoted by their stimulation, these α2-adrenoceptors, when stimulated by partial (clonidine) and full agonists (UK 14304 and epinephrine in the presence of propranolol), operate through a similar transducing mechanism to that of α2A-adrenoceptors, involving adenylate cyclase inhibition and reduction of intracellular cAMP levels. This receptor could be the putative α2D-subtype suspected in various tissues by some investigators using poorly adapted ligands such as [^{3}H]yohimbine and [^{3}H]rauwolscine, but further analyses are needed[43].

This α2-adrenoceptor subtype, labelled by [^{3}H]RX 821002 and having poor affinity for yohimbine, was also described in rat enterocytes[48]. Interestingly, it exhibits binding properties very similar to those of the rat α2-adrenoceptor subtype, which was recently cloned from a rat genomic library by the group of Lanier et al.[38]. This RG20 clone which encodes a protein of 457 amino acids possesses homology and common structural features with other α2-adrenoceptor proteins. The RG20 gene exhibits 87% homology with the α2-C10 in its nucleic acid sequence. The difference in binding properties between the RG20 and α2-C10 adrenoceptors are inconsistent with their classification as species homologues, while the degree of sequence homology between them is within the range of sequence identity observed for species homologues of other members of this receptor family. For the moment, it is difficult to state if it is a new gene family corresponding to the α2D-adrenoceptor subtype previously characterized in the submandibular gland of the rat[43] or a species homologue of the α2-C10 adrenoceptor exhibiting some differences with the human receptor in its binding properties i.e. "yohimbinophobic". In addition to this result, three of the subtypes encoding for the human α2-adrenoceptors have recently been characterized in various rat tissues although the fat cell was not investigated[39]. For the moment, the exact number of α2-adrenoceptor subtypes existing in a given species is still unknown.

Pharmacological strategies focusing on the adrenergic system: a critical appraisal

Apart from the pharmacological agents affecting appetite and the use of low calorie diets, one way to obtain greater and more prolonged weight loss could be the improvement of lipid mobilization and energy expenditure, a strategy which could reasonably be used in association with a hypocaloric diet. Although it is not intended to develop an exhaustive discussion of the possible pharmacological strategies, the main points should be noted concerning man and the animal models classically used.

The sympathetic nervous system (SNS) is a major regulator of adaptive thermogenesis in mammals; the latest results have recently been reviewed by Landsberg and Young[33]. Concerning the pharmacological approaches, focusing on the adrenergic system of the fat cell and tissues involved in energy expenditure, two major strategies can be proposed:

(1) The first one aims essentially at peripheral activities for the improvement of lipid mobilization and stimulation of energy expenditure. Beta-adrenoceptor agonists, acting as thermogenic agents, and reputed for their specific action at the "atypical" β-adrenoceptor of the brown fat cell of rodents, but also acting on white fat cells, have been used in animals and humans. Although recent data suggest that it may be possible to activate thermogenesis in adult man with such selective drugs, some of them suffer limitations since they have noticeable side-effects probably linked to a limited selectivity for various β-adrenoceptor subtypes. Some reports have mentioned stimulation of heart rate, insulin-secretory action, shaky hands and tremor[24]. Several questions about tissue targets justifying the utilization of these agents are still unsolved; they concern: (i) the clear determination of the extent of brown fat deposits in the adult man and of the nature of the β-adrenoceptor-dependent thermogenic action described in humans (as compared with rodent species having large amounts of brown fat); (ii) the demonstration of the presence of an "atypical" or β3-like adrenoceptor in white brown fat cells and other thermogenic tissues (muscle) of humans; (iii) the assessment of the absence of alteration of β-adrenoceptor-mediated effects after chronic administration of such exogenous β-agonist drugs.

(2) The second possible pharmacologic approach takes α2-adrenoceptors as targets. In the human fat, α2-adrenoceptors are heterogenously distributed in the various fat deposits and they could be involved in certain resistance to catecholamine-induced lipolysis when overexpressed in the fat cells.

Blockade of human fat cell α2-adrenoceptors with various selective α2-antagonists *in vitro* promotes enhancement of catecholamine-induced lipolysis and recent microdialysis studies of subcutaneous deposits *in situ* have demonstrated the mechanism of regulation of lipolysis in different fat deposits. It was shown that fat cell α2-adrenoceptors could be modulators of lipolysis at rest in humans[4]. Thus, α2-adrenoceptor antagonists which promote lipolysis may possibly be proposed to serve a therapeutic role in the treatment of obesity. In addition to their local role at the fat cell level, they can also be expected to be activators of the SNS and raise the sympathetic tone of a patient. Alpha2-adrenoceptors are located both centrally (in the brainstem where they control sympathetic and parasympathetic nerves) and peripherally (on the adrenergic and cholinergic nerve terminals where they are a key element in the local negative feedback system modulating neurotransmitter release).

The preliminary results obtained in humans indicate that the use of the α2-adrenoceptor antagonist, yohimbine, which is able to increase sympathetic activity during fasting or along with dieting therapy could be of interest to improve lipid mobilization by the activation of the SNS. It is noticeable that although promoting an activation of the sympathetic nervous system, yohimbine administration does not promote major effects on the cardiovascular system[5,22]. Recent experiments in dogs have demonstrated that α2-antagonist administration promotes sympathetic activation, lipid-mobilization and a thermogenic action without major cardiovascular effects (submitted for publication). The mechanisms involved in these effects have now been clarified. The α2-antagonists act: (i) by activation of the SNS through the blockade of central and presynaptic α2-adrenoceptors. At suitable concentrations an increment of circulating plasma noradrenaline is observed while plasma adrenaline levels are unchanged; (ii) by blockade of the antilipolytic α2-adrenoceptor on fat cell plasma membrane; (iii) by blockade of postjunctional α2-adrenoceptors on blood vessels which may offer an alternative for attenuating the pressor effects expected under elevation of sympathetic tone[33]; (iv) by the thermogenic effect which follows SNS activation.

To conclude, although the proposed indications for β-agonist and α2-adrenergic antagonist use in therapy are rare, the idea of their application for chemotherapy in obesity has gained ground. It is evident that such agents provoke an enhanced fat mobilization and utilization which should be expected to lead to diminished fat mass under chronic treatment The effects of β-agonists on increments of muscle mass and concomitant reduction of body fat also have very important implications in several areas including the meat industry; this aspect will not be considered here[58].

Nevertheless, concerning exploration of antiobesity therapies of such compounds, firstly, it is essential to keep in mind that noticeable species-specific differences exist in the expression of adrenoceptor subtypes in white fat cells and that the β- and α2-adrenoceptor equipment of the human fat cell is clearly different from that of the other commonly used mammal species. Secondly, in addition to the problems linked to the differences in fat cell adrenoceptors, it must not be forgotten that there are also striking species differences in the extent of the brown fat deposits and in the role they play in the thermogenic pathways. Brown fat plays a much more important role in small rodents than in man. In brown fat cells, in addition to stimulation of lipolysis, the role of adrenoceptors is to regulate thermogenesis. Brown fat exists in foetuses and most newborn animals, it rapidly regresses and even disappears with ageing in large mammals but still persists throughout the life-span in many small rodent species. Although brown fat cells exist in newborn children and play an important thermogenic role, most adult humans apparently have few brown fat cells in normal physiological conditions and muscle is quantitatively the major thermogenic tissue in man.

To sum up, all the pharmacological approaches referring to the classically used rodents should be interpreted very carefully. These striking differences focus attention on the care needed before extrapolating the results obtained in animals when a degree of clinical relevance is required.

References

1. Arch, J.R.S. (1989): The brown adipocyte β-adrenoceptor. *Proc. Nutr. Soc.* **48**, 215-223.
2. Arch, J.R.S., Ainsworth, A.T., Cawthorne, M.A., Piercy, V., Sennitt, M.V., Thody, V.E., Wilson, C. & Wilson, S. (1984): Atypical β-adrenoceptor on brown adipocytes as target for anti-obesity drugs. *Nature* **309**, 163-165.
3. Arner, P., Hellström, L., Wahrenberg, H. & Brönnegard, M. (1990): Beta-adrenoceptor in human fat cells from different regions. *J. Clin. Invest.* **86**, 1595-1600.
4. Arner, P., Kriegholm, E., Engfeldt, P. & Bolinder, J. (1990): Adrenergic regulation of lipolysis *in situ* at rest and during exercise. *J. Clin. Invest.* **85**, 893-898

5. Berlan, M., Galitzky, J., Rivière, D., Foureau, M., Tran, M.A., Flores, R., Louvet, J.P., Houin, G. & Lafontan, M. (1991): Plasma catecholamine levels and lipid mobilization induced by yohimbine in obese and non-obese women. *Int. J. Obesity* **15**, 305-315.
6. Bojanic, D., Jansen, J.D., Nahorski, S.R. & Zaagsma, J. (1985): Atypical characteristics of the β-adrenoceptor mediating cyclic AMP generation and lipolysis in the rat adipocyte. *Br. J. Pharmacol.* **84**, 131-137.
7. Buckland, P.R., Hill, R.M., Tidmarsh, S.F. & McGuffin, P. (1990): Primary structure of the rat beta2-adrenergic receptor gene. *Nucl. Acid Res.* **18**, 682.
8. Bylund, D.B. (1988): Subtypes of α2-adrenoceptors: pharmacological and molecular biological evidence converge. *Trends Pharmacol. Sci.* **9**, 356-361.
9. Carpene, C., Galitzky, J., Larrouy, D., Langin, D. & Lafontan, M. (1990): Non-adrenergic sites for imidazolines are not directly involved in the α2-adrenergic antilipolytic effect of UK 14304 in rat adipocytes. *Biochem. Pharmacol.* **40**, 437-445.
10. Carpene, C., Rebourcet, M.C., Guichard, C., Lafontan, M. & Lavau, M. (1990): Increased α2-adrenergic binding sites and antilipolytic effect in adipocytes from genetically obese rats. *J. Lipid Res.* **31**, 811-819.
11. Carruthers, A. (1990): Facilitated diffusion of glucose. *Physiol. Rev.* **70**, 1135-1176.
12. Collins, S., Bolanovski, M.A., Caron, M.G. & Lefkowitz, R.J. (1989): Genetic regulation of β-adrenergic receptors. *Ann. Rev. Physiol.* **51**, 203-215.
13. Degerman, E., Smith, C.J., Tornqvist, H., Vasta, V., Belfrage, P. & Manganiello, V. (1990): Evidence that insulin and isoprenaline activate the cGMP-inhibited low-K_m cAMP phosphodiesterase in rat fat cells by phosphorylation. *Proc. Natl. Acad. Sci. USA* **87**, 533-537.
14. Emorine, L., Feve, B., Pairault, J., Briend-Sutren, M-M., Marullo, S., Delavier-Klutchko, C. & Strosberg, D.A. (1991): Structural basis for functional diversity of β1, β2 and β3-adrenoeceptors. *Biochem. Pharmacol.* **41**, 853-859.
15. Emorine, L.J. & Strosberg, D.A. (1991): Molecular analysis of the three human β-adrenergic receptors. In *Adrenoceptors: structure, mechanisms, function*, eds. E. Szabadi & C.M. Bradshaw, pp. 79. Basel: Birkhauser Verlag.
16. Emorine, L.J., Marullo, S., Briend-Sutren, M.M., Patey, G., Tate, K., Delavier-Klutchko, C. & Strosberg, A.D. (1989): Molecular characterization of the human β3-adrenergic receptor. *Science.* **245**, 1118-1121.
17. Emorine, L.J., Marullo, S., Delavier-Klutchko, C., Kaven, S.V., Durieu-Trautmann, O. & Strosberg, A.D. (1987): Structure of the gene for the human β2-adrenergic receptor. Expression and promoter characterization. *Proc. Natl. Acad. Sci. USA.* **84**, 6995-6999.
18. Fève, B., Emorine, L.J., Briend-Sutren, M-M., Lasnier, F., Strosberg, D.A., & Pairault, J. (1990): Differential regulation of β1- and β2-adrenergic receptor protein and mRNA levels by glucocorticoids during 3T3-F442A adipose differentiation. *J. Biol. Chem.* **265**, 16343-16349.
19. Frielle, T., Collins, S., Daniel, K.W., Caron, M.G., Lefkowitz, R.J. and Kobilka, B.K. (1987): Cloning of the cDNA for the human β1-adrenergic receptor. *Proc. Natl. Acad. Sci. USA.* **84**, 7920-7924.
20. Galitzky, J., Larrouy, D., Berlan, M. & Lafontan, M. (1990): New tools for human fat cell alpha2A-adrenoceptor characterization. Identification on membranes and on intact cells using the new antagonist [^{3}H]RX821002. *J. Pharmacol. Exper. Ther.* **252**, 312-319.
21. Galitzky, J., Mauriege, P., Berlan, M. & Lafontan, M. (1989): Human fat cell α2-adrenoceptors. II. Comparative study of partial and full agonist binding parameters using [^{3}H]clonidine and [^{3}H]UK14304. *J. Pharmacol. Exp. Ther.* **249**, 591-600.
22. Galitzky, J., Taouis, M., Berlan, M., Rivière, D., Garrigues, M. & Lafontan, M. (1988): α2-antagonist compounds and lipid mobilization: evidence for a lipid mobilizing effect of oral yohimbine in healthy male volunteers. *Eur. J. Clin. Invest.* **18**, 587-594.
23. Harrison, J.K., Pearson, W.R. & Lynch, K.R. (1991): Molecular characterization of αl- and α2-adrenoceptors. *Trends Pharmacol. Sci.* **12**, 62-67.
24. Henny, C., Schutz, Y., Buckert, A., Meylan, M., Jequier, E. & Felber, J.P. (1987). Thermogenic effect of the new beta-adrenoceptor agonist RO 16-8714 in healthy male volunteers. *Int. J. Obesity.* **11**, 473-483.
25. Hollenga, C. & Zaagsma, J. (1989): Direct evidence for the atypical nature of functional β-adrenoceptors in rat adipocytes. *Br. J. Pharmacol.* **98**, 1420-1424.
26. Hollenga, C., Brouwer, F. & Zaagsma, J. (1991): Relationship between lipolysis and cyclic AMP generation mediated by atypical β-adrenoceptors. *Br. J. Pharmacol.* **102**, 577-582.
27. Hollenga, C., Haas, M., Deinum, J.T. & Zaagsma, J. (1990): Discrepancies in lipolytic activities induced by β-adrenoceptor agonists in human and rat adipocytes. *Horm. Metab. Res.* **22**, 17-21.

28. Kobilka, B.K., Dixon, R.A.F., Frielle, T., Dohlman, M.G., Bolanowsky, M.A., Sigal, I.S., Yang-Feng, T.L., Francke, U., Caron, M.G. & Lefkowitz, R.J. (1987): cDNA for the human β2-adrenergic receptor: a protein with multiple membrane spanning domains and encoded by a gene whose chromosomal location is shared with that of the receptor for platelet derived growth factor. *Proc. Natl. Acad. Sci. USA.* **84**, 46-50.
29. Lacasa, D., Mauriège, P., Lafontan, M., Berlan, M. & Giudicelli ,Y. (1986): A reliable assay for beta-adrenoceptors in intact isolated human fat cells with a hydrophilic radioligand, [^{3}H]CGP 12177. *J. Lipid Res.* **27**, 368-376.
30. Lafontan, M. & Berlan, M. (1981): α-Adrenergic receptors and the regulation of lipolysis in adipose tissue. *Trends Pharmacol. Sci.* **2**, 126-129.
31. Lafontan, M., Berlan, M. & Carpene, C. (1985): Fat cell adrenoceptors: inter and intraspecific differences and hormone regulation. *Int. J. Obesity.* **9** (Suppl. 1), 117-125.
32. Lafontan, M., Mauriège, P., De Pergola, G., Galitzky, J. & Berlan, M. (1987): Identification and quantification of β-and α2-adrenoceptors on membranes and intact adipocytes. In *Recent advances in obesity research V*, eds. E.M. Berry, S.H. Blondheim, H.E. Eliahou & E. Shafrir, pp. 212. London: John Libbey.
33. Landsberg, L. & Young, J.B. (1990): Obesity and the sympathetic nervous system. In *Obesity: towards a molecular approach*. eds, G.A. Bray, D. Ricquier & B.M. Spiegelman, pp. 81. New York: Wiley-Liss Inc.
34. Langin, D., Lafontan, M., Stillings, M.R. & Paris, H. (1989): [^{3}H]RX821002: a new tool for identification of α2A-adrenoceptors. *Eur. J. Pharmacol.* **167**, 95-104.
35. Langin, D., Paris, H. & Lafontan, M. (1990): Binding of [^{3}H]idazoxan and of its methoxy derivative [^{3}H]RX821002 in human fat cells: [^{3}H]idazoxan but not [^{3}H]RX821002 labels additional non-α2-adrenergic binding sites. *Mol. Pharmacol.* **37**, 876-885.
36. Langin, D., Paris, H., Dauzats, M. & Lafontan, M. (1990): Discrimination between α2-adrenoceptors and [^{3}H]idazoxan-labelled non-adrenergic binding sites in rabbit fat cells. *Eur. J. Pharmacol.- Mol. Pharmacol. Sec.* **188**, 261-272.
37. Langin, D., Portillo, M.P., Saulnier-Blache, J-S. & Lafontan, M. (1991): Coexistence of three β-adrenergic receptor subtypes in white fat cells of various mammal species. *Eur. J. Pharmacol.* **199**, 291-301.
38. Lanier, S.M., Downing, S., Duzic, E. & Homcy, C. (1991): Isolation of rat genomic clones encoding subtypes of the alphα2-adrenergic receptor: identification of a unique receptor subtype. *J. Biol. Chem.* **266**, 10470-10478.
39. Lorenz, W., Lomasney, J.W., Collins, S., Regan, J.W., Caron, M G. & Lefkowitz, R.J. (1990): Expression of three α2-adrenergic receptor subtypes in rat tissues: implications for α2-receptor classification. *Mol. Pharmacol.* **38**, 599-603.
40. Machida, C.A., Buzow, J.R., Searles, R.P., Van Tol, H., Tester, B., Neve, K.A., Teal, P., Nipper, V. & Civelli, O. (1990): Molecular cloning and expression of the rat β1-adrenergic receptor gene. *J. Biol. Chem.* **265**, 12960-12965.
41. Mauriège, P., De Pergola, G., Berlan, M. & Lafontan, M. (1988): Human fat cell β-adrenergic receptors β agonist-dependent lipolytic responses and characterization of β-adrenergic binding sites on human fat cell membranes with highly selective β1-antagonists. *J. Lipid Res.* **29**, 587-601.
42. Mauriège, P., Galitzky, J., Berlan, M. & Lafontan, M. (1987): Heterogenous distribution of beta and alpha2-adrenoceptor binding sites in human fat cells from various fat deposits: functional consequences. *Eur. J. Clin. Invest.* **17**, 156-165.
43. Michel, A.D, Loury, D.N. & Whiting, R.L. (1989): Differences between the α2-adrenoceptor in rat submaxillary gland and the α2A- and the α2B-subtype. *Br. J. Pharmacol.* **98**, 890-897.
44. Nahmias, C., Elalouf, J-M., Strosberg, D.A. & Emorine, L.J. (1991): Cloning and nucleotide sequencing of the murine β3-adrenergic receptor gene. *J. Cell Biochem.*, Suppl. 15B, Abstr. 218.
45. Nanoff, C., Freissmuth, M. & Schutz, W. (1987): The role of a low β1-adrenoceptor selectivity of [^{3}H]CGP12177 for resolving subtype-selectivity of competitive ligands. *Naunyn-Schmied. Arch. Pharmacol.* **336**, 519-525.
46. Neve, K.A., McGonigle, P. & Molinoff, P.B. (1986): Quantitative analysis of the selectivity of a radioligand for subtypes of β-adrenergic receptors. *J. Pharmacol. Exp. Ther.* **238**, 46-53.
47. O'Dowd, B.F., Lefkowitz R.J. & Caron, M.G. (1989): Structure of the adrenergic and related receptors. *Annu. Rev. Neurosci.* **12**, 67-83.
48. Paris, H., Voisin, T., Remaury, A., Rouyer-Fessard, C., Daviaud, D., Langin, D. & Laburthe, M. (1990): Alpha2-adrenoceptor in rat jejunum epithelial cells: characterization with [^{3}H]RX821002 and distribution along the villus-crypt axis. *J. Pharmacol. Exp. Ther.* **254**, 888-893.

49. Raasmaja, A. (1990): Alpha1- and beta-adrenergic receptors in brown adipose tissue and the adrenergic regulation of thyroxine 5'-deiodinase. *Acta Physiol. Scand.* **139**, Suppl. 590, 7-61.
50. Raymond, J.R., Hnatowich, M., Lefkowitz, R.J. & Caron, M.G. (1990): Adrenergic receptors: models for regulation of signal transduction processes. *Hypertension.* **15**, 120-131.
51. Revelli, J.P., Muzzin, P., Gocayne, J., Venter, J.C., Fraser, C.M. & Giacobino, J.P. (1991): Molecular characterization of an atypical rat β-adrenergic receptor. EASO Meeting 29 May – 1st June, Nice, Abstract
52. Saulnier-Blache, J.S., Carpéné, C., Langin, D. & Lafontan, M. (1989): Imidazolinic radioligands for the identification of hamster adipocyte α2-adrenoceptors. *Eur. J. Pharmacol.* **171**, 145-157.
53. Schütz, W., Nanoff, W. & Freissmuth, M. (1988): The fallacy of non-selectivity of radioactive ligands. *Trends Pharmacol. Sci.* **9**, 261-264.
54. Stillings, M.R., Chapleo, C.B., Butler, R.C.M., Davis, J.A., England, C.D., Myers, P.L., Tweddle, N., Wellbourn, A.P., Doxey, J.C. & Smith, C.F.C. (1985): α-Adrenoceptor reagents. 3. Synthesis of some 2-subsituted 1,4-benzodioxans as selective presynaptic α2-adrenoceptor antagonists. *J. Med. Chem.* **28**, 1054-1062.
55. Tan, S. & Curtis-Prior, P.B. (1983): Characterization of the β-adrenoceptor of the adipose cell of the rat. *Int. J. Obesity.* **7**, 409-414.
56. Taouis, M., Valet, P., Estan, L., Lafontan, M., Montastruc, P. & Berlan, M. (1989): Obesity modifies the adrenergic status of dog adipose tissue. *J. Pharmacol. Exp. Ther.* **250**, 1061-1066.
57. Vauquelin, G., De Vos, H. & De Backer, J-P. (1990): Identification of α2-adrenergic receptors in human frontal cortex membranes by binding of [^{3}H]RX821002, the 2-methoxy analog of idazoxan. *Neurochem. Int.* **17**, 537-546.
58. Yang, Y.T. & McElligot, M.A. (1989): Multiple actions of β-adrenergic agonists on skeletal muscle and adipose tissue. *Biochem. J.* **261**, 1-10.
59. Zaagsma, J. & Nahorski, R.S. (1990): Is the adipocyte β-adrenoceptor a prototype for the recently cloned atypical "β3- adrenoceptor"? *Trends Pharmacol. Sci.* **11**, 3-7.

Chapter 27

Identification and Analysis of an Adipose Specific Enhancer

Reed A. GRAVES, Peter TONTONOZ, Susan R. ROSS[1] and Bruce M. SPIEGELMAN

Dana-Farber Cancer Institute and the Department of Biological Chemistry and Molecular Pharmacology, Harvard Medical School, Boston, Massachusetts 02115 USA; [1]*Department of Biochemistry, University of Illinois Medical School, Chicago, Il 60612 USA*

We have evaluated the capacity of the 5'-flanking region of the aP2 gene to direct cell-type specific gene expression. Although the proximal promoter is capable of directing differentiation-dependent gene expression in cultured adipocytes, these constructs are essentially inactive in the tissues of transgenic mice. We found that –5.4 kb of the 5'-flanking region were required to direct heterologous gene (chloramphenicol acetyl transferase; CAT) expression to the adipose tissue of transgenic mice. By deletion analysis, we identified a 520 bp enhancer at –5.4 kb of the aP2 gene. We show that this enhancer can direct high levels of gene expression specifically to the adipose tissue of transgenic mice. This enhancer also functions in a differentiation-dependent manner in cultured adipocytes and is not transactivatable in preadipocytes by C/EBP. Molecular analysis indicates that several *cis*-acting elements contribute to the specificity and potency of this enhancer.

Introduction

The murine adipocyte P2 gene (aP2) encodes a member of the fatty acid binding protein family and is expressed specifically in adipose tissue[23]. The aP2 gene is regulated during the differentiation of preadipocytes in several cultured cell models systems and is also regulated by extracellular signals in terminally differentiated adipocytes[1,2,5,8,9,12,13,16,20]. The proximal promoter of the aP2 gene is capable of directing CAT gene expression in a differentiation-dependent fashion[11,12]. Molecular studies of the proximal promoter have defined two DNA elements, an AP1 site and a C/EBP binding site, that are important for this expression[6,11,15]. Mutation of either site severely reduces promoter activity. The AP1 site, which binds the proto-oncogenes *c-jun* and *c-fos*, is required for the cAMP responsiveness of the aP2 promoter[15]. Since the receptors for agents that increase the levels of cAMP are dramatically increased during the differentiation process, it seems reasonable to suggest that the apparent differentiation-dependent response of this element may merely reflect the increased responsiveness of adipocytes (compared to preadipocytes) to extracellular signals. C/EBP is also important for the differentiation-dependent activity of the proximal promoter[6,15]. The levels of mRNA for C/EBP are increased dramatically during adipocyte differentiation and C/EBP has been shown to transactivate the promoters of several fat cell genes (e.g. glut 4, stearoyl CoA desaturase)[6,15,17]. Thus, C/EBP has been proposed to play a central role in regulation of genes involved in energy metabolism and also as a differentiation-dependent switch[18].

Since the C/EBP gene is expressed in liver and several other tissues in addition to adipose tissue[3], we wanted to determine if the aP2 promoter was tissue-specific as well as differentiation-dependent. Surprisingly, the proximal promoter of the aP2 gene has no tissue-specificity and appears to be an extremely weak promoter in transgenic animals. This led us to search for regions of the aP2 gene that would direct both the potent and highly-specific transcriptional regulation observed with the endogenous gene. We report here our identification of the first enhancer with specificity for adipose tissue *in vivo*. This enhancer (520 bp fragment) is located at –5.4 kb of the aP2 gene and is able to confer potency and tissue-specificity to a minimal aP2 promoter lacking a C/EBP or AP1 site as well as to an enhancerless viral promoter (SV40 early). We also demonstrate that this enhancer is capable of directing differentiation-dependent gene expression in cultured cells and that the enhancer functions in the apparent absence of transactivatable C/EBP sites. We discuss a model for enhancer action and also discuss the discrepancies of the results obtained in cultured cells versus transgenic animals.

Methods

3T3-F442A cells were cultured and transfected as previously reported[14]. The conditions for transactivation with the C/EBP expression vector were as formerly established[15]. CAT assays from the tissues of transgenic mice were performed as described[19].

Results

Constructs containing different lengths of the aP2 5'-flanking region driving the CAT gene were evaluated for their ability to direct appropriate tissue-specific expression in transgenic mice. Four transgenes containing segments of the aP2 promoter varying from –5.4 kb to –168 bp were tested. Each promoter segment was terminated at the 3' end by the natural PstI site at position +21 of the aP2 mRNA. Promoter activity was assessed by quantitative CAT assay from various tissues of several strains of transgenic mice (Table 1). Previous results had shown that the proximal promoter (either –168 or –247) was sufficient to confer differentiation-dependent expression in cultured mouse adipocytes[8,11]. Strikingly, those small constructs and a construct extending to 1.7 kb were uniformly inactive in adipose tissue of any of the transgenic mice. Only when promoter activity was apparently forced by a huge copy number of the transgene (strain 3_{1a}; 1255 copies) was significant gene expression observed. However, in this case expression was an order of magnitude greater in spleen and thymus than adipose tissue.

By contrast, transgenic expression driven by the –5.4 kb aP2CAT construct was both highly potent and specific (Table 1). In these strains transgene expression in adipose tissue was at least four orders of magnitude greater than transgene expression directed by any of the smaller constructs. The specificity of transgenic expression for adipose tissue ranged from twofold to greater than 20-fold. It should be noted that the tissues (spleen and thymus) with the highest amounts of inappropriate transgene expression are also very likely to have been contaminated with fat when excised from the animal. Taken together, these results suggest that there is an element capable of conferring adipose-specific gene expression in the 3.7 kb fragment extending from –5.4 kb to –1.7 kb.

We next used cultured 3T3-F442A cells to rapidly scan this 3.7 kb DNA fragment for enhancing activity in adipocytes. As a basal promoter we have used either –63aP2CAT, which contains sequences from –63 to +21 of the aP2 gene and is deleted for the previously identified regulatory elements (C/EBP, AP1, CAAT box),[11] or the enhancerless SV40 promoter[4]. Both of these promoters are relatively inactive in preadipocytes and adipocytes. Several restriction fragments derived from the 3.7 kb fragment were ligated to –63aP2CAT and assayed for enhancing activity following transient transfection into cultured adipocytes. All of the results suggest that only one major enhancing activity is present in this fragment (data not shown). From this analysis we have identified a 520 bp "enhancer" extending from –5.4 kb to –4.9

kb. This enhancer was capable of stimulating CAT gene expression from the −63 aP2 promoter when transiently transfected into differentiated adipocytes (Fig. 1). By contrast, the same construct showed no stimulation when transiently transfected into preadipocytes (Fig. 1). Parallel control transfections with two CAT expression vectors driven by the viral RSV and AKV long terminal repeat promoter show that the transfection and efficiency of expression in the two cell types was similar (Fig. 1). Finally, we compared enhancer activity in a cell line consisting of a pool of 36 colonies that were stably transfected. CAT activity increased 15-fold following adipose differentiation (Fig. 1).

Table 1. CAT activity in the tissues of aP2CAT transgenic mice.

PART A		Specific activity in tissues (cpm/mg/min)						
Transgene	Copy number	Liver	Spleen	Thymus	Brain	Muscle	Lung	Adipose
168aP2CAT	50	0	0.033	0.017	0.001	nd	0.002	0
247aP2CAT	1255	0.012	1.351	3.295	0.305	0.107	0.051	0.07
247aP2CAT	21	0	0.009	0.012	0.024	nd	0.011	0.006
247aP2CAT	12	0.01	0.187	0.125	0.014	0.008	0.047	0.012
1700aP2CAT	5	0	0.456	0.241	nd	0	0.003	0.002
1700aP2CAT	45	0.004	0.814	0.402	0.006	0.003	0.007	0.034
1700aP2CAT	4	nd	0.484	0.001	0.425	0	0.019	0.008
5400aP2CAT	5	1	2200	4400	4	nd	1400	>11,000*
5400aP2CAT	5	8	450	360	29	43	73	860
5400aP2CAT	<5	27	93	130	0	nd	43	1300

PART B				% CAT conversion				
Transgene	Kidney	Liver	Spleen	Thymus	Brain	Muscle	Lung	Adipose
520/-63aP2	0.2	1.4	0.1	0.5	0.6	0.9	0.3	25.9
520/SV40	0.7	1.0	0.8	1.5	0.8	0.8	0.8	16.3

Transgenes in Part A contain from -168, -247, -1700 or -5400 by to +21 by of the aP2 gene promoter linked to CAT. In Part B transgenes contained the 520 bp aP2 enhancer linked to either the -63 aP2 promoter or to the enhancerless SV40 promoter. CAT assays were conducted with 2 mg of protein for 30 minutes at 37°C. The adipose samples in part A are derived from white fat while the adipose samples in part B are a combination of white and brown fat. *CAT activity was in the nonlinear range of the assay, so that accurate specific activities could not be determined and this value represents a minimal specific activity.

To determine if this enhancer was capable of directing tissue-specific gene expression, we made transgenic mice containing this construct. The results from three strains are shown in Table 1 part B. The specificity (i.e. adipose specific expression) of the enhancer is at least equivalent to the −5.4aP2CAT. These results clearly demonstrate that this 520bp enhancer is capable of directing high-levels of adipocyte specific gene expression in transgenic animals. Enhancer specificity (and activity) is independent of the aP2 promoter, since identical results in both cell culture and transgenic animals are obtained when the enhancer is ligated to the enhancerless SV40 promoter (Table 1, part B). These data clearly demonstrate that the C/EBP binding site at −140 bp of the aP2 promoter is not necessary for adipose-specific gene expression.

Since C/EBP has been shown to transactivate the promoter of several adipose cell genes (including the aP2 gene)[6,15], we wanted to determine whether the enhancer contained binding sites for C/EBP. We have not been able to identify a C/EBP binding site in the enhancer by either mobility-shift DNA binding or DNAase I footprinting assays (data not

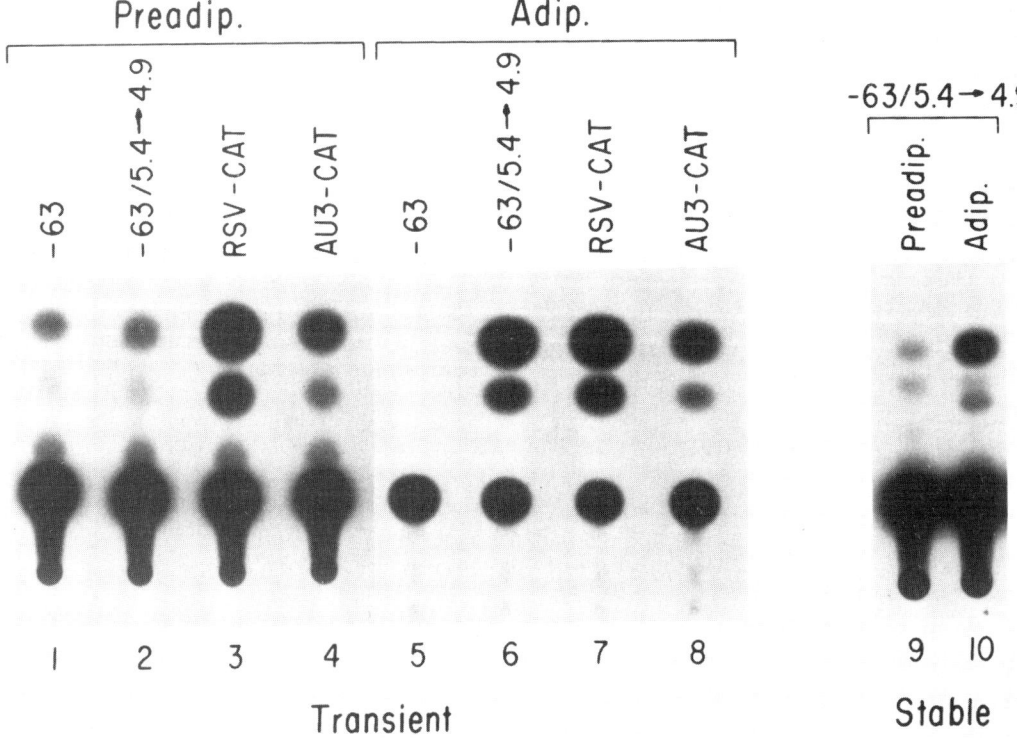

Fig. 1. Differentiation-dependent activation by the –5.4 to –4.9 kb fragment. The 500 bp fragment was inserted into the –63aP2CAT vector in an inverted orientation (i.e. in a 3' to 5' orientation relative to the endogenous gene). Preadipocytes (lanes 1–4) or adipocytes (lanes 5–8) were transiently transfected with 10 µg of –63aP2CAT (lanes 1 and 5); 10 µg of –63/5.4 → 4.9aP2CAT (lanes 2 and 6); 5 µg of RSVCAT (lanes 3 and 7); 1 µg of AU3CAT (lanes 4 and 8). CAT assays were performed as described[14]. The –63/5.4 → 4.9aP2CAT construct was stably introduced into preadipocytes and a pool of 36 colonies was expanded. Extracts from preadipocytes and adipocytes were prepared and assayed for CAT activity (lanes 9 and 10).

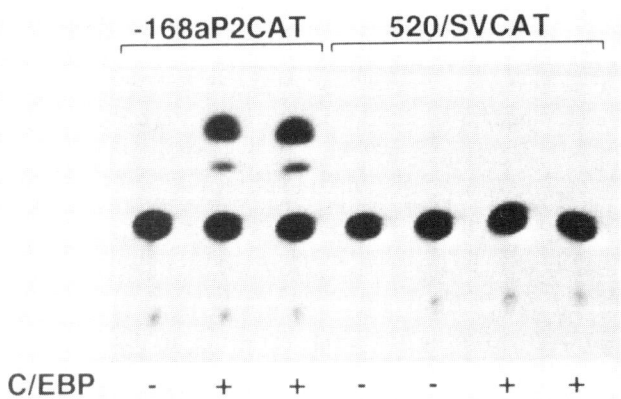

Fig. 2. C/EBP does not transactivate the aP2 enhancer. 3T3F442A preadipocytes were transfected with either –168aP2CAT or 520/SVCAT (the 520 bp enhancer ligated to the enhancerless SV40 promoter). Cotransfection with the C/EBP expression vector[15] is indicated by +.

shown). We also performed transactivation experiments in preadipocytes with a C/EBP expression vector. The results are shown in Fig. 2. C/EBP was able to transactivate the –168 aP2 CAT construct which contains a *bona fide* C/EBP binding site (Fig. 2). However, there was no transactivation by C/EBP of the 520 enhancer/SV40 promoter construct (Fig. 2). We conclude that C/EBP cannot activate the isolated aP2 enhancer in preadipocytes.

Discussion

We have identified the first enhancer with specificity for adipocytes in culture and in transgenic animals[14,19]. The ability to target high levels of gene expression to the adipose tissue of mice will be of importance in the fields of biology, pathophysiology and even agriculture. Pathological conditions that involve adipose tissue, such as obesity and lipodystrophy are associated with a variety of significant health problems, especially cardiovascular disorders and diabetes[7]. New experimental models of obesity or lipodystrophy might be brought about by overexpression of a variety of regulatory molecules, such as the β-adrenergic or α2-adrenergic receptors. Alternatively, the relationship between obesity and diabetes in several obese/diabetic mouse models could be probed by directly suppressing adipose cell formation and/or function through the delivery of toxins or other agents that suppress lipid accumulation. In the agricultural field, there has been considerable interest in developing genetic methods to alter the balance between lean and fat body mass in feed animals and the enhancer described here could open the door to such methods.

There are many genes whose transcription is regulated during the adipose differentiation process[2,5,8,12,20,21]. Some of these genes are also tissue specific (e.g. adipsin, aP2) while other differentiation-dependent genes are expressed in several tissues (e.g. glycerol-3-phosphate dehydrogenase). It is reasonable to suspect that there will be common *cis*-acting elements in the enhancer/promoter of these genes. Some of these *cis*-acting elements may play roles in determining its tissue-specificity as well as controlling differentiation-dependent gene expression. However, it is important to note that these phenomena represent fundamentally different processes. The tissue-specific enhancer that we have identified also functions in a differentiation-dependent fashion in cultured cells. Identification of sites in the enhancer that contribute to both differentiation-dependent and tissue-specific gene expression will allow us to determine the role of differentiation and cell-type specific transcription factors in regulating the specificity of gene expression. Our immediate goal is to identify the elements that determine tissue specificity since these elements are likely to play a role in the expression of many fat cell genes. Finally, it will be important to determine whether there exists a "master gene" for the adipogenic lineage parallel to that observed for another mesodermal lineage, muscle (e.g. myoD)[10].

One of the important conclusions for this work is that results from the cultured cell system do not always reflect the results obtained *in vivo*. For example, although the proximal promoter region of the aP2 gene is capable of directing differentiation-dependent gene expression, it is certainly neither sufficient nor necessary for tissue-specific expression. The proximal promoter constructs contain binding sites for two regulatory transcription factors. First, there is an AP-1 site that binds the proto-oncogenes c-*fos* and c-*jun*. This site is required for the cAMP responsiveness of –168aP2CAT constructs. Secondly, there is a C/EBP binding site. C/EBP has been proposed to play a regulatory role in the differentiation-dependent expression of several fat cell genes[6,17], since C/EBP is expressed only in differentiated adipocytes[6,15] and is able to transactivate the promoter of several different fat cell genes[6,17]. Our results do not contradict this data. However, it is clear that a C/EBP binding site is not required for differentiation-dependent gene expression. Clearly C/EBP plays some role in differentiation-dependent gene expression in cultured cells; however, it remains to be shown whether its role is as a key regulator or as an end product of differentiation. Moreover, our data show that C/EBP is neither sufficient nor necessary for tissue specific gene expression in adipose cells. One alternative explanation for the data is that C/EBP provides a mechanism to modulate adipose gene expression, perhaps in response to extracellular signals and that the apparent differentiation-dependent gene expression observed with the proximal promoter constructs merely reflects the heightened hormonal responsiveness of adipocytes compared to preadipocytes.

What factors bind to the adipocyte enhancer? By DNaseI footprinting and mobility-shift DNA binding assays, we can identify at least 4 different proteins that bind to the enhancer. One of these proteins is a member of the NF-1 family[14]. Although mutation of the NF-1 site reduces enhancer function dramatically, it remains to be determined whether the NF-1 site plays a regulatory (i.e. tissue-specific or differentiation-dependent) role in enhancer function. It is clear, however, that NF-1 is not the only site in the enhancer, since the enhancer with the NF-1 mutation retains significant differentiation-dependent activity. Thus there must be other positive *cis*-acting elements in the enhancer. The regulation of all of these factors in cell differentiation and obesity will be important subjects for further studies.

Acknowledgements

We thank Ms Adah Levens for help with the manuscript. We thank Dr Greg Robinson for advice in the use of the C/EBP expression vector. We thank members of the Spiegelman and Ross laboratories for helpful discussions.

References

1. Bernlohr, D.A., Bolanowski, M.A., Kelly, T.J.Jr. & Lane, M.D. (1985): Evidence for an increase in transcription of specific mRNAs during differentiation of 3T3-L1 adipocytes. *J. Biol. Chem.* **260**, 5563-5567.
2. Bernlohr, D.A., Angus, C.W., Lane, M.D., Bolanowski, M.A. & Kelly, T.J.J. (1984): Expression of specific mRNAs during adipose differentiation: identification of an mRNA encoding a homologue of myelin P2 protein. *Proc. Natl. Acad. Sci. USA* **81**, 5468-5472.
3. Birkenmeier, E.H., Gwynn, B., Howard, S., Jerry, J., Gordon, J.I., Landschulz, W.H. & McKnight, S.L. (1989): Tissue-specific expression and developmental and genetic mapping of the gene encoding C/EBP. *Genes Dev.* **3**, 1146-1156.
4. Celander, D. & Haseltine, W.A. (1984): Tissue-specific transcription preference as a determinant of cell tropism and leukaemogenic potential of murine retroviruses. *Nature* **312**, 159-162.
5. Chapman, A.B., Knight, D.M., Dieckman, B.A. & Ringold, G.M. (1984): Analysis of gene expression during differentiation of adipogenic cells in culture and hormonal control of the developmental program. *J. Biol. Chem.* **259**, 15548-15555.
6. Christy, R.J., Yang, V.W., Ntambi, J.M., Geiman, D.E., Landschulz, W.H., Friedman, A.D., Nakabeppu, Y., Kelly, T.J. & Lane, M.D. (1989): Differentiation-induced gene expression in 3T3-L1 preadipocytes: CCAAT/enhancer binding protein interacts with and activates the promoters of two adipocyte-specific genes. *Genes Dev.* **3**, 1323-1335.
7. Coleman, D.L. (1982): Diabetes-obesity syndromes. *The mouse in biomedical research*. New York: Academic Press.
8. Cook, J.S., Lucas, J.J., Sibley, E., Bolanowski, M.A., Christy, R.J., Kelly, T.J. & Lane, M.D. (1988): Expression of the differentiation induced gene for fatty acid binding protein is activated by glucocorticoid and cAMP. *Proc. Natl. Acad. Sci. USA* **85**, 2949-2953.
9. Cook, K.S., Hunt, C.R. & Spiegelman, B.M. (1985): Developmentally regulated mRNA in 3T3-adipocytes: analysis of transcriptional control. *J. Cell Biol.* **100**, 514-520.
10. Davis, R.L., Weintraub, H. & Lassar, A.B. (1987): Expression of a single transfected cDNA converts fibroblasts to myoblasts. *Cell* **51**, 987-1000.
11. Distel, R., Ro, H.-S., Rosen, B.S., Groves, D. & Spiegelman, B.M. (1987): Nucleoprotein complexes that regulate gene expression in adipocyte differentiation: direct participation of c-*fos*. *Cell* **49**, 835-844.
12. Djian, P., Phillips, M. & Green, H. (1985): The activation of specific gene transcription in adipose conversion of 3T3 cells. *J. Cell. Physiol.* **124**, 554-556.
13. Doglio, A., Dani, C., Grimaldi, P. & Ailhaud, G. (1986): Growth hormone regulation of the expression of differentiation-dependent genes in preadipocyte Ob1771 cells. *Biochem. J.* **238**, 123-129.

14. Graves, R.A., Tontonoz, P., Ross, S.R. & Spiegelman, B.M. (1991): Identification of a potent adipocyte-specificx enhancer: involvement of an NF-1-like factor. *Genes Dev.* **5**, 428-437.
15. Herrera, R., Ro, H.-S., Robinson, G.S., Xanthopoulos, K.G. & Spiegelman, B.M. (1989): A direct role for C/EBP and the AP-1-binding site in gene expression linked to adipocyte differentiation. *Mol. Cell Biol.* **9**, 5331-5339.
16. Hunt, C., Ro, J.H.-S., Min, H.-Y., Dobson, D.E. & Spiegelman, B.M. (1986): Adipocyte P2 gene: developmental expression and homology of 5'-flanking sequences among fat cell-specific genes. *Proc. Natl. Acad. Sci. USA* **83**, 3786-3790.
17. Kaestner, K.H., Christy, R.J. & Lane, M.D. (1990): Mouse insulin-responsive glucose transporter gene: characterization of the gene and transactivation by the CCAAT/enhancer binding protein. *Proc. Natl. Acad. Sci. USA* **87**, 251-255.
18. McKnight, S.L., Lane, M.D. & Gluecksohn, W.S. (1989): Is CCAAT/enhancer-binding protein a central regulator of energy metabolism? *Genes Dev.* **3**, 2021-4.
19. Ross, S.R., Graves, R.A., Greenstein, A., Platt, K.A., Shyu, H.-L., Mellovitz, B. & Spiegelman, B.M. (1990): A fat-specific enhancer is the primary determinant of adipocyte P2 (aP2) gene expression *in vivo*. *Proc. Natl. Acad. Sci. USA* **87**, 9590-9594.
20. Spiegelman, B.M., Frank, M. & Green, H. (1983): Molecular cloning of mRNA from 3T3-adipocytes. Regulation of mRNA content for glycerophosphate dehydrogenase and other differentiation-dependent proteins during adipocyte development. *J. Biol. Chem.* **258**, 10083-10089.
21. Spiegelman, B.M. & Green, H. (1980): Control of specific protein biosynthesis during the adipose conversion of 3T3 cells. *J. Biol. Chem.* **255**, 8811-8818.
22. Yang, V.W., Christy, R.J., Cook, J.S., Kelly, T.J. & Lane, M.D. (1989): Mechanism of regulation of the 422 (aP2) gene by cAMP during preadipocyte differentiation. *Proc. Natl. Acad. Sci. USA* **86**, 3629-3633.
23. Zezulak, K.M. & Green, H. (1985): Specificity of gene expression in adipocytes. *Mol. Cell. Biol.* **5**, 419-421.

Chapter 28

The Management of Obesity

John F. MUNRO and Nicola COLLEDGE
Medical Unit, Eastern General Hospital, Seafield Street, Edinburgh EH6 7LN, UK

Principles of management

The management principles of any medical condition encompass a number of facets. These include the treatment of the cause of the condition, the aggravating and precipitating factors, the condition itself, the complications of the condition, and finally the complications of the treatment. In some situations, such as essential hypertension, the underlying cause may be unknown but in spite of this treatment is available. The cause of obesity is clear cut; individual energy expenditure is exceeded by intake over a sustained time period. The reasons why this may occur are less easily defined. Although some subjects may be disadvantaged, for example by a small stature or by relatively low energy expenditure, it must be conceded that energy requirements rise with increase in the degree of obesity. Some subjects however find it hard to accept that they are not metabolically unique. As a consequence an initial component of treatment may involve "proving them wrong" either by measuring energy expenditure, or intake, or by asking a variety of questions designed to expose the difference between actual and assumed energy consumption. (For example, "What do you eat between meals and snacks?", and "When did you last binge?"). Unfortunately effort spent in establishing *what* the obese are doing may detract from the potentially more important management issue of *why* they are doing it. Few, if any, obese subjects with a normal hypothalamus overeat because of hunger. Some may do so because of the pleasure that they derive from food. More commonly food is used for comfort, changes in intake being associated with periods of tension or stress. Others may be overweight because they use obesity as a protective mechanism. It may be used to provide an explanation for feelings of self-reproach or inadequacy or to justify avoiding involvement in personal relationships. Sometimes the subject may be unaware of these factors; on other occasions they may relate them to unhappy experiences in childhood or in later life. Unless these issues are recognized and, where possible, resolved, the management of the consequences is likely to prove ineffective.

Management objectives

Those studies which report the consequences of treatment show a consistent tendency for weight loss to be regained in the longer term. This helps to explain the generally held view that the management of obesity is ineffective. Possibly however both the profession and the public have inappropriate expectations about management objectives with an excessive emphasis on the importance of weight loss. Clearly this is a central management objective but it is not the only one. The first prerequisite in any programme must the prevention of further weight gain. If a strategy could be developed to ensure this objective then clearly with time morbid obesity would be eradicated. For the individual this approach involves not only a shift in emphasis but also in attitude, replacing negative thinking ("this is pointless,

I have failed to lose weight in the last twelve months") with the positive ("this is very encouraging; I have not gained any extra weight in the last year").

Of equal importance is the treatment of the complications of obesity, be these medical or psychological. Weight reduction can an important component of the management of Type II diabetes mellitus, hypertension and hyperlipidaemia. However if these problems are of sufficient severity and if weight reduction is not occurring then they require treatment in their own right. Likewise the development of laparoscopic cholecystectomy has provided a method of treating cholelithiasis even in the morbidly obese. If a primary management aim is the reduction of medical risk factors then this objective encompasses not only the whole arena of "eating" but also the problem of other risk factors. In some circumstances stopping smoking or reducing alcohol consumption may be much more important than weight loss.

Weight loss – general principles

Every subject wishing to lose weight presents a unique management challenge. The magnitude of obesity, regional distribution of adiposity, and the presence and severity of obesity-related complications all influence therapeutic options. However there are three considerations which are common factors.

Realistic concepts

The magnitude of weight loss achieved by given energy deficit will depend upon how much is derived from fat and how much from the fat-free mass. A sustained energy deficit of 1000 k/cal per day will result in a weight loss of 1.0 kg of adipose tissue per week. It follows that the difference in weight loss achieved by daily intake of 1000 k/cal and of 500 k/cal converts to 0.5 kg. per week of adipose tissue. Any increase in the velocity of weight reduction can only be achieved by metabolizing fat free mass. Whether or not a realistic concept of the rate of weight loss improves outcome, it is only appropriate that subjects wishing to reduce should appreciate what is involved. Similarly, the target weight should be realistic. Indeed it is better to aim for a shape than for a weight. However many subjects set their sights on achieving "ideal weight", an actuarial concept sustained by cultural pressure rather than by medical means. A realistic target weight is often substantially greater than the ideal weight and should take into consideration the observation that few achieve and sustain a reduction in body weight greater than 20%.

Motivation

Obese subjects are in a sacrifice situation. Either they forego the benefits of weight reduction, be these medical or psychological, or they do without the pleasure and comfort that they obtain from their existing lifestyle. The therapist has a responsibility to provide the subject with a reasonable assessment of the medical risks involved, bearing in mind such factors as the degree of obesity, degree of disability, and the likely benefits of weight loss. These vary from one individual to another and only rarely are clear cut.

Permanency of change

There are some situations in which there may be a specific justification to achieve transient weight reduction, possibly as a prerequisite to surgery, for life insurance purposes, to help get a job or for more personal reasons such as going on holiday. Usually however short-term weight reduction is of very limited value. Weight loss will itself bring about a fall in energy expenditure. It follows that weight regain can be prevented *only* by making a permanent change in energy balance. Generally speaking the public are now well informed about the energy value of various foodstuffs. Some subjects however have little insight into the nature of their problem. Their energy intake is substantially greater than they recognize. The difference may lie in the energy value of fluids, both alcoholic and non-alcoholic, or of eating between meals and snacks, or of intermittent bingeing. An awareness of the problem is an important prerequisite to effective change. This may be achieved by the use of a "Food Diary", but therapist and subject alike require to be aware of the limitations as well as the advantages of recording even when undertaken at the time of eating.

The whole concept of "going on a diet" is potentially self-defeating as it almost intrinsically implies "coming off a diet" sooner or later. This may be particularly the case in subjects who binge, an eating disorder which is being more commonly recognized in North America, an observation in keeping with our own experience. Subjects who binge require to be identified because the initial management thrust is best directed at the bingeing problem where cognitive therapy may have a special value. Permanency of change in all subjects however involves as an initial step the awareness of what requires to be changed. Success then requires the ability to introduce changes step-by-step, and such changes may have to encompass not only what and how much is eaten but also alterations in the purchase and preparation of food, and in the time and situation of eating, as well as in the act of eating itself.

Specific treatment options

It has been customary to emphasize that dietary restriction is a sheet anchor of obesity management. Some subjects make the appropriate corrections in energy consumption without outside help. Other fail and these form the majority who look for support from self-help groups, commercial slimming organisations or medical practitioners. Although of the re-enforcement of dietary advice may be important it is often inadequate. Likewise, rigid behavioural modification programmes have serious limitations. Increasingly the tendency is to combine dietary advice with cognitive behavioural modification techniques so that subjects can develop a deeper understanding of the cause of their faulty eating, thereby learning to develop more effective ways of coping. For example, instead of making chocolate a forbidden food, it can be incorporated into acceptable eating patterns so that it no longer becomes a trigger to bingeing. Cognitive therapy is inevitably time consuming unless performed in a group setting. Additional treatment options include pharmacotherapy, VLCD and radical strategies.

Pharmacotherapy

Drug treatment can produce weight loss by either increasing energy expenditure or reducing the absorption of food from the GI tract, or by reducing food intake. At present those agents commercially available work primarily by reducing energy consumption. Because of their potential for drug abuse those with CNS stimulant properties have fallen into disfavour. Serotoninergic agent such as fenfluramine and d-fenfluramine are probably comparable in efficacy to the catacholaminergic drugs and can be expected to produce a mean additional weight loss of 0.25 kg per week over and above that obtained by "conventional" therapy. After a variable time interval this velocity of weight reduction will plateau. Thereafter if drug treatment is continued some subjects will regain weight and might reflect the development of drug tolerance. Others however appear to benefit throughout the duration of drug treatment. Indeed the mean weight changes mask very considerable person-to-person variations. Some lose substantial amounts, others nothing at all. Unfortunately there is no clear-cut method of distinguishing relative responders from non-responders. It follows that there is a natural tendency to restrict drug usage to those subjects who it is felt most require to lose weight.

The difficulty of selection of suitable subjects for pharmacotherapy is compounded in those countries where licensing authorities have restricted the duration of drug treatment. In the UK, both for fenfluramine and d-fenfluramine, this is for periods of up to three months. Such advice appears to be as logical as suggesting that oral hypoglycaemic agents can be given to improve diabetic control but must be stopped once good control has been achieved. Indeed, it would appear that either such drugs should be restricted to subjects in whom there is a justification for transient weight loss, or the prescribing practitioner should be prepared to breach the code of practice, an option rendered more hazardous because the relevant risks and advantages of long-term treatment can only be assessed by long-term usage. A compromise approach might be to use drugs either intermittently or alternating with an alternative drug with a different mode of action, or some other strategy such as VLCD. Such options require further critical analysis. Unfortunately our own experience with alternating phentermine and fenfluramine was disappointing, as has been the unpublished use of fluoxetine and VLCD. Alternating therapy however may be of advantage if combined with an adjustable waist cord, a regime that has been used with dental splinting and VLCD. An alternative approach, possibly more likely to prove acceptable to the licensing authorities would be the development of drugs which possess a dual efficacy. Current examples of such an approach include the use of metformin in the management of Type II diabetes mellitus, and of fluoxetine in the management of the obese depressed. The challenge to the pharmaceutical industry is the development of similar agents with greater weight reducing properties.

VLCD

The advantage of VLCD lies in the fact that some subjects find it easier in the short term to replace "kitchen food" with a liquid regime designed to provide adequate protein and other essential nutrients than to make a stepwise alteration in their "kitchen diet". The disadvantage is that the rigidity of the approach is in conflict with cognitive behavioural techniques. Recognition of this problem has resulted in increasing emphasis being placed on a comprehensive programme. Commercial organizations promoting products like the Cambridge Diet and Optifast are to be congratulated for this development but the specific value of the VLCD component of their programmes has become increasingly difficult to define. It may be that the long-term benefits are achieved in spite of, rather than because of, the VLCD component of the programme.

Radical therapies

Radical therapies include jaw wiring, gastric reduction operations and small-bowel bypass surgery. Jaw wiring is no more and no less than the rigid application of behavioural modification to a VLCD (or LCD) regime. It carries the same intrinsic advantages and disadvantages. The surgical options can produce very substantial weight reduction but the results are unpredictable and at best replace the hazards of severe obesity with some other problem, such as the small stomach syndrome. The inherent hazards of surgery should certainly restrict its use to a small proportion of subjects who fulfil carefully defined criteria.

Conclusion

(a) Often those subjects most wishing to lose weight are not at medical risk from their obesity, while those are high risk may have little desire to reduce.

(b) It is relatively easy to achieve weight loss but very difficult to prevent subsequent weight regain. Far more emphasis requires to be placed on weight maintenance (and obesity prevention) and possibly less on weight reduction.

(c) There are a number of effective methods of promoting weight reduction. At present however there is no reliable way of selecting those subjects most likely to benefit from any particular stratagem.

(d) At the end of the day, bearing these considerations in mind, it may be that what we try to do is less important than how we as individual therapists do it.

Chapter 29

Factors Influencing Completion and Attrition in a Weight Control Programme

R. RICHMAN, C.M. BURNS, K. STEINBECK and I. CATERSON
Department of Endocrinology, Royal Prince Alfred Hospital, Sydney, Australia

Attrition is a significant problem of weight control programmes. There are many possible factors that may influence attrition or completion of programmes. In a multidisciplinary weight control programme completers were significantly older than dropouts. They rated doctors' advice as more important in their decision to lose weight. The amount of weight lost by week 3 of the programme did not help identify completers or dropouts. Men lost more weight during the programme than women. Men nominated a desired goal weight that was significantly more than ideal weight (BMI 25), whereas women nominated a weight identical to ideal weight. This difference and the others studied failed to distinguish completers from dropouts. Demographic and weight variables are poor predictors of attrition in weight control programmes.

Introduction

Obesity is a major health problem in affluent Western communities and has adverse affects on the physical, psychological and social well-being of the individual. In 1989 the National Heart Foundation (NHF) of Australia conducted a follow-up study that indicated 60% of men and 50% of women aged 45 or over are overweight or obese[16]. The prevalence of obesity in Australia, contrary to expectations and despite public health and lifestyle promotions, has increased since the NHF study in 1983[15]. Obesity, through its associated morbidity and mortality, imposes a major financial cost to public health services. Obesity is a major risk factor in cardiovascular disease, non-insulin requiring diabetes, hypertension, hypercholesterolaemia, gall bladder disease and sleep apnoea[3,13].

Many treatment strategies have been adopted in the management of obesity[4,10]. The achievement of significant weight loss and maintenance of weight loss is difficult. However, programmes utilizing behaviour modification techniques have proven to be the most effective in the short and longer term[5,19,20]. Though programmes may be evaluated as being effective or successful the programme retention rate never reaches 100 per cent[17,20]. On examining reports of effectiveness of programmes, attrition rates are difficult to evaluate, as attrition is often dependent on the definition adopted by the particular study[11]. The reasons for attrition are unclear and probably multifactorial[2,12,14]. Reported attrition rates range from less than 10 per cent to more than 80 per cent[17,20]. Regardless of definition or reason for attrition, high attrition rates increase the relative cost of the programme and reduce the cost benefit of the programme.

The aim of this study was to identify factors that may influence completion or non-completion of a multidisciplinary behaviour-modification weight-control programme, with particular reference to weight-loss expectations and actual weight loss achieved.

Method

This is a descriptive study of 345 obese patients who enrolled in a 10-week structured behaviour-modification weight-control programme in 1989. The programme was based in a large inner-city teaching hospital. The programme emphasized change in eating and exercise patterns. The components of the programme were nutrition and exercise education, stress management techniques, methods of improving self-esteem, coping strategies and alternatives to overeating. The programme was administered on an individual basis by a primary therapist. The primary therapist was one of a multidisciplinary weight-control team, and each person in the team was available for consultation and cross-referral. Clinics were conducted in both hospital outpatient and community settings.

At the initial visit demographic, social and psychological data were collected. A brief medical, exercise and diet history was taken. Personal details were recorded and included age, sex, marital status, occupation, education level and the age of onset of obesity. It was noted if there was a family history of obesity. The number of previous attempts at weight loss was also recorded. Patients were asked "how much they would like to weigh" (desired goal weight) as well as their heaviest and lightest weight since the age of 18 years. Psychological status was assessed using Beck Depression Questionnaire (BDI)[1] and Locus of Control Questionnaire (LOC)[6].

Patients were asked to answer a 12 item questionnaire which related to reasons for enrolling in the weight control programme. Each item was rated on a scale of importance of 1 to 5 (1: not at all important; 2: slightly important; 3: somewhat important; 4: generally important; and 5: very important). The 12 items were 1: doctor's advice; 2: to improve health; 3: to improve looks; 4: to improve self-esteem; 5: to learn more about food and nutrition; 6: to learn more about exercise; 7: to learn to cope with stress; 8: to be more active; 9: to improve social interactions; 10: to improve sex life; 11: not to be different from thinner people; and 12: to improve chances of employment. These questionnaires were completed at the initial visit or returned at the second visit.

Weight was recorded using a digital platform scale with a capacity to 300 kg and accurate to 0.1 kg. Height was measured using a wall-mounted stadiometer and accurate to 0.5 cm.

Ideal weight and initial kilograms overweight were calculated from height and weight recorded at the initial visit. Ideal weight was calculated on a BMI of 25, i.e. Ideal weight = 25 x kg/m^2 and initial kilograms overweight was initial weight – ideal weight.

Patients who attended for 8 to 10 weeks of the programme were considered to have completed the programme and are referred to as completers. Patients who attended for less than 8 weeks were considered to be dropouts.

Early dropouts were those who attended only once. Patients who dropped out of the programme between the 4th and 7th week were considered late dropouts.

Statistical analysis was performed utilizing the BMDP statistical software package. Data was analysed using ANOVA, chi squared statistic, Student's t-test, simple linear correlation and multiple linear regression. Observations are mean ± SEM.

Results

One hundred and fourteen patients completed and 231 failed to complete 8 to 10 weeks of the programme. Completers, dropouts and late dropouts were similar for demographic and psychological parameters. Completers achieved a weight loss of 3.2 ± 0.4 kg during the programme, weight loss for males was 4.3 ± 0.63 kg and for females was 2.9 ± 0.41; $P < 0.05$. Completers were significantly older than dropouts. Early dropouts (n = 71) were significantly younger (36.9 ± 1.67 years) than completers (45.5 ± 1.53 years; $P < 0.001$), dropouts (41.9 ± 0.97 years; $P < 0.01$) and late dropouts (43.8 ± 1.60 years; $P < 0.01$). Early dropouts were significantly heavier (BMI 37.6 ± 1.00; $P < 0.05$) than completers (BMI 35.0 ± 0.65) and late dropouts (BMI 35.0 ± 0.80).

Table 1. Demographic variables of programme completers and dropouts

	Completers	Dropouts
Age (yr)	45.5 ± 1.53* (114)	41.9 ± 0.97 (231)
BMI (kg/m^2)	35.0 ± 0.65 (114)	36.2 ± 0.52 (224)
Age of onset of obesity (yr)	25.9 ± 1.7 (101)	24.2 ± 1.1 (38)
BDI score	9.7 ± 1.56 (30)	10.5 ± 1.54 (38)
LOC score	24.3 ± 2.02 (28)	28.2 ± 1.67 (39)
Attempts at weight loss	3.8 ± 0.48 (83)	4.5 ± 0.37 (156)

Student's t-test. *$P < 0.05$; (n) = observations.

Gender differences

Males were heavier than females but females had significantly more previous attempts at weight loss than males in both completer and dropout groups. Male completers and dropouts showed a significant difference between desired goal weight and ideal weight ($P < 0.05$), whereas for female completers and dropouts desired goal weight and ideal weight were similar.

There was not a difference in weight loss at week 3 for completers and late dropouts but there was a gender difference; females lost only half that of males at week 3. Male completers (n = 20) lost 2.29 ± 0.29 kg and female completers (n = 85) lost 1.21 ± 0.14 kg; $P < 0.01$. Similarly male (n = 13) and female dropouts (n = 80) lost 2.53 ± 0.42 kg and 0.99 ± 0.14 kg; $P < 0.001$ respectively at week 3. Weight loss was not significantly different for female completers and female dropouts.

Goal weight

Desired goal weight for completers (n = 114), dropouts (n = 224) and late dropouts (n = 76) was similar, 68.9 ± 1.22 kg, 68.7 ± 0.98 kg and 68.0 ± 1.39 kg respectively. Male completers desired goal weight was 82.2 ± 2.39 kg and ideal weight was 76.3 ± 1.61 kg; $P < 0.05$. Desired goal weight and ideal weight was 85.4 ± 2.23 kg and 75.6 ± 1.07 kg; $P < 0.05$ for male dropouts. There was a significant positive correlation for desired goal weight and ideal weight for completers (n = 92, r = 0.59; $P < 0.001$) and dropouts (n = 166, r = 0.53; $P < 0.001$). In addition, a significant positive correlation was evident for desired goal weight and initial kilograms overweight.

Table 2. Weight characteristics of male and female completers and dropouts

	Male completers	Female completers	Male dropouts	Female dropouts
BMI (kg/m^2)	36.2 ± 1.49 (25)	34.7 ± 0.72* (89)	39.2 ± 0.54 (40)	35.5 ± 0.54* (184)
Initial overweight (kg)	33.8 ± 4.17 (25)	25.0 ± 1.81†‡ (89)	42.4 ± 4.34 (40)	27.2 ± 1.40†‡ (184)
Desired goal weight (kg)	82.2 ± 2.39 (25)	65.3 ± 1.21†‡ (89)	85.4 ± 2.23 (26)	65.8 ± 0.74†‡ (147)
Ideal weight (kg)	76.3 ± 1.61 (25)	65.3 ± 0.62†‡ (89)	75.6 ± 1.07 (40)	64.8 ± 1.07†‡ (184)
Attempts at weight loss	2.6 ± 0.63 (20)	4.2 ± 0.59 (27)	2.8 ± 0.76 (24)	4.8 ± 0.41** (132)

ANOVA, (n) = observations; †$P < 0.05$, *$P < 0.05$ against male dropouts.
‡$P < 0.001$, **$P < 0.001$ against male completers.

Weight change

In completers (n = 83), using multiple regression analysis, three factors, age, degree of obesity (expressed in terms of BMI), and change in BMI at week 3 explained 29% of the variance in BMI at completion of the programme.

Even though there was no difference in weight loss at week 3 between completers and late dropouts, the independent variables age, ideal healthy weight and initial kilograms overweight accounted for 29% of the variance in weight loss at week 3 in late dropouts (n = 89) and only 15% in weight loss at week 3 in completers.

Rating of 12 item questionnaire

Doctors advice to enrol in the clinic was rated differently by completers and dropouts (χ^2 = 10.99; P = 0.03) and completers and late dropouts (χ^2 = 11.60; P = 0.02). There was not a difference in distribution of ratings for the remaining 11 items. A higher percentage of completers rated doctors advice as very important than did dropouts and late dropouts. 82.5% of completers rated doctors advise as generally or very important whilst only 56.6% of dropouts and 54.2% of late dropouts responded in this way. 81.3% of female completers rated doctor's advice as generally or very important whilst 48% of female dropouts and 48.4% female late dropouts responded in the same way.

Discussion

Numerous studies have analysed psychological, physical and social factors in an attempt to identify dropout or completer profiles[8,9,14]. The overall conclusion from such studies is that prospective identification of programme completers or non-completers is difficult and this current study has reached similar conclusions. However, most studies have found that those who complete the programme as opposed to those who dropout, are usually older[12,14]. Programme completers in this study were significantly older than dropouts and early dropouts were younger than late dropouts. This study is consistent with other reports in that the older, more overweight individual achieved a better weight loss[18].

Even though western societies appear to promote the svelte "ideal shape", this study suggests that overall, obese individuals have realistic weight-loss expectations. Desired goal weight was well correlated with ideal weight for both completers and dropouts. The nominated desired goal weight of men was some 6 to 10 kg more than ideal weight, whereas women nominated a desired goal weight identical to ideal weight. These trends may be a reflection of perceived social acceptability of greater size and weight for men[7]. Furthermore, women who dropped out of treatment had attempted weight loss on more previous occasions than men who completed the programme. Weight loss expectations influenced by social and medical norms coupled with higher attrition among younger age groups should be of major concern as these trends may be reflected in extra health care costs at a later stage.

It is obvious that many factors influence attrition and weight loss. Furthermore compliance and application are influenced by many complex issues[17]. A major area of research continues to be identification of factors which may influence programme completers and conversely non-completers. Factors such as those that may influence compliance (perceived importance of weight loss, health beliefs), attrition (age, social acceptability) and weight loss (degree of obesity, metabolic rate, age, application) are major areas of concern[17]. In this group of obese individuals, doctors' advice to lose weight appeared to be more important to those who completed the programme compared to those who did not and therefore may be of significance. Women, in particular, who dropped out of the programme rated "doctor's advice" as less important than women who completed the programme.

Consistent with other studies, this study demonstrates the difficulty in prospective identification of programme completers and non-completers by demographic and weight variables.

Conceptual models which focus on sociopsychological variables such as intention, environmental, personal, programme, demographic and attitudinal[17], may facilitate prospective identification of programme completers and non-completers.

References

1. Beck, H.T., Ward, C.H., Mendelson, M, *et al.* (1961): An inventory for measuring depression. *Arch. Gen. Psych.* **4**, 53-63.
2. Bennett, G.A. & Jones, S.E. (1986): Dropping out of treatment for obesity. *J. Psychosom. Res.* **30**, 5, 567-673.
3. Black, D. (1983): A report of the Royal College of Physicians. *J. Roy. Coll. Phys.* **17**, 5-63.
4. Bray, G.A. & Gray, D.S. (1988): Treatment of obesity: an overview. *Diabetes/Met. Rev.* **4**, 7, 653-679.
5. Brownell, K.D. & Jeffery, R.W. (1987): Improving long-term weight loss: pushing the limits of treatment. *Behav. Ther.* **18**, 353-374.
6. Craig, A.R., Franklin, J.A. & Andrew, G. (1983): A scale to measure locus of control. *Brit. J. Med. Psy.* **57**, 173-180.
7. Craig, P.L. & Caterson, I.D. (1990): Weight and perceptions of body image in women from a Sydney sample. *Comm. Health Studies* **14**, 373-383.
8. Edell, B.H., Edington, S., Herd, B., *et al.* (1987): Self efficacy and self motivation as predictors of weight loss. *Addict. Behav.* **12**, 63-66.
9. Fowler, J.L., Follick, M.J., Abrams, D.B. & Rickard-Figueroa, K. (1985): Participant characteristics as predictors of attrition in worksite weight loss. *Addict. Behav.* **10**, 445-448.
10. Garrow, J.S. (1988): *Obesity and related diseases.* London: Churchill Livingstone.
11. Kaplan, R.M. & Atkins, C.J. (1987): Selective attrition causes overestimates of treatment effects in studies of weight loss. *Addict. Behav.* **12**, 297-302.
12. Kolotkin, R.C. & Moore, J.M. (1983): Attrition in a behavioural weight control programme: a comparison of dropouts and completers. *Int. J. Eating Disorders* **2**, 93-100.
13. Kopelman, P.G., Apps, M.C.P., Cope, T., *et al.* (1986): Nocturnal hypoxia and sleep apnoea in asymptomatic obese men. *Int. J. Obesity* **10**, 211-17.
14. Mitchell, C. & Stuart, R.B. (1983): Effect of self-efficacy on dropout from obesity treatment. *J. Consult. Clin. Psych.* **52**, 6, 1100-1101.
15. National Heart Foundation of Australia. (1985): Risk factor prevalence study survey No. 2, 1983, Canberra.
16. National Heart Foundation of Australia. (1990): Risk factor prevalence study survey No. 3, 1989, Canberra.
17. Pratt, C.A. (1990): A conceptual model for studying attrition in weight reduction programs. *J. Nutr. Educ.* **22**, 4, 177-182.
18. Stein, P.M., Hassanein, R.S. & Lukert, B.P. (1981): Predicting weight loss success among obese clients in a hospital nutrition clinic. *Am. J. Clin. Nut.* **34**, 2039-2044.
19. Stunkard, A.J. (1985): Behavioural management of obesity. *MJA.* **142**, 513-520.
20. Wilson, G.T & Brownell, K.D. (1980): Behaviour therapy for obesity: an evaluation of treatment outcome. *Adv. Behav. Ther.* **3**, 49-86.

Chapter 30

Increased Resting Respiratory Quotient A Predictor of Weight Relapse in Post-obese Women

Paolo M. SUTER, Yves SCHUTZ and Eric JEQUIER
Institute of Physiology, University of Lausanne, 7 rue du Bugnon, 1005 Lausanne, Switzerland

Many factors are known to influence weight relapse after a successful weight loss programme. These risk factors for weight relapse can be arbitrarily summarized into five major groups: (a) metabolic factors, (b) nutritional factors, (c) life-style factors, (d) psychological factors and (e) miscellaneous factors (Table 1). There is growing evidence that the individual's lipid oxidizing capacity (as reflected partly in the respiratory quotient assessed during a basal metabolic or resting metabolic rate measurement) and the composition of food are major determinants in weight maintenance and weight relapse[1,6], respectively. The present study was designed to compare the effect of a high carbohydrate, high fibre diet *versus* an isocaloric mixed diet on the maintenance of weight in post-obese women.

Methods

Twenty-six post-obese women (mean ± SEM, body weight 69.3 ± 1.8 kg, BMI 26.1 ± 0.6 kg/m^2, 31.3 ± 1.1% body fat mass, were studied in a 6-month prospective study following a mean weight loss of 11.6 ± 0.9 % of predieting weight. They were randomly assigned to either a high carbohydrate, high fibre diet (65 per cent carbohydrates, 15 per cent protein, 20 per cent fat) or to a mixed diet group (40 per cent carbohydrate, 15 per cent protein and 45 per cent fat). The women were instructed to eat the assigned diet *ad libitum* and no specific energy restriction was imposed. The subjects were told to try to maintain their body weight and they were motivated to do so by frequent visits to the institute where they receive advice from a trained dietitian. Before the study and once a month during the first 4 months and at the 6th month, indirect calorimetry measurements using a ventilated hood system, body weight and body composition (using four skinfolds, bioelectrical impedance and body circumferences) were carried out[3,4]. The overall study design is summarized in Fig. 1.

Results

No significant differences in the anthropometric and metabolic characteristics between the two groups of subjects were found, neither at the start of the study, nor at the end 6 months later. Therefore the subjects were pooled for the present data analysis. Despite the dietetic intervention, body weight increased slightly but steadily during the study period and was significantly different from zero after 6 months (1.45 ± 0.64 kg, $P < 0.05$); percentage body fat showed the same trend and increased significantly until the end of the 6 month period (net change in percentage body fat: 1.71 ± 3.49%, $P < 0.05$). As expected, resting energy

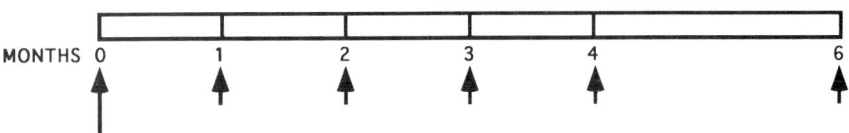

```
2 GROUPS :
  A. HIGH-CHO/FIBER DIET    n=16    65% CHO, 15% Protein, 20% Fat
  B. MIXED DIET             n=10    40% CHO, 15% Protein, 45% Fat
```

MEASUREMENTS : INDIRECT CALORIMETRY (hood)
               BODY WEIGHT
               BODY COMPOSITION (4-Skinfolds / Circumferences / Bioelectrical Impedance)

Fig. 1. Study design.

expenditure paralleled the changes in body weight and was slightly but significantly increased after 6 months (net change in resting energy expenditure: 0.07 ± 0.06 kJ/min, $P < 0.001$). Overall, there was no significant change in the respiratory quotient during the 6 month study. However, the individual changes in the respiratory quotient between the beginning and the end of the study were significantly correlated with the individual changes in body weight over the same time period ($r = 0.43$, $P < 0.05$).

Table 1. Risk factors for weight relapse

METABOLIC RISK FACTORS	BMR/RMR level
	Postprandial thermogenesis
	Endocrine factors
	Weight cycling (?)
	Low lipid oxidizing capacity
NUTRITIONAL RISK FACTORS	Dietary strategy used for weight loss and maintenance
	Food composition
LIFE STYLE FACTORS	Changes in physical activity habits
	Changes in smoking habits
PSYCHOLOGICAL RISK FACTORS	Psychological well being
	Motivation
	Compliance
MISCELLANEOUS	Sex
	Age
	Initial weight
	Duration of weight loss programme
	Type of obesity syndrome
	Eating frequency
	Genetics (?)
	Drugs

Discussion

This study revealed once more that losing weight is much easier than maintaining the weight loss. The reasons for weight relapse after a successful weight loss programme are manifold

(Table 1) and usually hard to come by in any therapeutic setting. Our subjects represented a rather heterogenous group so that no single factor for weight relapse could be identified. However, the prescribed high carbohydrate, high fibre diet (65% carbohydrate) was difficult to follow in practice and presumably compliance was achieved only with difficulty confirming previous investigations[2,5].

The data of the present study show that metabolic risk factors for weight relapse can be identified in post-obese women. The positive correlation between the individual changes in the respiratory quotient (RQ) between the study onset and the endpoints and the changes in body weight (kg) over the same time period – although weak – reveal that those subjects who demonstrated an increase in the RQ during this period had a definite tendency to increase their weight; by contrast the subjects whose RQ remained stable or whose RQ had a tendency to fall (suggesting an increased lipid oxidation) could maintain their weight and/or even showed a decline in body weight. Evidence suggests that obesity might result in part from the individuals decreased capacity to oxidize enough fat relative to glucose[1]. The latter metabolic condition might be reflected in part in a higher respiratory quotient, as in the women who gained weight.

The present study suggests that a net increase in the respiratory quotient measured in resting post-absorptive conditions during the post-dieting period, which is indicative of a diminished fat oxidation rate, may represent one predictive index among others of weight relapse in post-obese women.

References

1. Flatt, J.P. (1988): Importance of nutrient balance in body weight regulation. *Diabetes Metab. Rev.* **4**, 571-581.
2. Heaton, K.W. (1983): Dietary fiber in perspective. *Hum Nutrition: Clin Nutrition.* **37C**, 151-170.
3. Jequier, E., Acheson, K. & Schutz, Y. (1987): Assessment of energy expenditure and fuel utilization in man. *Ann. Rev. Nut.* **7**, 187-208.
4. Lukaski, H.C. (1987): Methods for the assessment of human body composition: traditional and new. *Am. J. Clin. Nutr.* **46**, 537-556.
5. Ryttig, K.R., Tellnes, G., Egh, L.H., Boe, E. & Fagerthun, H. (1989): A dietary fiber supplement and weight maintenance after weight reduction: a randomized, double blind, placebo-controlled long-term trial. *Int. J. Obes.* **13**, 165-171.
6. Van-Itallie, T.B. (1978): Dietary fiber and obesity. *Am. J. Clin. Nutr.* **31**, S43-S52.

Chapter 31

Contribution of Low Intensity Exercise Training to Treatment of Abdominal Obesity Importance of "Metabolic Fitness"

Jean-Pierre DESPRÉS, Denis PRUD'HOMME, Angelo TREMBLAY and Claude BOUCHARD

Physical Activity Sciences Laboratory, PEPS, Laval University, Ste-Foy, Quebec, Canada, G1K 7P4

It is now well established that the regional distribution of body fat is a significant risk factor for non-insulin-dependent diabetes mellitus and cardiovascular disease. In abdominal obese subjects, aerobic exercise training of low intensity and of long duration will improve insulin sensitivity and plasma lipid transport, despite modest changes in body composition and in maximal aerobic power (VO_2 max). However, our results indicate that total and abdominal fat losses are significant correlates of changes in carbohydrate and lipid metabolism in response to aerobic exercise training. These results suggest that exercise training *per se* can potentially improve metabolism in abdominal obese patients but that the exercise training related loss of body fat will be associated with further metabolic improvements. The increased insulin sensitivity appears to play a central role in improving plasma lipid transport in exercise trained individuals. From the results of several exercise training studies that we have conducted over the years, it is clear, however, that an increased cardiorespiratory fitness (as assessed by the VO_2 max test) is not required to improve indicators of "metabolic fitness", such as insulin sensitivity and plasma lipid transport, and therefore, to reduce the risk of cardiovascular disease in abdominal obese individuals. These results suggest that the improvement in VO_2 max should not be considered as an important objective of an exercise program designed for the abdominal obese patient. From a practical standpoint, it is suggested that walking at a brisk pace (about 50% of maximal aerobic power), probably represents the best exercise prescription for the treatment of the metabolic complications of abdominal obesity.

Introduction

Several studies published in the eighties have re-emphasized Vague's[35,36] notion that the regional distribution of body fat is a very significant component of the association between obesity and cardiovascular disease, and prospective studies have shown that a high proportion of abdominal fat is associated with an increased risk of cardiovascular disease and related mortality[18,19,26,27,33]. Abdominal obesity has also been associated with insulin resistance, hyperinsulinaemia, glucose intolerance, dyslipoproteinaemias, and hypertension[2-5,22-25,32,35,36].

The development of computed tomography (CT) as a means of assessing the amount of deep and subcutaneous abdominal fat at any site of the body[30] has substantially improved our ability to precisely and reliably assess the regional deposition of body fat. We have studied the potential associations between the accumulation of deep abdominal fat measured by CT and metabolism in a sample of obese premenopausal women and we have reported, in concordance with results of others[20,28,29,31] that the amount of deep abdominal fat was the best correlate of glucose tolerance[10] and of lipoprotein ratios[12] used in the estimation of the risk of coronary heart disease. Furthermore, obese women with low levels of deep abdominal fat only showed moderate changes in metabolism, suggesting that they were not substantially more at risk for CHD than non-obese women[14]. We have obtained essentially similar results in men (Pouliot et al., unpublished observations). These results emphasize the importance of deep abdominal fat accumulation as opposed to obesity *per se* as a risk factor for diabetes and CHD[15].

Effects of exercise on body fat distribution and related metabolism

As endurance exercise has beneficial effects on insulin sensitivity[1] and on plasma lipid transport[21], we have studied the adaptation of body composition, body fat distribution, and metabolism to prolonged aerobic exercise training. When no control over energy intake was performed, we have systematically found that men are more sensitive to exercise training-induced weight loss than women[6,11,34]. When weight loss occurs, fat-free mass is generally preserved by endurance exercise training and the loss of body weight is mainly explained by the reduction in body fat mass[6,11,34]. In both sexes, there seems to be a preferential mobilization of abdominal fat in comparison with femoral fat. However, changes in plasma lipid transport induced by aerobic exercise training appear to be dissociated from changes in cardiorespiratory fitness as assessed by the response of $\dot{V}O_2$ max, whereas changes in plasma cholesterol levels are proportionate to the amount of weight and central fat losses (Després et al., unpublished observations).

In another exercise training study in which subjects exercised 2 h/day for 22 consecutive days[7], we reported that the greater the amount of central fat loss during exercise training, the greater were the reductions in plasma cholesterol, apoprotein B, LDL-cholesterol, and insulin levels at the end of the training programme. Furthermore, the greater was the increase in insulin sensitivity, the greater were the decreases in plasma cholesterol, LDL-cholesterol and apoprotein B levels[7]. These results are the first to indicate that changes in the amount of abdominal fat produced by prolonged endurance training are a significant component of the effects of endurance exercise training on metabolism.

We have also studied the effects of endurance exercise training in a group of obese premenopausal women who performed 90 min exercise sessions, 4–5 times per week[8]. After 6 months, although no significant change in body composition had occured, significant changes in plasma lipid transport were noted, especially in women with initially high levels of abdominal fat[16]. These results indicate that exercise training *per se* may have beneficial effects on the metabolic profile of abdominal obese subjects even under circumstances where no loss of body fat is noted. We have also used a similar exercise training protocol for a longer period of time (14 months) in order to induce significant changes in body composition in obese women[17]. However, changes in metabolism induced by the exercise training programme were, once again, not correlated with changes in $\dot{V}O_2$ max, but were significantly correlated with losses of total, abdominal and visceral fat[17]. Two conclusions can be derived from these observations. First, no change in body composition is necessary to observe beneficial effects of exercise training on metabolism. However, when losses of total and abdominal fat are noted, further improvements in insulin sensitivity and in plasma lipid transport will be observed. Secondly, the improvement in cardiorespiratory fitness does not appear to determine the adaptation of carbohydrate and lipid metabolism to endurance exercise training[9].

This last notion has substantial implications for the treatment of the metabolic complications of abdominal obesity as it implies that emphasis should be placed on the improvement of "metabolic fitness" rather than on cardiorespiratory fitness. To test this last notion further, we have exercise trained moderately obese men for a period of 100 days, during which they exercised at low intensity (about 50% of their $\dot{V}O_2$max) 2 h per day, for a period of 100 days[13].

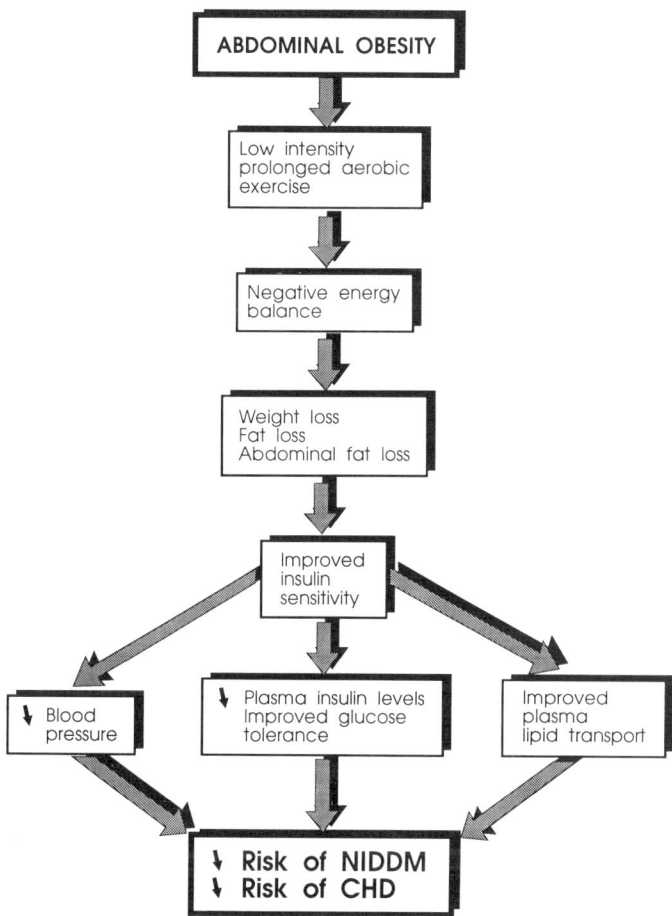

Fig. 1. Effects of low intensity, prolonged aerobic exercise training (1 h/session, at about 40–50% VO_2 max, 5-6 sessions/week) on body composition, the level of abdominal fat, and on related metabolism in abdominal obese patients. From the model presented, it is suggested that emphasis should be placed on exercise duration rather than intensity when aiming at the reduction of the risk of non-insulin-dependent diabetes mellitus (NIDDM) and coronary heart disease (CHD) in these individuals.

The exercise intensity was such that, at the end of the training programme, no significant increase in maximal oxygen uptake was noted. A substantial weight loss was, however, observed which was accompanied by substantial improvements in insulin sensitivity and in plasma lipid transport[13]. These results clearly support the notion that the metabolic and cardiorespiratory adapatations to aerobic exercise training are dissociated.

Effects of low intensity aerobic exercise training on CHD risk in abdominal obese patients: importance of "metabolic fitness"

As summarized in Fig. 1, results that we have obtained in our laboratory support the use of low-intensity prolonged exercise, performed regularly, in the treatment of the metabolic complications associated with abdominal obesity. Doubts can be raised, however, on the ability of endurance exercise alone to normalize body weight in most obese individuals. However, endurance exercise can potentially improve carbohydrate and lipid metabolism in the obese patient, even in situations where body weight is far from being normalized. In this regard, it appears that regular exercise, performed at an intensity corresponding to walking at a brisk pace (about 50% VO_2max) has very significant metabolic effects, despite the lack of substantial improvement in cardiorespiratory fitness. We believe that our results provide evidence that the improvement of "metabolic fitness" (insulin sensitivity, plasma lipid transport) rather than cardiorespiratory fitness should be the main objective when aiming at the reduction of CHD risk by aerobic exercise training in abdominal obese patients. Prolonged vigorous walking, performed on an almost daily basis, probably represents the best and most tolerable exercise prescription for the treatment of the metabolic complications of abdominal obesity.

Acknowledgements

Supported by the Quebec Heart Foundation, the Canadian Diabetes Association, the Medical Research Council of Canada, the National Institutes of Health, the Natural Sciences and Engineering Research Council of Canada, the Canadian Fitness and Lifestyle Research Institute, and by the Fonds de la Recherche en Santé du Québec (FRSQ). J.P. Després is a FRSQ research scholar.

References

1. Björntorp, P. (1981): The effects of exercise on plasma insulin. *Int. J. Sports Med.* **2**, 125-129.
2. Björntorp, P. (1985): Obesity and the risk of cardiovascular disease. *Ann. Clin. Res.* **17**, 3-9.
3. Björntorp, P. (1988): Abdominal obesity and the development of non-insulin-dependent diabetes mellitus. *Diabetes Metab. Rev.* **4**, 615-622.
4. Björntorp, P. (1990): Portal adipose tissue as a generator of risk factors for cardiovascular disease and diabetes. *Arteriosclerosis* **10**, 493-496.
5. Bouchard, C., Bray, G.A. & Hubbard, V.S. (1990): Basic and clinical aspects of regional fat distribution. *Am. J. Clin. Nutr.* **52**, 946-950.
6. Després J.P., Bouchard, C., Savard, R., Tremblay A., Marcotte M. & Thériault, G. (1984): Effect of a 20 week endurance training program on adipose tissue morphology and lipolysis in men and women. *Metabolism* **33**, 235-239.
7. Després, J.P., Moorjani, S., Tremblay, A., Poehlman, E.T., Lupien, P.J., Nadeau, A. & Bouchard, C. (1988): Heredity and changes in plasma lipids and lipoproteins after short-term exercise training in men. *Arteriosclerosis* **8**, 402-409.
8. Després, J.P., Tremblay, A., Nadeau, A. & Bouchard, C. (1988): Physical training and changes in regional adipose tissue distribution. *Acta Med. Scand.* **723**, 205-212.
9. Després, J.P. (1989): Physical activity and the risk of coronary heart disease. *Can. Med. Assoc. J.* **141**, 939.
10. Després, J.P., Nadeau, A., Tremblay, A., Ferland, M., Moorjani, S., Lupien, P.J., Thériault, G., Pinault, S. & Bouchard, C. (1989): Role of deep abdominal fat in the association between regional adipose tissue distribution and glucose tolerance in obese women. *Diabetes* **38**, 304-309.
11. Després, J.P., Tremblay A. & Bouchard, C. (1989): Sex differences in the regulation of body fat mass with exercise training. In *Obesity in Europe I*, eds. Björntorp, P. & S. Rossner, pp. 297-304. London: John Libbey & Co. Ltd.
12. Després, J.P., Moorjani, S., Ferland, M., Tremblay, A., Lupien, P.J., Nadeau, A., Pinault, S., Thériault, G. & Bouchard, C. (1989): Adipose tissue distribution and plasma lipoprotein levels in obese women: importance of intra-abdominal fat. *Arteriosclerosis* **9**, 203-210.
13. Després, J.P., Tremblay A., Moorjani S., Lupien P.J., Thériault, G., Nadeau, A. & Bouchard, C. (1989): Long-term exercise-training with constant energy intake. 3: Effects on plasma lipoprotein levels. *Int. J. Obesity* **14**, 85-94.
14. Després, J.P., Moorjani, S., Lupien, P.J., Tremblay, A., Nadeau, A. & Bouchard, C. (1990): Regional distribution of body fat, plasma lipoproteins, and cardiovascular disease. *Arteriosclerosis* **10**, 497-511.

15. Després, J.P. (1991): Obesity and lipid metabolism: relevance of body fat distribution. *Curr. Op. Lipidol.* **2**, 5-15.
16. Després, J.P. (1991): Obesity, regional adipose tissue distribution and metabolism: effect of exercise. *Proceedings of the International Symposium on Diet and Obesity*, Tsukuba, Japan, ed. M. Suzuki (in press).
17. Després, J.P., Pouliot, M.C., Moorjani, S., Nadeau, A., Tremblay, A., Lupien, P.J., Thériault, G. & Bouchard, C. (1991): Loss of abdominal fat and metabolic response to exercise training in obese women. *Am. J. Physiol. (Endocrinol. Metab.)*, **261**, E159-E167.
18. Donahue, R.P., Abbott, R.D., Bloom, E., Reed, D.M. & Yano, K. (1987): Central obesity and coronary heart disease in men. *Lancet* **i**, 822-824.
19. Ducimetière, P., Richard, J. & Cambien, F. (1986): The pattern of subcutaneous fat distribution in middle-aged men and the risk of coronary heart disease: The Paris Prospective Study. *Int. J. Obesity* **10**, 229-240.
20. Fujioka, S., Matsuzawa, Y., Tokunaga, K. & Tarui, S. (1987): Contribution of intra-abdominal fat accumulation to the impairment of glucose and lipid metabolism in human obesity. *Metabolism* **36**, 54-59.
21. Haskell, W.L. (1984): Exercise-induced changes in plasma lipids and lipoproteins. *Prevent. Med.* **13**, 23-26.
22. Kissebah, A.H., Evans, D.J., Peiris, A. & Wilson, C.R. (1985): Endocrine characteristics in regional obesities: role of sex steroids. In *Metabolic complications of human obesities.* eds. J. Vague, P. Björntorp, B. Guy-Grand, M. Rebuffé-Scrive & P. Vague, pp. 115-130. Amsterdam: Elsevier Science Publishers.
23. Kissebah, A.H., Peiris, A.N. & Evans, D.J. (1988): Mechanisms associating body fat distribution to glucose intolerance and diabetes mellitus: a window with a view. *Acta Med. Scand.* **S723**, 79-89.
24. Kissebah, A.H., Freedman, D.S. & Peiris, A.N. (1989): Health risks of obesity. *Med. Clin. North Am.* **73**, 111-138.
25. Kissebah, A.H. & Peiris, A.N. (1989): Biology of regional body fat distribution: relationship to non-insulin-dependent diabetes mellitus. *Diabetes Metab. Rev.* **5**, 83-109.
26. Lapidus, L., Bengtsson, C., Larsson, B., Pennert, K., Rybo, E. & Sjöström, L. (1984): Distribution of adipose tissue and risk of cardiovascular disease and death: a 12 year follow-up of participants in the population study of women in Gothenburg, Sweden. *Br. Med. J.* **289**, 1261-1263.
27. Larsson, B., Svärdsudd, K., Welin, L., Wilhemsen, L., Björntorp, P. & Tibblin, G. (1984): Abdominal adipose tissue distribution, obesity and risk of cardiovascular disease and death: 13 year follow-up of participants in the study of men born in 1913. *Br. Med. J.* **288**, 1401-1404.
28. Peiris, A.N., Sothmann, M.S., Hennes, M.I., *et al.* (1989): Relative contribution of obesity and body fat distribution to alterations in glucose insulin homeostasis: predictive values of selected indices in premenopausal women. *Am. J. Clin. Nutr.* **49**, 758-764.
29. Peiris, A.N., Sothmann, M.S., Hoffmann, R.G., *et al.* (1989): Adiposity, fat distribution, and cardiovascular risk. *Ann. Intern. Med.* **110**, 867-872.
30. Sjöström, L., Kvist, H., Cederblad, A. & Tylen, U. (1986): Determination of total adipose tissue and body fat in women by computed tomography, ^{40}K, and tritium. *Am. J. Physiol.* **250**, E736-E745.
31. Sparrow, D., Borkan, G.A., Gerzof, S.G., Wisniewski, C. & Silbert, C.K. (1986): Relationship of body fat distribution to glucose tolerance. Results of computed tomography in male participants of the normative aging study. *Diabetes* **35**, 411-415.
32. Stern, M.P. & Haffner, S.M. (1986): Body fat distribution and hyperinsulinemia as risk factors for diabetes and cardiovascular disease. *Arteriosclerosis* **6**, 123-130.
33. Stokes, J. III, Garrison, R.J. & Kannel, W.B. (1985): The independent contributions of various indices of obesity to the 22-year incidence of coronary heart disease: The Framingham heart study. In *Metabolic complications of human obesities.* eds. J. Vague, P. Björntorp, B. Guy-Grand, M. Rebuffé-Scrive & P. Vague, pp. 49-57. Amsterdam: Elsevier Science Publishers.
34. Tremblay, A., Després, J.P., Leblanc, C. & Bouchard, C. (1984): Sex dimorphism in fat loss in response to exercise-training. *J. Ob. Weight Regul.* **3**, 193-203.
35. Vague, J. (1947): La différenciation sexuelle, facteur déterminant des formes de l'obésité. *Presse Méd.* **30**, 339-340.
36. Vague, J. (1956): The degree of masculine differentiation of obesities: a factor determining predisposition to diabetes, atherosclerosis, gout, and uric calculous disease. *Am. J. Clin. Nutr.* **4**, 20-34.

Chapter 32

Long Term Result of Surgical Treatment of Obesity with Vertical Banded Gastroplasty

A. LAURENT-JACCARD[1], C. WYSS[1], P. BURCKHARDT[2] and A. JAYET[3]
[1]Medical Policlinic, [2]Department of Internal Medicine, [3]Service of Surgery, University Hospital, CHUV, 1011 Lausanne, Switzerland

For evaluation of long term results of vertical banded gastroplasty, 51 patients (four men, 47 women) were investigated by a computerized interview 56.3 (± 3.3 SEM) months after the operation. Their mean preoperative BMI was 41.4 (± 0.7 SEM) kg/m^2. Mean age was 37.5 years. Success was defined as a loss of at least 40 per cent of excess body weight, with good quality of life and without reoperations. Before operation, the mean BMI of the 31 successes was not different from that of the 20 failures (41.5 vs 41.4). At 12 months, it was 26.9 (± 1.3) vs 30.8 (± 1.3). At the time of the interview, it was 27.4 (± 0.6 SEM) vs 34.8 (± 0.8 SEM). Failures were due to reoperation because of excessive weight loss[4], to incomplete weight loss[13], and to insufficient gain in quality of life despite sufficient weight loss[2]. Postoperative morbidity (more than one unrelated diseases) was higher in the failure group (7/19, vs 5/32). There were no significant differences in snacking, number of meals, and food preferences. In conclusion, VBG is an effective treatment of morbid obesity (but not of superobesity), even if this is less evident in the long term than in short term studies.

Introduction

As with all other operations for morbid obesity, vertical banded gastroplasty (VBG) does not guarantee that the individual patient will have successful weight loss with a good quality of life. Few studies present results of VBG for more than 3 years after the operation[6,3]. The aim of this retrospective study was to assess the effect of VBG on body weight and on quality of life for several years.

Patients and method

Of 63 consecutive patients with BMI > 35.5 kg/m^2 who underwent VBG between December 1981 and December 1988, 51 were revisited 56.3 $\pm$ 3.3 months (24–95) post-operative, eight could not be found, one had left the country, and three refused to participate in the study. The mean age of these four men and 47 women was 37.5 years (17–58).

Vertical banded gastroplasty was performed with a double staple line according to the technique described by Mason[7]. Patients were investigated by a computerized interview. Their mean preoperative body weight was 194.4 per cent (± 3.4 SEM) of the mean ideal weight determined by the use of Metropolitan Life Insurance tables[9] and their mean BMI was 41.4 (± 0.7 SEM). Success was defined as a loss of at least 40 per cent of excess body weight, with good quality of life, and without reoperations. The data are expressed as the mean $\pm$ SEM or as a percentage. Comparisons were made by the Fisher test.

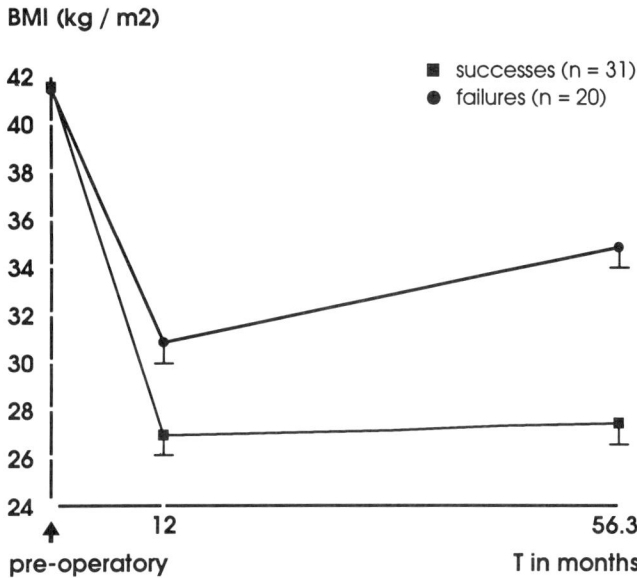

Fig. 1. Post-operative mean body weight evolution.

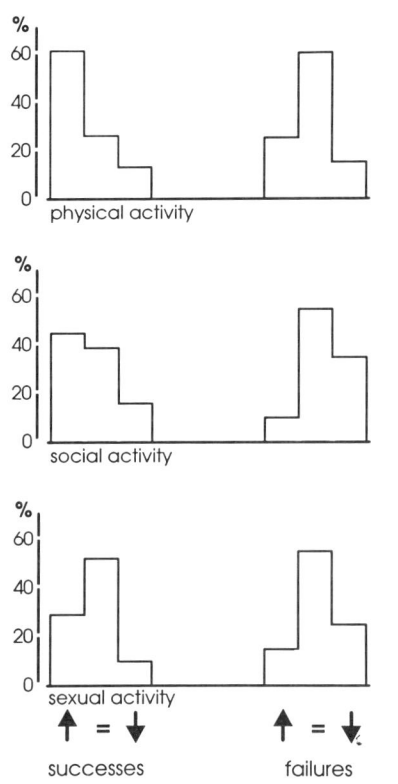

Fig. 2. Long-term effect of the VBG on physical, social and sexual activity.

Results

Thirty-one patients were defined as successes (loss of at least 40 per cent of excess body weight, with good quality of life, and without reoperations), 20 as failures (14 for incomplete weight loss, four for reoperation because of excessive weight loss, two for insufficient gain in quality of life). The psychosocial profile of the two groups was similar. Both had a prevalence of parental obesity. The frequency of child onset and adult onset of obesity was identical in the two groups. The maximum weight loss was reached after a median time of 12 months (Fig. 1). Table 1 gives the mean body weight in per cent of the ideal weight and the mean BMI preoperative, 12 months postoperative and at the moment of the interview. Of the 51 patients, 29 returned to a BMI below 30, 21 to a BMI between 30 and 35. Four patients had a superobesity (BMI > 50) before the operation. Three of them could not reach a BMI under 30. One patient in the failure group did not lose any weight and had had a failed jejunoileal bypass which had been converted to a gastroplasty. This evolution of weight is similar to the one described by Pessa et al.[10].

In the early postoperative period, gastroplasty was complicated in the success group by one pulmonar embolism (four in the failure group), two wound dehiscence (three in the failures), one wound infection (one in the failures), one rupture of the staple line (none in the failures).

Table 2 shows the long-term complications observed in both groups. The only significant difference ($P < 0.05$) between successes and failures concerns oesophagitis and gastritis, more frequent in the failure group. Table 3 shows the concomitant diseases existing before and after gastroplasty in the two groups.

Table 1. Mean body weight evolution post VBG in per cent of the ideal weight and in BMI

Body weight	Before gastroplasty	After 12 months	At follow up
Successes			
% Ideal weight	194.5 ± 4.5 SEM	126 ± 6.1 SEM	128.6 ± 2.9 SEM
BMI (kg/m^2)	41.5 ± 1 SEM	26.9 ± 1.3 SEM	27.4 ± 0.6 SEM
Failures			
% Ideal weight	194.5 ± 5.1 SEM	144.3 ± 6 SEM	163.6 ± 3.8 SEM
BMI (kg/m^2)	41.4 ± 1.1 SEM	30.8 ± 1.3 SEM	34.8 ± 0.8 SEM

Table 2. Long-term complications after VBG

Long term complications	failures 20	successes 31
Deficiencies		●●●●
Abdominal pain	■■■■	
Cholelithiasis	■■■	●●
Nausea, vomiting	■■■■■■■■■■	●●●●●●●●●●●●●●●
Oesophagitis, gastritis	■■■■■■■	●●●
Duodenal ulcer	■	●●
Constipation	■■■■■	●●●●●●●

Table 3. Concomitant diseases existing before and after VBG

Diseases	before gastroplasty		after gastroplasty	
	successes 31	failures 20	successes 31	failures 20
Arthritis	●●●●	■■	●●●●	■■■■
Back pain	●●●●●●●●●●	■■■■■■■■■■	●●●	■■■■■
Digestive troubles	●●●●	■■	●●●●●●	■■■■■■■
Hypertension	●●●●●●●	■■■■■	●	■■■■■■
Diabetes	●●●	■■■		
Depression	●●●●●●●●●●●●●●●●	■■■■■■■	●●	■

The long term effect of the gastroplasty on physical, social and sexual activity are shown in Fig. 2. Of the 10 singles in the success group, six got married, but none of the four singles in the failure group did.

There were no significant differences in snacking, number of meals and food preferences. Seventy-three per cent of the patients answered positively to the question if they would still accept gastroplasty, once they knew its consequences.

Discussion

Our definition of success is restrictive; the need for revisional surgery has been classified as a treatment failure, as in other studies[6]; in addition, quality of life was considered as an essential criteria of success. Fifty-seven per cent of the patients returned to a BMI below 30, but only one of the four patients with superobesity, as already observed by Mason[8]. Sugerman and co-workers[11] have noted a correlation between patients addicted to sweets and failures after VBG. We could not find any significant difference in our two groups regarding the preference for sweets.

In the long-term complications after gastroplasty, we have four cases of anaemia, which can occur after gastroplasty, as well as after gastric bypass. The incidence of postoperative cholelithiasis is similar to that reported in the literature[2]. Frequent vomiting was reported by Haydock and McIntosh[5]; our study shows that this symptom is still present after several years. Four patients were reoperated for stenotic outlet; this number is comparable with the literature[6].

Bull et al.[1] did not find alterations in eating habits studied after gastric surgery in 114 patients, except a decrease in quantity of food eaten. But in our patients only four could tolerate free access to all food items. The decrease in the number of depressions observed in both groups, is reported by Hawke and collaborators[4]. Haydock and Jarvie mention an improvement of libido and sexual relationships after gastroplasty[12] as also observed in the success group of this study.

Conclusion

The vertical banded gastroplasty is an efficient treatment of morbid obesity, but not in superobesity. However, the persistence of some complications for several years, such as nausea, vomiting, oesophagitis, gastritis and anaemia, suggests the necessity for a life-long medical follow-up at regular intervals.

References

1. Bull, R.H., Engels, W.D., Engelsmann, F. & Bloom, L. (1983): Behavioural changes following gastric surgery for morbid obesity: a prospective controlled study. *J. Psychosom. Res.* **27**, 457-467.
2. Deitel, M. & Petrov, I. (1987): Incidence of symptomatic gallstones after bariatric operations. *Surg. Gynecol. Obstet.* **164**, 549-552.
3. Hall, J.C., Watts, J.M., O'Brien, P.E., Dunstan, R.E., Walsh, J.F., Slavotinek, A.H. & Elmslie, R.G. (1990): Gastric surgery for morbid obesity. The Adelaide study. *Ann. Surg.* **211** (4), 419-427.
4. Hawke, A., O'Brien, P.E., Watts, J.M., Hall, J.C., Dunstan R.E., Walsh, J.F., Slavotinek, A.H. & Elmslie, R.G. (1990): Psychosocial and physical activity changes after gastric restrictive procedures for morbid obesity. *Aust. N. Z. J. Surg.* **60** (10), 755-758.
5. Haydock, C.A., McIntosh M.K. & Rupp, W.M. (1990): Vertical banded gastroplasty : follow up assessment of weight loss and nutritional status. *J. Am. Diet. Assoc.* **90** (9), A-69.
6. MacLean, L.D., Rhode, B.M. & Forse, R.A. (1990): Late results of vertical banded gastroplasty for morbid and super obesity. *Surgery* **107** (1), 20-27.
7. Mason, E.E. (1982): Vertical banded gastroplasty for obesity. *Arch. Surg.* **117**, 701-706.
8. Mason, E.E., Doherty, C., Maher, J.W., Scott, D.H., Rodriguez, E.M. & Blommers, T.J. (1987): Superobesity and gastric reduction procedures. *Gastroenterol. Clin. North Am.* **16**, 495-502.
9. Metropolitan Life Foundation (1983): Height and weight tables. New York: Metropolitan Life Insurance Company.
10. Pessa, M., Robertson, J. & Woodward, E. (1986): Surgical management of the failed jejunoileal bypass. *The Am. J. of Surg.* **151**, 364-367.
11. Sugerman, H.J., Londrey, G.L., Kellum, J.M., Wolf, L., Liszka, T., Engle, K.M., Birkenhauer, R. & Starkey, J.V. (1989): Weight loss with vertical banded gastroplasty and Roux-Y gastric bypass for morbid obesity with selective versus random assignment. *Am. J. Surg.* **157** (1), 93-102.
12. William, R.C. & Jarvie, G.J. (1986): Psychological sequelae of bariatric surgery: assessment of psychosocial effects of vertical banded gastroplasty patients. Presented at Southwestern Psychological Association, March 1986.

Chapter 33

Treatment of Abdominal Obese Men with Testosterone

Per MÅRIN, Sten HOLMÄNG*, Göran HOLM, Lars JÖNSSON and Per BJÖRNTORP

Departments of Medicine I and Urology, Sahlgren's Hospital, University of Göteborg, Sweden*

Testosterone in a preparation by-passing the liver or placebo was given in a double-blind randomized manner to 23 middle-aged men with abdominal type of obesity during 8 months. Before and after treatment the following examinations were performed: euglycaemic glucose clamps at submaximal insulin levels, anthropometric measurements, including sagittal diameter (indicating intra-abdominal fat mass), estimations of body fat and lean body mass from measurements of whole body potassium, fasting glucose and insulin concentrations, cholesterol and triglyceride concentrations, liver function tests, blood pressures and physical examination including the prostate.

The body weight did not change in either group during the study but the sagittal diameter decreased significantly in both groups, more pronounced in the testosterone group. Diastolic blood pressure, serum cholesterol and fasting glucose decreased in the testosterone group with no change in the placebo group. In parallel, insulin sensitivity was improved in the testosterone group compared to the placebo group. Those men with the lowest initial serum testosterone showed greatest improvement of insulin resistance. A feeling of psychological comfort was reported by 30 per cent in the testosterone group and by 10 per cent in the placebo group. Routine blood measurements including liver parameters were followed throughout the study. No side-effects were noted. The prostate volume increased 10 per cent in volume in the testosterone group but no subjective changes in voiding were noted.

We conclude that middle-aged men with abdominal obesity, especially those with low plasma testosterone, can successfully be improved metabolically by testosterone substitution.

Section VI
Obesity and related disorders

Chapter 34

Obesity and Related Disorders

H. DITSCHUNEIT
Department of Internal Medicine II, University of Ulm, D-7900 Ulm, Germany

Obesity is characterized by a disturbed ratio between "lean body mass" and fat body mass with an abnormal increase of the latter. The exact assessment of fat body mass requires sophisticated methodologies, which are not suitable for epidemiological and clinical studies. These studies usually rely on the determination of body mass index (BMI) on the basis of weight and height. For scientific purpose different methodologies are available for the assessment of body fat mass; in our experience, densitometry is the most reliable[27]. With this method the determination of body fat mass is precise with a mean error less than 100 g.

Insufficient grading of obesity by body weight and height

In a practical example I would like to point out the unreliability of BMI for the exact assessment of obesity. Two male patients had a BMI of 31.77 and 32.17 respectively, almost no difference. By densitometry we calculated 13.9 kg of fat, corresponding to 14.1 per cent of the body weight in one, and 37.2 kg corresponding to 33 per cent of the body weight in the other. This example emphasizes how a 1.3 per cent higher BMI may correspond to a 2.6-fold higher fat body mass (Fig. 1).

In juvenile patients and children, calculations on the basis of body weight and height are almost useless. By measuring skinfold thickness we recognized that girls have a much higher body fat mass as compared to boys. If "obesity" is defined as a twofold increase of fat body mass above normal controls and "overweight" as a 20% increase above the percentiles for body weight and height then a considerable proportion of obese children have normal weight (34 per cent of girls and 41 per cent of boys) and a considerable proportion of children with overweight are lean (62 per cent of girls and 38 per cent of boys)[3] (Fig. 2).

It is my intention to start my talk with these examples to depict the uncertainties of metabolic investigations based on fat body mass calculated by indirect means. In the individual case, the health risk related to obesity cannot be based on body weight and body height. And all studies intended to discover the relationship of metabolic disturbances and obesity which are based simply on height and weight are critical.

A further point in the evaluation of obesity as cause of secondary metabolic disorders arises from the fact that the regional disposition of fatty tissue plays a differential role in causing metabolic disturbances. This observation was first made by Vague[26]. In the meanwhile the number of publications on this topic is enormous. All these later studies confirmed the original clinical observation made by Vague.

Clinically we distinguish two types of obesity, the android and gynoid type, which are also nominated central or peripheral obesity. A fundamental metabolic aspect of these two types of obesity is the difference in insulin sensitivity, as shown by the oral glucose tolerance test[2,15]. Metabolically, android type obesity with increased fat mass in the abdominal region is of the greatest importance. The abnormal fat increase in obesity is primarily due to

		patient K.N. 176 cm, 98,4 kg	patient P.H. 187 cm, 112,5 kg
BMI	(kg × m^{-2})	31,77	32,17
overweight above ideal weight *	(%) (kg)	44,5 30,3	48,0 36,5
density	(g/cm^3)	1,0666	1,0247
body fat mass **	(%) (kg)	14,1 13,9	33,0 37,2
fat-free body mass **	(%) (kg)	85,9 84,5	67,0 75,3

* tables of Metr. Life Ins. Co., 1959
calculated by $y_1 = 0{,}9$ g/cm^3 and $y_2 = 1{,}1$ g/cm^3 according the Archimedic principle.

Fig. 1. Body density and composition of two patients with comparable overweight.

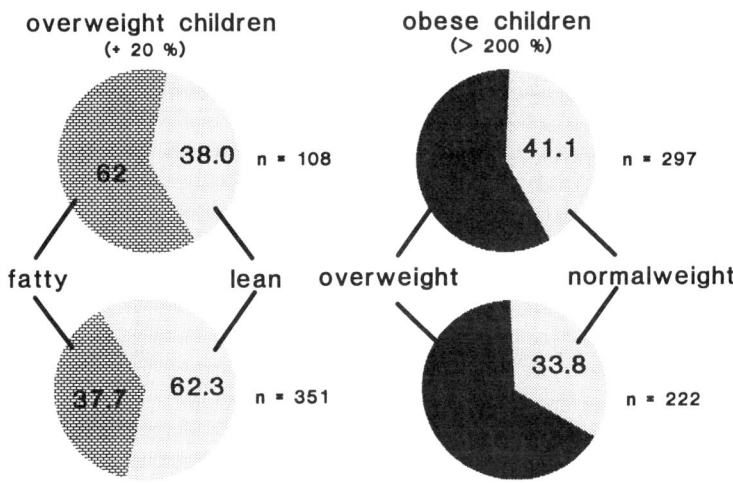

Fig. 2. Prevalance of fatty and lean boys (n=108) and girls (n=351), 4–16 year old, in overweight children and overweight and normalweight boys (n=297) and girls (n=222) in obese children (>200% of normal fat mass).

hypertrophy of adipocytes and only when the weight exceeds 60 per cent of the ideal body weight and the diameter of adipocytes increases above 100 μm does hyperplasia takes place also[6].

Fat cell size and intensified lipolysis, the base for metabolic disorders in obesity

The size of adipocytes in the abdominal region and obesity are closely correlated and this confirms that the increase in fat body mass in adults as well as in children is generally associated with cell hypertrophy[2,6]. With gynoid type obesity, by contrast, hyperplasia of adipocytes in the lower body is the dominating morphological appearance[15].

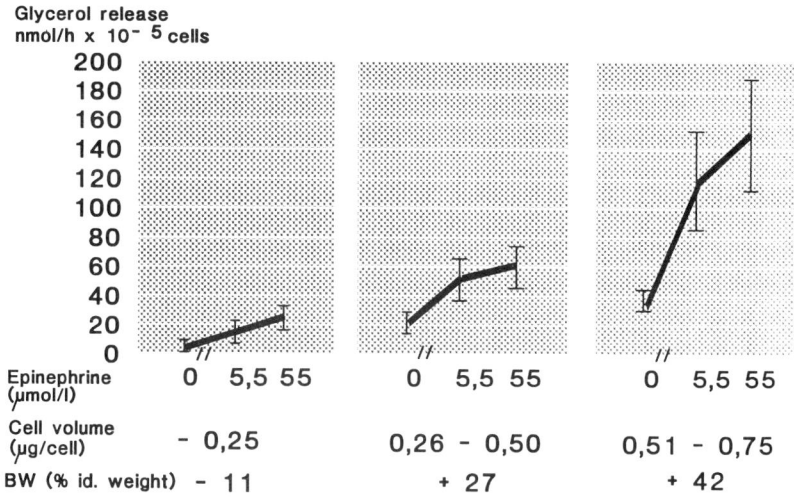

Fig. 3. Epinephrine-induced lipolysis in human fat cells of different size.

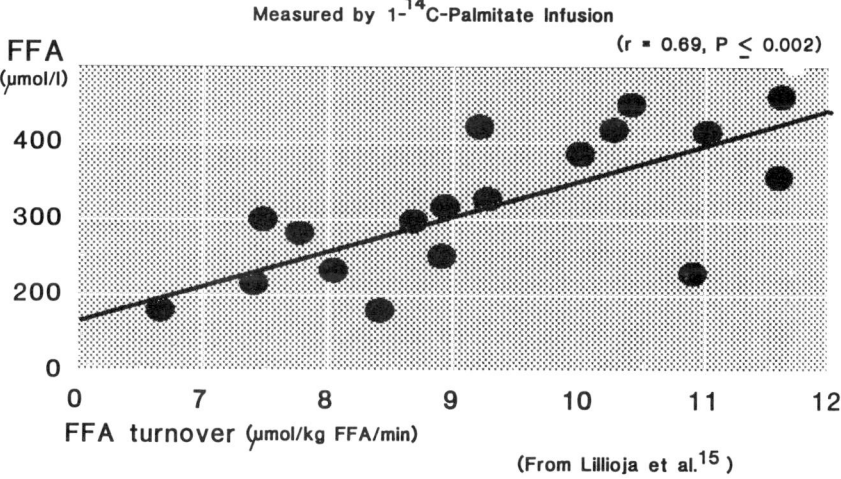

(From Lillioja et al.[15])

Fig. 4. Correlation of basal FFA concentration and basal FFA turnover.

The cell size of adipocytes is of primary importance for all metabolic disturbances. With the increasing size of these cells there is an increase in the basal and catecholamine-stimulated rate of lipolysis[2,7]. In subjects with a body weight reduced to −11 per cent of mean body weight, adipocytes release 3.18 nmol/h x 10^{-5} cells of glycerol, while adipocytes of control subjects with a mean weight of +27 per cent above normal show an increase in the rate of lipolysis up to 20.44; finally in patients with obesity of +42 per cent the lipolysis is further increased up to 33.56 nmol. Stimulation with 0.1 µg/ml epinephrine induces an expotential increase of lipolysis (Fig. 3). A threefold increase in cell size leads to a nine- to 10-fold increase in the rate of lipolysis. The antilipolytic effect of insulin is significantly decreased in large adipocytes[2,7].

These *in vitro* results agree very well with clinical observations. Obese patients, especially those with android type obesity, have increased serum concentrations of free fatty acids.

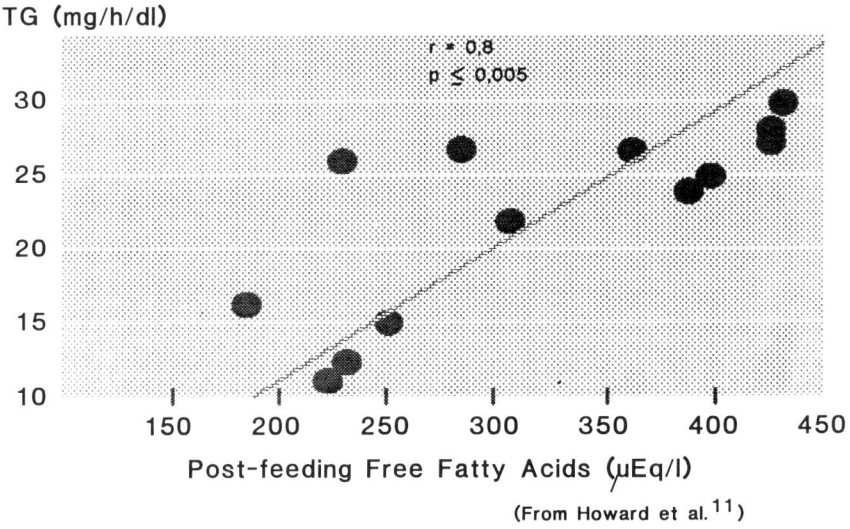

Fig. 5. Relation between VLDL-TG synthesis and FFA.

Patients with android type obesity have a twofold higher free fatty acid serum concentration during the night as compared to patients with gynoid type obesity, despite a comparable body mass index. In patients with android type obesity, hyperinsulinaemia and an abnormal oral glucose tolerance test, lipolysis increases during physical exercise much more than in slim persons. The increased oxidation of free fatty acids in these patients is shown by an increase of β-oxybutyric acid, as we always observed in our studies[2].

Free fatty acids, that are derived from lypolysis of adipocytes, are either oxidized or used for the hepatic synthesis of triglycerides. Consequently an increased rate of lipolysis is equivalent to an increased synthesis of triglycerides and also increased lipid oxidation. A large body of evidence for this pathway is derived from clinical experiments, and animal models as well as from studies on isolated tissues and organs. Researchers in Phoenix, Arizona[16] reported on a close positive correlation between serum concentrations of free fatty acids and their metabolism (Fig. 4). As already mentioned, part of the metabolic degradation of free fatty acids occurs by oxidation, but a much higher proportion of free fatty acids are used for the hepatic synthesis of triglycerides, released from the liver as VLDL into the blood. The concentration of free fatty acids correlates with the size of adipocytes and also with the degree of obesity[23] and finally also with the concentration of serum triglycerides (Fig. 5)[12,21].

Glucose and free fatty acids are competitive substrates in energy metabolism

Randle and co-workers[9] first reported in 1963 on reciprocal interactions between lipids and carbohydrates in the intermediary energy metabolism of cells. These interactions were formally nominated "glucose/fatty-acid cycle". The authors demonstrated on the isolated heart and diaphragm of rats that fatty acids (NEFA) and ketone-bodies inhibit glucose uptake, glycolysis and pyruvate oxidation. This result led to the hypothesis that NEFA and ketone-bodies inhibit glucose catabolism in muscles under conditions of prolonged starvation, warranting sufficient amounts of glucose for energetically glucose-dependent tissues. Inhibition of pyruvate oxidation as a consequence of an increased acetyl CoA does not inhibit glucose uptake but does inhibit glycogenolysis, a mechanism saving carbohydrates. On the other hand, glucose is an alternative and competitive substrate to lipids for energy metabolism. In this way a reduction of lipid oxidation can be observed with increasing insulin

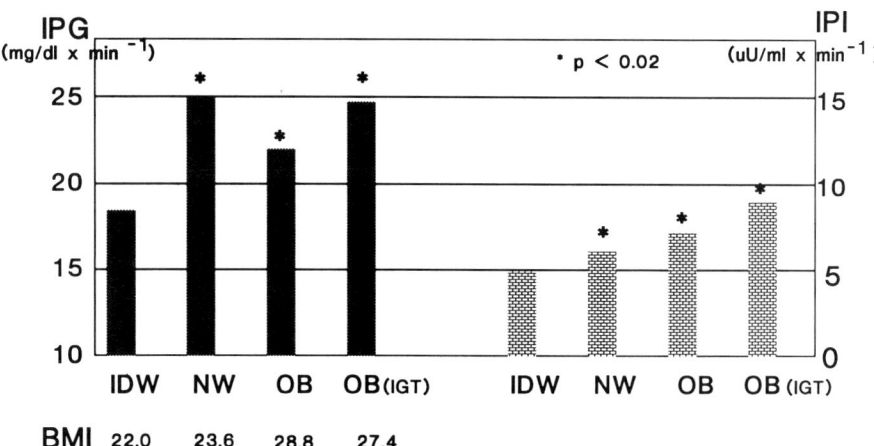

Fig. 6. Integrated plasma-glucose (IPG) and plasma-insulin (IPI) measured continuously over 4 h following lunch and exercise in subjects with ideal, normal and obese (IGT and non-IGT) body weight.

secretion secondary to hyperglycaemia. Insulin reduces triacylglycerol lipolysis and β-oxidation thereby promoting synthesis of fatty acids and their esterification to triglycerides.

The metabolic situation in obesity is completely opposite to conditions of fasting, acute hyperinsulinism, experimental diabetes, increased dietary fat intake, or even physical training. In obesity there is absence of net carbon loss, carbohydrate metabolism is balanced and the glycogen content in muscles is normal, but the influx of free fatty acids is constantly increased. As a consequence of this metabolic imbalance with increased fat oxidation, one can observe impairment of the non-oxidative glucose metabolism due to substrate inhibition[22].

The non-oxidative glucose uptake in the muscle-system (glycogen formation) determines glucose tolerance and consequently the insulin sensitivity of the total organism. Impaired insulin sensitivity is therefore constantly associated with increased serum concentrations of free fatty acids and obesity. An impaired glucose tolerance with increased serum glucose levels leads to hyperinsulinism as long as β-cells of the pancreas are normally functioning. This tight relationship is already evident as one compares individuals with normal body weight to individuals with ideal body weight (Fig. 6). Serum profiles in individuals with *normal* weight show significantly higher glucose and insulin concentrations as compared to individuals with *ideal* body weight.

For many years glucose metabolism is compensated by an increased insulin secretion induced by hyperglycaemia. Progressive impairment of β-cells resulting in impaired insulin secretion leads to more pronounced carbohydrate intolerance. With a certain degree of hyperglycaemia during fasting as well as after oral carbohydrate intake we are faced with frank diabetes mellitus. There is no way for a bimodular distribution curve for any parameter of a distinct group of obese subjects, even including diabetics, parameters such as glycaemia following glucose load, insulin, free fatty acids, degree of obesity, or any other metabolic enzymes, to be used as a sign for a specific defect responsible for diabetes mellitus. Currently there is much research going on for detecting the genetic determinant for type II diabetes. Personally, I have my doubts concerning the success of such scientific efforts. Children of diabetic parents, who were found to have a reduced insulin sensitivity showed in parallel a higher degree of overweight or obesity (BMI) as compared to children of healthy parents[10]. We strongly believe therefore that obesity, not impaired insulin sensitivity, is the primary disorder. Obesity and diabetes mellitus type II are linked together as the chicken and the egg but they do not represent for the individual subject an escapable destiny. The genetics are not the problem, problematic as our environment is today!

Intensified lipolysis, an important factor for arteriosclerosis mediated by triglyceridesynthesis

An important clinical problem of obesity is arteriosclerosis. Obese patients have increased triglyceride plasma concentrations and therefore an increased risk for arteriosclerosis[13,20]. Most of the patients with diabetes type II die as a consequence of arteriosclerosis[18]. What is the reason for that?

We recently completed a study which again emphasizes the close correlation of obesity and triglyceride plasma concentration (Fig. 7); we reported corresponding data from patients in childhood too[4]. Studies from Howard and coworkers on Pima indians in Phoenix, Arizona, clearly showed that increased triglyceride plasma concentrations are due to an increased

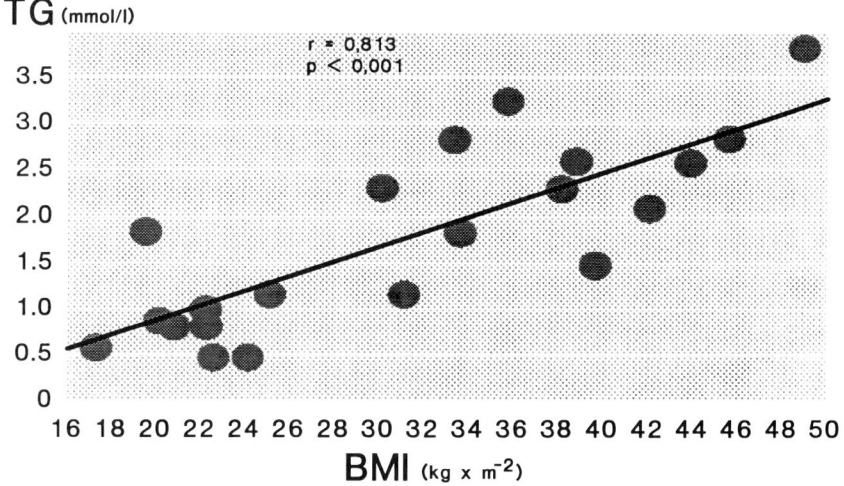

Fig. 7. Relationship of BMI to triglyceridaemia.

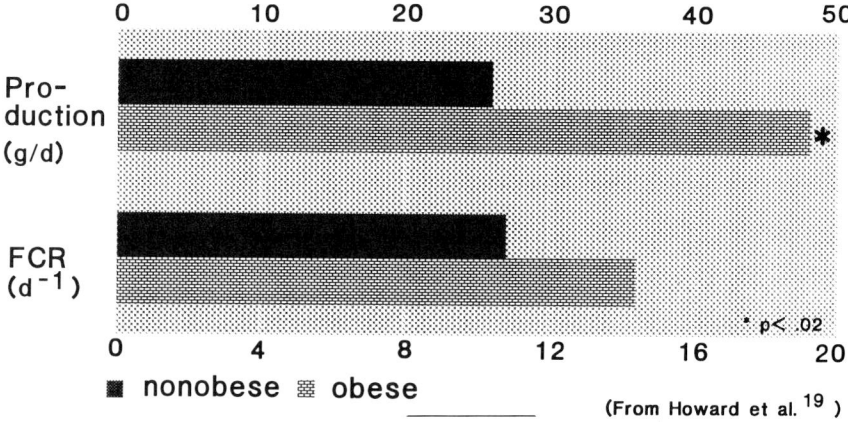

Fig. 8. Production and catabolic rates (FCR) of VLDL-triglyceride.

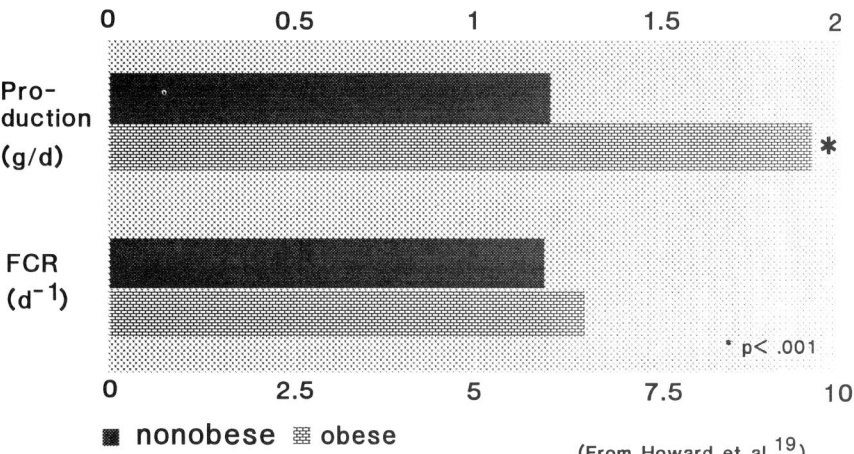

Fig. 9. Production and catabolic rate (FCR) of VLDL-apo B.

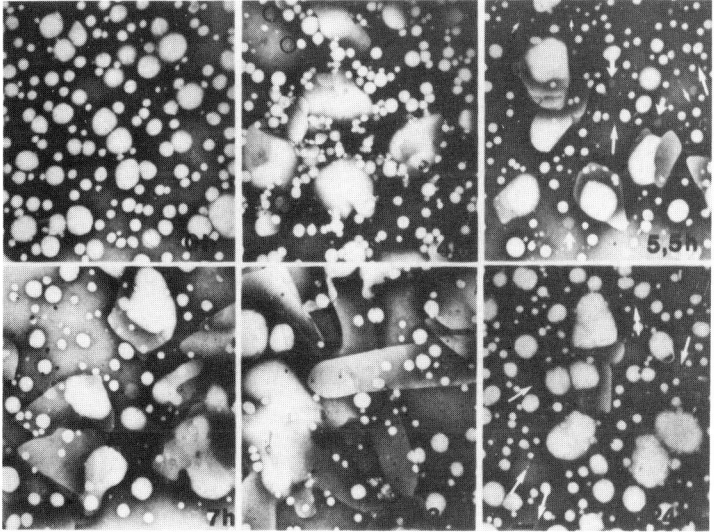

Fig. 10: Triglyceride rich particles 4, 5, 7, 13 and 24 hours following oral fat load (150 g) in a hyperlipemic patient (Typ III). Maximum generation of cholesterol-crystals after 13 hours.

rate of synthesis (Fig. 8)[11]. The parallel increase of trigylceride synthesis and synthesis of VLDL-apo B suggests that the release of VLDL particles from the liver into the circulation is increased (Fig. 9). Since the catabolism of these particles by IDL and LDL are not increased, it results in increased triglyceride plasma concentrations and a prolonged persistence of VLDL particles in the circulation. This condition is comparable to dyslipoproteinaemia of type III in which a disturbed receptor mediated elimination of VLDL is known. In type III hyperlipoproteinaemia, which is associated with a high risk for arteriosclerosis, Bode and Klör from our laboratory detected numerous cholesterol crystals in the blood during the isolation of fractions of triglyceride-rich particles[1]. These crystals disappear by lowering the triglyceride plasma concentrations, but reappear and persist for up to 24 h following an oral fat load (Fig. 10). From scanning electron microscopic studies we have gathered evidence that these lipoproteins "armed" with cholesterol crystals may cause damage to the endothelium of arteries and thereby initiate the process of arteriosclerosis.

In another recent study on patients with angiographically confirmed sclerosis of the coronary arteries we observed an abnormal increase and delayed clearance of serum triglyceride and VLDL after 6 h following an oral fat load. As in the previous study we could again demonstrate the formation of cholesterol crystals. We believe that these abnormal lipid serum patterns, neccessarily associated with the decrease in HDL-cholesterol[9], may be an early event in the process of arteriosclerosis and explain the early appearance of vascular damage in type II diabetes. Since the saturation kinetics of lipoprotein lipase for VLDL-triglycerides *in vivo* have a hyperbolic pattern with consistent interindividual variations, hypertriglyceridaemia in patients with obesity of a similar degree and with similar triglycerides synthesis is quite inhomogenous with respect to the individual risk[9,17]. Following an oral fat load all obese patients show a prolonged half-life of triglycerides and therefore obviously hypertriglyceridaemia. We think that the abnormal dynamics in triglyceride metabolism are the key for our current understanding of the significant correlation of increased fat intake and prevalence of coronary heart disease.

Preferential fatty acid oxidation, a promotor of glucose intolerance and evolution of diabetes mellitus

Increased free fatty acids lead to an increased consumption of free fatty acids in the oxidative energetic metabolism. Contemporaneously a decrease of glucose oxidation takes place. With high concentrations of insulin the increased oxidation of lipids can be reduced with a shift towards an increase in glucose oxidation[16]. Under experimental conditions this phenomenon can be simulated by lipid infusions – whereby the shift in substrate consumption between lipids and carbohydrates becomes apparent[24].

On the contrary a reduction in fat oxidation with a simultaneous increase in carbohydrate oxidation can be achieved by lowering free fatty acids using antilipolytic substances as Acipimox – a nicotinic acid analogue. A decrease in free fatty acids leads to a decrease of serum glucose concentration – this is achieved by a reduction of lipid oxidation and an increase in glucose oxidation[8]. Lowering of fatty acids also enhances the effect of insulin on the overall glucose metabolism including the non-oxidative glucose consumption[25].

When does the diabetic carbohydrate intolerance become evident? Diabetes becomes manifest when after many years insulin secretion is impaired. This condition is preannounced by an abnormally elevated 2 h serum glucose concentration following the oral glucose tolerance test. At this point glucose oxidation and glucose storage are slightly impaired. With progression of disturbed glucose tolerance following a progredient reduction in insulin secretion, glucose oxidation and glucose storage are further impaired. Evidence for the evolution from normal glucose tolerance to an impaired glucose tolerance and finally to an overt diabetic syndrome is reported by Jallut *et al.*[14] in a longitudinal study on obese patients for a period of 6 years only. The progressively decreasing glucose consumption following intravenously injected glucose with increasing age in 650 of our obese subjects, together with a reduction of the reactive insulin release is a further hint of the important link of the duration of obesity and for the evolution of diabetes[2].

Conclusions

(1) Obesity leads to hypertrophy of adipocytes, which are associated with an increased basal and stimulated rate of lipolysis.

(2) The increased rate of lipolytic activity induces a disturbed glucose tolerance and consequently an increased insulin secretion, i.e. hyperinsulinaemia.

(3) Increased lipolytic activity induces a higher synthesis of triglycerides and leads to dyslipoproteinaemia, which in turn promotes arteriosclerosis.

(4) Finally diabetes appears when the secretory capacity of the β-insulinar cells is exhausted. The time of onset of diabetes is dependent on the duration of obesity and an individual functional capacity of the insular cell system.

References

1. Bode, G., Klör, H.U. & Ditschuneit, H. (1978): Lipoproteine morphology in some LCAT-deficient states. *Scand. J. Clin. Lab. Invest.* **38**, Suppl. 150, 199-207.
2. Ditschuneit, H. (1971): Obesity and diabetes mellitus. 7th Congress International Diabetes Federation, 1970, pp. 526-541. Amsterdam: Excepta Medica.
3. Ditschuneit, H. (1980): Definition und Ursachen der Fettsucht. Möglichkeiten und Grenzen der Adipositastherapie, eds. H. Ditschuneit, J.G. Wechsler, pp. 14-21. Baden-Baden, Köln, New York: Witzstrock Verlag.
4. Ditschuneit, H.H., Klör, H.U., Jäger, H., Jung, F., Homoki, J.U. & Ditschuneit, H. (1979): Untersuchungen an Kindern bei eiweiß und fettreicher, kohlenhydratarmer Ernährung. *Ernährungs-Umschau* **26**, 253-258.
5. Dolderer, M., De la Fuente, A., Kerner, W., Zier, H. & Pfeiffer, E.F. (1991): Dynamic ambulatory continuous glucography: normal weight, non-diabetic subjects already show postprandial/post exercise hyperglycaemia, hyperinsulinism as nondiabetic obese persons. (In press).
6. Faulhaber, J.D. (1974): Size, number and function of adipose tissue cells in human obesity, discussion. lipid metabolism, obesity, and diabetes mellitus: impact upon atherosclerosis. *Horm. Metab. Res.*, Suppl. 4, 83-86.
7. Faulhaber, J.D., Petruzzi, E.N., Eble, H. & Ditschuneit, H. (1969): *In vitro* Untersuchungen über den Fettstoffwechsel isolierter menschlicher Fettzellen in Abhängigkeit von der Zellgröbe: Die durch Adrenalin induzierte Lipolyse. *Horm. Metab. Res.* **1**, 80.
8. Fulcher, G.R., Walker, M., Catalano, C. & Alberti, K.G.M.M. (1989): Overnight suppression of lipolysis with acipimox increases carbohydrate oxidation and lowers fasting blood glucose in Type II diabetes 25th EASD Annual meeting, Lisbon.
9. Grundy, S.M. & Vega, G.L. (1988): Hypertriglyceridemia: causes and relation to coronary heart disease. *Semin. Thromb. Hemost.* **14**, 149-164.
10. Haffner, S.M., Stern, M., Hazuda, H.P., Mitchell, B.D. & Patterson, J.K. (1988): Increased insulin concentrations in nondiabetic offsprings of diabetic parents. *N. Engl. J. Med.* **319**, 1297-1301.
11. Howard, B.V., Abbott, W.G., Egusa, G. & Taskinen, M.R. (1987): Coordination of very low-density lipoprotein triglyceride and apolipoprotein B metabolism in humans: effects of obesity and non-insulin-dependent diabetes mellitus. *Am. Heart J.* **113**, 522-526.
12. Howard, B.V., Zech, L., Davis, M., Bennion, L.J., Savage, P.J., Nagulesparan, M., Bilheimer, D., Bennett, P. & Grundy, S.M. (1980): Studies of very low density lipoprotein triglyceride metabolism in obese population with low plasma lipids: lack of influence of body weight or plasma insulin. *J. Lip. Res.* **21**, 1032-1041.
13. Hubert, H.B. (1986): The importance of obesity in the development of coronary risk factors and disease: the epidemiologic evidence. *Annu. Rev. Public Health* **7**, 493-502.
14. Jallut, D., Munger, G.R., Frascarolo, P., Schutz, Y., Jequier, E. & Felber, J.P. (1990): Impaired glucose tolerance and diabetes in obesity: a 6-year follow-up study of glucose metabolism. *Metab.* **39**, 1068-1075.
15. Kissebah, A.H., Vydelingum, N., Murray, R., Evans, D., Hartz, J., Kalkhoff, R.K. & Adams, P.W. (1982): Relation of body fat distribution to metabolic complications of obesity. *J. Clin. Endocrin. Metab.* **54**, 254-260.
16. Lillioja, S., Bogardus, C., Mott, D.M., Kennedey, A., Knowler, W.C. & Howard, B. (1985): Relationship between insulin-mediated glucose disposal and lipid metabolism in man. *J. Clin. Invest.* **75**, 1106-1115.
17. Nikkila, E.A. & Kekki, M. (1971): Polymorphism of plasma triglyceride kinetics in normal human adult subjects. *Acta Med. Scand.* **190**, 49.
18. Panzram, G. (1987): Epidemiologie der Arteriosklerose bei Diabetes mellitus. *Dtsch Ges. Inn Med.* pp. 427-432. München: Bergmann Verlag.

19. Randle, P.J.E., Garland, P.B., Hales, C.N. & Newsholm, E.A. (1963): The glucose fatty-acid cycle. its role in insulin sensitivity and the metabolic disturbances of diabetes mellitus. *Lancet* **i**, 785-789.
20. Schafer, E.J., McNamara, J.R., Genest, J. & Ordovas, J.M. (1988): Clinical significance of hypertriglyceridemia. *Semin. Thromb. Hemost.* **14**, 143-148.
21. Stern, M.P., Olefsky, J., Farquhar, J.W. & Reaven, G.M. (1973): Relationship between fasting plasma lipid levels and adipose tissue morphology. *Metabolism* **22**, 2311-1317.
22. Sugden, M.C. & Holness, M.J. (1990): Substrate interactions in the development of insulin resistance in Typ II diabetes and obesity. *J. Endocrinol.* **127**, 187-190.
23. Taskinen, M.R., Bogardus, C., Kennedey, A. & Howard, B.V. (1985): Multiple disturbances of free fatty acid metabolism in noninsulin-dependent diabetes. Effect of oral hyperglycaemic therapy. *J. Clin. Invest.* **76**, 637-644.
24. Thiébaud, D., DeFronzo, R.A., Golay, A., Acheson, K., Macher, E., Jequier, E. & Felber, J.P. (1982): Effect of long chain triglyceride infusion on glucose metabolism in man. *Metabolism* **31**, 1128-1136.
25. Vaag, A., Skott, P., Damsbot, P., Gall, M.A., Richter, E.A. & Beck-Nielsen, H.: Effect of the Anti-lipolytic nicotinic acid analogue acipimox on whole body and skeletal muscle glucose metabolism in patients with non-insulin dependent diabetes mellitus (NIDDM). In preparation.
26. Vague, J. (1947): La differenciation sexuelle, facteur determinant des formes de l'obesite. *Presse Med.* **65**, 339-340.
27. Wenzel, H., Schimming, H., Wechsler, J.G. & Ditschuneit, H. (1974): Die Messung der Korperdichte des Menschen – Ziel, Verfahren und Anwendung. *Ergebnisse der Adipositasforschung*, eds. H. Ditschuneit, J.G. Wechsler, pp. 52-69. Erlangen: Perimed Verlag.

Chapter 35

Normal Feedback Inhibition of Insulin Secretion by Insulin but Reduced Metabolic Clearance Rate of the Hormone in Obese Subjects

A.J. SCHEEN, M. CASTILLO, G. PAOLISSO, B. JANDRAIN and
P.J. LEFEBVRE

Division of Diabetes, Nutrition and Metabolic Disorders, Department of Medicine, CHU Liège, Sart Tilman, B-4000 Liège, Belgium

In order to better understand the pathophysiology of hyperinsulinism in obesity, we compared the feedback inhibition of insulin secretion by insulin and the metabolic clearance rate (MCR) of insulin during a euglycaemic hyperinsulinaemic glucose clamp (insulin delivery rate: 100 mU.kg^{-1}.h^{-1} from 0 to 120 min) in 12 obese (BMI: 33.0 ± 0.9 kg/m^2) and 10 lean (BMI: 19.8 ± 0.6 kg/m^2) female subjects. Insulin secretion kinetics was estimated by deconvolution analysis of the plasma C-peptide levels throughout the test while insulin MCR was calculated by dividing the constant insulin delivery rate by the net increase in plasma insulin levels during the clamp, after correction for simultaneous changes in endogenous insulin secretion. During the clamp, insulin secretion rates decreased progressively and parallelly in both groups (from 156 ± 11 to 72 ± 15 pmol/min in the obese and from 124 ± 9 to 55 ± 14 pmol/min in the lean subjects), to reach final rates which were about 45 per cent of the initial values. The plasma insulin plateau reached during the clamp was 30 per cent higher ($P < 0.02$) and the MCR of insulin was significantly lower (633 ± 41 *versus* 771 ± 46 ml.min^{-1}.m^{-2}; $P < 0.05$) in the obese than in the lean subjects. In conclusion, the hyperinsulinism associated with obesity is present despite a normal feedback inhibition of insulin secretion by insulin itself and may be, at least in part, explained by a decreased MCR of the hormone.

Introduction

Obesity is characterized by insulin resistance and hyperinsulinism (review in[15]). Hyperinsulinism may be due to either an increased insulin secretion rate or a decreased metabolic clearance rate (MCR) of insulin or to both mechanisms (review in[11]).

Controversial results have been published about the efficiency of the mechanism of feedback inhibition of insulin secretion by insulin itself in obesity. Elahi *et al.*[8] reported that this feedback inhibition was altered in obesity and, consequently, may contribute to the hyperinsulinism. However, this original finding was not confirmed later on[4,26].

Numerous data have suggested that the MCR of insulin is significantly reduced in obesity[3,7,9,16,17,21,25]. However, most of them[3,9,16,21,25] were derived from changes in the plasma molar ratio C-peptide/insulin, a method pertinently criticized by Polonsky and Rubenstein[18]. The data obtained after exogenous insulin infusion were by far more controversial, some studies showing a decreased MCR of insulin in the obese subjects[1,7,17] whereas others did not[6,8,20,22].

In order to understand better the pathophysiology of hyperinsulinism in obesity, the present study aimed at comparing the feedback inhibition of insulin secretion by insulin and the MCR of the hormone during a euglycaemic hyperinsulinaemic glucose clamp in lean and obese women.

Methods

Twelve obese women and ten lean controls participated to the study. Their characteristics are summarized in Table 1. All had a normal oral glucose tolerance test; none had a familial history of diabetes mellitus nor took any medication including oral contraceptives. We have previously demonstrated the absence of significant influence of the menstrual cycle on the various parameters studied[14].

Table 1. Clinical and biological characteristics of the two groups of subjects (fasting state)

Subjects	n	Age (yrs)	BMI (kg/m^2)	Blood glucose (mmol/l)	Plasma insulin (mU/l)	Plasma C-peptide (pmol/l)
Lean	10	22.0 ± 0.2	19.8 ± 0.6	4.21 ± 0.16	7.0 ± 0.5	342 ± 26
Obese	12	24.4 ± 1.5	33.0 ± 0.9	4.17 ± 0.09	10.4 ± 0.9	464 ± 33
$P <$		ns	0.001	ns	0.05	0.02

Each subject, having fasted overnight, was submitted to a euglycaemic hyperinsulinaemic glucose clamp (100 mU.kg^{-1}.h^{-1} for 120 min) using an artificial pancreas (Biostator^R, Miles Laboratories, Elkhart, Indiana, USA) as previously described[5,14,24]. Plasma insulin[12] and C-peptide[13] levels were measured every 15 or 20 min throughout the test. Endogenous insulin secretion was derived from the changes in plasma C-peptide levels using the deconvolution method[11] and the reference values of C-peptide kinetics parameters reported by Polonsky et al.[19] in lean and obese subjects respectively. The MCR of insulin was calculated by dividing the constant insulin delivery rate by the net increase in plasma insulin during the clamp (steady state 60–120 min minus basal values), after correction for the simultaneous changes in endogenous insulin secretion[8,10]. The MCR of glucose was obtained by dividing the mean glucose delivery rate during the last 60 min of the clamp by the mean plasma glucose levels during the same period[1].

The results were expressed as mean ± SEM. A statistical significance was considered at the 0.05 level using Student's t-test for non-paired data.

Results

Basal blood glucose concentrations were similar in both groups whereas basal plasma insulin and C-peptide levels were significantly higher in the obese than in the lean subjects (Table 1). As shown in Fig. 1 endogenous insulin secretion was significantly higher in the basal state when obesity was present (156 ± 11 versus 124 ± 9 pmol/min; $P < 0.05$). In both groups, plasma C-peptide levels and insulin secretion rates decreased progressively throughout the euglycaemic hyperinsulinaemic glucose clamp, despite plasma glucose levels being kept constant (coefficient of variation < 5 % in both groups). Insulin secretion rates fell to 72 ± 15 pmol/min in the obese and to 55 ± 14 pmol/min in the lean subjects (NS), rates which were about 45 per cent of the basal values in both groups (Fig. 1).

The steady-state plasma insulin levels reached during the clamp were almost 30 per cent higher in the obese subjects when compared to those of the lean controls (Table 2). The MCR of the hormone was significantly reduced by some 20 per cent in the obese population, whatever the mode of expression (per kg body weight or per m^2 corporeal surface). Finally, the MCR of glucose was also significantly reduced in the obese subjects when compared to the lean controls (Table 2).

Table 2. Plasma steady-state insulin levels, metabolic clearance rate (MCR) of insulin, and MCR of glucose measured during the last 60 min of a euglycaemic hyperinsulinaemic glucose clamp in lean (n = 10) and obese (n = 12) subjects

Subjects	Steady-state plasma insulin levels (mU/l)	MCR insulin		MCR glucose	
		ml/min.kg	ml/min.m^2	ml/min.kg	ml/min.m^2
Lean	98 ± 8	21.8 ± 1.2	771 ± 46	13.0 ± 1.5	450 ± 57
Obese	127 ± 8	13.5 ± 0.7	633 ± 41	5.1 ± 0.8	273 ± 49
P <	0.02	0.001	0.05	0.001	0.05

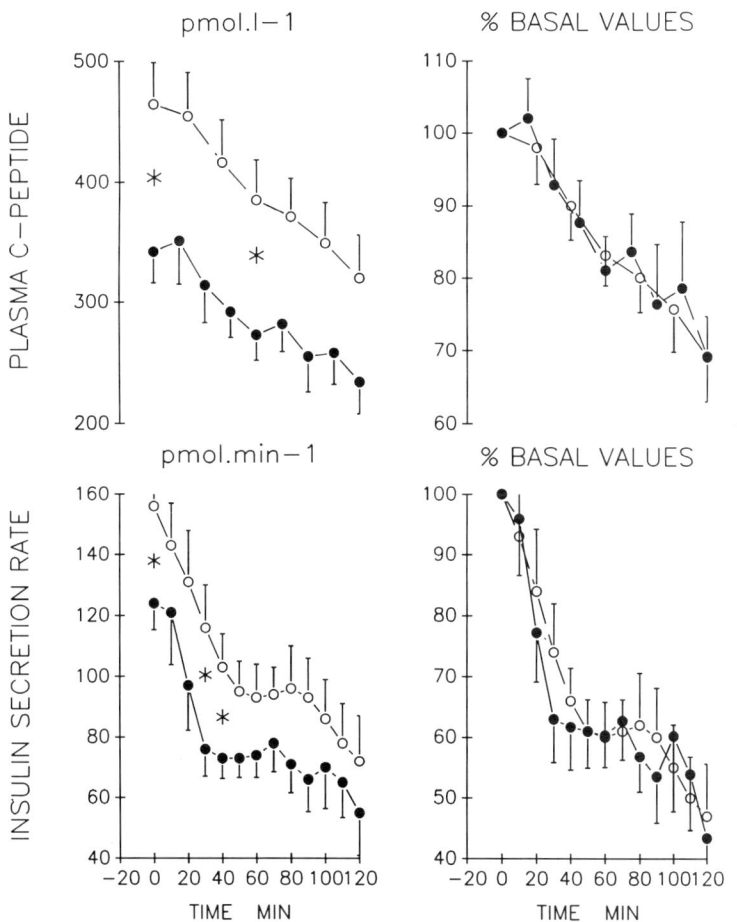

Fig. 1. Changes in plasma C-peptide levels and endogenous insulin secretion rates during a euglycaemic hyperinsulinaemic glucose clamp in lean (--- n = 10) and obese (--- n = 12) women. Results are expressed either in absolute values (left panel) or in percentage of basal levels (right panel). The asterisks indicate P < 0.05 between the two curves.

Discussion

As classically observed (review in[15]), our obese subjects had moderate basal hyperinsulinaemia. This is due, at least in part, to higher levels of endogenous insulin secretion[19]. Our data suggest that such enhanced insulin secretion is not due to a defect in the feedback inhibition of insulin secretion by insulin itself in the obese subjects. To this respect, our results are in agreement with those of Bratusch-Marrain and Waldhäusl[4] and of Zuniga-Guajardo et al.[26] and do not confirm that a defect of this inhibitory feedback loop may be related to the hyperinsulinaemia of obesity as previously reported by Elahi et al.[8].

Several studies suggested that the MCR of insulin is significantly reduced in obesity[3,7,9,16,21], more particularly the liver extraction in the subjects with abdominal or android obesity[17,25]. However, most of the available data[3,9,16,21,25] were derived from changes in the molar ratio plasma C-peptide to plasma insulin, assuming that there is an equimolar secretion of both compounds by the pancreas and that insulin only is cleared by the liver[11,18]. Nevertheless, as discussed in details by Polonsky and Rubenstein[18], this rationale has limitations and could lead to pitfalls, particularly in dynamic conditions.

The steady-state plasma insulin levels reached during the clamp were significantly higher in the obese than in the lean subjects, thus confirming numerous data of the literature as reviewed by Bergman et al.[1]. We, as others[7,17], found a significant reduction of the MCR of insulin measured during the clamp in the obese subjects when compared to the lean controls. Nevertheless, such abnormality was not found by all authors[6,8,20,22], or was observed only when the data were expressed per kg body mass[26]. All these negative results might be due to either insufficient weight excess[20], absence of correction for endogenous insulin secretion[20,22], or maybe heterogeneity of obesity[2,17,19,25].

Finally, the obese subjects were characterized by a significantly lower insulin-induced glucose disposal. These data confirm previous ones reported by our group[5,23,24] and by numerous others (review in[1,15]), thus demonstrating the presence of insulin resistance in obesity.

In conclusion, the hyperinsulinism associated with obesity is present despite a normal feedback inhibition of insulin secretion by insulin itself and may be, at least in part, explained by a decreased MCR of the hormone, presumably at the hepatic site.

References

1. Bergman, R.N., Finegood, D.T. & Ader, M. (1985): Assessment of insulin sensitivity *in vivo*. *Endocr. Rev.* **6**, 45-86.
2. Björntorp, P. (1988): Abdominal obesity and the development of non-insulin-dependent diabetes mellitus. *Diabetes Metab. Rev.* **4**, 615-622.
3. Bonora, E., Zavaroni, I., Bruschi, F., Alpi, O., Pezzarossa, A., Guerra, L., Dall'Aglio, E., Coscelli, C. & Butturini, U. (1984): Peripheral hyperinsulinemia of simple obesity: pancreatic hypersecretion or impaired insulin metabolism? *J. Clin. Endocrinol. Metab.* **59**, 1121-1127.
4. Bratusch-Marrain, P.R. & Waldhäusl, W.K. (1985): Suppression of basal, but not of glucose-stimulated insulin secretion by human insulin in healthy and obese hyperinsulinemic subjects. *Metabolism* **34**, 188-193.
5. Castillo, M., Scheen, A., Lefèbvre, P. & Luyckx, A. (1985): Insulin-stimulated glucose disposal is not increased in anorexia nervosa. *J. Clin. Endocrinol. Metab.* **60**, 311-314.
6. Cohen, P., Barzilai, N., Barzilai, D. & Karnieli, E. (1986): Correlation between insulin clearance and insulin responsiveness: studies in normal, obese, hyperthyroid, and Cushing's syndrome patients. *Metabolism* **35**, 744-749.
7. Davidson, M.B., Harris, M.D. & Rosenberg, C.S. (1987): Inverse relationship of metabolic clearance rate of insulin to body mass index. *Metabolism* **36**, 219-222.

8. Elahi, D., Nagulesparan, M., Hershcopf, R.J., Muller, D.C., Tobin, J.D., Blix, P.M., Rubenstein, A.H., Unger, R.H. & Andres, R. (1982): Feedback inhibition of insulin secretion by insulin: relation to the hyperinsulinemia of obesity. *N. Engl. J. Med.* **306**, 1196-1202.
9. Faber, O.K., Christensen, K., Kehlet, H., Madsbad, S. & Binder, C. (1981): Decreased insulin removal contributes to hyperinsulinemia in obesity. *J. Clin. Endocrinol. Metab.* **53**, 618-621.
10. Ferrannini, E., Wahren, J., Faber, O.K., Felig, P., Binder, C. & DeFronzo, R.A. (1983): Splanchnic and renal metabolism of insulin in human subjects: a dose-response study. *Am. J. Physiol.* **244**, E517-E527.
11. Ferrannini, E. & Cobelli, C. (1987): The kinetics of insulin in man. *Diabetes Metab. Rev.* **3**, 335-397.
12. Hales, C.N. & Randle, P.J. (1963): Immunoassay of insulin with insulin-antibody precipitate. *Biochem. J.* **88**, 137-146.
13. Heding, L.G. (1975): Radioimmunological determination of human C-peptide in serum. *Diabetologia* **11**, 541-548.
14. Jandrain, B., Scheen, A., Henrivaux, P., Paolisso, G., Luyckx, A.S. & Lefèbvre, P.J. (1985): Insulin sensitivity and glucose tolerance during the menstrual cycle. In *Metabolic complications of human obesities*, eds. J. Vague, P. Björntorp, B. Guy-Grand, M. Rebuffe-Scrive & P. Vague, ICS n°682, pp. 241-247. Amsterdam: Excerpta Medica.
15. Lillioja, S. & Bogardus, C. (1988): Obesity and insulin resistance: lessons learned from the Pima indians. *Diabetes Metab. Rev.* **4**, 517-540.
16. Meistas, M.T., Margolis, S. & Kowarski, A.A. (1983): Hyperinsulinemia of obesity is due to decreased clearance of insulin. *Am. J. Physiol.* **245**, E155-E159.
17. Peiris, A.N., Mueller, R.A., Smith, G.A., Struve, M.F. & Kissebah, A.H. (1986): Splanchnic insulin metabolism in obesity. Influence of body fat distribution. *J. Clin. Invest.* **78**, 1648-1657.
18. Polonsky, K.S. & Rubenstein, A.H. (1984): C-peptide as a measure of the secretion and hepatic extraction of insulin. Pitfalls and limitations. *Diabetes* **33**, 486-494.
19. Polonsky, K.S., Given, B.D., Hirsch, L., Shapiro, E.T., Tillil, H., Beebe, C., Galloway, J.A., Frank, B.H., Karrison, T. & Van Cauter, E. (1988): Quantitative study of insulin secretion and clearance in normal and obese subjects. *J. Clin. Invest.* **81**, 435-441.
20. Reaven, G.M., Moore, J. & Greenfield, M. (1983): Quantification of insulin secretion and *in vivo* insulin action in nonobese and moderately obese individuals with normal glucose tolerance. *Diabetes* **32**, 600-604.
21. Rossell, R., Gomis, R., Casamitjana, R., Segura, R., Vilardell, E. & Rivera F. (1983): Reduced hepatic insulin extraction in obesity: relationship with plasma insulin levels. *J. Clin. Endocrinol. Metab.* **56**, 608-611.
22. Savage, P.J., Flock, E.V., Mako, M.E., Blix, P.M., Rubenstein, A.H. & Bennett, P.H. (1979): C-peptide and insulin secretion in Pima indians and caucasians: constant fractional hepatic extraction over a wide range of insulin concentrations and in obesity. *J. Clin. Endocrinol. Metab.* **48**, 594-598.
23. Scheen, A.J., Castillo, M. & Lefèbvre, P.J. (1988): Insulin sensitivity in anorexia nervosa – A mirror image of obesity ? *Diabetes Metab. Rev.* **4**, 681-690.
24. Scheen, A.J., Paolisso, G., Salvatore, T. & Lefèbvre, P.J. (1991): Improvement of insulin-induced glucose disposal in obese patients with NIDDM after l-wk treatment with d-fenfluramine. *Diabetes Care* **14**, 325-332.
25. Van Gaal, L., Vansant, G., Van Acker, K. & De Leeuw, I. (1989): Effect of a long term very low calorie diet on glucose/insulin metabolism in obesity. Influence of fat distribution on hepatic insulin extraction. *Int. J. Obesity* **13**, Suppl. 2, 47-49.
26. Zuniga-Guajardo, S., Jimenez, J., Angel, A. & Zinman, B. (1986): Effects of massive obesity on insulin sensitivity and insulin clearance and the metabolic response to insulin as assessed by the euglycemic clamp technique. *Metabolism* **35**, 278-282.

Chapter 36

Does Hyperinsulinaemia Increase the Adrenocortical Androgen Secretion in Obese Hirsute Women?

J. LÉONET and J. KOLANOWSKI
Division of Endocrinology, University of Louvain (UCL) Medical School, Brussels, Belgium

To provide an additional insight into the mechanism(s) of idiopathic hirsutism of obese women, the relationship between plasma insulin and androgen levels was studied in 14 obese women (six with and eight without hirsutism). Androgen levels were measured either in baseline conditions or during an 8-h i.v. ACTH administration. Basal and ACTH-stimulated cortisol levels were normal and similar in both groups of patients. While no significant difference was observed for testosterone levels, which were within normal range in hirsute women, the hirsutism was associated with significant, two- to threefold increase in androstenedione, as well as in dehydroepiandrosterone (DHEA) and DHEA-sulphate (S) levels. In addition, the ACTH-induced increase in these androgens was enhanced in hirsute women, and only in these patients was insulinaemia positively correlated with baseline DHEA (r = 0.82) and DHEA-S (r = 0.89) levels. Thus the "idiopathic" hirsutism of obese women results in all likelihood from increased adrenal androgen secretion, and this form of hypersensitivity to ACTH may be promoted by hyperinsulinaemia.

Introduction

The idiopathic hirsutism, thus occurring in the absence of abnormally elevated plasma testosterone levels or of any detectable adrenocortical or ovarian pathology, is relatively frequent in young obese women. If the physiopathology of idiopathic hirsutism associated with obesity remains largely unknown, the hyperandrogenism due to the polycystic ovary disease, which is also frequently associated with obesity, is considered as at least partly related to the state of insulin resistance and hyperinsulinaemia[2,4,8]. Indeed, a stimulatory influence of insulin on ovarian androgen production has been demonstrated both *in vitro*[1] and *in vivo*[12]. In addition, hyperinsulinaemia induces a drop in plasma sex hormone-binding globulin[9,11], increasing thereby the levels of free androgens and their androgenic potency. While the steroidogenic abnormalities have never been extensively studied in obese women with idiopathic hirsutism, the role for hyperinsulinaemia in increased adrenocortical androgen secretion cannot be ruled out, since insulin may exert a permissive influence on adrenocortical steroidogenesis[6]. Therefore, the relationship between plasma insulin and androgen levels was evaluated in the present study in the obese women with and without "idiopathic" hirsutism.

Patients and methods

The study was performed on 14 obese women, six of them with idiopathic hirsutism (H; mean age 25.0 ± 2.2 (SE) years, mean BMI 32.3 ± 2.1 kg/m^2), while eight other obese women without hirsutism served as a control group (C; mean age 31.4 ± 5.4 years, mean BMI 40.5 ± 2.6 kg/m^2; $P < 0.05$ vs. H patients). Plasma glucose and insulin levels were measured after an overnight fast and following the ingestion of 75 g glucose. Plasma cortisol, 17-hydroxyprogesterone (17OHP), testosterone (T), androstenedione (A), dehydroepiandrosterone (DHEA) and DHEA-sulphate (DHEA-S) levels were measured in baseline conditions on two consecutive days, and then during an 8 h i.v. infusion of 0.25 mg ACTH$_{1-24}$ (Cortrosyn). In addition, urinary excretion of cortisol, androgen, and of their metabolites were measured in the baseline conditions. The results are provided as mean values $\pm$ SEM. The statistical significance of differences between hirsute and non hirsute women were analysed by the Student t-test for unpaired values.

Results and discussions

Fasting blood glucose levels were normal and very similar in both groups of patients (Table 1). The corresponding insulin levels were at the upper limit of the normal range, and the mean fasting insulinaemia was even slightly but not significantly higher in obese patients without hirsutism. Two hours after glucose ingestion glycaemia averaged 7.06 ± 0.71 mM in C and 6.20 ± 0.63 mM in H patients (ns) and insulinaemia 130 ± 34 and 164 ± 50 µU/ml, respectively (ns). Thus, fasting and glucose stimulated glycaemic and insulinaemic values were similar in both groups. The baseline plasma T levels were within normal range in both groups, with a mean value of total T concentration only slightly (ns) higher in H patients (Table 1). By contrast, the levels of A, DHEA and DHEA-S were two to three times higher in the hirsute patients ($P < 0.001$ vs. control).

Table 1. Fasting blood glucose and insulin concentrations, and the baseline androgen levels in obese non-hirsute (n = 8) and hirsute (n = 6) women (mean values $\pm$ SEM)

Patients	Non-hirsute	Hirsute	P
Glycaemia (mM)	4.55 ± 0.34	4.34 ± 0.13	ns
Insulinaemia (µU/ml)	27.6 ± 4.6	18.3 ± 2.3	ns
Testosterone (nM)	1.16 ± 0.16	1.68 ± 0.23	<0.1
Androstenedione (nM)	4.71 ± 0.50	8.11 ± 0.85	<0.005
DHEA (nM)	7.16 ± 1.28	19.90 ± 3.15	<0.005
DHEA-S (nM)	2.99 ± 0.70	8.02 ± 1.21	<0.005

While fasting or glucose-stimulated insulin levels were similar in patients with and without hirsutism, only in the obese hirsute women a strong positive correlation was found between fasting insulinaemia and baseline DHEA ($r = 0.82, P < 0.005$) or DHEA-S ($r = 0.89, P < 0.02$) levels (Fig. 1). It is noteworthy that this high degree of correlation was demonstrated despite a quite limited number of observations. By contrast, no significant correlation between insulinaemia and plasma T or A levels was found in both groups of patients.

Despite a similar excretion of creatinine (averaging 1.21 ± 0.12 g/24 h for C and 1.11 ± 0.11 g/24 h for H women) the excretion of 17-ketosteroids was significantly increased in hirsute group (13.4 ± 1.4 vs. 8.3 ± 0.9 mg/24 h in the control group; $P < 0.02$) confirming an increase in the androgen production rate. The excretions of free cortisol, as well as of 17-ketogenic steroids, DHEA, etiocholanolone and androsterone were also higher in hirsute group, but the differences did not reach statistical significance. As indicated on Fig. 2, the baseline plasma cortisol levels were quite similar and within normal range in both groups of patients. Likewise, the increase in response to ACTH infusion was quite normal and similar in H and C obese patients. The same conclusion applies to the baseline and ACTH-stimulated 17OHP levels, indicating a normal glucocorticoid secretion with the absence of even a partial deficiency of 21 hydroxylation. The ACTH-induced changes in plasma androgen levels are

Chapter 36 – Does Hyperinsulinaemia Increase the Adrenocortical Androgen Secretion in Obese

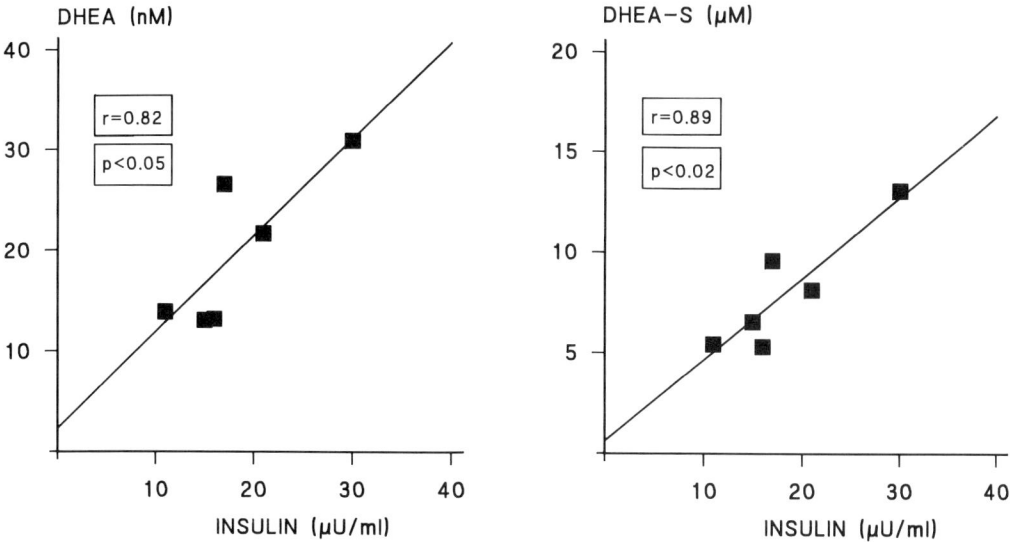

Fig. 1. Relationship between fasting insulinaemia and the baseline levels of DHEA (left) and DHEA-S (right) in obese women with idiopathic hirsutism.

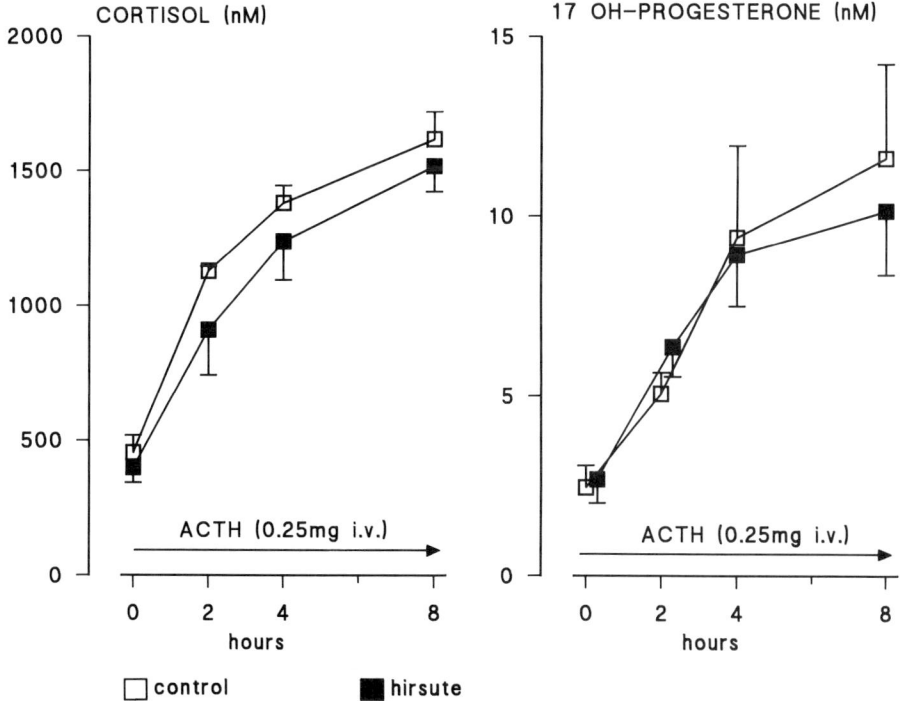

Fig. 2. Changes in levels of plasma cortisol (left) and 17-hydroxyprogesterone (right) levels induced by an 8-h ACTH infusion in obese women with (closed symbols; n = 6) and without (open symbols; n = 8) idiopathic hirsutism. Mean values ± SEM.

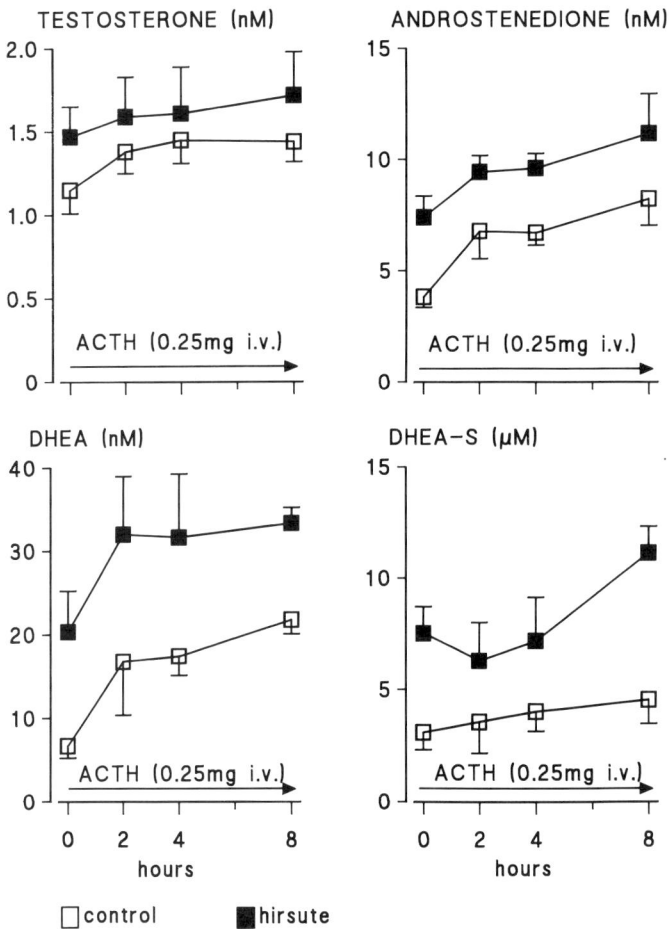

Fig. 3. Changes in levels of plasma total testosterone and androstenedione (upper panel) and in plasma DHEA and DHEA-S (lower panel) induced by an 8-h ACTH infusion in obese hirsute (closed symbols; n = 6) and non hirsute (open symbols; n = 8) women. Mean values ± SEM.

depicted in Fig. 3. No significant changes in T levels resulted from ACTH infusion, and the levels of this steroid were only barely (ns) increased in hirsute patients either before or during ACTH administration. While the baseline plasma A levels were higher ($P < 0.005$) in the hirsute women, the magnitude of ACTH-induced increase in A levels was similar in both groups. The pattern of changes in DHEA levels was also similar (Fig. 3, lower panel). By contrast, plasma DHEA-S levels, significantly higher in the hirsute women in baseline conditions, exhibited in these patients a delayed but significant ($P < 0.005$) increase upon ACTH infusion. Indeed, the ACTH-induced increment in plasma DHEA-S levels averaged 4.43 ± 0.93 µM in hirsute vs. 1.48 ± 0.36 µM in non-hirsute obese women ($P < 0.01$).

The results of the present study clearly indicate that the idiopathic hirsutism of obese women is associated with abnormally higher baseline androstenedione, DHEA and DHEA-S levels, while those of cortisol and testosterone remain within a normal range. In addition, only in obese hirsute women the DHEA-S levels rose significantly in response to ACTH administration. The latter observation is of particular interest since, as we also observed in the non-hirsute obese women, the circulating DHEA-S levels remain normally unchanged during an acute stimulation with ACTH[3,5,10,13]. It may therefore be concluded that idiopathic hirsutism is associated in obese women with an increased sensitivity to ACTH of the steroidogenic pathway involved in the adrenal androgen secretion, as it has been previously demonstrated in the non-obese women with idiopathic hirsutism[5]. Since androgen clearance rate is usually increased in obese women as a result of depressed SHBG levels[7], the increased circulating adrenocortical androgen levels observed in obese women with idiopathic hirsutism reflected in all likelihood an increased adrenocortical production of these steroids. This dissociation of steroidogenic influence of ACTH on cortisol and androgen secretion, already demonstrated in other pathological condition[3], was clearly present in the hirsute obese women studied here, since the baseline and ACTH-stimulated cortisol levels were normal contrasting with enhanced androgen concentrations. That the mechanism of this abnormally high sensitivity of adrenal androgen secretion to ACTH, demonstrated only in the obese hirsute women, may involve an effect of hyperinsulinaemia on the potency of the steroidogenic pathway leading to androgen production by the adrenocortical cells, is suggested by a strong positive correlation of circulating DHEA and DHEA-S levels with fasting insulinaemia (Fig.1). It should be noted, however, that fasting and glucose-stimulated insulin levels were comparable in hirsute and non-hirsute obese women. Thus, aside from the suggested role for insulin, other factors should be involved in this abnormally high sensitivity to ACTH of the steroidogenic pathway involved in adrenocortical androgen secretion.

References

1. Barbieri, R.L., Makris, A., Randall, R.W., Daniels, G., Kistner, R.W. & Ryan, K.J. (1986): Insulin stimulates androgen accumulation in incubations of ovarian stroma obtained from women with hyperandrogenism. *J. Clin. Endocrinol. Metab.* **62**, 904-910.
2. Burghen, G.A., Givens, J.R. & Kitabchi, A.E. (1980): Correlation of hyperandrogenism with hyperinsulinism in polycystic ovarian disease. *J. Clin. Endocrinol. Metab.* **50**, 113-116.
3. Cutler, G.B., Jr., Davis, S.E., Johnsonbaugh, R.E. & Loriaux, D.L. (1979): Dissociation of cortisol and adrenal androgen secretion in patients with secondary adrenal insufficiency. *J. Clin. Endocrinol. Metab.* **49**, 604-609.
4. Flier, J.S., Eastman, R.C., Minaker, K.L., Matteson, D. & Rowe, J.W. (1985): Acanthosis nigricans in obese women with hyperandrogenism. Characterization of an insulin-resistant state distinct from the type A and B syndromes. *Diabetes* **34**, 101-107.
5. Guthrie, G.P., Jr., Wilson, E.A., Quillen, D.L. & Jawad, M.J. (1982): Adrenal androgen excess and defective 11-B-hydroxylation in women with idiopathic hirsutism. *Arch. Intern. Med.* **142**, 729-735.
6. Ill, C.R., Lepine, J. & Gospodarowicz, D. (1984): Permissive effect of insulin on the adenosine 3',5'-monophosphate-dependent upregulation of low density lipoprotein receptors and the stimulation of steroid release in bovine adrenal cortical cells. *Endocrinology* **114**, 767-775.
7. Kirschner, M.A., Samojlik, E. & Silber, D. (1983): A comparison of androgen production and clearance in hirsute and obese women. *J. Steroid Biochem.* **19**, 607-614.
8. Nestler, J.E., Clore, J.N. & Blackard, W.G. (1989): The central role of obesity (hyperinsulinemia) in the pathogenesis of the polycystic ovary syndrome. *Am. J. Obstet. Gynecol.* **161**, 1095-1097.
9. Nestler, J.E., Powers, L.P., Matt, D.W., Steingold, K.A., Plymate, S.R., Rittmaster, R.S., Clore, J.N. & Blackard, W.G. (1991): A direct effect of hyperinsulinemia on serum sex hormone-binding globulin levels in obese women with the polycystic ovary syndrome. *J. Clin. Endocrinol. Metab.* **72**, 83-89.
10. Parker, L.N. & Odell, W.D. (1980): Control of adrenal androgen secretion. *Endocr. Rev.* **1**, 392-410.
11. Peiris, A.N., Sothmann, M.S., Alman, E.J. & Kissebah, A.H. (1989): The relationship of insulin to sex hormone-binding globulin: role of adiposity. *Fertil. Steril.* **52**, 69-72.
12. Stuart, C.A., Prince, M.J., Peters, E.J. & Meyer III, W.J. (1987): Hyperinsulinemia and hyperandrogenemia: *in vivo* androgen response to insulin infusion. *Obstet. Gynecol.* **69**, 921-925.
13. Vaitukaitis, J.L., Dale, S.L. & Melby, J.C. (1969): Role of ACTH in the secretion of free dehydroepiandrosterone and its sulfate ester in man. *J. Clin. Endocrinol. Metab.* **29**, 1443-1447.

Chapter 37

Microalbuminuria in the Non-diabetic Obese Patient

P. VALENSI, M. BUSBY, M.E. COMBES and J.R. ATTALI
*Service d'Endocrinologie-Diabétologie-Nutrition, Hôpital Jean Verdier,
Avenue du 14 juillet 93143 Bondy, France*

The present study was designed to evaluate the frequency of an increase in the urinary albumin excretion rate (UAER) and the factors involved in this parameter in obese patients. Eighty-four non-diabetic obese patients with BMI = 34.4 ± 0.6 (SEM) kg/m^2 were investigated. None had proteinuria or history of nephropathy or uropathy. Twenty-one of them had moderate hypertension. Compared with a group of 22 lean controls, UAER was significantly higher in the obese patients (21.6 ± 3.1 mg/24 h vs 3.2 ± 0.6 mg/24 h, $P < 0.001$). UAER was elevated (> 20 mg/24 h) in 21 patients (25 per cent), up to 151.2 mg/24 h. It was more frequently elevated in hypertensive than in normotensive patients (10/21 vs 11/63, $P < 0.01$). In patients with microalbuminuria, BMI was significantly higher (36.1 ± 1.0 kg/m^2 vs 33.3 ± 0.7 kg/m^2, $P < 0.05$), creatinine clearance was higher (148 ± 52 ml/min vs 112 ± 17 ml/min, NS), plasma albumin was significantly lower (38.2 ± 0.8 g/l vs 40.0 ± 0.4 g/l, $P < 0.05$) and the estimated value of fractional albumin clearance was significantly higher. These results show the high frequency of microalbuminuria in non-diabetic obese patients and particularly in hypertensive patients. They suggest a link between UAER and BMI via renal hyperfiltration and a widespread abnormality of the capillary permeability.

Introduction

Microalbuminuria is defined as an increase in urinary albumin excretion without the presence of proteinuria detected by the usual assessment methods.

In IDDs and NIDDs microalbuminuria predicts the occurrence of macroproteinuria and chronic kidney failure[6,7]. Moreover, in NIDDs microalbuminuria predicts a higher cardio-vascular mortality[4]. In essential hypertension, urinary albumin excretion is occasionally increased. In non-diabetic subjects microalbuminuria has been found in 9.4% of the cases, and this abnormality is independently associated with the occurrence of coronary heart disease[11].

Nephropathy is sometimes a complication in cases of massive obesity. Focal glomerulosclerosis is generally found. Thus, in a series of 17 obese non-diabetic subjects with nephropathy the kidney biopsy revealed this type of histological abnormality in nine cases[5]. Macroproteinuria, however, seems to be rare in obese subjects, as it has only been found in less than 2 per cent of the cases[3]. Possible pathophysiological explanations are an increase in glomerular filtration, but also abnormalities in the lipid metabolism (glomerular foam cells have been observed) or a frequently associated glucose intolerance.

The aim of this work was to determine the urinary albumin excretion rate (UAER) and the factors involved in this parameter in non-diabetic obese subjects.

Patients and methods

Patients

Eighty-four hospitalized obese patients were studied. Their BMI was above 27 kg/m^2 and its mean value ± ESM was 34.4 ± 0.6 kg/m^2. The patients were aged 41.6 ± 1.4. A glucose tolerance test with assays of fasting glycaemia and glycaemia 120 min after oral administration of 75 g of glucose was always normal, except for four patients presenting a glucose intolerance according to the criteria of the WHO 1985. Plasma fructosamine was normal (2.10 ± 0.03 mmol/l), as well as the haemoglobin A1c level (5.1 ± 0.2%). Twenty-one of the 84 patients had moderate hypertension. No patient had a urinary infection or heart failure, nor was taking an anticoagulant or antiagregant treatment. None had known uropathy or nephropathy.

The control group consisted of 22 hospitalized subjects of normal weight; they also had none of the above-mentioned abnormalities and treatments.

Methods

The proteinuria, assayed by sulphosalicylic acid turbidimetry, was lower than 0.10 g/l. The UAER was determined from 24 h urine samples by means of a immunonephelemetry laser method as previously described[8]. With this method the detection limit for albuminuria was 1.5 mg/l, and the intra-assay variation coefficient was 6.5 per cent.

A second test was performed in 20 of the 84 patients after 3 days of a low-calorie diet with a reduction of calorie intake of 30–40 per cent.

The creatinine clearance was calculated. The fractional albumin clearance was assessed with the formula (urinary albumin/creatinine ratio) × (plasma creatinine/albumin ratio).

The results were expressed in mean values ± SEM. Statistical analysis included variance analyses, chi-square tests and correlations according to a linear regression model.

Results

In the control group UAER = 3.2 ± 0.6 mg/24 h. We considered a UAER value above 20 mg/24 h to be abnormal and indicative of microalbuminuria.

In the obese subjects UAER was significantly higher than in the controls: 21.6 ± 3.1 mg/24 h ($P < 0.001$), ranging from 1.15 to 151.2 mg/24 h. Twenty-one patients had microalbuminuria.

The number of patients with microalbuminuria was significantly higher among the hypertensive patients than among the normotensive ones (10/21 vs 11/63, $\chi^2 = 7.75$, $P < 0.01$).

The age and the sex ratio were not significantly different between patients with microalbuminuria and those with a normal UAER. However, body weight and the BMI were significantly higher for patients with microalbuminuria (98.9 ± 4.4 kg vs 89.7 ± 2.3 kg, $P = 0.05$ and 36.1 ± 1.0 kg/m^2 vs 33.3 ± 0.7 kg/m^2, $P < 0.05$ respectively).

Creatinine clearance was higher in patients with microalbuminuria (148 ± 52 ml/min vs 112 ± 17 ml/min, NS). Fractional albumin clearance was significantly higher in patients with microalbuminuria (9.14 ± 1.89 vs 2.93 ± 0.32, $P < 0.001$). A significant positive correlation was found between this parameter and the UAER ($r = 0.843$, $P < 0.001$). The plasma triglyceride rate was not significantly different between patients with microalbuminuria and those with a normal UAER. However the plasma albumin was significantly lower in patients with microalbuminuria (38.2 ± 0.8 g/l vs 40.0 ± 0.4 g/l, $P < 0.05$), as was the plasma cholesterol (4.74 ± 0.23 mmol/l vs 5.50 ± 0.18 mmol/l, $P < 0.05$).

No significant correlation was found between the UAER and fasting glycaemia, glycaemia 120 min after oral glucose, the plasma fructosamine rate, HbA1c and plasma triglycerides.

Out of the 20 patients whose UAER was assessed twice, 13 had a normal UAER in both tests, five had a high UAER in both tests, but in the other two patients it was high in only one of the two tests performed.

Discussion

The long-term follow-up of diabetics has shown the unfavourable prognostic value of microalbuminuria in these patients[4,6,7]. In non-diabetics as well, microalbuminuria may have an unfavourable prognostic effect on the risk of coronary heart disease[11]The possibility that there is nephropathy present in massive obesity led us to study kidney function in obese subjects, using a very sensitive immunological assay for urinary albumin excretion. None of the patients studied here had diabetes. Microalbuminuria above the 20 mg/24 h threshold was found in 25 per cent of the patients. The incidence was particularly high in hypertensive obese patients (47.6 per cent).

The higher level of BMI in patients with microalbuminuria suggests that there is a link between excess weight and incipient nephropathy. Glomerular filtration was assessed by the creatinine clearance, which was found to be higher in patients with microalbuminuria, although the difference, compared to the group with a normal UAER, was not significant, probably because of scattered results. This finding, however, does suggest the glomerular origin of microalbuminuria and the role played by glomerular hyperfiltration.

The plasma albumin found to be significantly lower in patients with microalbuminuria cannot be explained solely by urinary albumin excretion. It is more likely that there is a widespread abnormality of the capillary permeability which causes albumin extravasation in the interstitial spaces. As other authors[1], we have found evidence of this abnormality in many obese patients complaining of swelling (unpublished data) as well as in obese NIDDs[9], by using an isotopic method. The mechanism of this abnormality of capillary permeability remains to be determined in obese patients.

The reversibility of microalbuminuria is under study. The results of the second test after a few days of low-calorie diet suggest that in some patients microalbuminuria is not permanent. This variability can be compared with the wide variability observed in diabetics (about 30 per cent) from day to day[2].

The prognostic value of microalbuminuria, particularly from the cardiovascular point of view, can only be assessed by means of longitudinal studies on obese subjects.

Finally, it should be emphasized that in NIDDs, most of whom are overweight, microalbuminuria has been observed in more than 15 per cent of the patients. In a series of 203 NIDDs we found it in 17 per cent of the cases[10]. The findings of the present study suggest that excess weight may contribute to incipient nephropathy in the NIDD.

In conclusion, microalbuminuria is frequent in the non-diabetic obese subjects. It probably results from a glomerular hyperfiltration mechanism. The possibility that excess weight plays a role in the microalbuminuria observed in NIDDs and also the non-diabetic population should therefore be considered.

Acknowledgements

The authors thank Mrs Marion Sutton-Attali for help in English translation and Mrs Anne-Marie Del Negro for secretarial assistance.

References

1. Creff, A.F., Behar, A. & Nathan, P. (1989): Les obesites "nutritionnellement" paradoxales. *Rev. Franc. Endocrinol. Clin.* **30**, 531-544.
2. Feldt-Rasmussen, B. & Mathiesen, E.R. (1984): Variability of urinary albumin excretion in incipient diabetic nephropathy. *Diab. Nephropathy* **3**, 101-103.

3. Goldszer, R., Irving, J., Lazarus, J.M. et al. (1984): Renal findings in obese humans. *Kidney Int.* **25**, 165.
4. Jarrett, R.J., Viberti, G.C. Argyropoulos, A., Hill, R.D., Mahmud, U. & Murrells, T.J. (1984): Microalbuminuria predicts mortality in non-insulin-dependent diabetes. *Diabetic Med.* **1**, 17-19.
5. Kasiske, B.L. & Crosson, J.T. (1986): Renal disease in patients with massive obesity. *Arch. Intern. Med.* **146**, 1105-1109.
6. Mogensen, C.E. (1987): Microalbuminuria as a predictor of clinical diabetic nephropathy. *Kidney Int.* **31**, 673-689.
7. Parving, H-H., Oxenboll, B., Svendsen, P.A., Christiansen J.S. & Andersen A.R. (1982): Early detection of patients at risk of developing diabetic nephropathy: a longitudinal study of urinary albumin excretion. *Acta Endocrinol. (Copenh)* **100**, 550-555.
8. Valensi, P., Ferrière, F., Attali, J.R., Erault, C., Modigliani, E., Delrieux, C. & Sebaoun, J. (1986): Microalbuminurie chez les diabetiques porteurs d'une hypertension arterielle modérée. *Arch. Mal. Coeur* **6**, 785-789.
9. Valensi, P., Attali, J.R., Behar, A. & Sebaoun, J. (1987): Isotopic test of capillary permeability to albumin in diabetic patients: effects of hypertension, microangiopathy and duration of diabetes. *Metabolism* **36**, 834-839.
10. Valensi, P., Jourdain, L., Ferriere, F., Modigliani, E. & Sebaoun, J. (1989): La néphropathie débutante des diabétiques non-insulinodépendants: ses facteurs de risque. *Diabète Métab.* **15**, XX.
11. Yudkin, Y.S., Forrest, R.D. & Jackson, C.A. (1988): Microalbuminuria as predictor of vascular disease in non-diabetic subjects. *Lancet* **ii,** 530-533.

Chapter 38

Possible Relationship Between Proteinuria and Obesity

A. SAIBENE, F. CAVIEZEL[1], F. ZILLI[1], L. GIANOLLI*, F. DOSIO* and G. POZZA

*Istituto Scientifico San Raffaele, Cattedra di Clinica Medica and *Servizio di Medicina Nucleare; [1]Istituto di Scienze Medico Chirurgiche San Donato, Cattedra di Endocrinologia e Medicina Costituzionale, Università di Milano, Milano, Italy*

Nephrotic syndrome or mild proteinuria have been reported in obesity; its precise prevalence in obese patients without diabetes mellitus and/or hypertension, however, is still unknown. Forty-two normotensive obese subjects without complications were therefore studied before and after weight loss, together with 20 healthy control subjects.

Overnight albumin excretion rate (AER) was assessed using a RIA method. Glomerular filtration rate (GFR) was also evaluated in 14 obese subjects using ^{51}Cr before and after weight loss. AER was found to be higher (about twice) in obese subjects, although not statistically different, compared to controls; after weight loss AER of obese became quite similar to that of controls. GFR was normal in basal conditions and showed a tendency to decrease following weight loss. Systolic and diastolic blood pressure significantly decreased following weight loss ($P < 0.01$ and $P < 0.025$, respectively).

In conclusion, although the presence of true nephropathy in uncomplicated obesity is not confirmed in our study population, obesity might facilitate at kidney level the occurrence of those haemodynamic alterations which, in the presence of diabetes or hypertension, may lead to the appearance of the nephrotic syndrome.

Introduction

In morbid obesity, one or more of the following organs or functions can be involved: cardio-vascular, respiratory, endocrine, metabolic, hepatic and biliary. As a matter of fact, it is well known that obesity can lead to various and often serious complications.

Nephrotic syndrome or mild proteinuria have also been reported in obesity, especially in the so-called morbid obesity[8,10]. However, the literature concerning the possible relationship between proteinuria and obesity is rather scanty and its pathophysiological meaning rather unclear. In addition, these previous studies mainly refer to obese subjects affected by non-insulin-dependent diabetes mellitus and/or by hypertension, two pathologies that may lead to renal complications *per se*[5].

Therefore, the aim of this study was to evaluate renal function in uncomplicated obese subjects, in order to assess whether or not proteinuria, even of minor degree, like microalbuminuria, could be related to obesity.

Patients and methods

We studied 42 obese women (mean age 43.3 ± 2 ($\pm$ SEM) yr: range from 18 to 65; mean weight

94.7 ± 2.4 kg; BMI 37.1 ± 0.9) and 20 non-obese women as a control group (mean age 32.2 ± 3.4 yr: range from 18 to 63; weight 55.0 ± 1.4 kg; BMI 20.8 ± 0.4). All subjects had normal blood pressure (< 140/90, according to WHO/ISH criteria)[1], normal glucose tolerance (according to NDDG)[4], normal hepatic and renal function, no history of menstrual alterations. None of them had macroproteinuria (Albustix negative). The following parameters were evaluated: systolic and diastolic blood pressure, measured at the admission (1st, 3rd and 5th day) and at the end of the diet period; 75 g OGTT, with plasma glucose and insulin determination at 0, 60, 120 min.

Microalbuminuria was measured by radioimmunoassay (H Albumin Kit, Sclavo, Milano, Italy) on overnight urine samples, collected three times after three days of isocaloric weight maintaining diet (CHO 50 per cent, protein 20 per cent, lipid 30 per cent). The same parameters were measured after three weeks of a hypocaloric diet (3344 J/day with the same nutrient distribution). In 14 obese subjects glomerular filtration rate (GFR) was also evaluated by means of ^{51}Cr before and after diet. Data were analysed by paired and unpaired Student's t-test and by multiple regression analysis.

Results

Albumin excretion rate (AER) in obese subjects was higher, although not significantly and still within the normal range, when compared to that of controls (601.2 ± 74.6 vs 459.4 ± 82.6 μg/h); it was slightly reduced after a mean weight loss of 6.5 kg in three weeks, and appeared to be quite similar to the value of control subjects (448.5 ± 69.7 μg/h) (Fig. 1).

There was also a significant reduction of systolic (from 131.7 ± 1.6 to 124.7 ± 1.4 mmHg), and diastolic blood pressure (from 84.3 ± 0.9 to 80.5 ± 1.0 mmHg), $P < 0.001$ and $P < 0.005$, respectively (Fig. 2). The GFR showed a trend to reduction after diet (from 96.7 ± 4.1 to 88.4 ± 2.34 ml/min, $0.1 < P > 0.05$) (Fig .3).

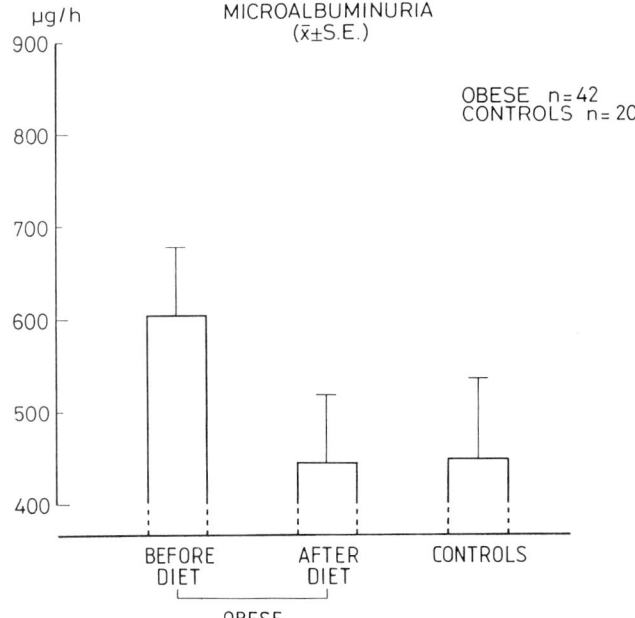

Fig. 1. Microalbuminuria in obese subjects (before and after weight loss) and in controls.

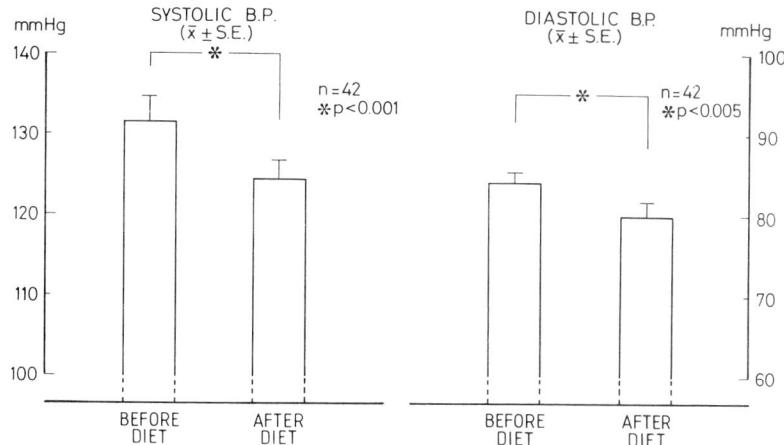

Fig. 2. Systolic and diastolic blood pressure in obese subjects before and after weight loss.

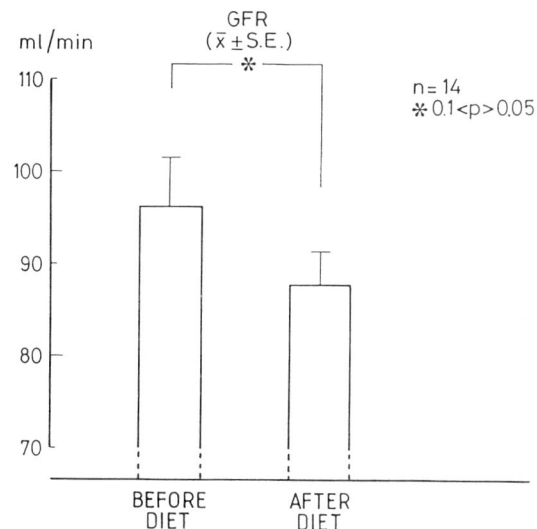

Fig. 3. Glomerular filtration rate in obese subjects before and after weight loss.

Discussion

Preble[5] in the 1920s pointed out the presence of protein-loosing nephropathy in almost 40 per cent of 1000 obese subjects. However most of these subjects were affected by other illnesses such as hypertension and diabetes mellitus.

Later, Weil[9] and then Weisinger et al.[10] described in eight obese patients with nephrotic syndrome the improvement of renal function after marked weight loss. Renal biopsy specimens obtained from obese proteinuric subjects, studied by Warnke and Kempson[8] and Kasiske and Crosson[3], showed the presence of focal glomerulosclerosis, together with accumulation of fibrillar material in the subendothelial part of glomerular capillary. These findings, however, were not observed in all proteinuric obese. Recently, the disappearance of proteinuria after weight loss in an obese subject whose renal biopsy was normal before dietary regimen has been reported[11]. Indeed, haemodynamic abnormalities could be responsible for the genesis of protein-loosing nephropathy in obesity, and they could be reversible after weight loss.

On the other hand haemodynamic alterations could be responsible for glomerular changes: in fact, experimental data suggest that a rise in capillary glomerular pressure and in glomerular plasma flow can cause focal glomerulosclerosis in animal models[2].

Moreover, glomerular filtration rate of markedly obese subjects was found to be higher than in controls and was reduced after weight loss obtained by means of intestinal by-pass[6,7].

However, it must be underlined that almost all previous studies mainly refer to obese subjects also affected by diabetes mellitus and/or hypertension. So, the existence of a pure protein-loosing nephropathy in uncomplicated obesity is still debatable. The aim of our study was then to check the presence of microalbuminuria, as a predictive factor for the development of macroproteinuria in obese subjects without impaired glucose tolerance, diabetes or hypertension. We studied also the effect of weight loss on microalbuminuria, GFR and arterial blood pressure: these two latter parameters have been intentionally examined since they represent crucial factors in determining proteinuria.

Briefly, microalbuminuria seemed to be slightly higher in obese subjects, although within the normal range, and it could be reduced by adequate weight loss. GFR, which was normal in basal conditions, showed the same behaviour. Both systolic and diastolic blood pressure were significantly decreased after weight loss. These changes altogether result in lower microalbuminuria, whose different values in comparison with the basal condition could be caused by the haemodynamic variations described here.

In conclusion, from our data, obesity *per se* does not seem to be complicated by nephrotic syndrome. Anyway, it could predispose to a more or less severe macroproteinuria which would become of relevance when the obesity is associated with diabetes mellitus and/or hypertension.

Acknowledgement: This work was supported in part by Grant No. 89.02486.04 from the Consiglio Nazionale delle Ricerche, Rome.

References

1. 1989 Guidelines for the management of mild hypertension: memorandum from a WHO/ISH Meeting (1989). *J. Hipert.* **7**, 689-693.
2. Kasiske, B.L., Cleary, M.P. & O'Donnell, M.P. (1986): Effects of carbohydrate restriction on renal injury in the obese Zucker rat. *Am. J. Clin. Nuir.* **44**, 56-65.
3. Kasiske, B.L. & Crosson, J.T. (1986): Renal disease in patients with massive obesity. *Arch. Intern. Med.* **146**, 1105-1109.
4. National Diabetes Data Group (1979): Classification and diagnosis of diabetes mellitus and other categories of glucose intolerance. *Diabetes* **28**, 1039-1057.
5. Preble, W.E. (1923): Obesity: observation in one thousand cases. *Boston Med. Surg. J.* **188**, 617-621.
6. Schteingart, D.E. & Conn, J.W. (1956): Characteristics of increased adrenocortical function observed in many obese patients. *Ann. N.Y. Acad. Sci.* **131**, 388-394.
7. Stockholm, K.M. & Brochner-Mortensen, J. (1980): Increased glomerular filtration rate and adrenocortical function in obese women. *Int. J. Obes.* **4**, 57-63.
8. Warnke, R.A. & Kempson, R.L. (1978): The nephrotic syndrome in massive obesity. *Arch. Pathol. Lab. Med.* **102**, 431-438.
9. Weil, M.H. (1955): Polycythemia associated with obesity. *J. Am. Med. Ass.* **159**, 1592-1595.
10. Weisinger, J.R., Kempson, R.C., Eldrige, F.L. & Swenson, R.S. (1974): The nephrotic syndrome: a complication of massive obesity. *Ann. Intern. Med.* **81**, 440-447.
11. Wesson, D.E., Kurtzman, N.A. & Frommer, J.P. (1985): Massive obesity and nephrotic proteinuria with a normal renal biopsy. *Nephron* **40**, 235-237.

Chapter 39

Radiological Osteoarthrosis, Subjective Symptoms and Clinical Findings in the Extremity Joints of Severely Obese and Control Subjects

T. RÖNNEMAA, H. ALARANTA and T. AALTO
Rehabilitation Research Centre of the Social Insurance Institution, Peltolantie 3, SF-20720 Turku, Finland

The prevalence of radiological osteoarthrosis and extremity joint symptoms was studied in 68 severely obese subjects and their age and sex-matched non-obese controls. Mean age of study subjects was 39 years and mean BMI (kg/m^2) was in obese men 40.9, in obese women 42.8, in control men 24.6 and in control women 22.3. In most subjects obesity had developed before the age 20. There was no consistent differences between obese and non-obese subjects in the prevalence of radiological arthrosis or symptoms or clinical findings in hand joints. In knee joints the prevalence of radiological arthrosis was higher in the obese subjects compared to controls (in men 21.7 per cent vs 4.0 per cent, P NS; in women 44.4 per cent vs 2.2 per cent, $P < 0.001$) and obese subjects also had rest pain, motion tenderness and restriction of joint movement more often in knees (for all variables $P < 0.01$ in both sexes). There was also a tendency towards a higher prevalence of symptoms and clinical findings in talocrural and metatarsophalangeal joints in obese subjects compared to controls. Male obese subjects had significantly more often radiological osteoarthrosis in forefoot joints compared to controls (26.1 per cent vs 4.0 per cent, $P < 0.05$). The prevalence of calcaneal spurs was 42.2 per cent in obese women and 2.2 per cent in control women ($P < 0.001$). Obese subjects with and without radiological arthrosis did not differ from each other in respect to serum uric acid concentration, glucose tolerance or plasma insulin concentration. Our data are in favour of the hypothesis that obesity is an important causative factor in osteoarthrosis by causing increased wear and tear of weight-bearing joints.

Introduction

The association between obesity and cardiovascular diseases and their risk factors has been studied extensively. However, musculoskeletal diseases are even a more common cause of disability in middle-aged subjects in Western societies but their association with obesity has received less attention. Obesity has generally been accepted as a contributory factor in the genesis of osteoarthrosis without questions[7]. However, it has not been totally excluded that obesity is a consequence rather than a cause of osteoarthrosis because of the sedentary life style that usually accompanies osteoarthrosis. Supposing that obesity is causally related to osteoarthrosis, two main explanations are possible: first, obesity may cause wear and tear leading to microtraumas and further to osteoarthrosis, or secondly, metabolic disturbances related to obesity, such as hyperuricaemia and abnormal glucose tolerance, might be operative in the genesis of osteoarthrosis[3]. Our aim was to assess the association between morbid obesity and musculoskeletal problems in terms of the prevalence of pain symptoms, clinical findings and radiological findings in weight-bearing and non-weight-bearing joints.

Subjects and methods

Obese subjects were participants in a weight reduction programme. The participants were collected by an announcement in a local newspaper. The only inclusion criteria were age between 22 and 54 years and body weight of at least 110 kg in women and 130 kg in men. None was excluded because of any disease. For each obese subject we selected an age- and sex-matched control subject from the local population register. A letter asking the height and weight was sent to the possible controls and all those within ± 15% of recommendable weight were accepted to the study. The participation rate of controls was 84%.

The mean age of both men and women was approximately 40 years (Table 1). The BMI in obese men and women was slightly above 40. According to the subjects' own estimation obesity had its onset before the age of 20 years in 76% of the women and in 50% of the men. An interview regarding musculoskeletal symptoms and a standardized clinical examination were performed by one and the same physician in both obese and non-obese subjects. Pain at rest was graded as mild or severe. Mild pain occurred at least monthly but did not disturb sleep or cause use of analgesics. Severe pain was defined as pain disturbing sleep or causing use of analgesics. Motion tenderness in clinical examination was graded as mild when the patient informed of pain in passive movement and as severe when signs of pain were visible during passive movement. Restriction in joint movement was graded according to the decrease from normal range of joint movement, mild representing a decrease by 0 to 10 degrees and severe a decrease by more than 10 degrees. Radiological osteoarthrosis was defined as definitive narrowing of the joint space and presence of osteophytes. All X-rays were analysed by one and the same radiologist. Regarding symptoms, clinical findings and X-ray findings, a subject was judged to have the disorder if he or she had the disorder on at least one side and in respect to hand and forefoot, in at least one joint.

Table 1. Anthropometric data

	Males			Females		
	Obese (n=23)	P	Non-obese (n=25)	Obese (n=45)	P	Non-obese (n=45)
Age (yr)	39 ± 9	ns	40 ± 9	38 ± 8	ns	38 ± 8
Height (cm)	183 ± 7	<0.01	177 ± 6	166 ± 6	<0.01	163 ± 6
Weight (kg)	137 ± 9	<0.001	77 ± 8	118 ± 10	<0.001	59 ± 6
BMI (kg/m^2)	40.9 ± 2.9	<0.001	24.6 ± 2.2	42.8 ± 4.5	<0.001	22.3 ± 1.9

Results

There was no consistent difference in the prevalence of symptoms or signs in hand joints between obese and non-obese subjects although obese men had more often mild rest pain and obese women had slightly more often marked restriction in joint movement compared to respective controls (Table 2). In hip joints obese subjects had consistently more often mild rest pain, motion tenderness and restriction in movement compared to controls although the difference was statistically significant only among women in respect to joint movement (Table 3). The most consistent difference between obese and non-obese subjects in the prevalence of symptoms and signs was observed in knee joints. In addition, one third of obese females showed valgus deformity in their knees. Regarding talocrural joints there was a tendency towards a higher occurrence of rest pain and motion tenderness in obese compared to non-obese subjects, the only statistically significant difference being observed in motion tenderness among women (Table 4). In both the first and other metatarsophalangeal joints obese women, but not men, had a higher prevalence of rest pain and motion tenderness compared to controls. The prevalence of radiological osteoarthrosis in hand joints did not

Chapter 39 – Radiological Osteoarthrosis, Joint Symptoms and Clinical Findings

differ between obese and non-obese subjects, whereas in knee joints and to a lesser extent in forefoot joints osteoarthrosis was more common among the obese subjects (Table 5). A remarkable finding was the striking difference in the prevalence of calcaneal spurs in women, probably indicating that obese women have more often had calcaneal periostitis[2].

Table 2. Clinical characteristics of hand joints in obese and non-obese subjects according to sex (%)

	Males			Females		
	Obese (n=23)	P	Non-obese (n=25)	Obese (n=45)	P	Non-obese (n=45)
Pain at rest						
severe	4.4	ns	0	6.7	ns	2.2
mild-severe	26.1	<0.05	4.0	20.0	ns	20.0
Motion tenderness						
severe	0		0	2.2	ns	2.2
mild-severe	13.0	ns	8.0	20.0	ns	13.3
Restriction of joint movement						
severe	13.0	ns	12.0	11.1	<0.05	0
mild-severe	39.1	ns	32.0	17.8	ns	6.7

Table 3. Clinical characteristics of hip and knee joints in obese and non-obese subjects according to sex (%)

	Males			Females		
	Obese (n=23)	P	Non-obese (n=25)	Obese (n=45)	P	Non-obese (n=45)
HIP JOINT						
Pain at rest						
severe	0		0	4.4	ns	4.4
mild-severe	13.0	ns	0	15.6	ns	6.7
Motion tenderness						
severe	0		0	0		0
mild-severe	21.7	ns	8.0	11.1	ns	4.4
Restriction of joint movement						
severe	8.7	ns	0	4.4	ns	0
mild-severe	26.1	ns	8.0	22.2	<0.01	2.2
KNEE JOINT						
Pain at rest						
severe	0		0	13.3	<0.05	0
mild-severe	26.1	<0.01	0	28.9	<0.001	6.7
Motion tenderness						
severe	4.4	ns	0	6.7	ns	0
mild-severe	56.6	<0.001	8.0	33.3	<0.01	6.7
Restriction of joint movement						
severe	8.7	ns	0	2.2	ns	0
mild-severe	39.1	<0.001	0	15.6	<0.01	0
Varus deformity (>5 cm)	4.4	ns	4.0	0	ns	4.4
Valgus deformity (>5 cm)	13.0	ns	0	35.6	<0.001	0

Table 4. Clinical characteristics of talocrural and metatarsophalangeal joints in obese and non-obese subjects according to sex (%)

	Males			Females		
	Obese (n=23)	P	Non-obese (n=25)	Obese (n=45)	P	Non-obese (n=45)
TALOCRURAL JOINTS						
Pain at rest						
severe	0	ns	0	2.2	ns	0
mild-severe	17.4	ns	4.0	17.8	ns	6.7
Motion tenderness						
severe	4.4	ns	0	0		0
mild-severe	17.4	ns	4.0	26.7	<0.001	0
Restriction of joint movement						
severe	0		0	4.4	ns	0
mild-severe	4.4	ns	4.0	6.7	ns	0
I MTP JOINT						
Pain at rest						
severe	0		0	6.7	ns	4.4
mild-severe	8.7	ns	4.0	17.8	ns	6.7
Motion tenderness						
severe	0		0	2.2	ns	2.2
mild-severe	8.7	ns	9.0	26.7	<0.05	8.9
II-V MTP JOINT						
Pain at rest						
severe	0		0	4.4	ns	0
mild-severe	0		0	11.1	<0.05	0
Motion tenderness						
severe	0		0	4.4	ns	0
mild-severe	4.4	ns	4.0	17.8	<0.01	0

Table 5. Radiological osteoarthrosis of various joints and calcaneal spurs in obese and non-obese subjects according to sex (%)

	Males			Females		
	Obese (n=23)	P	Non-obese (n=25)	Obese (n=45)	P	Non-obese (n=45)
Hand	17.4	ns	16.0	15.6	ns	8.9
Knee	21.7	ns	4.0	44.4	<0.001	2.2
Forefoot	26.1	<0.05	4.0	11.1	ns	2.2
Calcaneal spur	34.8	ns	16.0	42.2	<0.001	2.2

The mean (SD) concentration of fasting serum uric acid was 360 (83) µmol/l in obese subjects having radiological knee arthrosis and 391 (106) µmol/l in obese subjects without knee arthrosis (P = NS). The concentration of serum uric acid was also similar in obese subgroups with or without radiological arthrosis in the forefoot and in subgroups with or without a calcaneal spur. The mean (SD) concentration of fasting and 2 h blood glucose in a 75 g oral glucose tolerance test was 5.3 (1.3) and 6.6 (2.8) mmol/l in the obese subgroup with radiological knee arthrosis and 5.5 (1.6) and 6.5 (3.7) mmol/l in those without knee arthrosis (for both variables P = NS). Both fasting and 2 h glucose level was also similar in obese subgroups with or without other radiological findings. Fasting and 2 h plasma insulin concentration was also similar among obese subjects with or without radiological knee osteoarthrosis and in those with or without other radiological findings. The mean (SD) age of obese subjects with radiological knee arthrosis was 42.2 (8.4) years and of those without arthrosis 36.7 (7.6) years ($P = 0.01$). From obese subjects with rest pain in knees 53 per cent, and from obese subjects without rest pain 31 per cent had radiological knee osteoarthrosis ($P = 0.09$).

Discussion

The prevalence of joint symptoms and signs as well as radiological osteoarthrosis was more common in morbidly obese subjects compared to controls in weight-bearing joints, especially in knees. However, the prevalence of these symptoms and findings in hands was almost similar in the obese and non-obese subjects. These results are in accordance to those obtained in milder obesity[6] and are compatible with the hypothesis that obesity is related to osteoarthrosis through wear and tear mechanisms. This idea is strengthened by the fact that among obese subjects those with and without radiological arthrosis did not differ in the metabolic variables measured, i.e. uric acid concentration and glucose metabolism. This is in accordance with the NHANES study showing that obesity is associated with knee osteoarthrosis independently of metabolic factors[4].

One may argue that symptomatic arthrosis leads to sedentariness and consequently to obesity. Our results do not support this idea because obesity had had its onset in most subjects before the age of 20, an age before which osteoarthrosis is very unlikely to occur. Our obese study population was not collected from a population-based survey but was a group of subjects willing to participate in a weight-reduction programme. This may have had some influence on the results of our cross-sectional study, because obese subjects with joint symptoms might have been more eager to seek help to lose weight compared to asymptomatic obese subjects. However, longitudinal population-based studies in milder obesity favour the concept that overweight is really causally related to radiological osteoarthrosis[5].

All previous studies have not confirmed the association between obesity and musculoskeletal morbidity in lower extremities. For example, Aro and Leino[1], using relative weight of ≥ 120 per cent as the criterion for overweight, found no increased 10-year incidence of musculoskeletal complaints in weight-bearing joints of obese subjects. In our study, compared to controls, both symptoms and radiological osteoarthrosis were more common in the obese group with a mean BMI above 40 kg/m^2 indicating that at least severe obesity is clearly associated with increased musculoskeletal morbidity of lower extremities.

References

1. Aro, S. & Leino, P. (1985): Overweight and musculoskeletal morbidity: a ten-year follow-up. *Int. J. Obesity* **9**, 267-275.
2. Bordelon, R.L. (1983): Subcalcaneal pain. A method for evaluation and plan for treatment. *Clin. Orthopaed. Rel. Res.* **177**, 49-53.
3. Cimmino, M.A. & Cutolo, M. (1990): Plasma glucose concentration in symptomatic osteoarthritis: a clinical and epidemiological survey. *Clin. Exp. Rheumatol.* **8**, 251-257.
4. Davis, M.A., Ettinger, W.H. & Neuhaus, J.M. (1990): Obesity and osteoarthritis of the knee: evidence from the National Health and Nutrition Examination Survey (NHANES I). *Semin. Arthritis Rheum.* **20**, 34-41.
5. Felson, D.T., Anderson, J.J., Naimark, A., Walker, A.M. & Meenan, R.F. (1988): Obesity and knee osteoarthritis. The Framingham Study. *Ann Intern. Med.* **109**, 18-24.

6. vonHunecke, I. & Reuter, W. (1975): Degenerative Gelenkveränderungen bei Adiposen unter Berücksichtigung des Lebensalters. *Beitr. Orthop. u. Traumatol.* **22**, 575-579.
7. Sokoloff, L. (1979): Pathology and pathogenesis of osteoarthritis. In *Arthritis and allied conditions*, 9th edn, ed. D.J. McCarty, pp. 1149. Philadelphia: Lea & Febiger.

Chapter 40

Disturbances in Respiratory Function in Obese Subjects

J. RAISON*, D. CASSUTO*, E. ORVOEN-FRIJA**, M.F. DORE**,
J. ROCHEMAURE** and B. GUY-GRAND*

*Service de Médecine et Nutrition, Hôtel Dieu, 75004 Paris, France**; Service de Pneumologie, Hôtel Dieu, 75004 Paris, France

Respiratory function was studied in 191 non-selected obese subjects (121 females and 70 males) of mean age 48 ± 13 and of mean BMI 42 ± 10, attending the Nutrition Clinic from 1988 to 1990. The consistent reduction in expiratory reserve volume, functional residual capacity and hypoxaemia were related to the degree of obesity. Abdominal fat distribution contributed to alteration in functional reserve capacity and in lung volumes only in moderate obesity. Additional alterations in total lung capacity and in vital capacity were seen in severe obesity. These alterations in lung volumes were less pronounced in female than in male obese subjects.

Introduction

The most consistent disturbances in respiratory function that have been associated with obesity are the reduction in functional residual capacity, expiratory residual volume and hypoxaemia[1,2,5,7]. The total lung capacity and vital capacity have been variously reported as normal or decreased[5,7]. These abnormalities have been mainly related to the adverse effect of obesity on chest and respiratory muscles mechanics[5,7]. The increase in abdominal fat mass acting on the diaphragm might also be expected to alter respiratory function. In an attempt to identify factors which contribute to abnormalities in functional reserve capacity and in static lung volumes, we reviewed respiratory function of a large number of obese male and female subjects.

Methods

Respiratory function was studied in 191 non-selected obese subjects (121 females and 70 males) of mean age 48 ± 13 years and of mean BMI 42 ± 10 kg/m^2, attending the Nutrition Clinic from 1988 to 1990.

Obese patients were of BMI > 27 and were divided into two groups by BMI: group 1 with 27 < BMI < 40 and group 2 with BMI equal or > to 40.

Body fat distribution was assessed by the measurement of minimal waist circumference in standing position divided by body surface area in m^2.

In all subjects, vital capacity (VC), expiratory reserve volume (ERV) and forced-expiratory volume in one second (FEV1) were measured by spirometry (Pulmonet III) in a sitting position. FRC was measured by the helium dilution technique. Residual volume was calculated as FRC − ERV. Total lung capacity (TLC) was calculated as VC + RV. The results were expressed in percentage of reference values determined for men and women from regression equations including age and standing height[8]. Arterial blood gas measurements were made in the semi-recumbent position in 149 obese subjects.

Results

In all 191 obese subjects, ERV and FRC were below the reference values and should be considered as abnormal. RV, VC, FEV1 and TLC were within the accepted limits of normal values. A moderate hypoxaemia and a normocapnia were observed (Table 1).

Table 1. Clinical parameters and respiratory function tests in all obese subjects (mean ± SD)

Age (yr)	46 ± 13
BMI (kg/m^2)	42 ± 10
ERV (% ref)	48 ± 27
RV (% ref)	87 ± 25
FRC (% ref)	72 ± 18
VC (% ref)	101 ± 19
FEVI (% ref)	96 ± 20
FEVI/VC	77 ± 8
TLC (% ref)	96 ± 14
PaO$_2$ (Torr)	86 ± 13
PaCO$_2$ (Torr)	37 ± 5

Table 2. Comparison of respiratory function in obese with BMI < 40 and in obese with BMI > 40 (mean ± SD)

	BMI < 40	BMI > 40	P
n	102	89	
Age (yr)	47 ± 13	44 ± 11	< 0.05
ERV (%)	58 ± 28	36 ± 21	< 0.0001
RV (%)	88 ± 25	86 ± 25	
FRC (%)	78 ± 12	66 ± 18	< 0.0001
VC (%)	104 ± 17	96 ± 20	< 0.05
TLC (%)	99 ± 12	93 ± 15	< 0 02
PaO$_2$ (Torr)	88 ± 13	82 ± 12	< 0.001
PaCO$_2$ (Torr)	37 ± 5	38 ± 7	< 0.05

After grouping subjects by BMI, ERV and FRC were found to be more deeply reduced in obese subjects with BMI > 40 than in those with BMI < 40. VC and TLC were significantly decreased in obese subjects with BMI > 40. RV was similar in the two groups. PaO$_2$ was significantly lower and PaCO$_2$ significantly higher in obese subjects with BMI > 40 (Table 2).

Comparing male and female obese subjects, mean age and mean BMI were similar, ERV and FRV were not significantly different in male and female obese subjects. VC, TLC, PaO$_2$ were significantly decreased and PCO$_2$ significantly increased in male as compared to female obese subjects (Table 3).

In dividing the two groups of obese subjects by the mean of abdominal circumference/m^2, we found that in obese subjects with BMI < 40, ERV, RV, FRC, VC, TLC, were significantly lower in obese subjects with waist > 55 cm/m^2 than in those with waist < 55 cm/m^2. In obese subjects with BMI > 40, the reduction in ERV, FRC, VC and TLC was not significantly different according to waist/m^2 values (Table 4).

Table 3. Comparison in respiratory function in male and female obese subjects

	Females (121)	Males (70)	P
Age (yr)	46 ± 13	44 ± 12	
BMI (kg/m^2)	42 ± 10	41 ± 9	
ERV (%)	48 ± 28	48 ± 25	
RV (%)	84 ± 23	92 ± 27	< 0.01
FRC (%)	71 ± 17	75 ± 20	
VC (%)	105 ± 18	92 ± 17	< 0.0001
TLC (%)	98 ± 14	93 ± 14	< 0.02
PaO$_2$ (Torr)	88 ± 12	82 ± 12	< 0.01
PaCO$_2$ (Torr)	36 ± 4	38 ± 4	< 0.05

Table 4. Comparison in respiratory function in obese subjects grouped by BMI and waist/m^2 circumference

	n	ERV %	FRC %	VC %	TLC %	PaO$_2$	PaCO$_2$
BMI < 40							
Waist < 55 cm/m^2	17	70 ± 43**	87 ± 19**	112 ± 19*	107 ± 13*	87 ± 16	36 ± 5
Waist > 55 cm/m^2	17	42 ± 16**	66 ± 18**	106 ± 12*	99 ± 9*	86 ± 10	35 ± 3
BMI > 40							
Waist < 55 cm/m^2	14	42 ± 21	66 ± 20	94 ± 19	90 ± 19	84 ± 11	38 ± 4
Waist > 55 cm/m^2	24	33 ± 20	63 ± 17	103 ± 21	96 ± 18	82 ± 10	39 ± 4

*$P < 0.05$; **$P < 0.01$.

Discussion

In this population of non-selected obese male and female subjects, the reduction in ERV and FRC was observed in all obese subjects, while CV and TLC were only altered in severe obesity with BMI over 40. The reduction in ERV and FRC was more marked in severe obesity and associated with decreasing PaO$_2$. These findings corroborate the close inverse relationship between ERV and degree of obesity which has been shown both in moderate and in morbid obesity before and after weight loss[1,2,5,7]. The arterial hypoxaemia has been correlated with the reduced ERV in moderate obesity and attributed to ventilation-perfusion mismatching.[5,7] However, the increment in hypoxaemia of severely obese subjects may require further explanations. One can suggest that the FRC and consequently ERV are so reduced in severe obesity that they could be associated with small airway closure and supplemental impairment of gas exchange[5,7].

The decrease in TLC and VC only in severe obesity remains unclear. The decrease in TLC seemed to be due to the decrease in VC since RV was close to normal values and unchanged with increasing BMI. Since a few studies have documented that inspiratory capacity was nearly normal in obese subjects, it can be assumed that the loss in TLC and VC was largely the result of a low FRC[7]. The alterations in these lung volumes have been previously described in a small number of subjects with extreme obesity or with hypoventilatory syndrome, and have not been consistently improved after weight loss[5,7]. The variations in TLC and CV only in severe obesity and the lack of such variations with weight loss suggest that other factors than obesity itself may be involved. The few studies including severely obese subjects indicated that additional factors such as alteration in thoracic compliance, inefficacy of respiratory muscles, chest and abdominal wall limitations in obesity could contribute to these disturbances in VC and TLC[4,5,6]. In this study, for the same reduction in

ERV and FRC, alterations in VC and TLC were found in male but not in female obese subjects of same age and BMI, suggesting that factors linked to sex should be considered. According to the way of expression of the results either in absolute or in normalized values, sex differences in lung volumes have been found or not[2,5]. Nevertheless, some reasons could have overestimated the sex differences in lung volumes in this study. The differences in percentage reference values could be partly due to male/female differences in body fatness or fat-free mass, since these parameters were not included in the regression equation of reference values. Pathological pulmonary factors or tobacco consumption which were not described in this study could have influenced lung volumes specially in male subjects. The findings of a decreasing TLC and VC with increasing abdominal obesity suggest that FRC and lung volumes may be also influenced by the increase in intra-abdominal fat acting on diaphragm or by other muscular, haemodynamic or hormonal disorders associated with this type of obesity[3]. Nevertheless, the inverse relationship between VC, TLV and abdominal fat predominance was not true in severe obese patients in whom the effect of massive overweight on respiratory function was more important than that of body fat distribution. Although this data may keep a clinical significance, errors in measurement of abdominal circumference in severe obesity could have weakened these relationships.

In conclusion, the consistent reduction in expiratory reserve volume, functional residual capacity and hypoxaemia were related to the degree of obesity. Abdominal fat distribution contributed to alteration in functional reserve capacity and in lung volumes only in moderate obesity. Additional alterations in total lung capacity and in vital capacity were seen in severe obesity. These alterations in lung volumes were less pronounced in female than in male obese subjects.

References

1. Babb, T.G., Buskirk, E.R. & Hodgson, J.L. (1989): Exercise end-expiratory lung volumes in lean and moderately obese women. *Int. J. Obesity* **13**, 11-19.
2. Barlett, H.L. & Buskirk, E.R. (1983): Body composition and the expiratory reserve volume in lean and obese men and women. *Int. J. Obesity.* **7**, 339-343.
3. Björntorp, P. (1985): Obesity and the risk of cardiovascular disease. *Ann. Clin. Res.* **17**, 3-9.
4. Burki, N.K. & Baker, R.W. (1984): Ventilatory regulation in eucapnic morbid obesity. *Am. Rev. Respir. Dis.*, **129**, 538-543.
5. Ray, C.S., Sue, D.Y., Bray, G., Hansen J.E. & Wasserman, K. (1983): Effects of obesity on respiratory function. *Am. Rev. Respir. Dis.* **128**, 501-506.
6. Refsum, H.E., Holter, P.H., Lovig, T., Haffner, J.F.W. & Stadaas, J.O. (1990): Pulmonary function and energy expenditure after marked weight loss in obese women: observations before and one year after gastric banding. *Int. J. Obes.* **14**, 175-183.
7. Rochester, D.F. & Enson, Y. (1974): Current concepts in the pathogenesis of the obesity-hypoventilation syndrome. Mechanical and circulatory factors. *Am. J. Med.* **57**, 402-420.
8. Quanjer, Ph.H. (1983): Standardization of lung function tests. *Bull. Eur., Physiopathol. Respir.* **19** (supp. 5), 7-10.

Section VII
CNS-Periphery relationships

Chapter 41

New Aspects of the Physiopathology of Obesity and Insulin Resistance in Rodents

**B. JEANRENAUD, I. CUSIN, C. GUILLAUME-GENTIL,
F. ASSIMACOPOULOS-JEANNET, J. TERRETTAZ and
F. ROHNER-JEANRENAUD**

*Laboratoires de Recherches Métaboliques, 64, Avenue de la Roseraie, 1211 Geneva 4,
Switzerland*

The present work was undertaken in an attempt to study the relationship between hyperinsulinaemia or hypercorticosteronaemia, and glucose uptake by white adipose tissue and by various muscles. The rationale for doing so is that the genetically obese (*fa/fa*) rats are not only continuously exposed to considerable hyperinsulinaemia but, as is described below, to an excess of corticosterone. To impose hyperinsulinaemia or hypercorticosteronaemia on normal rats is a way to define, separately, the effects of the two hormonal abnormalities. For this purpose, normal rats were infused with saline or insulin (both delivered by minipumps) and compared. Other normal rats were infused with corticosterone *via* subcutaneously implanted pellets delivering the hormone. At the end of the respective saline, insulin or corticosterone administration, euglycaemic-hyperinsulinaemic clamps associated with the labelled 2-deoxy-D-glucose (2DG) method were performed to measure *in vivo* insulin-stimulated overall glucose utilization, as well as that of individual tissues (*via* the 2DG method) notably in white adipose tissue as well as in several muscles. During the clamps the hepatic glucose production process was also investigated.

Insulinization of normal rats: impact on glucose handling *in vivo*

Treatment of normal rats with insulin plus glucose (glycaemia of 6.3 ± 0.3 mM) for 4 days resulted in a mean hyperinsulinaemia of 230 ± 15 µU/ml compared to an insulinaemia of 54 ± 6 µU/ml for controls. Insulin treatment also produced, within the 4 experimental days, a delta increase in body weight gain of 18.8 ± 1.6 g compared to a delta of 10.6 ± 2.0 g for controls ($P < 0.05$)[3].

The glucose utilization index (i.e. the tissue responsiveness of this process to insulin) of white parametrial adipose tissue was *higher* in rats previously treated with insulin ("insulinized" rats) than in controls. In contrast, the glucose utilization index of several muscle types (soleus, extensor digitorum longus, epitrochlearis, tibialis, diaphragm) was *lower* in the insulin-treated ("insulinized") group than in the control one[4].

No intergroup difference was observed when the insulin-stimulated glucose utilization index was measured in non-insulin dependent tissues such as the skin, the gut and the brain. Note also that the ability of insulin to shut off hepatic glucose production was normal in both control and "insulinized" rats[4].

Liver and white adipose tissue *de novo* lipogenesis was also studied, during euglycaemic-hyperinsulinaemic clamps, in "insulinized" rats and saline-infused controls. It was observed that lipogenesis was higher in the liver of "insulinized" rats than in that of saline-infused controls. This was in keeping with the increased hepatic fat content measured in the insulin-treated group compared to controls. Similar increases in the *de novo* lipogenesis was observed in white adipose tissue of "insulinized" rats compared to that of saline-infused controls, an observation that was in keeping with increased total inguinal fat pad weight of insulin-treated rats[4].

The relative abundance of mRNA coding for the insulin-responsive glucose transporter Glut4 (assessed at the end of insulin or saline infusion) was measured by Northern blots[3]. It was found that Glut4 mRNA abundance was markedly increased in white adipose tissue and definitely decreased in muscles, compared to that measured in tissues from saline-infused controls. This was quantified by densitometry and expressed as ratio between the relative amount of Glut4 mRNA and that of actin mRNA. In insulin-treated rats, the amount of insulin-responsive glucose transporter (Glut4) detected by the 1F8 antibody was increased in the homogenates of white adipose tissue, while it was decreased in those of the tibialis, remaining unchanged in the diaphragm, compared to saline infused controls[3].

These data show that hyperinsulinaemia imposed for 4 days to normal rats ("insulinized" rats) results in an increased body weight gain. This is accompanied by increases in the insulin-stimulated glucose utilization index in white adipose tissue, by increased *de novo* adipose tissue lipogenesis, and by increased *de novo* liver lipogenesis. Furthermore, the induced hyperinsulinaemia increases the abundance of the insulin-responsive glucose transporter mRNA (Glut4) in white adipose tissue, while it decreases that in the two muscles studied, the diaphragm and the tibialis. These divergent changes of Glut4 mRNA levels produced by hyperinsulinaemia on white adipose tissue and muscles fit with the measurements of the *in vivo* glucose utilization index that is increased in white adipose tissue and decreased in muscles of the "insulinized" rats, relative to controls[3,4].

The increase in Glut4 mRNA abundance observed in white adipose tissue from hyperinsulinaemic rats is accompanied by an increase in the amount of the glucose transporter protein measured with a monoclonal antibody. The decrease in Glut4 mRNA abundance measured in muscles from hyperinsulinaemic rats is accompanied by an actual decrease in the glucose transporter protein in the tibialis, but not in the diaphragm. Thus, in the white adipose tissue and in tibialis of "insulinized" rats, the relationship between glucose transport, mRNA abundance and amount of glucose transporter protein is straightforward. It is less so in the diaphragm of "insulinized" rats, in which the observed decrease in the *in vivo* glucose utilization and amount of Glut4 mRNA is not accompanied by a decrease in the amount of the glucose transporter protein. It should be assumed – in this particular case – that other changes of the transporting protein (e.g. lack of activation, inadequate signal transduction) could play a role in the occurrence of insulin resistance.

These data together show that hyperinsulinaemia *per se* produces divergent changes in glucose transport and glucose transporter mRNA in white adipose tissue and muscles. They favour the view that a state of hyperinsulinaemia, even of short duration, can be one of the driving forces responsible for increased white adipose tissue and liver metabolic activity (increased lipogenic activity, hence beginning of obesity), together with incipient muscle insulin resistance, the hepatic glucose production process remaining unaltered[3,4].

Hypercorticosteronaemia and obesity

High corticosterone levels or high responsiveness to the hormone are also thought to play a role in the development and maintenance of the obesity syndrome of the genetically obese *fa/fa* rat. In fact, after adrenalectomy, the food intake and the rate of body weight gain of adult *fa/fa* rats are decreased to levels seen in lean rats[2,10], and their plasma insulin and triglyceride levels, lipoprotein lipase activity, fatty acid synthesis and fat cell size are reduced[2,5,9,10]. Adrenalectomy also brings the high energetic efficiency of obese animals back to values observed in lean rats[8].

The beneficial effects of adrenalectomy on most of the parameters just mentioned have been shown to be reversed by the replacement by corticosterone (e.g.[2,5]).

One of the aims of the study was therefore to unravel a possible hypercorticosteronaemic state in obese animals. Plasma corticosterone values (morning values) were statistically higher in both female and male obese rats than in their respective lean controls. The increase was about 1.5-fold for female and fourfold for male obese animals. Evening levels were higher than the respective morning ones. The evening plasma corticosterone levels were similar in lean and obese females, whereas they were statistically higher in obese males than in lean ones[6].

To substantiate further putative alterations in the regulation of the hypothalamo-pituitary-adrenal axis (HPA) of obese animals, various tests on stress were carried out. Plasma corticosterone responses to immobilization stress carried out in lean and obese male rats were measured. Higher levels of corticosterone were observed in the obese animals compared to the controls, after 1 h immobilization, as well as during the whole recovery period that lasted for 3 additional hours. The surface areas of corticosterone output during the stress and recovery period were much greater in obese male than in lean control rats. This abnormality, although present, was less marked in obese female rats[6].

Cold stress studies (2 h to 7 days at 6°C) were performed in male rats. Much greater levels of corticosterone were measured at 6°C in the obese group than in the lean one. Here again the surface areas over baseline calculated over the 7 day exposure to cold were much higher in obese males than in lean controls. Analogous defects (though less marked) were observed in obese female rats. Plasma ACTH levels measured 2 h after cold exposure were considerably higher in the obese males than in the lean group. The cold-induced increases in plasma ACTH levels were accompanied by corresponding increases in corticosteronaemia[6].

The dexamethasone suppression test carried out in male rats showed a complete inhibition of corticosterone in both lean and obese animals. However, obese male animals escaped the dexamethasone-induced suppressive effect more rapidly than normal rats[1].

The number of corticotrophin-releasing factor (CRF)-labelled median eminence (ME) axons, the intra-axonal area occupied by anti-CRF-labelled material, and the total CRF immunoreactivity were higher in male obese than in lean rats[1]. By immunocytochemistry, the number of corticotropes in the anterior lobe, the pituitary area occupied by anti-ACTH-labelled material, the total anti ACTH immunoreactivity, and the anti-ACTH immunoreactivity per μm^2 were higher in male obese than in lean animals[1]. The adrenal weight was higher in male obese than in lean rats and the light microscopical analysis of the adrenal cortex showed a hypertrophic zona fasciculata in the obese rats compared to that of controls.

As hyperinsulinaemia and hypercorticosteronaemia are concomitantly present in genetically obese rats it was decided to cause hypercorticism in otherwise normal rats, to define the abnormalities produced by hypercorticosteronaemia. To do so, normal rats were implanted subcutaneously for 2 days with pellets delivering stress levels of the hormone. At the end of this procedure and as mentioned above, corticosterone-treated rats were compared to controls during euglycaemic-hyperinsulinaemic clamps associated with the labelled 2-deoxyglucose technique[7]. It was observed that the insulin administered during the clamp (insulin responsiveness) stimulated the overall glucose utilization to a much lesser extent in corticosterone-treated rats than in controls. This was accompanied by a considerable decrease in the insulin-stimulated glucose utilization index in all muscle types studied, while the glucose utilization index of white adipose tissue was not modified. Furthermore, while the hepatic glucose production was normally suppressed by insulin in control rats, it was not in the corticosterone-treated group[7].

The data together are consistent with the presence, in the model of genetic obesity mentioned above, of a hypercorticism of central (hypothalamic) origin.

It is also shown that when hypercorticism (stress levels of the hormone) is imposed for 2 days on normal rats, it produces a marked insulin resistance of the overall glucose utilization process *in vivo*, with a marked insulin resistance of the glucose utilization of all muscles studied and no alteration in the glucose utilization of the white adipose tissue. Furthermore, hypercorticism imposed on normal rats also brings about insulin resistance at the level of the hepatic glucose production process. Although the underlying mechanisms of the defects just summarized remain to be defined at the cellular and molecular levels it may be concluded that corticosterone administration to normal rats produces both peripheral and hepatic insulin resistance, a basic feature of the *fa/fa* rat. Finally, increased levels of both insulin and corticosterone may explain most of the facets of the obesity syndrome, particularly in animal models, and possibly in humans[3,4,7].

Acknowledgements

This work was carried out thanks to grant No. 32-26405.89 of the Swiss National Science Foundation (Bern, Switzerland) and by a grant-in-aid of Nestlé S.A. (Vevey, Switzerland). It was also supported by the Swiss National Science Foundation Grants 3.034-0.84 and 3.028-0.87.

References

1. Bestetti, G.E., Abramo, F., Guillaume-Gentil, C., Rohner- Jeanrenaud, F., Jeanrenaud, B. & Rossi, G.L. (1990): Changes in the hypothalamo-pituitary-adrenal axis of genetically obese *fa/fa* rats: a structural, immunocytochemical, and morphometrical study. *Endocrinology* **126**, 1880-1887.
2. Castonguay, T.W., Dallman, M.F. & Stern, J.S. (1986): Some metabolic and behavioral effects of adrenalectomy on obese Zucker rats. *Am. J. Physiol.* **251**, R923-R933.
3. Cusin, I., Rohner-Jeanrenaud, F., Zarjevski, N., Assimacopoulos-Jeannet, F. & Jeanrenaud, B. (1990): Hyperinsulinemia increases the amount of GLUT4 mRNA in white adipose tissue and decreases that of muscles: a clue for increased fat depot and insulin resistance. *Endocrinology* **127**, 3246-3248.
4. Cusin, I., Terrettaz, J., Rohner-Jeanrenaud, F. & Jeanrenaud, B. (1990): Metabolic consequences of hyperinsulinemia imposed on normal rats on glucose handling by white adipose tissue, muscles and liver. *Biochem. J.* **267**, 99-103.
5. Freedman, M.R., Horwitz, B.A. & Stern, J.S. (1986): Effect of adrenalectomy and glucocorticoid replacement on development of obesity. *Am. J. Physiol.* **250**, R595-R607.
6. Guillaume-Gentil, C., Rohner-Jeanrenaud, F., Abramo, F., Bestetti, G.E., Rossi, G.L. & Jeanrenaud, B. (1990): Abnormal regulation of the hypothalamo-pituitary-adrenal axis in the genetically obese *fa/fa* rat. *Endocrinology* **126**, 1873-1879.
7. Guillaume-Gentil, C., Terrettaz, J., Assimacopoulos-Jeannet, F. & Jeanrenaud, B.: Corticosterone-induced insulin resistance. Submitted for publication.
8. Marchington, D., Rothwell, N.J., Stock, M.J. & York, D.A. (1983): Energy balance, diet-induced thermogenesis and brown adipose tissue in lean and obese *(fa/fa)* Zucker rats after adrenalectomy. *J. Nutr.* **113**, 1395-1402.
9. York, D.A. & Godbole, V. (1979): Effect of adrenalectomy on obese fatty rats. *Horm. Metab. Res.* **11**, 646.
10. Yukimura, Y. & Bray, G.A. (1978): Effects of adrenalectomy on body weight and the size and number of fat cells in the Zucker (fatty) rat. *Endocr. Res. Commun.* **5**, 189-198.

Chapter 42

Caloric Regulation in Liver-transplanted Rats

C. LARUE-ACHAGIOTIS*, A. MICHEL, J. BERNARBÉ, J. BOILLOT and J. LOUIS-SYLVESTRE
Neurobiologie de la Nutrition, Université P.M. Curie, 4 place Jussieu, 75252 Paris Cedex 05, France

It has been proposed that hepatic receptors are involved in the control of food intake. Various studies using hepatic denervation have been done, but the extent of liver denervation was uncertain. Orthotopic liver transplantation allows unambiguous total denervation. We have previously demonstrated that, in liver transplanted rats maintained on a familiar diet, only minor changes appeared in the *ad lib* feeding pattern. It was hypothesized that disturbances could become apparent in response to acute changes in the caloric content and/or the composition of the diet. In the present study the response of liver-transplanted (T) rats to caloric dilution was examined. Two months after transplantation, feeding patterns of male rats fed *ad lib* were continuously recorded and compared to those of normal (N) rats of the same body weight. Meal patterns and body weight changes were followed before, during (9 days) and after (5 days) caloric dilution. No significant differences were observed between the two groups of rats, even in the first 12 h of caloric dilution. Feeding patterns (24 h, night and day intakes, meal number and meal size) were identical in T and N rats. T rats do adjust like N rats. At the conclusion of the experiment, rats were killed, and liver samples were taken. Norepinephrine liver content was significantly smaller in T rats as compared to N rats indicating that no hepatic reinnervation had occurred at this time. Liver innervation is not necessary for caloric adjustment. This result questions the importance of hepatic receptors for energy-intake regulation. Liver signals may be redundant with other information.

Introduction

It has been suggested several years ago[5] that hepatic receptors were involved in the control of food intake. Various studies using hepatic denervation have been realized, but in these experiments the completeness of hepatic denervation has been questioned, because nerve fibres running in the muscular wall of the vessels were not severed by surgery. Orthotopic liver transplantation offers an alternative way to solve the problem. Reinnervation is theoretically possible, but practically it has not been observed even a long time after liver denervation[1]. The feeding pattern observed 2 months post operatively is the spontaneous pattern of animals deprived of hepatic nerve afferents and efferents.

We have demonstrated[3] that in liver-transplanted rats maintained on a familiar diet only minor changes appeared in the *ad lib* feeding pattern. It was shown that from days 15 to 25 after surgery, transplanted rats (T) gained significantly less body weight (BW) than normal rats (N) and their 24 h food intake (FI) was reduced: day-time FI increased while night-time FI decreased. Between days 50 and 60 the BW gain and the 24 h FI of group T were nearly identical to those of group N, and the ratio of day/night food intake was nearly the same. Only small (but not significant) long-lasting changes in the feeding patterns of T rats were observed. It was hypothesized that disturbances could become apparent in responses to acute changes in the diet. In the present study we chose to modify the caloric value of the standard diet. Moreover, to tentatively have a better understanding of the behaviour of these animals we decided to look for some metabolic and hormonal data.

Methods

Male, adult rats (F_1 DA x Lewis, C.S.E.A.L. Orléans) were used. There is no tissue rejection between those animals. Six rats received an orthotopic liver transplantation, five were sham-operated animals, and three intact rats were added for metabolic studies. Liver transplantation was realized according to the technique described by Kamada and Calme[2]. Sham-operated rats were laparotomized. Rats were individually housed in plexiglas cages placed in a quiet temperature-controlled room ($23° ± 1°C$) in which a 12-12 h light-dark cycle was maintained. Rats received water and food (stock powdered diet, UAR A04, 2.9 kcal/g) *ad lib*. The diet was diluted by adding 25 per cent cellulose to the diet (1 g = 2.18 kcal). The feeding patterns were automatically and continuously recorded on chart paper by means of pens connected to electric strain gauge balances[4].

Experimental design

The study was performed on T rats at least 80 days after surgery. Feeding patterns and BW data were recorded for T and N rats maintained on the standard diet (at least 4 days), then the diluted diet (9 days) and then again on the control diet (5 days). The diluted diet was introduced at the end of the diurnal period. At the end of the experiment the rats were sacrificed by anaesthesia: blood and liver samples were taken for metabolic and hormonal assays.

Assays

Plasma glucose levels were measured using a glucose oxidase method (Beckman Autoanalyser II); plasma insulin levels were measured with a rat insulin as standard and a charcoal separation (intra-assay reproducibility = 6 per cent). Plasma glucagon levels were measured using a radioimmunoassay with the "30K" antibody and separation with dextran-coated charcoal. Hepatic catecholamines: The concentrations of catecholamines present in tissues were measured by high performance liquid chromatography (HPLC) with electrochemical detection (Bioanalytical System).

Results

Body weights were nearly identical at the beginning of the observation period. There was no significant variation of body weight under caloric dilution or when the rats were returned to the control diet (Fig. 1). No significant difference was observed between T and N rats in 24 h food intake or in feeding pattern before caloric dilution. Under caloric dilution, both N and T rats increased their 24 h volume of food consumed but never compensated for the diminished caloric value. In group N, all rats increased the weight of food consumed, but sustained adjustment of caloric intake did occur in one rat only. In the other four rats intake was 12% lower for the whole period of caloric dilution. In group T, two rats compensated exactly for the diminished caloric value, while intake in the other four rats remained 12 per cent lower. The increase in FI appeared as early as the first meals of the night and was exactly the same in T and N rats. The augmented FI was due to an increase in meal size both during the day and the night. The mean caloric content of the meal during the dilution period was identical to that of the control period in N (night: $6.4 ± 0.3$ kcal *vs* $6.3 ± 0.4$ kcal; day: $3.6 ± 0.2$ kcal *vs* $3.7 ± 0.4$ kcal) and T rats ($6.1 ± 0.2$ *vs* $6.1 ± 0.3$ kcal; day: $3.7 ± 0.2$ *vs* $4 ± 0.3$ kcal). The number of meals was not significantly modified. At the restoration of the control diet, both N and T rats reduced the weight of food ingested as soon as the first night, but the caloric intake of this 24 h period remained higher than baseline intake. Norepinephrine liver content was significantly smaller in T rats as compared to N rats ($34.7 ± 4.5$ ng/g

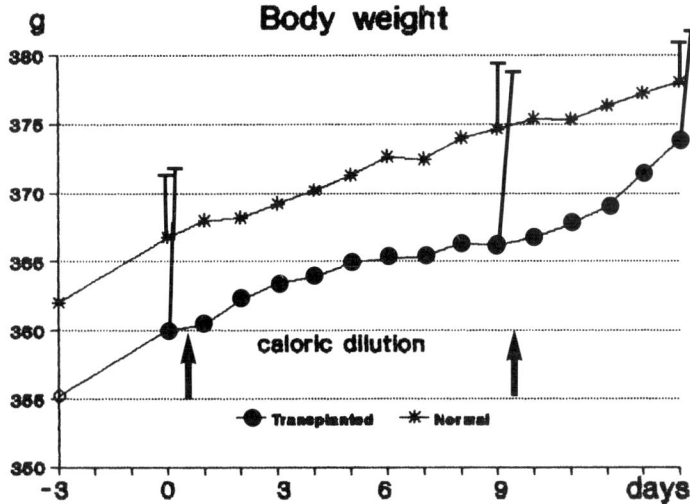

Fig. 1. Body weight in liver-transplanted and control rats.

vs 135.3 ± 7.7 ng/g fresh weight tissue, $P < 0.01$). Plasma glucose was significantly lower in T rats (= 96.2 ± 5.9 mg/100 ml vs n = 130.6 ± 2.7 mg/100 ml; $P < 0.01$), while plasma insulinaemia was not significantly modified (T = 185.5 ± 41.3 µU vs N = 164.4 ± 26.1 µU). Plasma glucagon remained significantly increased in T rats (754 ± 220 pg/ml vs 306 ± 30 pg/ml fresh weight tissue; $P < 0.05$).

Discussion

Liver transplantation is an unambiguous total hepatic denervation. Reinnervation was not demonstrated here since norepinephrine content of T rats liver is only 1/4 of that of N rats.

It is well known that when the energy content of a diet is decreased by dilution with a relatively inert material, animals adjust the amount of food consumed so that caloric intake remains constant. At 25 per cent dilution, the increased volume of food consumed compensates for the lowered caloric values of the diet offered. In the present study, T and N rats did not compensate ideally for the caloric dilution, but they did not lose body weight, and they maintained their BW gain. There is evidence suggesting that rats can digest part of the potential energy in cellulose. Yang et al.[6] reported digestibility of cellulose by rats of 30 to 40 per cent. Since T and N rats increase the volume of food consumed in the same way and there is no difference in their feeding patterns, it can be concluded that hepatic metabolic receptors are not the determining agents of caloric adjustment. It seems probable that intestinal receptors are mainly involved in this situation. However the variations of metabolic correlates observed here indicated that some defect remained in T rats. Further studies are required to give a clear-cut interpretation of the differences observed in liver glycogen content, blood glucose and glucagon levels.

References

1. Bellinger, L., Mendel, V.E., Williams, F.E. & Castonguay, T.W. (1984): The effect of liver denervation on meal patterns, body weight and body composition of rats. *Physiol. Behav.* **33**, 661-667.
2. Kamada, N. & Calne, R.Y. (1979): Orthotopic liver transplantation in the rat. *Transplantation* **28**, 47-50.

3. Louis-Sylvestre, J., Larue-Achagiotis, C., Michel, A. & Houssin, D. (1990): Feeding pattern of liver-transplanted rats. *Physiol. Behav.* **48**, 321-326.
4. Le Magnen, J. & Devos, M. (1980): Parameters of the meal pattern in rat: their assessment and physiological significance. *Neurosci. Biobehav. Rev.* **4** (suppl 1): 1-11.
5. Russek, M. (1963): Demonstration of the influence of hepatic glucoreceptors in the control of intake of food. *Nature* **197**, 7980.
6. Yang, M.S, Manoharan, K. & Young, A.K. (1969): Influence and degradation of dietary cellulose in cecum of rats. *J. Nutr.* **97**, 260-269.

Chapter 43

Control of Cephalic Thermogenic Phase of Feeding

J. LEBLANC[1], P. DIAMOND[1], M. GRIGGIO[3], A. NADEAU[2] and D. RICHARD[1]

[1]Department of Physiology and [2]Unit for Diabetic Research, School of Medicine, Laval University, Quebec City, Canada; [3]Department of Physiology, School of Medicine, São Paulo, Brazil

A cephalic phase of feeding has been reported for insulin and norepinephrine secretion, and for thermogenesis in humans, dogs and rats. Further investigation was undertaken on humans and mice. (A) Six male subjects were fed either a carbohydrate (sugar pie) or a protein-rich food (fish) while norepinephrine (NE) and oxygen consumption were measured before and during the 120 min after the meal. Both the carbohydrate and protein meal induced an early increase in NE and O_2 consumption independent of the composition of the meal. It is suggested that the palatability of the meal is involved in these actions. (B) The sympathetic nervous system activity was also investigated in the heart and BAT of mice either fed *ad libitum* or meal-fed by measuring dopamine accumulation following dopamine betahydroxylase inhibition by CHMI (cyclohexyl-2-mercapto-imidazole) injections. It was found that the ingestion of food produced an increased NE turnover in the heart and BAT of both *ad libitum* and meal-fed mice. This increase was also evident at the time of feeding (8 a.m.) in the meal-fed group even in the absence of food at that time. These studies further confirm the presence of an early cephalic phase of feeding on hormonal and metabolic responses to a meal and suggest it is induced by the sensory stimulation of food.

Introduction

The increased energy metabolism which is observed after the ingestion of food (TEF) accounts for approximately 12% of the total daily energy expenditure of sedentary persons[9]. The composition of the diet and the form in which the nutrients are transformed (protein, lipids or glycogen) are important modulators of this postprandial thermogenesis[6]. There is also evidence that sensory stimulations of feeding may have some influence, specially in the early post-meal thermogenic responses[2-6]. These studies were first made on the dog which proved to be an excellent animal model. In this species, during the 40 min following the beginning of a meal which subsequently was termed the cephalic phase of feeding, there is a marked increase in oxygen consumption which is twice as high as that found during the subsequent gastrointestinal phase, even if the absorption of food is larger during this latter phase as evidenced by plasma glucose and insulin variations. This finding is reaffirmed by results obtained when the animals were either sham-fed or tube-fed. Indeed when the food that the animal eats is diverted into an oesophageal fistula to prevent its absorption (sham-feeding) the initial cephalic response is as large as when food is ingested normally whereas the gastrointestinal response is absent as would be expected. Furthermore when the food is placed directly into the stomach with a tube, no cephalic phase is observed whereas the gastrointestinal phase response is comparable to that observed during normal meal feeding[10]. Studies on humans have also shown that tube-feeding reduces the early cephalic postprandial thermogenesis whereas sham-feeding, during which food is chewed, tasted and spited out, causes a very significant response during the cephalic phase[11,12].

The control of the cephalic postprandial thermogenesis by the autonomic nervous system remains a debated question. Studies have shown that propranolol has no effect following glucose ingestion in humans[20] or hay feeding in sheep[17]. It has also been reported that glucose ingestion produced an increase in plasma NA in man, but that protein and fat had no effect[18]. On the other hand a cafeteria diet was found to significantly increase the NA turnover in the heart and BAT of rats[19]. Experiments on dogs have also shown that feeding or sham-feeding palatable food to dogs caused a twofold increase in plasma NA which paralleled the increase in oxygen consumption[2]. When given propranolol, the early increased thermogenesis was blocked by 60 per cent[4]. It is then proposed that the conflicting evidence might be due to a difference in the palatability of the food which was used in the various studies. We proceeded to examine the response of mice to meal and sham-feeding, and of humans to a palatable meal composed of either carbohydrate or of protein exclusively.

Methods

Human studies

Six overnight fasting male volunteers participated in three experiments. In a first experiment they ate a portion of sugar pie containing 66 g of carbohydrate, 1 g of protein and 16 g of fat per 100 g of wet weight. In the second experiment, a portion of haddock fish was consumed which contained 18 g of protein, 0.2 g of fat and no carbohydrate per 100 g of wet weight. The weight of each meal was adjusted to contain 1260 kJ. In the third experiment the subjects were asked to mimic the hands and mouth movements of a meal for 4 min in the absence of food. For 30 min before and 120 min after the meal the subjects remained in a plastic metabolic chamber (1.02 m^3) which allowed continuous oxygen consumption measurements[11]. Blood sampling at 0, 2, 10, 30 and 90 min were used for NA determinations. At the end of the experiment the subjects were asked to rate palatability of the food on a 0 to 100 scale showing "extremely palatable" at one end and "not palatable at all" at the other.

Mice studies

Male albino mice with initial body weighty of 31 g were used. They were divided into two groups; one group was fed *ad libitum* and the other was meal fed between 09:00 and 11:00 h and between 21:00 and 22:00 h. SNS activity was estimated in the heart and BAT by measuring dopamine (DA) accumulation over 1 h after blocking with CHMI (Cl-cyclohexyl-2-mercapto-imidazole) injection the transformation of DA into NA. In this situation the higher the DA accumulation, the higher the SNS activity. Details of this procedure are reported elsewhere[8].

On the day SNS activity was assessed, continuously-fed (CF) or meal-fed (MF) mice were injected with either saline of CHMI 1 h before being killed. Immediately after the injection, half of the MF mice received their everyday meal whereas the remaining MF animals were not fed (MF no meal). This latter group of mice was used to assess the anticipatory effects of being fed on SNS activity; MF mice were obviously expecting food at the time CHMI was injected. Additional groups of CF and MF mice were not treated, and they were killed at the time of the injection in order to determine the basal levels of both DA and NA in the heart and BAT.

Results

Human study

Oxygen consumption (Fig. 1)

The resting oxygen consumption before eating the pie and the fish were respectively 3.58 ± 0.29 and 3.64 ± 0.41 ml/kg.min^{-1} and they were not statistically different. Previous studies have suggested two phases in postprandial thermogenesis, a cephalic phase, lasting about 40 min and a subsequent gastrointestinal phase[10]. In the present experiment a comparable increase ($P < 0.01$) above RMR was observed for carbohydrate and protein meal during the cephalic phase; the response to blank feeding was not significant. During the gastrointestinal phase (40 to 120 min) the thermogenic response to the fish meal was significantly larger than that to the pie. With blank feeding the response was not significant.

Plasma glucagon and norepinephrine (Fig. 2)

The pie meal caused a significant drop in plasma glucagon at 30 and 90 min and a significant increase was observed at 90 min following the fish meal. Basal plasma norepinephrine levels were not different for the two experiments and averaged 185 ± 22 ng/ml. A significant

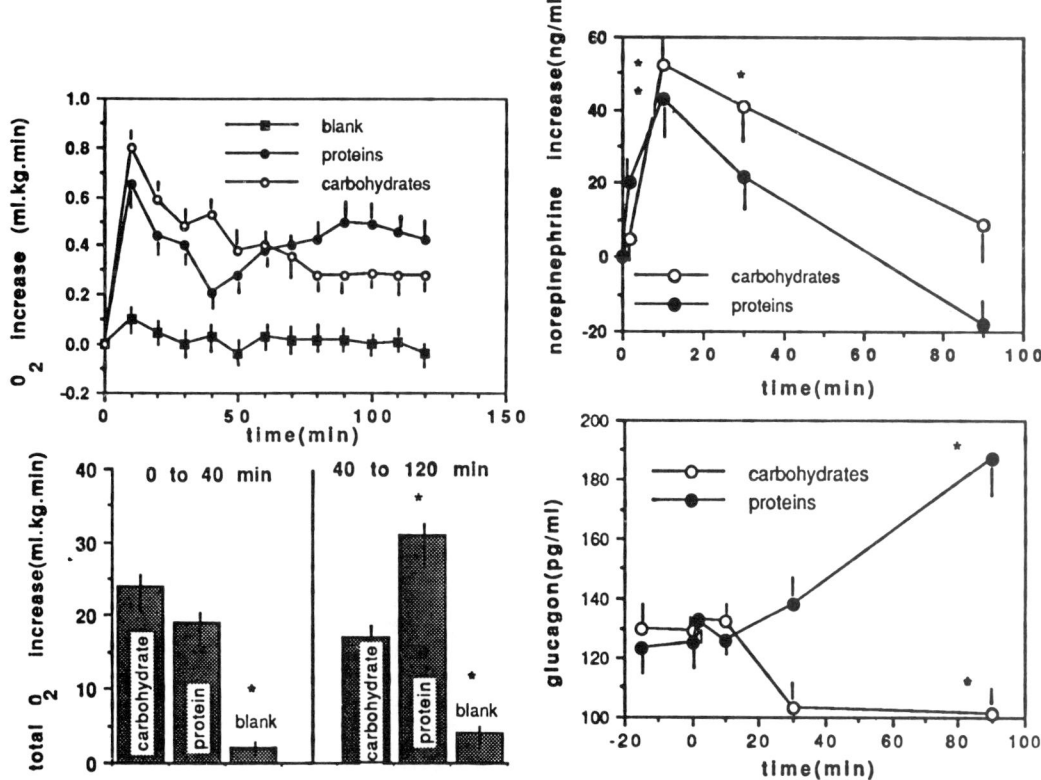

Fig. 1 (left). Increase in oxygen consumption following a protein (fish), carbohydrate (pie) or blank (no food) meal. The lower panel shows the total increase over the initial 40 min and the subsequent 80 min period. * $P < 0.05$.

Fig. 2 (right). Plasma glucagon and norepinephrine increase before and 90 min after the ingestion of a carbohydrate (pie) or protein (fish) meal.

elevation was observed at 10 min after both the pie and the fish meal. This elevation remained significant at 30 min after the pie meal only.

Subjective rating of palatability

Both food items were rated as palatable with a median scoring of 82 for the carbohydrate-rich meal and 76 for the protein meal. The application of the Wilcoxon matched-pairs signed-ranks test indicated that the palatability was the same for both meals.

Mice study

Results on DA accumulation are summarized in Fig. 3. Regardless of whether mice were CF, MF or MF no-meal, DA accumulations in both heart and BAT were higher in CHMI-injected mice than in either saline or non-injected mice. DA accumulated more in tissues of MF groups of mice than in those of CF mice. There was no difference in both heart and BAT DA accumulation between MF mice and MF no-meal mice. The concentrations of DA were higher in BAT than in heart, irrespective of the various conditions to which the animals were subjected in the present study.

The tissue NA contents are shown in Fig. 4. ANOVA did not reveal any significant effects regardless of the factors evaluated.

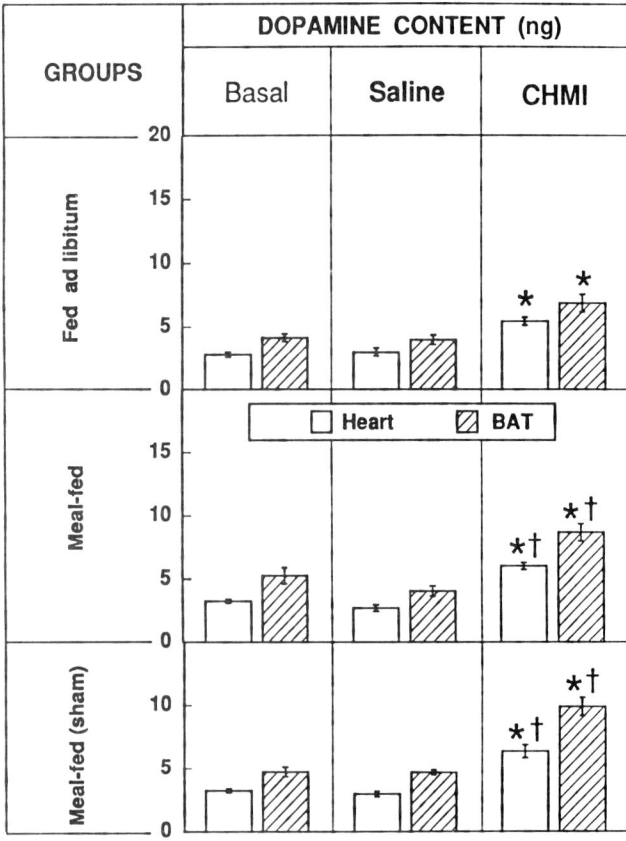

Fig. 3. *Dopamine content of heart and BAT of rats either fed ad libitum, meal-fed or sham meal-fed before and 1 h after inhibition of dopamine transformation into norepinephrine with CHMI (Cl-cyclohexyl-2-mercapto-imidazole).*

Discussion

The maximum increase in oxygen consumption following pie or fish ingestion is observed within 10 min, that is even before the nutrients are absorbed and reach the circulation[13]. This finding suggest that factors other than the specific dynamic action of food are at play. In addition the fact that blank feeding has no significant effect on oxygen consumption indicates that the early postprandial thermogenesis is not due to the bodily movements which accompany food intake. This first study adds evidence for the existence of an early cephalic thermogenesis and confirm previous studies on humans[11], dogs[2] and rats[1].

It was also shown that the high carbohydrate and protein meals which were rated as highly palatable caused an elevation of plasma NA during the early phase of feeding. Mixed meals had the same effect[14] and the fact that propranolol significantly reduced the increase in oxygen consumption[4] suggest a causal relationship between sympathetic activity and early postprandial thermogenesis. The same relationship is suggested with the pie or fish meal and it is proposed that these actions are due to the palatability of the food rather than exclusively to their composition. Recently Welle et al.[18] measured oxygen consumption and plasma norepinephrine with different nutrients and their study indicates that the possible

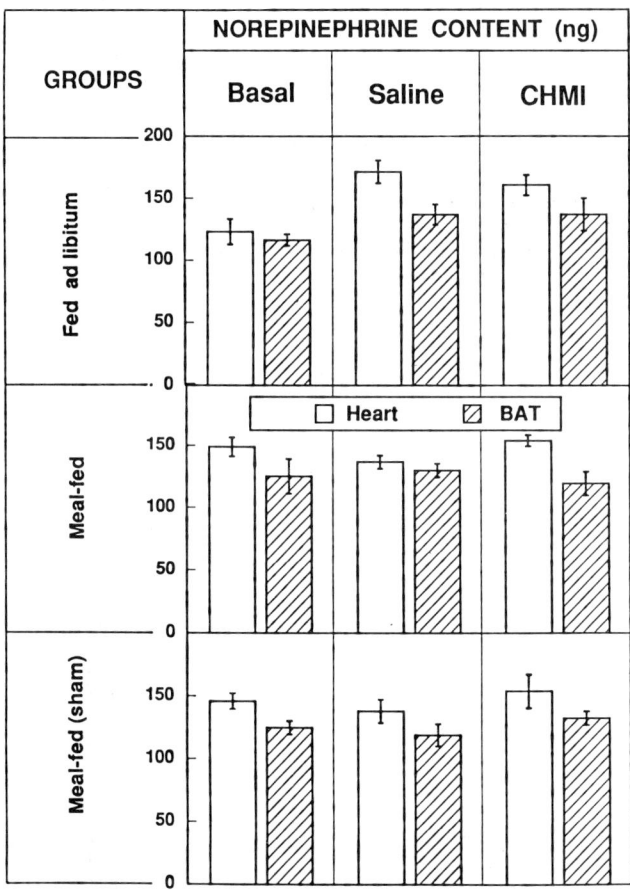

Fig. 4. Norepinephrine content of heart and BAT of rats either fed ad libitum, meal-fed or sham meal-fed before and 1 h after inhibition of dopamine transformation into norepinephrine with CHMI (Cl-cyclohexyl-2-mercapto-imidazole).

involvement of the sympathetic system in postprandial thermogenesis is supported for carbohydrate but not for protein or fat. It would seem possible that the lack of response to the protein meal that they reported was caused by the unpalatability of the food as stated by authors themselves. Indeed, in order to be able to drink the 200 ml collagen hydrolysate, the subjects had to take a lidocaine mouth rinse to temporarily eliminate taste aversion. In our study the protein meal which was rated by the subjects as very palatable, caused an increase in plasma norepinephrine. These results suggest that the palatability of food, either rich in carbohydrates or proteins, is involved in the activation of the sympathetic nervous system observed after feeding.

In the study on mice it was shown that 1 h after the CHMI injection, DA concentrations in both heart and BAT increased significantly above both the basal levels and those measured in saline-injected mice. DA accumulation was higher in MF groups of mice than in CF animals, a finding suggesting that meal intake stimulates SNS activity. In fact, the measurements were made in the morning, when CF mice were inactive and showing little feeding activity, whereas MF mice were at this time strongly expecting food. Interestingly, the present results provide evidence that the effect of meal intake on SNS activity relates largely to the anticipation of being fed; indeed fasting MF mice exhibited an increase in SNS activity similar to that of MF mice that received a meal. Some studies have documented a SNS-mediated cephalic phase in meal-induced thermogenesis that is partly anticipatory and cognitive[2,11,12]. On the other hand, other authors have recognized that the expectation of food may increase energy expenditure but that the increase in expenditure was not mediated by SNS. In a study carried out by Rothwell et al.[15], the use of propranolol did not block the anticipatory increase in expenditure that occurred before a meal. It is worth pointing out that this latter study of Rothwell was conducted in rats, in which the expectation of food may not be as marked as in mice. Indeed, mice show a large increase in energy expenditure while anticipating a meal (Richard, D., unpublished observations). Glick and Raum[7] also did not observe any increase in noradrenaline turnover in meal-fed rats that were not fed the day NA turnover was investigated. In addition to relate to species particularities, the difference between the above-mentioned results and those of the present study may be linked to the length of the period over which NA turnover was determined. Glick and Raum estimated postprandial NA turnover over a period of 3 h as compared to 1 h in the present study. The SNS activation associated with the anticipation of receiving a meal may not last long, and therefore, it is possible that it may be masked in the case where NA turnover is estimated over a long period.

The present study shows that the intake of food increases SNS activity in both heart and BAT and that such an effect is largely cephalic. SNS activation of thermogenic effectors such as BAT should not be underrated as it may promote futile energy dissipation. BAT is a tissue with a considerable heat producing capacity, and its repeated activation may lead to permanent changes liable to increase energy expenditure. In naturally overfed rats, in which BAT undergoes adaptive changes susceptible to increase its thermogenic activity and capacity, energy expenditure is higher than in normally fed rats[16]. The cephalic SNS activation of BAT may therefore contribute to the adaptive mechanisms promoting energy expenditure in overfed rats.

The results reported on humans and on dogs along with those of the present investigation indicate that the anticipation of a meal, without effective food intake, produces an activation of the SNS and parallel increase in oxygen consumption suggesting that these two activities are related to sensory stimulations (cognitive, olfactory and gustatory) induced by palatable food. There is also evidence that palatable food, whether it is fed in the form of mixed meal or as high carbohydrate (pie) or a high protein (fish) food, causes an early postprandial thermogenesis as a result of SNS activation. Other investigations on the dog have indicated the related participation of insulin and NA in the cephalic phase of meal-thermogenesis. Indeed atropine or selective pancreatic vagal denervation not only blocked the cephalic insulin release, but also diminished that of NA by about 65 per cent, with an inhibition of 50 per cent of the oxygen consumption increase[3]. The whole of these findings, associated with the results of the present investigation suggest a metabolic cephalic phase of feeding having the following sequence of events. The sensory stimulations of feeding, caused by the palatability of food, produce a central activation of vagal efference to the pancreas causing an enhanced insulin release which in turn is partly related to an SNS activation. As a result, the oxygen consumption is increased during the early phase of feeding, but this effect is significantly reduced by beta-blockade.

References

1. Allard, M. & Leblanc, J. (1987): Effects of cold acclimation, cold exposure and palatability of food on postprandial thermogenesis in rats. *Int. J. Obesity* **12**, 169-178.
2. Diamond, P. & Leblanc, J. (1987): Hormonal control of postprandial thermogenesis in dogs. *Am. J. Physiol.* **252**, E719-E726.
3. Diamond, P. & Leblanc, J. (1987): A role for insulin in the cephalic phase of postprandial thermogenesis in dogs. *Am. J. Physiol.* **254**, E625-E632.
4. Diamond, P. & Leblanc, J. (1987): Role of the autonomic nervous system in postprandial thermogenesis in dogs. *Am. J. Physiol.* **252**, E719-E726.
5. Diamond, P., Brondel, L. & Leblanc, J. (1985): Palatability and postprandial thermogenesis in dogs. *Am. J. Physiol.* **248**, E75-E79.
6. Flatt, J.P.(1977): The biochemistry of energy expenditure. In *Recent advances in obesity research II"*, ed. G. Bray, pp. 211-228, Washington, D.C.: Newman.
7. Glick, Z. & Raum, W.J. (1986): Norepinephrine turnover in brown adipose tissue is stimulated by a single meal. *Am. J. Physiol.* **251**, R13-R17.
8. Griggio, M.A., Richard, D. & Leblanc, J. The involvement of the sympathetic nervous system in meal-induced thermogenesis in mice. *Int. J. Obesity*, in press.
9. Jequier, E.T. (1981): Thermogenic regulation in man. In *Obesity: pathogenesis and treatment*, ed. Enzi, et al, pp. 44-55. New York: Academic Press.
10. Leblanc, J. & Diamond (1986): Effect of meal size and frequency on postprandial thermogenesis. *Am. J. Physiol.* **250**, E144-E147.
11. Leblanc, J., Cabanac, M. & Samson, P. (1984): Reduced postprandial heat production with gavage as compared with meal feeding in human subjects. *Am. J. Physiol.* **246**, E95-E101.
12. Leblanc, J. & Cabanac, M. (1989): Cephalic postprandial thermogenesis in human subjects. *Physiol. Behav.* **46**, 479-482.
13. Leblanc, J., Diamond, P. & Nadeau, A.: Thermogenic and hormonal responses to palatable protein and carbohydrate rich food. *Horm. Met. Res.*, in press.
14. Leblanc, J. & Brondel, L. (1985): Role of palatability of meal-induced thermogenesis in human subjects. *Am. J. Physiol.* **248**, E333-E338.
15. Rothwell, N.J., Saville, M.E. & Stock, M.J. (1982): Factors influencing acute effect of food on oxygen consumption in the rat. *Int. J. Obesity* **6**, 53-59.
16. Rothwell, N.J. & Stock, M.J. (1986): Brown adipose tissue and diet-induced thermogenesis in BAT. In *Brown adipose tissue*, eds. P. Trayhurn & D.G. Nicholls, pp. 269-298. London: Edward Arnold.
17. Webster, A.J.F. & Hays, F.L. (1968): Effects of beta-adrenergic blockade on energy expenditure of sheep. *Can. J. Physiol. Pharmacol.* **46**, 577-583.
18. Welle, S., Lilavivat, U. & Campbell, R.G. (1981): Thermic effect of feeding in man. Increasing plasma norepinephrine levels following glucose but not protein or fat consumption. *Metabolism* **30**, 353-358.
19. Young, J.B., Saville, E., Rothwell, N.J., Stock, M. & Landsberg, L. (1982): Effect of diet and cold exposure on norepinephrine turnover in brown adipose tissue in the rat. *J. Clin. Invest.* **69**, 1061-1071.
20. Zwillich, G.W., Sahn, S.A. & Weil, J.V. (1973): Effects of hypermetabolism on ventilation and chemosensitivity. *J. Clin. Invest.* **60**, 900-906.

Chapter 44

Does Insulin Play a Role in Cephalic Postprandial Thermogenesis in Human Subjects?

Laurent BRONDEL, Geneviève VAILLANT, Michel GUIGUET and Marc FANTINO

Laboratoire de Physiologie, Faculté de Médecine, Université de Bourgogne, 7 Bd Jeanne d'Arc, F-21033 Dijon Cedex, France

To study the role of insulin in the development of the cephalic phase of the thermic effect of food, two sets of experiments were performed.

In the first, nine insulin-dependent diabetic subjects in whom there was no possible secretion of insulin, on different days, either: (1) ate a meal containing 2580 kJ, (2) saw, smelt and tasted the same meal, or (3) saw, smelt and tasted non-alimentary substances. Oxygen consumption (VO_2) was then recorded by indirect calorimetry over a 20 min rest period then for 90 min. VO_2 increased after normal meal ingestion ($P < 0.01$) but not after presentation of the sensory stimuli (alimentary or not). Then, in the absence of insulin secretion, cephalic postprandial thermogenesis did not appear.

In the second experiment, the same tests were performed in four healthy male subjects, but blood samples were also collected for measurement of glucose and plasmatic insulin levels. VO_2 increased after meal ingestion as well as after alimentary sensory stimulation. The increment after normal ingestion was greater ($P < 0.01$) than that after alimentary sensory stimulation; which in turn was greater than that after non-alimentary sensory stimulation ($P < 0.05$). In contrast, glucose and insulin increased only after the true meal and then 90 min after the start of ingestion (during intestinal absorption). Thus, the cephalic phase of postprandial thermogenesis has been well observed in contrast to the cephalic secretion of insulin.

In conclusion, insulin could play a role in the development of cephalic postprandial thermogenesis since the latter, noted in normal subjects, was not observed in insulin-dependent diabetics, i.e. in absence of insulin secretion. As no changes in plasmatic insulin were observed during the cephalic phase in normal subjects, it may be assumed that those changes are small, that other factors could modify insulin activity or that the plasmatic changes of insulin were not noted due to technical reasons.

Introduction

In animals[3,9,12] as well as in humans[6,7,8] it has been observed that the early phase of postprandial thermogenesis depends on both metabolic and sensory events linked to food intake.

Recently, we observed in nine healthy male subjects that sensory stimulation (sight, smell and taste of a meal) increases resting oxygen consumption (VO_2), contrary to non-alimentary sensory stimulation (sight, smell and taste of non-alimentary stimuli). Conversely, by introducing the meal directly into the stomach, and thus by-passing the oral sensory stimuli, resting VO_2 did not increase as much as after normal ingestion of the same meal (unpublished).

In order to examine the role of insulin in the development of the sensory component in human subjects, two sets of experiments were performed. In the first, the changes in VO_2 after alimentary sensory stimulation were studied in insulin-dependent diabetic subjects. In the second experiment, performed in normal subjects, blood samples were taken during the VO_2 assessment to measure plasmatic insulin both during and after alimentary sensory stimulation.

Experiment one

To evaluate the role of insulin in the mechanism of cephalic thermogenesis, nine insulin-dependent diabetic subjects, in whom there was no possible cephalic reflex secretion of insulin, were tested. The early phase of their postprandial thermogenesis was then examined.

Methods

All the diabetic subjects (four females, five males), aged 21 to 41, had a normal body weight (Body Mass Index (BMI) ranging from 19.5 to 25.6 kg/m^2). None of them had any degenerative diabetic complications. They were all treated by exogenous insulin which, for five of them, was injected by a pump. In all the tests, the rate of injected insulin was maintained constantly, thus avoiding changes in plasmatic insulin.

The three randomized tests were conducted at 2–3 day intervals, as follows:

(1) ingestion of a four course meal (2580 kJ) composed of: mixed vegetables in a mayonnaise sauce; bacon and eggs; flan; cookies and jam.

(2) presentation of the same four course meal but without ingestion (the subjects only saw, smelt and tasted the meal).

(3) presentation of four non-alimentary substances: Hexitidine (Hextril^R, Substancia-France); toothpaste; aluminium gel phosphate; siam benzoin tincture.

On each of the test days, the subjects, who had eaten a lighter breakfast than usual without tea or coffee, came to the laboratory at 10.00 a.m. For a further 90 min, they rested in a room at 22°C ($\pm$1°C). At the end of this period (at 11.30 a.m.), after micturition and body weighing, oxygen consumption was measured in one of the three tests.

VO_2 was measured for 20 min to evaluate the resting metabolic rate. Then, the meal or the sensory stimuli (alimentary or not) were administered in the subsequent 40 min period. During this period, VO_2 was measured over the 7 min intervals between each ingestion of a course (each ingestion lasted 3 min) or, between each alimentary or non-alimentary sensory stimuli. VO_2 was subsequently measured for a further 50 min to evaluate postprandial oxygen consumption (the postprandial period was limited to 50 min due to the diabetic condition). VO_2 was continuously measured by indirect calorimetry using a mouthpiece and a mass spectrometer (MGA 2000, Airspec-England). The volume of expired air was calculated using the argon dilution technique[2,5].

Statistical comparisons were performed by general linear analysis of variance for randomized data followed *post hoc*, by the Newman-Keul's multiple comparison test.

Results

Mean resting VO_2 values were close in all three tests (meal: 241.6 $\pm$ 43.8 ml/min; alimentary sensory stimulation: 238.8 $\pm$ 35.1 ml/min; non-alimentary sensory stimulation: 243.9 $\pm$ 38.0 ml/min). After meal ingestion, VO_2 rose progressively. After alimentary sensory stimulation as well as after non-alimentary sensory stimulation it remained similar to resting values. Thus, there was a significant increase in VO_2 for the whole 90 min period in meal ingestion test (+8.9 per cent of the resting VO_2; $P < 0.01$) and no changes in resting VO_2 for the other two tests (+1.2 per cent after alimentary stimulation and −1.3 per cent after non-alimentary stimulation).

These results indicate that the cephalic component in the early phase of postprandial thermogenesis was not observed in diabetic subjects, in contrast to normal subjects. Thus, the absence of the cephalic postprandial thermogenesis in diabetics could be a consequence of the absence of the cephalic insulin secretion reflex normally induced by feeding.

In order to understand better the role of insulin in the development of cephalic thermogenesis in normal subjects, a second experiment was performed with evaluation of the plasmatic changes of insulin.

Experiment two

Methods

Four healthy male subjects, aged 26 to 28 and with a BMI ranging from 20.9 to 24.6 kg/m^2, were submitted to the previous tests but this time, blood samples were also drawn. The randomized tests were:

(1) ingestion of a meal (identical to that previously described),

(2) presentation of the meal without ingestion,

(3) presentation of non-alimentary substances.

The same temporal pattern was used as in experiment one, except that, when the subjects arrived (at 10.00 a.m.), a catheter was inserted into an antecubital vein.

Blood samples were drawn at t = −5 min (i.e. during the resting period, 5 min before the start of the meal or sensory stimulation), then at t = +5 and t = +25 min (i.e. during the meal or sensory stimulation), then at t = +45 and t = +90 min (*i.e.* during the postprandial period). Glucose (Astra 8, Beckman instruments-USA) and insulin, assayed with radio immunoassay kit (SB-INSI, Sorin Biomedica-Italy)[14], were measured in the blood samples.

Statistical analyses were performed as before.

Results

During the resting period, nearly identical resting VO_2 values were observed in the three tests (meal: 240.0 ± 22.2 ml/min; alimentary sensory stimulation: 238.4 ± 28.5 ml/min non-alimentary sensory stimulation: 241.1 ± 17.1 ml/min). Over the whole 90 min experimental period (after resting period), the mean changes in VO_2 from resting values were in percentage terms +11.5, +4.6 and −1.9 respectively (meal *vs* alimentary stimulation: $P < 0.01$; alimentary stimulation vs non-alimentary stimulation: $P < 0.05$).

No changes were observed in the concentrations of plasma insulin and plasma glucose as compared to resting values after the alimentary or non-alimentary sensory stimulation procedures, but a significant increase was noted 90 min after the beginning of the meal ingestion ($P < 0.05$) (Fig. 1 a, b).

These results indicate that the cephalic component in the early phase of postprandial thermogenesis observed in normal subjects, was not associated with an increase in plasmatic insulin, in contrast to other studies[4,6].

General discussion

The results obtained in normal subjects indicate that alimentary sensory stimulation led to significant thermogenesis.

On the other hand, in insulin-dependent diabetic subjects, alimentary sensory stimulation had no effect on thermogenesis. As it is well known that secretion of insulin is not possible

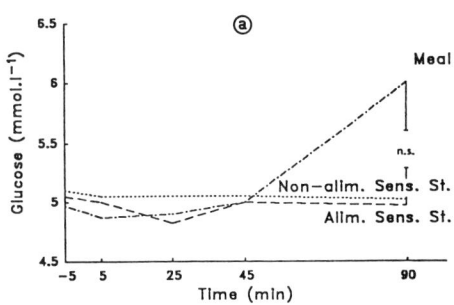 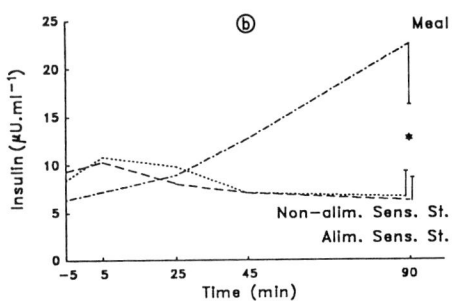

*Fig. 1. Mean plasma levels of glucose (a) and insulin (b) after meal ingestion (•–•), alimentary sensory stimulation (– –) and non-alimentary sensory stimulation (••••) in four normal subjects. *P < 0.05 by ANOVA test, n.s.: non-significant.*

by insulin-dependent diabetics, and as a cephalic postprandial increase in insulin secretion has been described[10,11], we may suggest that insulin plays a role in the development of cephalic postprandial thermogenesis. The absence of the cephalic component in diabetics may be a consequence of the absence of the cephalic secretion reflex of insulin.

In favour of the role of insulin in the development of the cephalic postprandial thermogenesis, other studies indicate that insulin has a thermic effect during the postprandial period[1,13]. An associated increase in plasmatic insulin and cephalic postprandial thermogenesis has also been reported in both animals[4] and humans[6]. Furthermore, preliminary results reveal that injection of insulin to insulin-dependent diabetics during meal ingestion restores their postprandial thermogenesis.

Now we must ask why no changes were noted in normal subjects for plasmatic insulin levels after alimentary sensory stimulation as well as during the cephalic phase of normal meal ingestion. The answer could be that there was an insufficient number of blood samples or simply due to the fragmentation of the meal. Nevertheless, other determining factors may play a role alongside that of insulin in the development of the cephalic component, in particular an increase in norepinephrine secretion as indicated by others[6,7].

In conclusion and according to the results obtained in diabetic subjects, there is some evidence that insulin plays a role in the development of cephalic thermogenesis. In fact, cephalic thermogenesis was not observed in the diabetic subjects and their postprandial thermogenesis was reduced when compared to normal subjects.

Acknowledgements

This work was supported by a Grant-In-Aid for the Ministère de la Recherche et de la Technologie and Benjamin Delessert Foundation.

References

1. Christin, L., Nacht, C.-A., Vernet, O., Ravussin, E., Jequier, E. & Acheson, K.J. (1986): Insulin. Its role in the thermic effect of glucose. *J. Clin. Invest.* **77**, 1747-1755.
2. Davies, N.J.H. & Denison, D.M. (1979): The measurement of metabolic gas exchange and minute volume by mass spectrometry alone. *Respir. Physiol.* **36**, 261-267.
3. Diamond, P., Brondel, L. & Leblanc, J. (1985): Palatability and postprandial thermogenesis in dogs. *Am. J. Physiol.* **248**, E75-E79.
4. Diamond, P. & Leblanc, J. (1988): A role for insulin in cephalic phase of postprandial thermogenesis in dogs. *Am. J. Physiol.* **254**, E625-E632.

5. Hughes, S.W., Lanigan, C., Moxham, J. & Ponte, J. (1985): Continuous measurement of oxygen consumption and carbon dioxide production in man. *J. Physiol. (Lond.)* **371,** 233P.
6. Leblanc, J. & Brondel, L. (1985): Role of palatability on meal-induced thermogenesis in human subjects. *Am. J. Physiol.* **248,** E333-E336.
7. Leblanc, J. & Cabanac, M. (1989): Cephalic postprandial thermogenesis in human subjects. *Physiol. Behav.* **46,** 479-482.
8. Leblanc, J., Cabanac, M. & Sampson, P. (1984): Reduced postprandial heat production with gavage as compared with meal feeding in human subjects. *Am. J. Physiol.* **246,** E95-E101.
9. Leblanc, J. & Diamond, P. (1986): Effect of meal size and frequency on postprandial thermogenesis in dogs. *Am. Physiol.* **250,** E144-E147.
10. Louis-Sylvestre, J. (1976): Preabsorptive insulin release and hypoglycemia in rats. *Am. J. Physiol.* **230,** 56-60.
11. Nicholaidis, S. (1969): Early systemic responses to orogastric stimulation in the regulation of food and water balance: functional and electro-physiological data. *Ann. NY Acad. Sci.* **178,** 1176-1200.
12. Rothwell, N.J. & Stock, M.J. (1978): A paradox in the control of energy intake in the rat. *Nature London* **273,** 146-147.
13. Rothwell, N.J. & Stock, M.J. (1981): A role for insulin in the diet-induced thermogenesis of cafeteria-fed rats. *Metabolism* **30,** 673-678.
14. Wilson, M.A. & Miles, L.E.M. (1977): Radioimmunoassay of insulin. In *Handbook of radioimmunoassay*, ed. G.E. Abraham, p. 275. New York: Dekker.

Chapter 45

The Influence of Meal Composition on Plasma Serotonin and Norepinephrine Concentrations

I. BLUM*, Y. VERED, E. GRAFF, Y. GROSSKOPF, R. DON**, A. HARSAT and O. RAZ

Tel-Aviv Medical Center, The Sackler School of Medicine, Tel-Aviv University, Ramat Aviv, Israel

Reports concerning changes in plasma neurotransmitter values as a result of dietary manipulations, have not been published so far. The influence of various meal compositions on platelet poor plasma (PPP) serotonin (5-HT) and norepinephrine (NE) levels was investigated. Healthy volunteers were subjected to three test meals: a carbohydrate-rich meal (86 per cent carbohydrates), a protein-rich meal (70 per cent protein) and a fat-rich meal (92 per cent fat). After a carbohydrate-rich meal PPP 5-HT values increased significantly (4.47-fold, $P < 0.02$) whereas a smaller increase (1.66 fold, P = N.S.) was observed after a fat rich meal. These effects on PPP 5-HT values could be correlated with insulin plasma levels. A protein-rich meal significantly reduced (P = 0.0011) PPP 5-HT to 28 per cent of initial values despite an increase in plasma insulin levels.

In conclusion, in this study it has been shown that: (a) changes in meal compositions influence PPP 5-HT and to a lesser extent NE values; (b) the resulting changes in PPP 5-HT levels parallel those reported for brain neurotransmitters; (c) these results seem to indicate that PPP 5-HT levels may be a model for its brain synthesis and release.

Introduction

Changes in meal composition have been shown to influence brain monoamine synthesis and release in animals[5,6] and in humans[3]. Changes in plasma neurotransmitter levels as a result of dietary manipulations have not been reported. The aim of the present study is to examine the effect of dietary manipulations on platelet-poor plasma (PPP) serotonin and norepinephrine levels.

Materials and methods

A group of nine (four men and five women, aged 28–53) healthy, drug-free volunteers participated in this study. The volunteers were given test meals at weekly intervals, after a 14 h fast and at a set time (8 a.m.). In this way possible changes induced by circadian variation or by previous meals were minimized.

Test meal no.1 (carbohydrate-rich) with a caloric value of 837.2 kJ consisted of 86 per cent carbohydrates, 12 per cent proteins, < 0.1 per cent fat. Test meal No.2 (protein-rich) had a caloric value of 837.2 kJ, 70 per cent proteins, 29 per cent fat and 0.2 per cent carbohydrates. Meal No.3 (fat-rich) had a caloric value of 1883.7 kJ, 92 per cent fat, 3.5 per cent proteins and 4.5 per cent carbohydrates. In each case venous blood was drawn before the meal and at hourly intervals thereafter for a period of 3 h. The parameters measured were glucose, insulin, NE and 5-HT.

Platelet poor plasma (PPP) was prepared by centrifugation at 1500 **g** for 15 min at 4°C. Each PPP sample was divided into two separate tubes and stored at −20°C until analysed.

Glucose was measured by autoanalyser by a glucose oxidase method. Insulin was measured by RIA. PPP concentrations of serotonin[8] and NE (BAS Application Note No. 14) were determined by an HPLC-ECD method.

Results

The basal serum levels of glucose and insulin were in the range of 3.9–5 mmol/L and 6.1–12.7 µU/ml respectively. Platelet-poor plasma values of serotonin and norepinephrine were in the range of 10–220 nmol/L and 0.46–2.36 nmol/L respectively.

All three test meals enhanced serum insulin levels (Fig. 1). The most significant increase was produced by the carbohydrate meal (test meal #1). The protein-rich meal and the fat-rich meal (test meals #2 and #3 respectively) raised serum insulin levels although serum glucose levels remained unchanged (Fig. 1). The most conspicuous and significant raise in PPP serotonin ($447 \pm 1.4\%$, $P < 0.001$) was observed after the administration of the carbohydrate-rich meal (test meal #1) (Fig. 2). The peak value of serotonin was reached 3 h after meal administration in most subjects (seven out of nine). A smaller non-significant raise in PPP serotonin values was observed 3 h after ingestion of the fat-rich meal (test meal #3) (Fig. 2). This raise paralleled the increase in the serum insulin level[5]. The protein-rich meal (test meal #2) produced a significant reduction in PPP serotonin levels ($28 \pm 0.02\%$, $P = 0.0011$) (Fig. 2). The maximal reduction was observed 3 h after meal administration. The caloric value of the meals had no influence on PPP 5-HT.

PPP NE values increased significantly ($P < 0.002$) 1 h after the fat-rich meal (test meal #3). The other test meals produced no significant changes in plasma NE values. No correlation was found between the changes produced in the values of the measured parameters by the test meals and the age, sex and BMI of the subjects.

Discussion

The results presented by us in this study, show that dietary manipulations cause changes in plasma neurotransmitters. These changes are consistent with those previously reported for brain 5-HT and NE synthesis as a response to their precursors availability[3,5,6].

The increase in PPP 5-HT levels reached its peak 3 h after carbohydrate-meal administration. The late onset of PPP serotonin elevation after carbohydrate consumption, argues against a gut-mediated effect[1,4,7]. These changes in serotonin PPP levels, reflecting newly synthesized 5-HT, parallel changes occurring in the CNS[11], and the plasma insulin increase.

Plasma serotonin changes paralleling those occurring in the brain[11] have been also produced by the protein meal. The significant increase in PPP 5-HT after the carbohydrate meal and the significant decrease after the protein meal suggest that PPP 5-HT may reflect centrally occurring processes. However, since PPP 5-HT reflects newly synthesized serotonin[2], and since platelet uptake and release play an important role in maintaining it within limits[9], it might be argued that changes in meal composition act by influencing these processes.

The significant increase in plasma norepinephrine after a fat-rich meal, might be due to an excess of calories[10] or an excess of acetylcholine synthesis[11] accompanied by secondary norepinephrine secretion. Since it has been shown that plasma may serve as an indicator for brain adrenergic activity, it is conceivable that PPP 5-HT might be also a useful *"in vivo"* peripheral model for processes occurring in human brains.

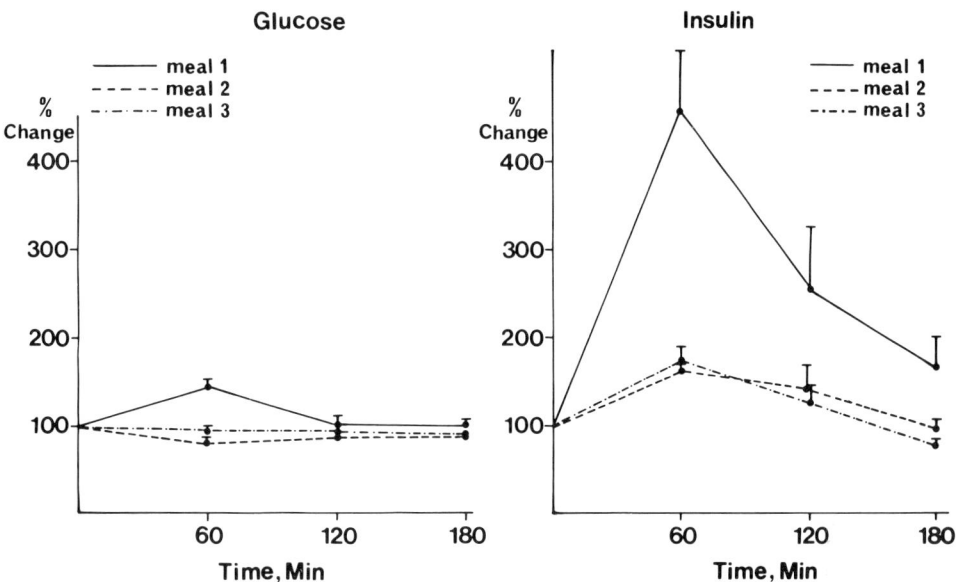

Fig. 1. Percentage change observed in serum values of glucose and insulin after the administration of test meals

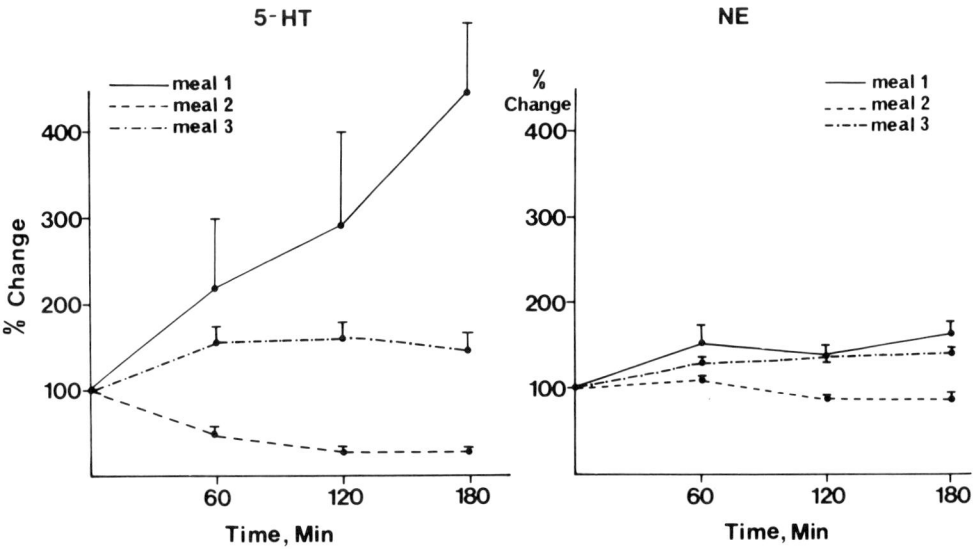

Fig. 2. Percentage change observed in platelet-poor plasma (PPP) values of serotonin (5-HT) and norepinephrine (NE) after the administration of test meals.
(meal no.1 = carbohydrate-rich; no.2 = protein-rich; no.3 = fat-rich)

Acknowledgements

We wish to thank Dr Frank Meyer, Tel-Aviv Medical Center for fruitful discussions.

The full version of this paper has been accepted for publication in *Metabolism*, and this abstract is printed with permission.

References

1. Blett, R.F, MacMillan, M., Sole, M.J., Toal, C.B. & Anderson, G.H. (1984): Free tyrosine levels of rat brain and tissues with sympathetic innervation following administration of L-tyrosine in the presence of large neutral amino acids. *J. Nutr.* **114**, 835-839.
2. Artigas, F., Sarrias, M.J., Martinez, E. & Gelpi, E. (1985): Serotonin in body fluids: characterization of human plasmatic and cerebrospinal fluid pools by means of a new HPLC method. *Life Sci.* **37**, 441-447.
3. Ashley, V.M.D. & Leathwood, P.D.(1983): Meals which may influence brain serotonin metabolism in man. *Int. J. Vitam. Nutr. Res.* **53**, 26.
4. Carlson, H.E, Hyman, D.B. & Blitzer, M.G.(1990): Evidence for an intracerebral action of phenylalanine in stimulation of prolactin secretion: interaction of large neutral amino acids. *J. Clin. Endocrinol. Metab.* **70**, 814-816.
5. Fernstrom, J.D. & Wurtman, R.J. (1972): Brain serotonin content: physiological regulation by plasma amino acids. *Science* **178**, 414-416.
6. Fernstrom, J.D. & Faller, D.V. (1978): Neutral amino acids in the brain: changes in response to food ingestion. *J. Neurochem.* **30**, 1531-1538.
7. Hargraves, K.M. & Partridge, W.M.(1988): Neutral amino acid transport at the human blood brain barrier. *J. Biol. Chem.* **23**, 19392-1937.
8. Tagari, P.C., Boullin, D.J. & Davies, C.L. (1984): Simplified determination of serotonin in plasma by liquid chromatography. *Clin. Chem.* **30**, 131-135.
9. Vanhoutte, P.M. (ed). (1985): *Serotonin and the cardiovascular system*. New York: Raven Press.
10. Wells, S., Lilawathma, U. & Campbell, R.G. (l980): Increased plasma NE concentrations and metabolic rates following glucose ingestion in man. *Metabolism* **29**, 806-809.
11. Wurtman, R.J. (1988): Effect of their nutrient precursors on the synthesis and release of serotonin, the catecholamines and acetylcholine: implications for behavioral disorders. *Clin. Neuropharmacol.* **11**, s187-s193.

Chapter 46

Glucocorticoid Hormone Effects on Visceral Adipose Tissue Metabolism and Distribution

M. REBUFFÉ-SCRIVE, A. MOYER and J. RODIN
Department of Psychology, Yale University, P.O. Box 11A Yale Station, New Haven, CT 06520-7447, USA

Regional effects of glucocorticoid hormones on subcutaneous adipose tissues have been observed, however no data are available concerning visceral fat. In this report, visceral and subcutaneous adipose tissue morphology and metabolism have been studied in male rats which received high doses of the physiological hormone, corticosterone. It was shown that fat was preferentially accumulated in visceral fat tissues while fat mobilization seemed to be preferentially stimulated in the subcutaneous depots. It was suggested that these mechanisms might explain the central redistribution of fat observed in patients with Cushing's syndrome.

Introduction

The recent findings of an important relationship between abdominal, particularly visceral, fat accumulation and prevalent diseases have made it important to study the factors which regulate fat distribution and metabolism. *In vitro* studies by Cigolini and Smith[2] have shown that a fourfold increase in abdominal lipoprotein lipase (LPL) activity can be induced by glucocorticoids in the presence of insulin. *In vivo* studies have shown that patients with Cushing's syndrome[8] have a two to three times higher LPL activity in subcutaneous abdominal adipose tissue in comparison with obese or non-obese controls. Thus, it has been suggested[1] that glucocorticoid hormones might favour fat accumulation in subcutaneous abdominal adipose tissue, *via* stimulation of LPL activity, the key enzyme regulating fat storage. However, in these studies visceral adipose tissues were not assessed. Similarly, several authors[3,5] have suggested that glucocorticoid hormones have a permissive effect on fat mobilization, but no data on potential regional specificity are available.

There are however, some indications that visceral adipose tissues might be even more responsive to glucocorticoid hormones than subcutaneous fat. Measurements of visceral fat, by computerized tomography, in patients with Cushing's syndrome have shown[7] that they have five times more visceral fat than controls while only a twofold increase in subcutaneous fat was observed. Determination of glucocorticoid hormone receptors in human[8] and rat[4] adipose tissues have shown a higher density of receptors as well as receptor mRNA[9] in visceral fat in comparison with subcutaneous adipose tissues.

In the following, the effects of high doses of corticosterone on visceral and subcutaneous fat cell morphology and metabolism were studied in male rats.

Methods

Twenty-seven male Sprague-Dawley rats were randomly assigned to three groups and received various doses of corticosterone *via* subcutaneous implantation of corticosterone pellets. The first group was sham-operated while the two other groups received respectively two and four pellets containing 100 per cent pure corticosterone. All animals were pair-fed in order to control for the effect of corticosterone on food intake[6]. After 14 days, all animals were sacrificed. Four fat pads (three internal depots (epidydimal, retroperitoneal, mesenteric) and one subcutaneous (inguinal)) were dissected, weighed and sampled for determination of fat cell size, LPL activity and basal and norepinephrine (NE)-stimulated lipolysis. Blood was collected at days 1, 6 and 13 after surgery for determination of corticosterone.

The results were analysed with a one-way analysis of variance followed by *post-hoc* contrasts using Tukey's test for comparisons between control and experimental animals receiving different doses of corticosterone.

Results

Plasma corticosterone raised dramatically just after the implantation of the pellets, then decreased over time but still remained elevated 13 days after the surgery (25–30 µg/100 ml). There were significant group differences in body weight, showing a decrease in body weight with increasing doses of corticosterone ($P < 0.0001$). As expected, insulin was elevated in the both experimental groups ($P < 0.001$).

There were significant group differences for fat pad weight, only in the mesenteric fat depot ($P < 0.002$) and for fat cell size in epidydimal ($P < 0.05$), retroperitoneal ($P < 0.05$) and mesenteric ($P < 0.01$) regions. Significant group differences in LPL activity were shown in all regions, epidydimal ($P < 0.01$), retroperitoneal ($P < 0.05$), mesenteric ($P < 0.01$) and inguinal ($P < 0.05$). Basal and NE-stimulated lipolysis were not changed in retroperitoneal and mesenteric depots while significant group differences were observed at maximal NE concentration (10^{-4} M) in epidydimal fat ($P < 0.01$) and at basal as well as at all NE concentrations utilized, in inguinal fat ($P < 0.01$).

Table 1. Regional adipose tissue changes in LPL activity, NE-stimulated glycerol release (lipolysis) and fat cell size after corticosterone administration in male rats

	EPI	RET	ING	MES
Lipoprotein lipase activity, U/10^6 cells	++	+	+	++
NE-stimulated glycerol release, nmol/10^5 cells	+	/	++	/
Fat cell size, µg lipid cell	++	+	/	++

EPI = epidydimal, RET = retroperitoneal, ING = inguinal, MES = mesenteric, + = $P < 0.05$, ++ = $P < 0.01$, / = no changes.

Conclusions

These results show, as summarized in Table 1, that when supraphysiological doses of corticosterone are administrated to male rats, LPL activity is increased in all regions but that this increase is more pronounced in mesenteric and epidydimal depots. In contrast, fat mobilization was stimulated at the highest NE concentration in epididymal fat and was elevated at all NE concentrations in the subcutaneous inguinal depot. Thus, the end results of these metabolic activities, namely fat cell sizes, were increased in all visceral fat tissues particularly in the epidydimal and mesenteric regions. It is interesting to note that in both these regions a higher density of glucocorticoid receptors were earlier demonstrated[4]. No changes were observed in inguinal fat-cell size.

These data have shown that high doses of glucocorticoid hormones seem to lead to a redistribution of fat towards the internal fat regions. Furthermore, it is suggested that these mechanisms might explain the central (particularly visceral) redistribution of fat observed in Cushing patients.

Acknowledgements

This work has been supported by the John D. and Catherine T. MacArthur Foundation Health and Behavior Network (mid-career fellowship to M. Rebuffé-Scrive).

References

1. Björntorp, P., Ottoson, M., Rebuffé-Scrive, M. & Xu, X. (1990): Regional obesity and steroid hormone interactions in human adipose tissue. In *Obesity: towards a molecular approach.* eds. G. Bray, B. Spiegelman & D. Ricquier, pp. 147-157. New York: Alan Liss Inc.
2. Cigolini, M. & Smith, U. (1979): Human adipose tissue in culture: VIII. Studies on the insulin antagonistic effect of glucocorticoids. *Metabolism* **28**, 502-510.
3. Fain, J.N. & Czech M.P. (1974): Glucocorticoid effects on lipid mobilization and adipose tissue metabolism. In *Handbook of physiology.* **4**, eds. H. Blasschko, G. Sayers & A.D. Smith, pp. 169-178. Baltimore: Waverby.
4. Feldman, D. & Loose, D. (1977): Glucocorticoid receptors in adipose tissue. *Endocrinology* **100**, 398-405.
5. Giudicelli, Y., Lacasa, D., de Mezancourt, P., Pasquier, Y.N. & Pecquery, R. (1988): Steroid hormones and lipolysis regulation. In *Obesity in Europe 88.* eds. P. Björntorp & S. Rössner, pp. 185-194. John Libbey: London.
6. Krotkiewski, M., Krotkiewska, J. & Björntorp, P. (1970): Effects of dexamethasone on lipid mobilization in the rat. *Acta Endocrinol.* **63**, 185-192.
7. Mayo-Smith, W., Hayes, C., Biller, B., Klibanski, A., Rosenthal, H. & Rosenthal,D. (1989): Body fat distribution measured with CT: correlations in healthy subjects, patients with anorexia nervosa and patients with Cushing syndrome. *Radiology* **170**, 515-518.
8. Rebuffé-Scrive, M., Krotkiewski, M., Elfverson, J. & Björntorp P.(1988): Muscle and adipose tissue morphology and metabolism in Cushing's Syndrome. *J. Clin. Endocrinol. Metab.* **67**, 1122-1128.
9. Rebuffé-Scrive, M., Lundholm, K. & Björntorp, P. (1985): Glucocorticoid hormone binding to human adipose tissue. *Eur. J. Clin. Invest.* **15**, 267-271.
10. Rebuffé-Scrive, M., Nilsson, A., Bronnegard, M., Eldh, J., Gustafsson, J.A. & Björntorp, P. (1990): Steroid hormones receptors in human adipose tissues. *J. Clin. Endocrinol. Metab.* **71**, 1215-1219.

Chapter 47

Increased Pancreatic Islet Blood Flow in Obese Zucker Rats

Nadia ATEF, Alain KTORZA, Luc PICON and Luc PENICAUD
Laboratoire de Physiopathologie de la Nutrition, CNRS URA 307, Université Paris VII, Tour 23-33, 2 Place Jussieu, 75251 Paris Cedex 05 France

Hyperinsulinaemia, a main feature of human and animal obesity, has been demonstrated to be due to both an increased sensitivity to nutrient secretagogues and an increased parasympathetic activity. Recent studies have shown that pancreatic islets blood flow increased under conditions associated with an enhanced insulin secretion. The aim of this study was to determine whether or not changes in islets blood flow (IBF) could participate in the hyperinsulinaemia of obese Zucker rats and if this could be related to an increased parasympathetic activity. We showed an IBF higher in obese than in lean rats. Bilateral subdiaphragmatic vagotomy had no effect on IBF of lean rats whereas it decreased it significantly in obese Zucker rats. It is concluded that obese Zucker rats exhibit increased pancreatic islets blood flow which may result, at least in part, from higher than normal parasympathetic activity.

Introduction

Jansson and Hellerström have recently demonstrated that an increase in blood glucose concentration led to a specific enhancement of islet blood flow and that this increase was mediated by vagal cholinergic fibres[1-3]. Although several studies have dealt with the regulatory mechanisms involved in the hyperinsulinaemia observed in obesity, to our knowledge, none concerning the relationship between islet blood flow and oversecretion of insulin in obese animals or humans is available.

The present work was undertaken in order to quantify the pancreatic islet blood flow in obese rats and to investigate the possible role of the parasympathetic nervous system in the control of this variable.

Materials and methods

Genetically obese (*fa/fa*) or lean (*Fa/Fa*) female Zucker rats 11–12 weeks old were bred in our laboratory. Animals were housed in cages in a room in which the temperature was maintained at 24°C with light from 7 a.m. to 7 p.m. They had free access to water and laboratory chow pellets (UAR, Villemoisin, France, 53 per cent carbohydrates, 5 per cent lipids, 22 per cent proteins).

Blood flow measurements were performed on anaesthetized rats (pentobarbital 0.8 mg/kg) as described by Jansson et al.[2-4]. 1–1.5 x 10^5 nonradioactive microspheres (New England Nuclear Cop., Boston, MA, USA) with a diameter of 10 µm were injected *via* an intracardiac catheter. Simultaneously, an arterial blood sample was withdrawn with a peristaltic pump (0.6 ml/min) from a catheter placed in the abdominal aorta. Then 500 µl of blood were quickly sampled, centrifuged and the plasma frozen. Plasma glucose and insulin concentrations were determined using respectively a glucose analyser (Glucose analyser 2, Beckman, Fullerton, CA, USA) and a radioimmunoassay (Kit INSIK 1, CEA, Saclay, France).

The rats were killed by cervical dislocation and the pancreas and both adrenal glands were removed, blotted and weighed. The organs and the reference sample were further processed and examined for microspheres content, as previously described[3,4]. The microspheres content of the adrenal gland was used as a measure of the mixing of the microspheres with the blood. A difference of more than 10 per cent between the two glands excluded the animal from the study.

In another series of experiments, the two branches of the vagus nerve were cut just under the diaphragm 30 min before the microspheres injection.

Results are expressed as mean ± SEM. Statistical significance of differences between means were evaluated using Student's unpaired t-test.

Results

In obese rats, the plasma glucose level was significantly lower whereas plasma insulin concentrations and islet blood flow (IBF) were significantly higher than in lean rats (Table 1).

Table 1. Plasma glucose and insulin concentrations and islets blood flow (IBF) in obese or lean Zucker rats. Effect of bilateral subdiaphragmatic vagotomy

		Lean (Fa/Fa)	Obese (fa/fa)
Plasma glucose, mg/dl	Basal	115 ± 2	105 ± 2*
	Vagotomized	121 ± 6	134 ± 4†
Plasma insulin, µU/ml	Basal	34 ± 3	121 ± 3*
	Vagotomized	38 ± 5	48 ± 5†
IBF, µl/min/g pancreas	Basal	58 ± 5	160 ± 7*
	Vagotomized	70 ± 10	83 ± 8†

Data are means ± SEM of 4 to 7 measurements.
* Significantly different from lean rats. † Significantly different from intact rats.

In lean rats, vagotomy did not change significantly either the plasma glucose or plasma insulin concentrations. In obese rats, section of the vagus nerves induced a significant increase of plasma glucose concomitant with a 2.5-fold decrease of plasma insulin. Vagotomy had no significant effect on IBF in lean rats but it reduced IBF by a factor of 2 in obese rats. As a consequence, IBF was no more different in vagotomized lean and obese rats.

Discussion

The present data show that obese rats have a higher islet blood flow than lean rats. Although this cannot strictly imply a relationship between both variables, this suggests that a high islet blood flow could be involved in insulin oversecretion of obese rats.

Insulin secretion is under the influence of stimulatory vagal nerves. On the other hand, several studies indicate that in obese rodents, hyperinsulinaemia is mediated *via* an increased parasympathetic activity[5,6]. In an order to determine whether or not these changes in the autonomic nervous function could be involved in the increased islet blood flow observed in the obese rats, we performed a bilateral subdiaphragmatic vagotomy.

In lean rats, vagotomy had no significant effect on IBF and plasma insulin concentrations. This absence of effect in lean Zucker rats is in good agreement with previous results obtained in normal Wistar rats[3]. In vagotomized obese rats, IBF and plasma insulin concentrations were significantly decreased. This suggests an involvement of the parasympathetic system in the increased IBF observed in the Zucker rats.

Taken together the data indicate that the high islet blood flow in obese rats could participate in the hyperinsulinaemia observed in obesity. Furthermore, they demonstrate that this increased IBF is related to the exaggerated parasympathetic activity.

References

1. Jansson, L. & Hellerström, C. (1983): Stimulation by glucose of the blood flow to the pancreatic islets of the rat. *Diabetologia* **25**, 45-50.
2. Jansson, L. (1984): The blood flow to the pancreas and the islets of Langerhans during an intraperitoenal glucose load in the rat. *Diabet. Res.* **1**, 111-114.
3. Jansson, L. & Hellerström, C. (1986): Glucose-induced changes in pancreatic islet blood flow mediated by central nervous system. *Am. J. Physiol.* **251**, E644-E647.
4. Jansson, L. & Hellerström, C. (1981): A rapid method of visualizing the pancreatic islets of studies of islet capillary blood flow using nonradioactive microspheres. *Acta Physiol. Scand.* **113**, 371-374.
5. Rohner-Jeanrenaud, F., Hochstrasser, A.C. & Jeanrenaud, B. (1983): Hyperinsulinemia of preobese and obese *fa/fa* rats is partly vagus nerve mediated. *Am. J. Physiol.* **244**, E317-E319.
6. Jeanrenaud, B. (1985): An hypothesis of the aetiology of obesity: dysfunction of the central nervous system as a primary cause. *Diabetologia* **28**, 502-513.

Section VIII
Enzymatic and metabolic regulation of adipose tissue

Chapter 48

The Role of Gut Hormones in the Adipose Tissue Metabolism of Lean and Genetically Obese (*ob/ob*) Mice

J. OBEN, R. ELLIOTT, L. MORGAN, J. FLETCHER* and V. MARKS
*School of Biological Sciences, University of Surrey, Guildford, Surrey GU2 SXH, UK and *Unilever Research, Colworth House, Sharnbrook, MK44 1LQ, UK*

The insulinotropic gut hormones, gastric inhibitory polypeptide (GIP) and glucagon-like-polypeptide (7–36) amide (tGLP-1) have direct anabolic actions on adipose tissue. This study measured tissue and plasma tGLP-1 in lean and obese (*ob/ob*) mice and investigated the effects of GIP and tGLP-1 on omental adipose tissue metabolism. Plasma tGLP-1 levels showed a slight but significant ($P < 0.05$) elevation in obese animals compared with lean littermates; intestinal tGLP-1 concentrations were not significantly different. Adipose tissue fatty acid synthesis was stimulated by GIP, tGLP-1 and insulin in lean mice, but in obese mice fatty acid synthesis was only stimulated by tGLP-1. Adipose tissue lipoprotein lipase (LPL) activity in lean mice was stimulated by insulin (5 nM) and GIP (4 nM) ($P < 0.01$) but not by tGLP-1. LPL activity was four- to fivefold higher in obese animals. The ability of insulin to stimulate LPL activity was impaired, but LPL activity was stimulated by tGLP-1 ($P < 0.01$) in obese mice. The anabolic action of GIP and tGLP-1 on adipose tissue and their higher circulating levels in obese mice suggests a role in the development of their obesity. In addition, differences in their responsiveness to these hormones may contribute to some of the metabolic abnormalities of the obese state.

Introduction

The hormonal control of nutrient accumulation in adipose tissue is complex and a key role has been ascribed to insulin. An "entero-insular" axis has been well established providing a mechanism by which hormonal peptides from the gut, notably gastric inhibitory polypeptide (GIP) and glucagon-like polypeptide-1 (7–36)amide have the potential indirectly to influence adipose metabolism by their facilitation of glucose-mediated insulin secretion[7]. In addition, direct actions of gut hormones on adipose tissue have also been described; GIP stimulates both the synthesis and secretion of lipoprotein lipase by pre-adipocytes[6] and the incorporation of fatty acids into adipose tissue[3]. We have recently shown that both GIP and tGLP-1 exert direct anabolic effects on rat adipose tissue *in vitro* whereas glucagon and glucagon-like peptide 2 (GLP-2) were without effect[10].

In addition to hyperphagia and hyperinsulinaemia, the genetically obese mouse (*ob/ob*) has higher intestinal and circulating concentrations of GIP than lean animals[2]. The present study has measured the tissue and plasma concentrations of tGLP-1 in lean and obese mice and investigated the effects of GIP and tGLP-1 on adipose tissue metabolism in these animals.

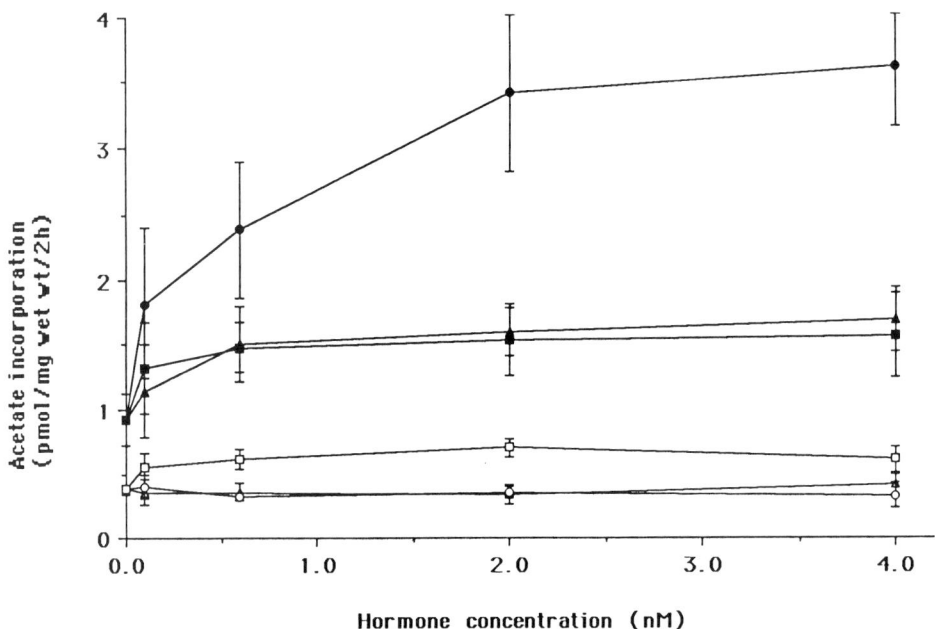

Fig. 1. The effect of hormones on fatty acids synthesis in omental adipose tissue in obese (ob/ob) and lean mice. ●–● = insulin/lean, ○–○ = insulin/obese, ▲▶▲ = GIP/lean, △–△ = GIP/obese, ■–■ = tGLP-1/lean, ❏–❏ = tGLP-1/obese (mean ± SEM, n = 6).

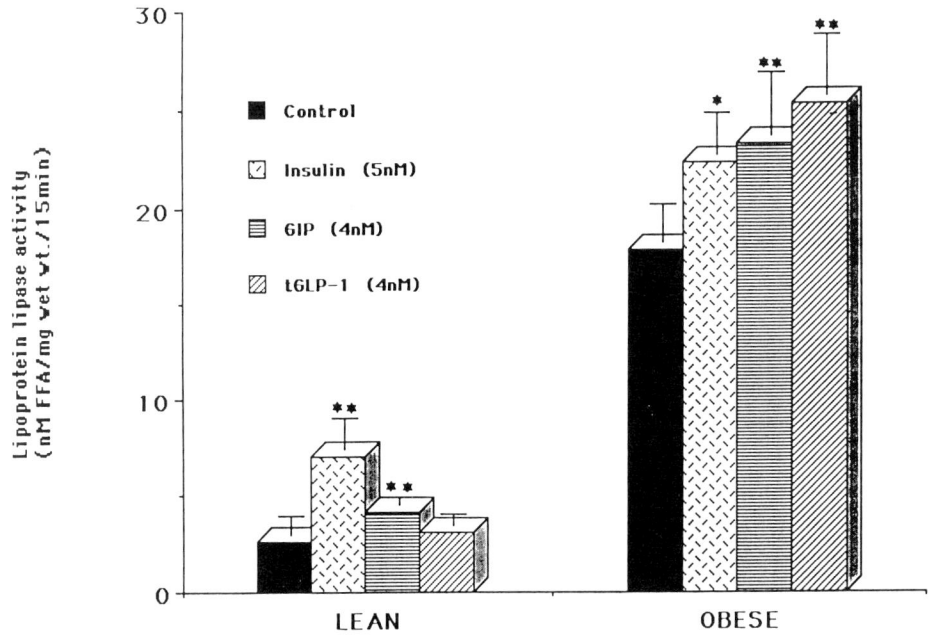

Fig. 2. The effect of hormones on lipoprotein lipase activity in omental adipose tissue of obese (ob/ob) and lean mice (mean ± SEM, n = 10 for all lean animals, obese/basal and obese/insulin, n = 6 for GIP/obese, n = 5 for tGLP-1/obese). *$P < 0.05$, **$P < 0.01$ compared with basal.

Methods

Animals and preparation of adipose tissue explants

Obese (*ob/ob*) mice and lean litter-mates on the Aston background aged 16–20 weeks were studied. The origin and characteristics of these mice have been described in[1]. Mice were killed by cervical dislocation between 08.00 h and 10.00 h on the day of the experiment. Omental adipose tissue was excised and transferred into Medium 199. Explants (0.4–0.6 mg) of adipose tissue were prepared as described by Dils[5]. Explants, six per well, were transferred to multiwell dishes containing Medium 199, supplemented with various concentrations of the hormone under investigation, after an initial recovery period of 90 min. The explants were incubated for 2 h, after which fatty acid synthesis was determined by measuring sodium [^{14}C] acetate incorporation into saponifiable fat. Lipoprotein lipase activity was measured in homogenates of adipose tissue explants previously cultured in hormone-containing Medium 199. The assay for lipoprotein lipase was as described by Nilson-Ehle[9], using triolein as substrate.

Measurement of gut and plasma GIP and tGLP-1

Blood was obtained from obese (*ob/ob*) and lean mice by cardiac puncture, after an overnight fast, or from animals with free access to food. The blood was transferred into heparinized tubes containing aprotinin (100 KIU) the plasma separated immediately and stored at 20°C until assay. Guts were removed immediately after sacrifice, washed with ice-cold distilled water and extracted using acid ethanol (50:16:1, v/v/v EtOH/water/37 per cent HCl). Plasma GIP and tGLP-1 were measured by double antibody radioimmunoassay[8]. Synthetic tGLP-1 and porcine GIP were used for the preparation of standards and of ^{125}I-tracers.

Statistical analyses

Results were compared by ANOVA followed by Duncan's range analysis to locate differences. Hartley's F-test was used to check for heteroscediscity of data. Values of $P < 0.05$ were taken as statistically significant.

Results

Fatty acid synthesis was stimulated by insulin, GIP and tGLP-1 in adipose tissue from lean mice (Fig. 1). In obese mice, fatty acid synthesis was however only stimulated by tGLP-1 ($P < 0.01$).

Basal adipose tissue lipoprotein lipase activity was four- to fivefold higher in obese mice compared to lean littermates (Fig. 2). In lean mice this activity was significantly stimulated by insulin (5 nM) and GrP (4 nM) ($P < 0.01$) but not by tGLP-1 (4 nM). The ability of insulin to stimulate LPL activity was reduced in the obese group. However, tGLP-1 caused a significant stimulation of LPL activity in obese animals ($P < 0.01$), in contrast with their lean littermates.

tGLP-1 was located throughout the length of the small and large intestines, with highest concentrations found in ileum and colon. There were no significant differences between lean and obese animals (Table 1). Plasma tGLP-1 levels were not affected by the nutritional status of the animals (Table 2). However, obese animals as a group had higher circulating levels of tGLP-1 than their lean littermates (44.8 ± 5.0 *vs.* 62.3 ± 5.7 pmol/L for lean and obese animals respectively, $P < 0.05$).

Discussion

Obese (*ob/ob*) mice on the Aston background have been shown to exhibit a marked elevation in circulating GIP and insulin with levels more than 10-fold higher than their lean counterparts[2]. In contrast, we have found that circulating tGLP-1 levels are only slightly raised in obese animals and that their gut tGLP-1 levels are similar to lean animals. The inability of insulin and GIP to stimulate fatty acid synthesis in adipose tissue from obese mice, and the partial attenuation of the tGLP-1 response could be due to down-regulation or masking of the hormone receptors by elevated circulating levels of these hormones. Obese mice also show differences in the sensitivity of LPL to hormones. tGLP-1 stimulated LPL activity in obese animals in contrast with their lean littermates, although caution should be exercised in view of the small number of animals studied. This finding has parallels in studies of Zucker fatty rats, where obese animals do not show marked elevations in circulating GIP, but exhibit an increased sensitivity to its actions[4]. The direct anabolic effects of GIP and tGLP-1 as well as their higher circulating levels in obese mice, suggest a role in their development of obesity. In addition, differences in their sensitivity to GIP and tGLP-1 may contribute to some of the metabolic abnormalities of the obese state.

Table 1. Immunoreactive tGLP-1 concentrations in lean and obese (ob/ob) mouse gut (mean ± SEM, n = 4)

tGLP-1 (pmol/g)	Stomach	Duodenum	Jejunum	Ileum	Caecum	Colon
Lean	ND	34.5±10	56.2±15	99.5±24	48.1±4.7	79.3±23
Obese	ND	22.2±4.9	51.9±8.2	106±32	20.8±1.6	67.1±1.6

ND = None detected.

Table 2. Plasma immunoreactive tGLP-1 concentrations in lean and obese (ob/ob) mice (mean ± SEM, n = 6)

	tGLP-1 (pmol/l)	
	Fasted	Fed
Lean	47.5±8.2	42.2±6.5
Obese	70.5±3.4	54.2±10.2

References

1. Bailey, C., Flatt, P.R. & Atkins, T.W. (1982): Influence of genetic background and age on the expression of the obese hyperglycaemic syndrome in Aston ob/ob mice. *Int. J. Obes.* **6**, 11-21.
2. Bailey, C., Flatt, P., Kwasowski, P., Powell, C. & Marks, V. (1986): Immunoreactive gastric inhibitory polypeptide and K-cell hyperplasia in obese hyperglycaemic mice fed high fat and high carbohydrate cafeteria diets. *Acta Endocrinol.* **112**, 224-229.
3. Beck, B. & Max, J. (1983): Gastric inhibitory polypeptide enhancement of the insulin effect of fatty acid incorporation into adipose tissue in the rat. *Regul. Pept.* **7**, 3-8.
4. Beck, B. & Max, J. (1986): Increased effect of GIP on lipid metabolism in adipose tissue of obese Zucker (fa/fa) rats. In *Proceedings of the 6th International conference on gastrointestinal hormones*, pp.53. Vancouver, BC., Ottawa: National Research Council of Canadian Research Journals.
5. Dils, R. & Forsyth, I. (1981): Preparation and culture of mammary gland explants. *Methods Enzymol.* **72**, 724-742.
6. Eckel, R., Fujimoto, W. & Brunzell, J. (1978): Gastric inhibitory polypeptide enhances lipoprotein lipase activity in cultured pre-adipocytes. *Diabetes*, **28**, 1141-1142.
7. Morgan, L., Flatt, P. & Marks, V. (1988): Nutrient regulation of the entero-insular axis and insulin secretion. *Nutr. Res. Rev.* **1**, 79-97.
8. Morgan, L., Morris, B. & Marks, V. (1978): Radioimmunoassay of gastric inhibitory polypeptide. *Ann. Clin. Biochem.* **15**, 172-177.
9. Nielson-Ehle, P., Garfinkel, A., Schotz, M. (1976): Lipolytic enzymes and plasma lipoprotein metabolism. *Ann. Rev. Biochem.* **49**, 667-693.
10. Oben, J., Morgan, L., Fletcher, J. & Marks, V. (1991): The effect of the entero-pancreatic hormones gastric inhibitory polypeptide and glucagon-like polypeptide-1 (7–36) amide on fatty acid synthesis in explants of rat adipose tissue. *J. Endocrinol.* (in press).

Chapter 49

Activation of Multiple Insulin Effectors in White Adipose Tissue of 1 Week VMH-lesioned Rats

Béatrice COUSIN, Karen AGOU, Anne Françoise BURNOL*, Armelle LETURQUE*, Jean GIRARD* and Luc PENICAUD

Laboratoire de Physiopathologie de la Nutrition, CNRS URA 307, 2 Place Jussieu, 75251 Paris Cedex 05 and *Centre de Recherche sur l'Endocrinologie Moléculaire et le Developpement, CNRS, 9 rue Jules Hetzel, 92130 Meudon, France

We have shown in white adipose tissue of rats 1 week after VMH lesion an increase (1) in insulin receptor kinase activity, (2) in glucose transport and protein concentration of insulin sensitive glucose transporter and (3) in lipogenesis. Thus the increased glucose utilization previously described *in vivo* in white adipose tissue from rats at the onset of VMH obesity is related to both receptor and post receptor changes.

Introduction

We have previously shown that rats made obese by lesion of the ventromedial hypothalamus nuclei present 1 week after injury, a hyperresponsiveness to insulin in regard to whole body glucose utilization, this being mainly due to an increased glucose uptake in white adipose tissue[8,9]. The aim of the present work was to study further the insulin effectors involved in this increase. We measured respectively tyrosine kinase activity of the insulin receptor, glucose transport, expression of the insulin responsive glucose transporter (Glut 4), and glucose metabolism.

Methods

Animals

Female Wistar rats received a bilateral electrolytic lesion under ketalar anaesthesia as described previously[8]. They were fed *ad libitum* and maintained in a room in which a dark-light cycle was monitored. The lesion was considered as successful when body weight gain was greater than 5 g/day. Experiments were done 1 week after the lesion.

Insulin receptor kinase activity

The preparation of WAT insulin receptors and the measurement of their tyrosine kinase activity was performed as described by Burnol *et al.*[1]. Preparations from lean and obese rats were always run in parallel, and were equalized to the same insulin binding capacity, determined by Scatchard analysis. Insulin receptor preparations were incubated in the absence or presence of 10^{-7} M insulin and used for either determining autophosphorylation or phosphorylation of exogenous substrate poly (Glut4: Tyr1).

Glucose transport and metabolism in isolated adipocytes

White adipocytes were isolated as described previously by Rodbell[11]. Glucose transport studies were performed by measuring the cell-associated radioactivity after a rapid incubation of white adipocytes with 50 μM [6-^{14}C] glucose and insulin [^{3}H]. Isolated adipocytes, at a final concentration of 2×10^5 cells/ml, were preincubated during 1 h, in the absence or the presence of 6 nM insulin, in Krebs-Ringer phosphate containing 2 mM pyruvate. The assays were ended after 20 s by rapidly centrifuging 200 μl aliquots of cell suspension with dinoyl-phtalate oil. The cell layer was removed and the radioactivity was counted.

Isolated white adipocytes, at a concentration of 10^5 cells/ml, were incubated for 2 h with 5 mM [U-^{14}C] glucose, in the absence or the presence of 6 nM insulin. Glucose incorporation into CO_2, total lipids, fatty acids, glycerol and lactate were measured as described elsewhere[1].

Glucose transporter quantification

The amount of Glut 4 protein was determined by Western blot analysis[7] of white adipose tissue homogenate using a specific monoclonal antibody. Quantification was performed by scanning densitometry. Results were expressed as mean ± SEM. Statistical analysis was performed by Student's t-test for unpaired data.

Table 1. Insulin receptor kinase activity in white adipose tissue of control rats and rats 1 week after lesion of the VMH, in the absence (basal) or the presence of 10^{-7} M insulin (maximal)

	Controls	VMH	
Autophosphorylation, % max			
Basal	4.9 ± 3	42 ± 12	
Maximal	100	236 ± 13	$P < 0.05$
Exogenous substrate phosphorylation, % max			
Basal	35 ± 8	66 ± 20	
Maximal	96 ± 1	260 ± 44	$P < 0.05$

Results are mean ± SEM of 4 experiments.

Table 2. Glucose transport and glucose incorporation into CO_2 and total lipids in white adipocytes of control rats and rats 1 week after lesion of the VMH, in the absence (basal) or the presence of 6 nM insulin (maximal)

	Controls	VMH	
Glucose transport, nmol/min/10^6 cells			
Basal	0.24 ± 0.02	0.48 ± 0.08	$P < 0.01$
Maximal	0.55 ± 0.04	1.07 ± 0.15	$P < 0.01$
Incorporation of glucose into CO_2, nmol/min/10^6 cells			
Basal	47 ± 11	1660 ± 208	$P < 0.001$
Maximal	234 ± 55	3883 ± 262	$P < 0.001$
Incorporation of glucose into lipids, nmol/min/10^6 cells			
Basal	129 ± 43	1119 ± 143	$P < 0.001$
Maximal	389 ± 72	3207 ± 431	$P < 0.001$

Results are mean ± SEM of 4–8 experiments.

Results

Receptor kinase activity

As shown in Table 1, in the basal state, insulin receptor kinase activity (autophosphorylation and exogenous substrate phosphorylation), in control and VMH rats was not statistically different. However, at maximal insulin concentration, autophosphorylation and phosphorylation of exogenous substrate were 2.5-fold higher in receptors from obese rats compared to controls.

Glucose transport and glucose transporter protein

The rate of glucose transport was increased twofold both in the absence and the presence of insulin, in adipocytes from VMH rats when compared to controls (Table 2). We then measured the protein concentration of insulin-sensitive glucose transporter, Glut 4. The enhancement of glucose transport was parallel to a threefold increase in Glut 4 protein concentration in obese rats compared to controls.

Glucose metabolism

In order to determine if a glucose metabolic pathway was specifically affected in VMH rats, we measured glucose metabolism in the isolated adipocytes. Both glucose incorporation in CO_2 and total lipids were significantly higher in presence of maximal insulin concentration in adipocytes from obese rats (Table 2). The incorporation of glucose into lipids is the pathway which is the most stimulated by insulin in VMH rats. This is due to a higher incorporation into fatty acids, the incorporation into glycerol not being different in control and VMH lesioned rats (results not shown). Incorporation into lactate was similar in the two groups of rats (results not shown).

Discussion

These results show that the tyrosine kinase activity of the insulin receptor from adipose tissue of obese VMH rats is increased 1 week after surgery. This is in contrast to what is usually described in obese humans and rodents. However, it should be underlined that these later results were obtained when obesity is well established and when white adipose tissue has been reported to be resistant to insulin. The present results, in agreement with a study performed in young genetically obese Zucker rats[4], indicate that during the first stage of obesity, insulin receptor autophosphorylation and phosphorylation of substrate are increased.

Apart from increased insulin receptor activity, we have shown that white adipose tissue of 1 week VMH rats also presents changes in glucose transport and metabolism. Thus, glucose transport, insulin-sensitive glucose transporter protein concentration and the lipogenic pathway are all higher in adipocytes from VMH rats than in those from controls. This once again is reminiscent of what was observed in the young obese *fa/fa* rats[6,10]. There is also an increased conversion of glucose into CO_2, which is probably due to an increased activity of the pentose shunt.

Such an increase in glucose transport, glucose transporter protein concentration and lipogenesis has been reported in white adipose tissue of normal rats made hyperinsulinaemic for a short period of time (1 to 4 days)[3,13]. This tissue in such rats has also been shown to be hyperresponsive to insulin *in vivo*[2,12]. Since VMH rats oversecrete insulin very soon after the lesion[9], it is tempting to speculate that insulin plays a major role in the changes in insulin effectors of white adipose tissue from VMH rats described in the present paper.

References

1. Burnol, A.F., Ebner, S., Kandé, J. & Girard, J. (1990): Insulin resistance of glucose metabolism in isolated brown adipocytes of lactating rats. Evidence for a post-receptor defect in insulin action. *Biochem. J.* **265**, 511-517.
2. Cusin, I., Terrettaz, J., Rohner-Jeanrenaud, F. & Jeanrenaud, B. (1990): Metabolic consequences of hyperinsulinaemia imposed on normal rats on glucose handling by white adipose tissue, muscles and liver. *Biochem. J.* **267**, 99-103.
3. Cusin, I., Terrettaz, J., Rohner-Jeanrenaud, F., Assimacopoulos-Jeannet, F. & Jeanrenaud, B. (1990): Hyperinsulinaemia increases the amount of Glut 4 mRNA in white adipose tissue and decreases that of muscles: a clue for increased fat depot and insulin resistance. *Endocrinology* **127**, 3246-3247.
4. Debant, A., Guerre-Millo, M., Le Marchand-Brustel, Y., Freychet, P., Lavau, M. & Van Obberghen, E. (1987): Insulin receptor kinase is hyperresponsive in adipocytes of young obese Zucker rats. *Am. J. Physiol.* **252**, E273-E278.
5. Goldman, J. & Bernardis, L. (1974): Metabolism of glucose, fructose and pyruvate in tissues of weanling rats with hypothalamic obesity. *Horm. Metab. Res.* **6**, 370-375.
6. Hainault, I., Guerre-Millo, M., Guichard, C. & Lavau, M. (1991): Differential regulation of adipose tissue glucose transporters in genetic obesity (fatty rats). Selective increase in the adipose cell/muscle glucose transporter (Glut 4) expression. *J. Clin. Invest.* **87**, 1127-1131.
7. Leturque, A., Postic, C. & Girard, J. (1991): Nutritional regulation of glucose transporter in muscles and adipose tissue of weaned rats. *Am. J. Physiol.* **260**, E588-E593.
8. Pénicaud, L., Rohner-Jeanrenaud, F. & Jeanrenaud, B. (1986): *In vivo* metabolic changes as studied longitudinally after ventromedial hypothalamic lesions. *Am. J. Physiol.* **250**, E662-E668.
9. Pénicaud, L., Kinebanyan, M. F., Ferré, P., Morin, J., Kandé, J., Smadja, C., Marfaing-Jallat, P. & Picon, L. (1989): Development of VMH obesity: *in vivo* insulin secretion and tissue insulin sensitivity. *Am. J. Physiol.* **257**, E255-E260.
10. Pénicaud, L., Ferré, P., Assimacopoulos-Jeannet, F., Perdereau, D., Leturque, A., Jeanrenaud, B., Picon, L. & Girard, J. (1991): Increased gene expression of lipogenic enzymes and glucose transporter in white adipose tissue of suckling and weaned obese Zucker rats. *Biochem. J.* (in press).
11. Rodbell, M. (1964): Metabolism of isolated fat cells. Effects of hormones on glucose metabolism and lipolysis. *J. Biol. Chem.* **239**, 375-380.
12. Takao, F., Laury, M. C., Ktorza, A., Picon, L. & Pénicaud, L. (1990): Hyperinsulinaemia increases insulin action *in vivo* in white adipose tissue but not in muscles. *Biochem. J.* **272**, 255-257
13. Trimble, E., Weir, G., Gjinovci, A., Assimacopoulos-Jeannet, F., Benzi, R. & Renold, A. (1984): Increased insulin responsiveness *in vivo* and *in vitro* consequent to induced hyperinsulinaemia. *Diabetes* **34**, 444-449.

Chapter 50

Late Expression of the α_2-adrenergic Mediated Antilipolysis during Adipocyte Differentiation of Hamster Preadipocytes

Jean Sébastien SAULNIER-BLACHE[1], Michèle DAUZATS[1], Danielle DAVIAUD[1], Danielle GAILLARD[2], Gérard AILHAUD[2], Raymond NÉGREL[2] and Max LAFONTAN[1]

[1]INSERM U317, Institut de Physiologie, 2 rue François Magendie, 31400 Toulouse, France; [2]Centre de Biochimie (CNRS UPR 7300), Faculté des Sciences, Université de Nice, Sophia Antipolis, Parc Valrose, 06034 Nice Cédex, France

Catecholamine-dependent lipolysis in white adipocytes relies on the balance between β- and α_2-adrenergic responsiveness. Whereas the β-adrenergic receptor (β-AR) mediates activation of lipolysis through a cAMP-dependent phosphorylation of a hormone-sensitive-lipase (LHS), the α_2-adrenergic receptor (α_2-AR) activation promotes an antilipolytic effect which counteracts the β-adrenergic-mediated responses.

Previous studies have focused attention upon the major role played by the adipocyte α_2-AR in human adipose tissue. An over-expression of this receptor has been shown to be involved in the resistance to the lipolytic action of catecholamines in the femoral adipose tissue of women[5]. However, the reason for this over-expression remains actually unknown.

In animal models, it has been demonstrated that the expression of the adipocyte α_2-AR is positively correlated to the adipose tissue enlargement (in relation to fat cell hypertrophy) as observed during animal growth or on animals submitted to nutritional manipulations[1]. Moreover, recently, an androgenic control of the α_2-AR expression has been described *in vivo* in the hamster and appears to be independent of fat-mass modifications[7]. So, it clearly appears that the adipocyte α_2-AR can be subjected to both fat mass-dependent and fat mass-independent regulation of its expression.

In order to determine the neuro-humoral and/or nutritional factors involved in the fat mass-dependent or the fat mass-independent control of the adipocyte α_2-AR, an *in vitro* adipocyte model appears really necessary to explore more deeply the cellular mechanism of α_2-AR regulations observed *in vivo*.

For several years, preadipocytes isolated from the adipose tissue of various species as well as cells from established preadipocyte clonal lines, have been extensively used to delineate the main events involved in adipose cell differentiation and have appeared appropriate for long-term regulation studies. In these cells, the β-adrenergic control of lipolysis, as well as the effects of insulin, adenosine or prostaglandins have already been studied, but no data regarding the α_2-adrenergic control of lipolysis were shown. However it is noticeable that most of the preadipocyte models so far described were established from rat or mouse, in which the α_2-adrenergic control of lipolysis in mature adipocytes is poorly efficient when compared to man, dog, rabbit or hamster.

Thus, in order to delineate the ontogenesis of the α_2-adrenergic control of lipolysis during adipose conversion as well as to define an *in vitro* model of adipose cells on which α_2-AR regulation studies could be performed, we decided to develop a model of hamster cultured preadipocytes isolated from the stromal-vascular fraction of the adipose tissue. Indeed, conversely to the rat, the hamster fat cells express a fully efficient α_2-AR which has already been defined with appropriate pharmacological tools[6]. In the present work, optimal culture conditions allowing induction of adipose conversion of hamster preadipocytes were defined. The β- and α_2-adrenergic control of lipolysis was explored by a pharmacological approach at different steps of the differentiation and was compared to that of mature adipocytes isolated from adipose tissues from young or adult hamsters.

Fibroblast-like cells isolated from the stromal-vascular fraction of hamster adipose tissue were grown to reach confluence in a Dulbecco's modified Eagles-HamF12 medium supplemented with 10 per cent foetal calf serum and 850 nM insulin. Confluent cells exposed to an ITT medium (850 nM insulin, 10 µg/ml transferrin, 200 pM triiodotyronine)[2] were able to differentiate into adipose-like cells as revealed by the G3PDH activity increment and the accumulation of triacylglycerol droplets. In order to avoid cell detachment which was observed after 15 to 17 days post-confluence (due to increased cellular triacylglycerol content), the ITT medium was supplemented with 2 per cent foetal bovine serum and 1.5 mg/ml bovine serum albumin, a supplementation which was without any influence on the process of the adipose conversion. Under these conditions, the cells could be maintained until 25–30 days after confluence at a stage where the cells reached a size ranging between 15 and 20 µm which is close the size of mature adipocytes from very young animals.

In 8-day post-confluent differentiating cells the half-maximal lipolytic concentrations, EC_{50} (nM), of different β-adrenergic agonists were equivalent to those defined on isolated mature hamster adipocytes and the following order of potency was defined: BRL 37344 > norepinephrine = isoproterenol > epinephrine > fenoterol. This pharmacological profile which is characteristic of an "atypical" β-AR[4] is also found in differentiated BFC-1 and Ob17 adipose like cells[3]. These results confirm the early expression of the adipocyte β-adrenoceptors during the process of adipose conversion.

Concerning the α_2-adrenergic control of lipolysis, our study gives evidence of a different developmental pattern as compared to the β-AR. The α_2-adrenergic control of lipolysis was defined by exploring the antilipolytic activity of two α_2-adrenergic agonists (UK14304 and clonidine) by comparison with effectors known to act through other antilipolytic receptors such as the A1-adenosine receptor (phenylisopropyladenosine: PIA) and the prostaglandin E1 (PGE1) receptor. Whereas 10^{-6} M PIA and 10^{-6} M (PGE1) were able to suppress completely the lipolysis induced by 4 µg/ml adenosine deaminase (ADA), in both 8 days and 20–25 days post-confluent differentiating adipose-like cells, the antilipolytic effect of clonidine and UK 14304 was only detectable in 20–25 day post-confluent cells. Their antilipolytic activity was dose-dependent and was blocked in the presence of 10^{-5} M RX821002, a highly selective α_2-adrenergic antagonist. Dose-dependent blockade (induced by increasing concentrations of three α_2-adrenergic antagonists) of the antilipolytic effect of 10^{-6} M UK14304, revealed the same order of potency (RX821002 > phentolamine >> yohimbine) than that defined in mature hamster fat cells. This specific pharmacology is suspected to correspond to a variant of the α_2A-AR subtype (α_2D-AR ?) and is characterized by a low affinity for the classical α_2-adrenergic antagonist yohimbine[6].

Radioligand binding studies performed with the antagonist [³H]RX821002 using 200 µM epinephrine for the definition of the nonspecific binding, revealed a high affinity for this radioligand (K_d = 1 nM) with a saturable specific binding in 8 days as well as in 20–25 days differentiating preadipocytes. Determination of B_{max} values revealed a significant increase in the density of α_2-adrenoceptors between 8 days and 20–25 days post-confluent differentiating preadipocytes (19 ± 1 vs 30 ± 1 fmol/mg protein: $P < 0.01$) without significant modification of the affinity (0.9 ± 0.1 vs 1.1 ± 0.1 nM). However, the α_2-AR density of 20–25 days post-confluent differentiating preadipocytes was lower than that determined on 30 µm mature adipocytes isolated from young hamsters (179 ± 54 fmol/mg protein) itself lower than that determined in 80 µm mature adipocytes isolated from adult hamsters.

Identification of the Gi proteins by ADP-ribosylation revealed the presence of the same two αi subunits (αi_1 and/or αi_3, plus αi_2) than in mature adipocytes. Quantification of Gi proteins revealed a slight but significant increase in their amount between 8 days and 20–25 days differentiating preadipocytes (31 ± 4 vs 43 ± 4 per cent of the ADP-ribosylated Gi amount present in mature adipocytes isolated from adult hamsters: $P < 0.05$).

These data show that conversely to the β-adrenergic, A1-adenosine and PGE1 mediated control of lipolysis, the α_2-adrenergic dependent control of lipolysis appeared in the later steps of the hamster adipose conversion (20–25 days after confluence) with a pharmacological profile similar to that defined in mature adipocytes. It can be attributed to both an increase in the α_2-AR density and an increase in the amount of Gi proteins. To our knowledge, it is the first demonstration of the existence of α_2-adrenoceptors on a cultured preadipose cell model. It must be pointed out that no specific binding of [^{3}H]RX821002 could be detected in the differentiated 3T3F442A preadipose cell line (12 days post-confluence) (not shown). Since previous studies have presented evidence in favour of a relationship between α_2-AR expression and fat mass enlargement (correlated to adipose cell size, i.e. triacylglycerol content), our observations may have physiological relevance. It is therefore proposed that the very late expression of the α_2-AR during the adipose conversion can be considered as a marker of adipose cell hypertrophy. But the existence of fat mass-independent regulation of the adipocyte α_2-AR expression which have been demonstrated with androgens[7] revealed that the increase of α_2-AR expression with fat cell size increment can be considered as a consequence rather than a cause of the fat cell hypertrophy.

So, the hamster preadipocyte model described herein appears to be a valuable model for the study of the ontogenesis of both the β- and the α_2-AR during adipose conversion as well as for exploring the fat mass-dependent and the fat mass-independent regulations of the adipocyte α_2-AR expression.

References

1. Carpéné, C., Galitzky, J., Saulnier-Blache, J.S. & Lafontan, M. (1990): Selective reduction of (α2-adrenergic responsiveness in hamster adipose tissue during prolonged starvation. *Am. J. Physiol.* **259**, E80-E88.
2. Deslex, S., Négrel, R. & Ailhaud, G. (1987): Development of a chemically defined serum-free medium for differentiation of rat adipose precursor cells. *Exp. Cell Res.* **168**, 15-30.
3. Forest, C., Doglio, A., Ricquier, D. & Ailhaud, G. (1987): A preadipocyte clonal line from mouse brown adipose tissue. Short and long-term responses to insulin and β-adrenergics. *Exp. Cell Res.* **168**, 218-232.
4. Langin, D., Portillo, M.P., Saulnier-Blache, J.S. & Lafontan, M. (1991): Coexistence of three β-adrenoceptor subtypes in white fat cells of various mammalian species. *Eur. J. Pharmacol.* (in press).
5. Mauriège P., Galitzky, J., Berlan, M. & Lafontan, M. (1987): Heterogenous distribution of alpha2-adrenoceptor binding sites in human fat cells from various fat deposits: functional consequences. *Eur. J. Clin. Invest.* **17**, 156-165.
6. Saulnier-Blache, J.S., Carpéné, C., Langin, D. & Lafontan, M. (1989): Imidazolinic radioligands for the identification of hamster adipocyte α2-adrenoceptors. *Eur. J. Pharmacol.* **171**, 145-157.
7. Saulnier-Blache, J.S., Larrouy, D., Carpéné, N., Quideau, Dauzats, M. & Lafontan, M. (1990): Photoperiodic control of adipocyte α2-adrenoceptors in Syrian Hamsters: role of testosterone. *Endocrinology* **127**, 1245-1253.

Chapter 51

In situ Investigations of Adipose Tissue Metabolism

Peter ARNER
Karolinska Institute at the Department of Medicine and Research Center, Huddinge Hospital, Stockholm, Sweden

Several methods are now available for the study of adipose tissue metabolism *in situ*. Using arteriovenous cannulation we can observe the substrate turnover in adipose tissue *in vivo*. The extracellular space in adipose tissue may be investigated in different ways. A single metabolite (usually glucose) can be continuously monitored using electrochemical sensors which are implanted in adipose tissue. Microdialysis of the tissue permits continuous simultaneous monitoring of several metabolites in the extracellular space. In addition, microdialysis may be used for the *in situ* manipulation of adipose tissue, which is very useful for investigations of metabolism regulation. A problem with most of the *in situ* methods is that they cannot distinguish between changes in cell metabolism and changes in the circulation. This problem can be overcome by combining *in situ* metabolic analysis with *in situ* flow measurements.

Introduction

White adipose tissue plays a major role in regulating the energy balance. Through esterification, glucose and fatty acid are stored in fat cells as triacylglycerols, energy is released from fat cells through lipolysis, when triacylglycerols are broken down to free fatty acids and glycerol. The adipose tissue is under intense hormone regulation and alterations in fat cell metabolism are of pathophysiological importance for common disorders such as obesity, diabetes and dyslipoproteinaemia.

Most of our knowledge of adipose tissue metabolism is derived from *in vitro* studies. A major breakthrough in this respect was the development of methods to isolate fat cells from the surrounding stroma by collagenase treatment[28]. Obviously, there is also a need to study fat cell metabolism in its natural environment *in vivo*. Usually this is done by investigating circulating lipid metabolites. However, such methods give only indirect information about fat cell metabolism.

During recent decades several methods have been developed to study adipose tissue metabolism directly *in situ*. In this paper I shall review such past and current methods and discuss their respective advantages and disadvantages.

There are at least three methods for the study of adipose tissue metabolism *in situ* (Table 1). They entail the use of nuclear magnetic resonance (NMR) or arteriovenous cannulation or monitoring of the extracellular fluid space. These methods will be dealt with separately.

Table 1. Methods for study of adipose tissue metabolism *in situ*

Method	Adipose region
Nuclear magnetic resonance	All adipose deposits
Arteriovenous cannulation	Inguinal subcutaneous fat pads in dogs. Abdominal subcutaneous region in humans.
Monitoring of the extracellular space (wick technique, electrochemical sensors, microdialysis)	All subcutaneous adipose deposits

Table 2. Steady-state levels of metabolites in the extracellular space of human adipose tissue

Metabolite	Level in comparison to that in blood
Glucose	Same
Pyruvate	Same
Lactate	Same or somewhat higher
Adenosine	50% lower
Glycerol	2–3 times higher

NMR

The NMR technique can be used for selective *in vivo* investigations of glucose and lipid metabolism in all tissues including adipose tissue. NMR methods have been described concerning the study of glucose metabolism in human skeletal muscle and rat liver *in vivo*[33,34].

As regards adipose tissue, NMR has hitherto been used only for *in vitro* metabolic studies[35]. In theory, NMR can be used to investigate glucose and lipid metabolism in all adipose depots, bearing in mind the important regional differences in fat cell metabolism[5]. This is a major advantage over other *in situ* methods. However, NMR is less useful than other methods in kinetic studies. Moreover, it is very expensive.

Arteriovenous cannulation

This is the first method which was used for the study of adipose tissue metabolism *in situ*. Twenty-five years ago a technique was worked out in dogs to isolate the inguinal subcutaneous fat pad from the surrounding tissues leaving intact one artery, one vein and (sometimes) one nerve to supply the tissue[29]. With this method one can study arteriovenous differences across adipose tissue and alter adipose tissue metabolism by the direct administration of active drugs or by local manipulation of blood flow and nerve activity, respectively. Several major discoveries regarding the *in vivo* function of adipose tissue have been made using the cannulated inguinal fat pad. These discoveries involve the importance of adrenergic innervation[4] as well as the role of acidosis[20], adenosine[16] and blood flow[11], in lipolysis regulation. However, there are several problems connected with this method. First, it seems suitable only for studies in dogs, which today represents a major ethical problem in many countries. Secondly, it can only be performed during general anaesthesia which may markedly affect adipose tissue metabolism. Thirdly, it cannot be used for detailed pharmacological investigations of potent agents, such as catecholamines, because the administration of high doses induce generalized effects. Perhaps for these reasons the inguinal cannulation method is rarely used for *in vivo* studies of adipose tissue at present.

Recently, a cannulation method has been developed for *in situ* investigations of human subcutaneous adipose tissue metabolism[15]. A superficial vein of the abdominal wall is cannulated in an antegrade direction. Blood is sampled from this vein which primarily drains subcutaneous adipose tissue. An antecubital vein is cannulated retrogradely and blood is thereby collected from the deep tissues. In addition, arterialized blood is collected from a vein which drains the contralateral hand. Using the above-mentioned method it is possible to calculate arteriovenous differences across deep (mainly muscle) and superficial (mainly subcutaneous fat) tissues. It has been used to study the influx and efflux of carbohydrates and lipids in the fasting[10] and fed[8] states, during ethanol ingestion[14], as well as in connection with insulin infusion[9]. By comparing net uptake and release of glycerol and free fatty acids over the subcutaneous adipose tissue it is also possible to study the re-esterification of fatty acids *in situ*[8,9].

The major advantage with the "human cannulation method" is that it facilitates the estimation of substrate turnover in adipose tissue. This may be the only method now available which allows *in situ* studies of the potentially important re-esterification phenomenon in man[27]. On the other hand, there are several problems in the human cannulation technique which limit its clinical use. The contribution of metabolism from tissues surrounding adipose tissue is unknown, in particular from the skin and, to some extent, from the abdominal muscles. It cannot distinguish changes in substrate fluxes that are induced by tissue metabolism, from those that are induced by tissue blood flow. The method cannot be used for local manipulation of adipose tissue, such as direct exposure of the tissue to metabolically active agents. Finally, it is elaborate and not suitable for investigations of regional variations in adipose tissue metabolism.

Monitoring of the extracellular space

An attractive way to study tissue metabolism *in situ* is to make direct measurements of the extracellular fluid space. As regards adipose tissue, this method has been approached in three ways: the sampling of extracellular fluid, direct measurements with electrochemical sensors and microdialysis.

Sampling of extracellular fluid

Several attempts have been made in the past to obtain a reliable sample from the extracellular space. The problem of obtaining analytical fluid can be reduced to the equilibration of a concentration between the interstitial space and an analytical compartment, which consists of a wick. The wick technique for sampling interstitial fluid was described over 20 years ago[30] but has only recently been used for *in situ* studies of adipose tissue metabolism[13].

Cotton threads are implanted in the subcutaneous adipose tissue. After an appropriate interval the wicks are removed and centrifuged. The chemical composition of the resulting fluid sample is analysed. The advantage of the wick technique is that it probably measures accurately the concentration of a particular substance in the extracellular space and can therefore be used as a reference method for other assays of the latter compartment.

The concentrations of proteins, potassium and glucose in the extracellular fluid of the subcutaneous adipose tissue in the dog have been determined by the wick technique[30]. However, the method can only be used for steady-state measurements. For example, it is unreliable for the kinetic analysis of subcutaneous adipose tissue glucose concentrations following glucose loads or insulin injections[30].

Electrochemical sensors

Implantable biosensors are being developed in experimental and clinical medicine because they allow continuous measurements of rapidly varying analytes without the need for other reagents or withdrawal of body fluids. As regards adipose tissue, such sensors have been developed to monitor the glucose levels in the extracellular space of adipose tissue. Needle-shaped electrodes coated with immobilized glucose oxidase are implanted in the subcutaneous tissue. The interaction between the electrochemical sensor and glucose in the extracellular fluid generates an electric signal, which is collected by an external receiver.

Results with animals[7,31] as well as humans[26,32] indicate that the kinetics of adipose tissue glucose closely mirror those in blood after insulin injections or glucose loading. Thus, biosensors are probably useful for continuous monitoring of metabolites in subcutaneous adipose tissue. However, electrochemical sensors have several disadvantages. As stated[25], they are difficult to calibrate, usually showing artificially low values and large inter- and intra-individual variability. Furthermore, they can solely be used to monitor one metabolite, because the electrode can be coated only with a single detection enzyme.

Microdialysis

Among the methods for studying the extracellular fluid space of adipose tissue, microdialysis has the greatest potential. This technique was originally worked out for studies of brain function in rats[12]. Recently, it has been applied to adipose tissue. A small probe, containing a semipermeable dialysis membrane, is implanted in adipose tissue and the probe is perfused with isotonic dialysis solvent (usually saline or Ringer's solution) with the aid of precision pumps. Metabolites are collected from the extracellular space and analysed in the perfusate. Because of the small sample volume and sometimes incomplete recovery (see below), it is often necessary to use ultrasensitive analytical methods, such as high-pressure liquid chromatography or enzymatic luminometric assays.

The most suitable molecular cut-off point of the dialysis membrane is between 5000 and 30,000. Any molecule of a size less than 10 per cent of the cut-off point can easily pass through the membrane. This means that most metabolites of interest, such as carbohydrates, amino acids, glycerol and electrolytes, can be measured using standard dialysis membranes.

The microdialysis of adipose tissue has many advantages. It causes little discomfort and can therefore be used in clinical studies of children and/or critically ill subjects. The tissue damage caused by the probe is relatively minor and only transient[6]. Several metabolites can be monitored simultaneously. A unique feature of microdialysis is that metabolically active agents can be delivered to the extracellular space through the microdialysis probe at the same time as metabolites are collected from this compartment. Since it is possible to expose adipose tissue locally to very high concentrations of such agents without causing generalized effects detailed pharmacological investigations of adipose tissue metabolism can be performed *in situ* using microdialysis.

Recovery problems can at least partly be overcome by increasing the length of the dialysis membrane and by reducing the perfusion speed. It should, however, be borne in mind that *in vivo* recovery is lower than *in vitro* recovery. Therefore, the probes cannot be calibrated by simple *in vitro* testing against standard solutions with known amounts of the metabolites of interest. An equilibrium technique has been developed to estimate the true recovery and thereby the actual concentration of a substance in the extracellular space[24]. Using this method, adipose tissue is perfused with increasing concentrations of the substance of interest and the equilibrium concentration is determined, which is the same concentration as that in the extracellular space.

Two different probes have been used for microdialysis of adipose tissue. There is a commercially available needle-shaped probe[36] that consists of a double-steel cannula. On top of the probe is glued a dialysis tube. The dialysis solvent enters the probe through the inner cannula and leaves it through the outer one. The other probe consists of a single dialysis tube glued to a nylon tube and implanted in adipose tissue by the use of a steel cannula[24].

By the aid of the equilibrium technique described above, steady-state levels of various metabolites have been determined in human adipose tissue (Table 2). The levels of glucose, pyruvate and lactate are in the same range in adipose tissue as in blood[18,21,24]. The concentration of glycerol is higher and that of adenosine lower in adipose tissue than in blood[22,23].

The kinetics of glucose and glycerol (lipolysis index) have been investigated in human adipose tissue. The changes in adipose tissue glucose levels mirror closely the changes in blood glucose following carbohydrate loading and insulin infusion in normal, obese and diabetic subjects[6,17,19]. Lipolysis has been monitored in different subcutaneous adipose regions during exercise[3]. Regional variations in lipolysis activity have been demonstrated, the abdominal site being more active than the gluteal one.

With the use of *in situ* manipulation of adipose tissue, several new findings regarding adrenergic regulation of lipolysis have been made. This has been achieved by the local administration of adrenergic agents to the tissue through the probe in combination with simultaneous measurements of glycerol in the tissue perfusate. It appears that the adrenergic regulation of lipolysis in man and rat differs. In humans very low concentrations of catecholamines are lipolytic, but the effect is transient due to tachyphylaxia[2]. In the rat, more prolonged lipolytic effects are observed but at higher doses[1]. In humans α2-adrenergic inhibitor receptors modulate lipolysis at rest whereas β-adrenergic receptors modulate lipolysis during exercise[3].

The major disadvantage of microdialysis is that it cannot distinguish between cell metabolism and blood flow. A change in the concentration of a metabolite in the extracellular space of adipose tissue is the net sum of uptake or release from fat cells and removal or input from the circulation. Therefore, the method is not suitable for the quantitative estimation of substrate turnover. It may, however, be quantitative when used together with specific measurements of blood flow. When kinetic experiments are believed to be influenced by circulatory factors, it may also be desirable to perform microdialysis with solvents containing vaso-active substances.

Conclusion

In order to study adipose tissue function better there is a need for increased knowledge of fat cell metabolism *in vivo*. In this context several methods are available for the study of adipose tissue metabolism *in situ*. All have advantages and disadvantages. Arteriovenous cannulation techniques are most suitable for the quantitative estimation of substrate turnover. Microdialysis is the best method for kinetic experiments and *in situ* manipulation of adipose tissue. A problem with most methods is the difficulty of distinguishing between fat cell metabolism and blood flow. In this respect, the microdialysis method seems to have the greatest potential if it can be combined with specific flow measurements.

Acknowledgements

This study was supported by grants from the Swedish Medical Research Council, Karolinska Institute and Medicus Bromma AB.

References

1. Arner, P., Bolinder, J., Eliasson, A., Lundin, A. & Ungerstedt, U. (1988): Microdialysis of adipose tissue and blood for *in vivo* lipolysis studies. *Am. J. Physiol.* **255**, E737-E742.
2. Arner, P., Kriegholm, E. & Engfeldt, P. (1990): *In situ* studies of catecholamine-induced lipolysis in human adipose tissue using microdialysis. *J. Pharm. Exp. Ther.* **254**, 284-288.
3. Arner, P., Kriegholm, E., Engfeldt, P. & Bolinder, J. (1990): Adrenergic regulation of lipolysis *in situ* at rest and during exercise. *J. Clin. Invest.* **85**, 893-98.
4. Belfrage, E. & Rosell, S. (1976): The role of neuronal uptake at alpha- and beta-adrenoceptor sites in subcutaneous adipose tissue. *Naunyn Schmiedebergs Arch. Pharmacol.* **294**, 9-15.
5. Björntorp, P. (1987): Fat cell distribution and metabolism. *Ann. NY Acad. Sci.* **499**, 66-72.
6. Bolinder, J., Hagstrom, E., Ungerstedt, U. & Arner, P. (1989): Microdialysis of subcutaneous adipose tissue *in vivo* for continuous glucose monitoring in man. *Scand. J. Clin. Lab. Invest.* **49**, 465-74.
7. Claremont, D.J., Sambrook, I.E., Penton, C. & Pickup, J.C. (1986): Subcutaneous implantation of a ferrocene-mediated glucose sensor in pigs. *Diabetologia* **29**, 817-821.

8. Coppack, S.W., Fisher, R.M., Gibbons, G.F., Humphreys, S.M., McDonough, M.J., Potts, J.L. & Frayn, K.N. (1990): Postprandial substrate deposition in human forearm and adipose tissue *in vivo. Clin. Sci.* **79**, 339-348.
9. Coppack, S.W., Frayn, K.N., Humphreys, S.M., Dhar, H. & Hockaday, T.D.R. (1989): Effects of insulin on human adipose tissue metabolism *in vivo. Clin. Sci.* **77**, 663-670.
10. Coppack, S.W., Frayn, K.N., Humphreys, S.M., Whyte, P.L. & Hockaday, T.D.R. (1990): Arteriovenous differences across adipose and forearm tissues after overnight fast. *Metabolism* **39**, 384-390.
11. Croke, R.P., Longo, M.B. & Skinner, N.S. (1977): Effect of reflex stimuli on vascular resistance and glycerol release in *in vivo* dog subcutaneous adipose tissue. *Pflügers Arch.* **369**, 49-54.
12. Delgado, J.M.R., Feudis, F.V., Roth, R.H., Ryugo, D.K. & Mitruka, B.M. (1972): Dialytrode for long-term intravertebral perfusion in awake monkeys. *Arch. Int. Pharmacodyn. Ther.* **198**, 9-21.
13. Fischer, U., Ertle, R., Abel, P., Rebrin ,K., Brunstein, E., Hahn von Dorsche, H. & Freyse, E.J. (1987): Assessment of subcutaneous glucose concentration: validation of the wick technique as a reference for implanted electrochemical sensors in normal and diabetic dogs. *Diabetologia.* **30**, 940-945.
14. Frayn, K.N., Coppack, S.W., Walsh, P.E., Butterworth, H.C., Humphreys, S.M. & Pedrosa, H.C. (1990): Metabolic responses of forearm and adipose tissues to acute ethanol ingestion. *Metabolism.* **39**, 958-966.
15. Frayn, K.N., Coppack, S.W., Whyte, P.L. & Hymphreys, S.M. (1989): Metabolic characteristics of human adipose tissue *in vivo. Clin. Sci.* **76**, 509-516.
16. Fredholm, B.B. & Sollevi, A. (1977): Antilipolytic effect of adenosine in dog adipose tissue *in situ. Acta. Physiol. Scand.* **99**, 254-256.
17. Hagström, E., Arner, P., Engfeldt, P., Rössner, S. & Bolinder, J. (1990): *In vivo* subcutaneous adipose tissue glucose kinetics after glucose ingestion in obesity and fasting. *Scand. J. Clin. Lab. Invest.* **50**, 129-136.
18. Hagström, E., Arner, P., Ungerstedt, U. & Bolinder, J. (1990): Subcutaneous adipose tissue – a source of lactate production following glucose ingestion in man. *Am. J. Physiol.* **258**, E888-93.
19. Hagström-Toft, E., Arner, P., Näslund, B., Understedt, U, & Bolinder, J. (1991): Effects of insulin deprivation and replacement on *in vivo* subcutaneous adipose tissue substrate metabolism in man. *Diabetes* (in press).
20. Hjelmdahl, P. & Fredholm, B.B. (1974): Comparison of the lipolytic activity of circulating and locally released noradrenaline during acidosis. *Acta. Physiol. Scand.* **92**, 1-11.
21. Jansson, P.A., Smith, U. and Lönnroth, P. (1990): Evidence for lactate production by human adipose tissue *in vivo. Diabetologia* **33**, 253-256.
22. Jansson, P-A., Smith, U. & Lönnroth, P. (1990): Interstitial glycerol concentration measured by microdialysis in two subcutaneous regions in humans. *Am. J. Physiol.* **258**, E918-E922.
23. Lönnroth, P., Jansson, P.A., Fredholm, B.B. & Smith, U. (1989): Microdialysis of intercellular adenosine concentrations in subcutaneous tissue in humans. *Am. J. Physiol.* **256,** E250-E255.
24. Lönnroth, P., Jansson, P.A. & Smith, U. (1987): A microdialysis method allowing characterization of the intercellular water space in humans. *Am. J. Physiol.* **253**, E228-E231.
25. Pickup, J.C. (1989): Biosensors: a clinical perspective. *Lancet* **ii**, 817-820.
26. Pickup, J.C., Shaw, G.W. & Claremont, D.J. (1989): *In vivo* molecular sensing in diabetes mellitus: an implantable glucose sensor with direct electron transfer. *Diabetologia* **32**, 213-217.
27. Rabinowitz, D. & Zierler, K.L. (1962): Role of free fatty acids in forearm metabolism in man quantitated by use of insulin. *J. Clin. Invest.* **41**, 2191-2197.
28. Rodbell, M. (1964): Metabolism of isolated fat cells. *J. Biol. Chem.* **239**, 375-380.
29. Rosell, S. (1966): Release of free fatty acids from subcutaneous adipose tissue in dogs following sympathetic nerve stimulation. *Acta Physiol. Scand.* **67**, 343-351.
30. Scholander, P.F., Hargens, A.R. & Miller, S.L. (1968): Negative pressure in the interstitial fluid of animals. *Science* **161**, 321-328.
31. Shichiri, M., Kawamori, R., Goriya, Y., Yamasaki, Y., Nomura, M., Hakui, N. & Abe, H. (1983): Glycaemic control in pancreatectomized dogs with a wearable artificial endocrine pancreas. *Diabetologia* **24**, 179-184.
32. Shichiri, M., Kawamori, R., Yamasaki, Y., Hakui, N. & Abe, H. (1982): Wearable artificial endocrine pancreas with needle-type glucose sensor. *Lancet.* **ii**, 1129-1130.

33. Shulman, I., Rothman, D.L., Jue, T., Stein, P., DeFronzo, R.A. & Shulman, R.G. (1990): Quantitation of muscle glycogen synthesis in normal subjects and subjects with non-insulin-dependent diabetes by ^{13}C nuclear magentic resonance spectroscopy. *N. Engl. J. Med.* **322**, 223-228.
34. Siegfried, B.A., Reo, N.V., Ewy, C.S., Shalwitz, R.A., Ackerman, J.J.H. & McDonald, J.M. (1985): Effects of hormone and glucose administration on hepatic glucose and glycogen metabolism *in vivo*. *J. Biol. Chem.* **260**, 16137-16142.
35. Sillerud, L.O., Han, C.H., Bitensky, M.W. & Francendese, A.A. (1986): Metabolism and structure of triacylglycerols in rat epididymal fat pad adipocytes determined by ^{13}C nuclear magnetic resonance. *J. Biol. Chem.* **261**, 4380-4388.
36. Tossman, U. & Ungerstedt, U. (1986): Microdialysis in the study of extracellular levels of amino acids in the rat brain. *Acta Physiol. Scand.* **128**, 9-14.

Chapter 52

Anti-obesity Action of ICI D7114 is Associated with the Appearance of Active Brown Adipose Tissue in Adult Dogs

B.R. HOLLOWAY+, O. CHAMPIGNY*, O. BLONDELL*, D. RICQUIER*, R.M. MAYERS+ and M.G. BRISCOE+

Centre De Recherches Sur La Nutrition, 9 rue Jules Hetzel, 92190 Meudon-Bellevue, France; +ICI Pharmaceuticals, Mereside, Alderley Park, Macclesfield, Cheshire, SK10 4TG, UK

Brown adipose tissue (BAT) is present in neonates of larger mammals including dogs[1], cats[8], sheep[4], cattle[3] and man[7]. However, it is undetectable or present in only small quantities in the adults of these species. We have investigated the effects of treatment of adult dogs with a novel β3-adrenoceptor agonist (ICI D7114) which has thermogenic and anti-obesity properties[6]. The results suggest that in the dog, chronic stimulation of β3-adrenoceptors leads to a reduction in body weight coupled with the reactivation of dormant BAT or to the recruitment of fully differentiated BAT from pre-adipocyte precursor cells.

Methods

Female beagle dogs were given free access to water and fed 400 g of pelleted chow, daily. The dogs were weighed and measurement made of girth (immediately in front of the hind legs) once every week. Four dogs were dosed with a placebo preparation twice daily for 27 weeks. Four other dogs were also dosed with placebo for 5 weeks and then with capsules containing 0.03 mg/kg ICI D7114 for the next 9 weeks, followed by a period of 13 weeks with 0.1 mg/kg ICI D7114. After 27 weeks the treatments were crossed-over and the dogs treated for a further 8 weeks. The purpose of this protocol was to assess the effects of D7114 on weight gain and girth in dogs. Adipose tissue samples were also taken. Further samples were taken from untreated age-matched control dogs. Adipose tissue was also taken from dogs which had been treated with 1.0 or 10.0 mg/kg ICI D7114 twice daily for 2 weeks and from a group dosed with 1.0 mg/kg, twice daily for 4 weeks.

A crude mitochondrial fraction was prepared by differential centrifugation of homogenates prepared from samples of perirenal adipose tissue. Mitochondrial protein was determined by the method of Lowry[9], GDP-binding by a minor modification of the method of Nicholls[10] and cytochrome oxidase by the method of Yonetani et al.[12]. For detection of mitochondrial uncoupling protein (UCP) 50 µg of mitochondrial protein was run in 10 per cent polyacrylamide-SDS gels. Western blots were performed and dog UCP detected using antibodies raised against rat UCP[11]. Isolated adipose tissue RNA (20 µg) was fractionated on 1 per cent formaldehyde-agarose gels and transferred to a nylon membrane (Hybond). The Northern blot was probed with a randomly-primed H-UCP-0.5 kilobase fragment[12] corresponding to the central domain of the human UCP gene. The blot was washed to low stringency and exposed for 3 days. The same blot was also hybridized with a nick-translated plasmid containing whole mouse mitochondrial DNA.

Results and discussion

Administration of ICI D7114 increases whole body oxygen consumption and BAT activity with little increase in heart rate in the rat[5]. *In vitro* both ICI D7114 and its acid metabolite were potent stimulants of oxygen consumption in isolated brown fat cells but had only low potency effects on isolated atria (β_1) and trachea (β_2)[5]. This and other data suggest that ICI D7114 is a selective agonist of the rat BAT β_3-adrenoceptor.

In an experiment to investigate the effects of ICI D7114 in a higher mammal, dogs were dosed chronically with the compound. In the first phase of this experiment groups of dogs were dosed twice daily with capsules containing ICI D7114 or a placebo preparation. Treatment with ICI D7114 decreased abdominal girth and body weight gain. In the second phase of the experiment the treatments were crossed over; dogs which had initially been dosed with placebo were treated with capsules containing ICI D7114 and vice versa. Those dogs which were dosed with ICI D7114 in the second phase of the experiment rapidly lost weight (–0.6 kg) and decreased their girth (–5.2 cm), whilst dogs dosed with placebo gained weight (+0.9 kg) and girth (+5.5 cm).

In those dogs which had been treated with ICI D7114 in the final phase of the experiment to assess the effects of the drug on weight gain, adipose tissue collected from several sites appeared light brown in colour whilst that from the same sites in placebo-treated dogs and in age-matched controls was white. Although the weight of perirenal adipose tissue was similar in drug- and placebo-treated dogs, greater amounts of mitochondrial protein were isolated from the former group (Fig. 1). Also, in those dogs in which the final treatment was ICI D7114, levels of total but not specific mitochondrial GDP-binding and of cytochrome oxidase were higher than in tissue from placebo-treated or age-matched control dogs although these differences did not achieve statistical significance. Similar changes were apparent in adipose tissue of dogs treated for shorter periods with higher doses of ICI D7114.

It is possible that these results could reflect differences in the recovery of mitochondria from

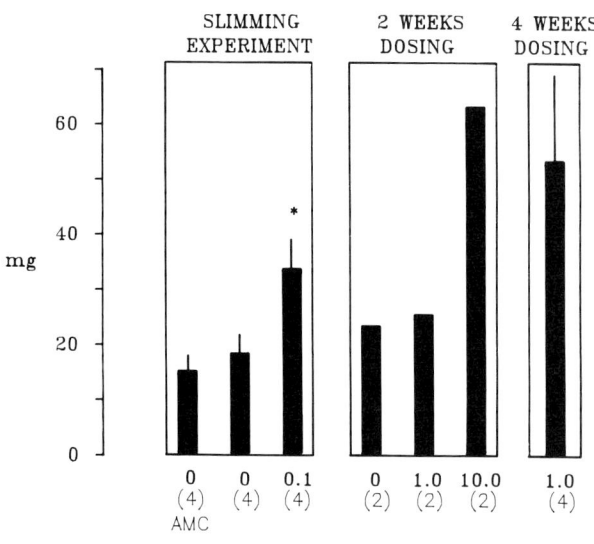

Fig. 1. Mitochondrial protein content in perirenal adipose tissue from treated and control dogs. Results are the mean and standard error of the number of observations indicated. AMC = Age matched control.

homogenates of adipose tissue. However, there was clear immunological evidence for the presence of UCP in adipose tissue mitochondria prepared from a number of sites in the treated dogs but not in mitochondria from placebo-treated animals. RNA extracted from adipose tissue from treated but not control dogs hybridized to the cDNA probe for the central domain of the human UCP gene. Although there was clearly mRNA for UCP in dogs treated with 0.1 mg/kg ICI D7114 the strongest signals were in animals treated with 1.0 and 10.0 mg/kg of the drug (Fig. 2). Strong signals corresponding to UCP mRNA were seen in extracts of perirenal, peribladder and pericardiac adipose tissue, whilst weaker signals were apparent in extracts of subcutaneous and omental adipose tissue. Treatment with the drug was also associated with an increase in signal when extracted RNA was hybridized with a nick-translated plasmid containing whole mouse mitochondrial DNA.

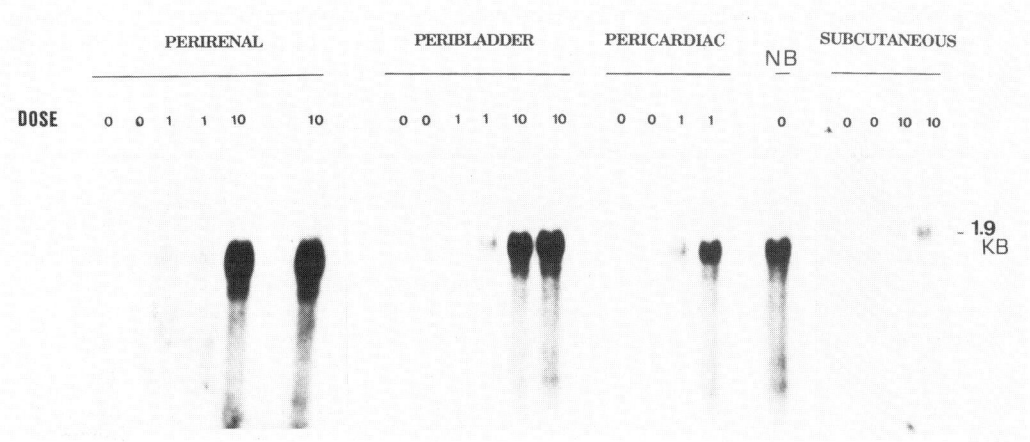

Fig. 2. UCP mRNA in Northern blots of dog adipose tissue from an experiment in which dogs were treated with 0, 1.0 or 10.0 mg/kg ICI D7114 for 2 weeks (two dogs/treatment). A sample of adipose tissue (NB) from a new-born dog was included as a positive control.

The results indicate that chronic treatment with ICI D7114 leads to a decrease in weight and abdominal girth. The chronic effects of the drug are associated with the appearance of BAT. Active BAT is present in neonatal dogs but not in control adult dogs. One possible explanation for these results is that the activity of BAT decreases with age in the dog and develops a phenotypic resemblance to white adipose tissue. Although UCP and its messenger RNA are undetectable in such tissue, it may be that levels are below the limits of detection. It is also possible that that active neonatal BAT is replaced by white adipose tissue in adult dogs. β_3-adrenoceptor stimulation may reactivate dormant BAT or lead to the recruitment of fully differentiated BAT cells from pre-adipocytes. Some evidence for the latter has recently come from experiments in which the active, acid metabolite of ICI D7114 was added to cultures of pre-adipocytes isolated from rat or mouse BAT (Champigny, personal communication). In these experiments, inclusion of the compound in the culture media led to expression of the UCP gene which was not expressed in control cultures.

References

1. Ashwell, M., Stirling, D.M., Freeman, S. & Holloway, B.R. (1987): Immunological, histological and biochemical assessment of brown adipose tissue activity in neonatal, control and β-stimulant treated adult dogs. *Int. J. Obes.* **11**, 357-365.

2. Bouillaud, F., Villarroya, F., Hentz, E., Raimbault, S., Cassard, A. & Ricquier, D. (1988): Detection of brown adipose tissue uncoupling protein mRNA in adult patients by a human genomic probe. *Clin. Sci.* **75**, 21-27.
3. Casteilla, L., Champigny, O., Bouillaud, F., Robelin, J. & Ricquier, D. (1989): Sequential changes in the expression of mitochondrial protein mRNA during the development of brown adipose tissue in bovine and ovine species. *Biochem. J.* **257**, 665-671.
4. Gemmel, R.T., Bell, A.W. & Alexander, G. (1972): Morphology of adipose tissue cells in lambs at birth and subsequent transition of brown to white adipose tissue in cold and warm conditions. *Am. J. Anat.* **133**, 143-164.
5. Holloway, B.R., Briscoe, M., Growcott, J.W., Wilson, C. & Stock. M.J. (1991): *In vitro* and *in vivo* selectivity of ICI D7114 for brown fat and thermogenesis. adrenoceptors: structure, mechanisms, function. *Advances in pharmacological sciences*, ed. E. Szabodi. Basel: Birkhauser Verlag.
6. Holloway, B.R., Howe, R., Rao, B.S. & Stribling, D. ICI D7114: A novel selective β-adrenoceptor agonist of brown fat and thermogenesis. *Am. J. Clin. Nutr.* (in press).
7. Lean, M.E.J., James, W.P.T., Jennings, G. & Trayhurn, P. (1986): Brown adipose tissue uncoupling protein content in human infants, children and adults. *Clin. Sci.* **71**, 291-297.
8. Loncar, D., Bedrica, L., Mayer, J., Cannon, B., Nedergard, J., Afzelius, B.A. & Svajger. A. (1986): The effect of intermittent cold treatment on the adipose tissue of the cat – apparent transformation from white to brown adipose tissue. *J. Ultr. Mol. Struc. Res.* **97**, 119-129.
9. Lowry, O.H., Rosenbrough, N.J. & Farr, A.L. (1951): Protein measurement with the folin-phenol reagent. *J. Biol. Chem.* **193**, 265-27S.
10. Nicholls, D.G. (1976): Hamster brown adipose tissue mitochondria. Purine nucleotide control of the ion conductance of the inner membrane, the nature of the nucleotide binding site. *Eur. J. Biochem.* **62**, 223-228.
11. Ricquier, D., Barlet, J., Garel, J., Combes-George, M. & Dubois, M.P.(1983): An immunological study of the uncoupling protein of brown adipose tissue mitochondria. *Biochem. J.* **210**, 859-866.
12. Yonetani, T. & Ray, G.S. (1965): Studies on cytochrome oxidase VI. Kinetics of the aerobic oxidation of ferro-cytochrome C by cytochrome oxidase. *J. Biol. Chem.* **240**, 3392-3398.

Chapter 53

Fatty Acid-binding Protein (FABP) in Rat Brown Adipose Tissue

Asim K. DUTTA-ROY*, Yiming HUANG and Paul TRAYHURN

Division of Biochemical Sciences, Rowett Research Institute, Bucksburn, Aberdeen AB2 9SB, Scotland, UK

A fatty acid-binding protein (FABP) has been identified and purified from brown adipose tissue of the rat. The molecular weight of the protein was found to be 14,400 daltons. Scatchard analysis of oleate binding to purified FABP showed a K_d value of approximately 0.8 µM. The FABP concentration in brown adipose tissue was twice that of FABP in white adipose tissue. Fatty acid analysis of FABP from brown adipose tissue reveals that the endogenous arachidonic acid content is much higher than that present in FABP of either rat liver or white adipose tissue.

Introduction

Fatty acid-binding proteins (FABP) belong to a family of small molecular weight cytosolic proteins (MW 14–15000 daltons) which are found in abundance in a number of mammalian tissues. FABPs play an important role in intracellular fatty acid metabolism, such as energy delivery and the synthesis of membrane lipids and lipid mediators (e.g. prostaglandins, leukotrienes and thromboxanes)[11,15]. In addition to their fatty acid-binding activity, FABPs also bind various heterogeneous ligands including haem, prostaglandin E_1, and the lipoxygenase metabolites of arachidonic acid (15 and 5 hydroperoxyeicosatetraenoic acid)[4,14,17]. It has recently been suggested that FABPs may be involved in cell growth and regulation by virtue of their affinity for ligands associated with these processes[11].

FABPs have been isolated and purified from several mammalian tissues, including white adipose tissue of humans, rats and pigs, as well as from the 3T3-L1 adipocyte cell line[1,8,11,12,15]. These proteins are also present in fatty acid-mobilizing tissues of birds, fishes and insects[7,11,15]. The concentration of FABP is influenced by diet, developmental stage and by drugs[5,7,15]. An increase in fat content of the diet has been reported to increase the FABP concentration of liver, heart, distal intestine, and the mammary gland[11,15]. The induction of FABP content closely correlates *in vivo* with the induction of peroxisomal β-oxidation[16]. A number of drugs that affect lipid metabolism cause a marked change in FABP level, indicating a direct relationship between the protein and intracellular fatty acid metabolism. The significance of FABP for fatty acid oxidation is demonstrated by the correlation of FABP level and fatty acid oxidizing capacity of liver, heart, kidney and skeletal muscle of fed rats under normal conditions and after clofibrate treatment[11,15].

The phosphorylation and dephosphorylation of FABP in response to insulin by preadipocyte 3T3 cells suggests that besides its general involvement in intracellular fatty acid metabolism, the protein may also serve a tissue-specific function by acting as a second messenger in white adipocytes[10]. The turnover of the phosphoryl group of FABP is coupled to signal transduction in the glucose transport system in white adipose tissue[2].

In contrast to white adipose tissue, no information is available on whether FABP is present in the other form of adipose tissue, namely brown adipose tissue. Brown adipose tissue is the major site of non-shivering thermogenesis in mammals and free fatty acids are used as the main fuel, even in the presence of glucose[9]. It has been suggested that the level of free fatty acids controls the function of the uncoupling protein responsible for thermogenesis. FABP could play, in principle, an important role in regulating fatty acid pools and thus thermogenesis in brown adipose tissue; here we report the identification and isolation of FABP from brown fat of the rat.

Materials and methods

Preparation of FABP

FABP was purified following the procedures described previously[4]. In brief, interscapular brown adipose and epidymal white adipose tissue were collected from male Hooded Lister rats (150–160 g). The tissues were washed in ice-cold saline to remove blood. The tissues were then homogenized in 20 mM Tris-HCl buffer, pH 7.4, containing 1 mM EDTA, 1 mM PMSF and 0.25 mM sucrose. After homogenization, the homogenate was centrifuged at 5000 **g** for 15 min at 4°C. The supernatant was then recentrifuged at 110,000 **g** for 1 h 20 min at 4°C. The supernatant obtained after the second centrifugation was subjected to 70 per cent ammonium sulphate saturation, after which it was centrifuged at 20,000 **g** for 20 min. The supernatant was then dialysed against 10 mM Tris-HCl buffer, and concentrated by ultrafiltration (Amicon Diaflow, MW cut off 3500 daltons). The protein was finally purified by ion exchange and gel filtration column chromatography. The purity of the protein was assessed by SDS-polyacrylamide gel electophoresis, under reducing conditions. The purified protein was kept at –70°C for further studies.

Fatty acid binding assay

The fatty acid binding assay was performed as described previously[4] using the Lipidex method. Typically, 10–20 µg of protein in 50 mM Tris-HCl buffer, pH 7.4, was incubated with 1 µM [^{14}C]oleate for 20 min at 37°C. After incubation, the assay mixture was cooled and 100 µl of Lipidex 1000 suspension was added to remove the unbound radioligand. After further incubation for 10 min at 4°C, it was centrifuged. One hundred µL of supernatant was used for the determination of radioactivity in a scintillation counter. Non-specific binding was determined in the presence of a 1000-fold excess of unlabelled oleate. A Scatchard analysis was performed by incubating 20 µg of protein with various concentrations of radioligand (0.1–1 µM).

Fatty acid analysis

Both the tissue lipids and the fatty acids from the FABP were extracted according to the method of Folch[6]. The fatty acid composition was then analysed by gas liquid chromatography, after methylation of fatty acids by H_2SO_4-methanol[3].

Fluorescence assay

The fluorescence assay of FABP was performed according to the method described previously[10]. Fluorescence measurements were carried out in a Perkin-Elmer Luminescence spectrophotometer LS-5B at 22°C. Fluorescence intensity was measured at 500 nm after excitation at 350 nm, with a slit width of 10 nm for both excitation and emission.

Results

A FABP was identified in brown adipose tissue and purified to homogeneity using the combinations of ion exchange and size exclusion chromatography. The FABP showed a single band following 15 per cent SDS-polyacrylamide gel electophoresis. The molecular weight of the purified FABP appeared to be 14,400 daltons (Fig. 1). A Scatchard analysis showed a K_d value for oleate binding of around 0.8 ± 0.02 µM, with a single binding site.

Fig. 1. SDS-polyacrylamide gel electrophoresis (15 per cent) of purified FABP from brown adipose tissue and marker protein (α lactalbumin, MW 14,400 daltons).

After 70 per cent ammonium sulphate treatment of the homogenate, and subsequent dialysis, the protein fraction was concentrated. The binding of radiolabelled oleate to FABP fractions from white adipose tissue was compared to brown adipose tissue. The binding of oleate to the FABP fraction appeared to be 1.9-fold higher in brown adipose tissue than with white fat. The increased binding of fatty acid was found to be correlated with the amount of FABP in the samples. This suggests that the increase is not due to a differential increase in affinity for oleate binding to FABP from brown adipose tissue, but is due to a higher concentration of FABP in brown fat relative to white adipose tissue.

The behaviour of FABP towards the fluorescence probe, dansylamino undecanoic acid (UDA), was also examined. FABP from brown adipose tissue did not enhance the fluorescence intensity significantly on binding to UDA in comparison to that of FABP from liver or white adipose tissue. This suggests that the probable fine structure of the hydrophobic binding sites is different in FABP of brown than in white adipose tissue and the liver.

Analysis of the endogenous fatty acids bound to FABP indicated differences between the proteins from the two forms of adipose tissue. A particularly notable difference was the relatively high level of arachidonic acid bound to FABP from brown adipose tissue (at least one-third more than in FABP of white adipose tissue).

Discussion

This paper reports for the first time the identification and preliminary characterization of FABP from brown adipose tissue of rats. Brown adipose tissue is recognized to play a major role in non-shivering thermogenesis with free fatty acids being used as the primary fuel. At present it is not clear as to how precisely FABP contributes to fatty acid metabolism in brown adipose tissue; this requires further investigation. The available data suggest, however, the existence of structure- and tissue-specific specialization of function among different members of the FABP gene family[15]. FABP is reported to be present in abundance in a number of tissues, but in general its concentration is found to be much higher in those tissues which are known to use free fatty acids as the major fuel – with the exception of the liver[3,5,11,15].

The concentration of FABP in rat brown adipose tissue was found to be almost twofold higher than that in white adipose tissue, suggesting that there may be an increased requirement for FABP for handling free fatty acid metabolism in brown adipose tissue. Fatty acid analysis reveals the presence of an increased arachidonic acid content compared to that of FABP of liver[17]. This intriguing observation merits further consideration. Further detailed study of FABP in brown adipose tissue is needed to establish the role of the protein in fatty acid metabolism, including the response to cold acclimatization, i.e. the long-term stimulation of thermogenesis.

References

1. Armstrong, M.K., Bernlohr, D.A., Storch, J. & Clarke, S.D. (1990): The purification and characterisation of a fatty acid-binding protein specific to (*Mus domesticus*) adipose tissue. *Biochem. J.* **267**, 373-378.
2. Bemier, M. Laird, D.M. & Lane, M.D. (1988): Effect of vanadate on the cellular accumulation of pp15, an apparent product of insulin receptor tyrosine kinase action. *J. Biol. Chem.* **263**, 13626-13634.
3. Dutta-Roy, A.K., DeMarco, A.C., Raha, S.K., Shay, J., Garvey, M. & Horrobin, D.F. (1990): Effects of linoleic and gamma-linolenic acids (evening primrose oil) on fatty acid binding proteins of rat liver. *Mol. Cell. Biochem.* **98**, 177-182.
4. Dutta-Roy, A.K., Gopalswamy, N. & Trulzsch, D.V. (1987): Prostaglandin E$_1$ binds to Z protein of rat liver. *Eur. J. Biochem.* **162**, 615-619.
5. Dutta-Roy, A.K., Trinh, M.V., Sullivan, T.S. & Trulzsch, D.V.(1988): Choline deficient diet increases Z protein concentration in rat liver. *J. Nutr.* **118**, 1116-1119.
6. Folch, L., Lees, M. & Sloane-Stanely, G.H. (1957): A simple method for isolation and purification of total lipids from animal tissues. *J. Biol. Chem.* **226**, 89-95.
7. Haunerland, N.H. & Chrishlom, J.M. (1990): Fatty acid binding protein in flight muscle of the locust, *Schistocerca gregaria*. *Biochim. Biophys. Acta.* **1047**, 233-238.
8. Haq, R.-L., Christodoulides, L., Ketterer, B. & Shrago, E. (1982): Characterization and purification of fatty acid-binding protein in rat and human adipose tissue. *Biochim. Biophys. Acta.* **713**, 193-198.
9. Himms-Hagen, J. (1989): Brown adipose tissue thermogenesis and obesity. *Prog. Lipid Res.* **28**, 67-115.
10. Hresko, R.C., Bernier, M., Hoffman, R.D., Flores-Riveros, J.R., Liao, K., Laird, D.M. & Lane, M.D. (1988): Identification of phosphorylated 422 (aP2) protein as pp15, the 15-kilodalton target of the insulin receptor tyrosine kinase in 3T3-Ll adipocytes. *Proc. Natl. Acad. Sci. USA* **85**, 8835-8839.
11. Kaikaus, R.M., Bass, N.M. & Ockner, R.K. (1990): Functions of fatty acid binding proteins. *Experientia* **46,** 617-630.
12. Matarese, V. & Bernlohr, D.A. (1988): Purification of murine adipocyte lipid-binding protein. Characterization as a fatty acid and retinoic acid binding. *J. Biol. Chem.* **263**, 14544-14551.
13. Paulussen, R.J.A., Geelen, M.J.H, Beynen, A.C. & Veerkamp, J.H. (1989): Immunochemical quantitation of fatty acid-binding proteins; I. Tissue and intracellular distribution, postnatal development and influence of physiological conditions on rat heart and liver FABP. *Biochim. Biophys. Acta.* **1001**, 201-209.
14. Raza, H., Pongubala, J.R. & Sorof, S. (1989): Specific high affinity binding of lipoxygenase metabolites of arachidonic acid by liver fatty acid binding-protein. *Biochem. Biophys. Res. Commun.* **161,** 448-455.
15. Veerkamp, J.H., Peters, R.A. & Maatman, R.G.H.J. (1991): Structural and functional features of different types of cytoplasmic fatty acid-binding proteins. *Biochim. Biophys. Acta.* **1081**, 1-24.
16. Veerkamp, J.H. & Van Moerkerk, H.T.B. (1986): Peroxisomal fatty acid oxidation in rat and human tissues: effect of nutritional state, clofibrate treatment and postnatal development in the rat. *Biochim. Biophys. Acta.* **875**, 301-310.
17. Vincent, S.H. & Muller-Eberhard, U. (1985): A protein of the Z class of liver cytosolic proteins in the rat preferentially binds heme. *J. Biol. Chem.* **260**, 14521-14528.

Section IX
Control of energy expenditure

Chapter 54

Swedish Obese Subjects, SOS. An Intervention Study of Obesity
A selected description of the obese state and relationships between adipose tissue distribution and metabolic aberrations in the first 1006 subjects examined

Lars SJÖSTRÖM
Department of Medicine, Sahlgren's Hospital, University of Gothenburg, S-413 45 Gothenburg, Sweden

Obesity and risk

Obesity is associated with an increased prevalence of cardiovascular risk factors such as hypertension[7,46,48], lipid disturbances[10,46,48] and diabetes mellitus[46,48]. These risk factors are improved by weight reduction[1,8,9,11,12,13,16,17,36].

In contrast to prevalence and risk factor studies, considerable inconsistencies have been reported for the relationship of obesity to the incidence of cardiovascular disease and total mortality. Several reviewers have found that approximately 40 per cent of all population, community and employee studies fail to find a relationship between obesity and these incidences[2,23,40]. Suggested reasons for these inconsistencies have been misclassifications, confusions, unknown protective factors and surrogate risk factors[2]. However, the single most important explanation for the deviating results is that far-reaching conclusions have been drawn from small (n < 7000), relatively short (15 years and less) studies ([40] and Fig. 1). Insurance studies[4,5] and all other studies with cohorts larger than 7000 and follow-up periods longer than 5 years[6,14,18,25,26,30-32,34,35,45,49,50] have found a U- or J-shaped relationship between body weight on the one hand and incidence of cardiovascular disease and/or mortality on the other. Several long-term (more than 15 years), relatively small, studies have also been able to identify obesity as a cardiovascular risk factor ([47] men but not women[15,33]). A large fraction of these positive studies have been published during the last 10 years and four studies[14,26,35,50] since 1988. Today, the scientific community has probably more or less unanimously accepted the statistical relationship between obesity and cardiovascular risk.

Although two uncontrolled studies indicate a risk reversibility induced by weight reduction[27,28], the causal relationships between obesity, cardiovascular incidence and mortality have not been definitely proved however, since no controlled intervention studies of obesity have been undertaken. Hopefully, "Swedish Obese Subjects, SOS"[37,41-44] and other intervention studies that may be started will elucidate the question whether obesity is or is not a cardiovascular risk factor.

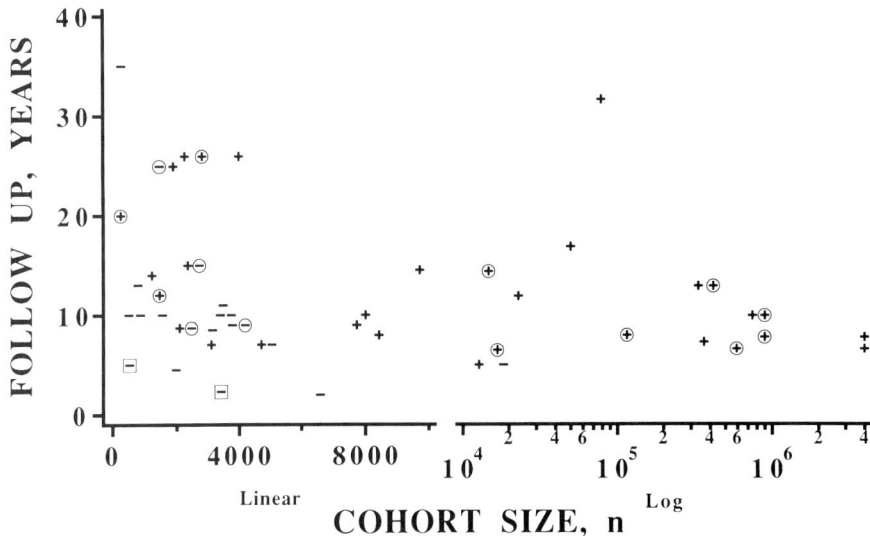

Fig. 1. Cohort size and follow up period in relation to 40 employee, community, insurance or random population studies finding (+) or not finding (−) a positive relationship between obesity and mortality. Encircled signs represent female cohorts and squares around signs indicate that men and women were analysed together. For layout reasons seven cohorts have been plotted in positions deviating as little as possible from the true values. Each study can be identified in[40].

Study design of SOS

SOS is an ongoing project which consists of a Register study and an Intervention Study of severely obese subjects. The study has been described in detail elsewhere[43].

In the Register study 7000–10,000 obese subjects will participate in a health examination at about 700 primary health care centres all over Sweden. The patients are recruited by advertisements in newspapers, radio and television. Before the health examination the patients have to complete extensive questionnaires covering information on weight development, diseases, psychological characteristics, medication, ethnic origin, education, socio-economic conditions, utilization of medical care, sleep patterns, physical activity, food, alcohol and smoking habits, weight of relatives and quantitative information on social contacts with them. In the Register examination weight, height, blood pressure, ECG and a number of anthropometric measurements including the sagittal diameter at L_{4-5} of recumbent subjects[19,37-39] are collected. Blood glucose, serum lipids, insulin and several other biochemical determinations are performed[43].

The inclusion criteria of the Register study are age 37–57 years and BMI ≥ 34 in men and BMI ≥ 38 in women. No exclusion criteria are used in the Register study

In the Intervention study one surgically treated group (n = 2000) and one matched conventionally treated control group (n = 2000) will be compared over 10 years. Accepted surgical techniques are gastric banding, vertical banded gastroplasty and gastric bypass. The surgical group is recruited from the register study and from pre-existing waiting lists at participating surgical departments. For each surgical case a computerized matching procedure selects the optimal control among eligible controls of the register study. For several reasons discussed elsewhere a randomized study was not possible[43]. The surgical cases will be operated on at 26 county or university hospitals in Sweden while the control cases are followed at the 750 primary health care centres.

The inclusion and exclusion criteria are identical for surgical cases and control cases of the intervention study. The inclusion criteria are the same as in the Register study. Ten (categories of) exclusion criteria are described elsewhere[43].

The main aims of the study are to examined if long-term weight reduction (obtained by surgery) decreases total mortality and mortality and morbidity of specific diseases. Attempts will be made to answer some 15 other interdisciplinary oriented questions[43].

Material and methods

For the purpose of the current presentation the first 1006 health-examined subjects of the Register study will be used (Table 1)[43] and compared with population studies of men[20,23,24] and women[3] going on in Gothenburg, Sweden. Results on 383 surgical cases and the same number of matched controls will also be briefly mentioned.

Table 1. Description of the first 1006 patients who were health-examined in the SOS project

	Males	Females
n	450	556
Age	48 ± 6	48 ± 6
BMI, kg/m^2	37.6 ± 4.0	41.0 ± 4.3
Weight, kg	119.3 ± 14.9	110.7 ± 13.6
Estimated LBM, kg	74 ± 6	46 ± 4
Estimated total AT, kg	45 ± 9	65 ± 11
Estimated subcutaneous AT, kg	37 ± 8	60 ± 10
Estimated visceral AT, kg	8.6 ± 2.6	5.0 ± 1.2

Means ± SD. Age, ns; otherwise $P < 0.0000$ between sexes.

In addition to methods mentioned under "Study design" above. a three-compartment model was used to estimate the weights of lean body mass, subcutaneous and visceral adipose tissue from body weight, height and sagittal trunk diameter. The estimates are based on CT calibrated equations (Fig. 2). Our original CT calibrated equations (and the cross-validation of them)[19] have now been further validated in larger materials[37-39] and it has turned out that the original equations are robust, even in cases with Cushing's disease and in subjects of Indian origin.

ANTHROPOMETRIC ESTIMATES

$$BW \rightarrow \begin{cases} \textbf{LBM} \\ \text{total AT} \rightarrow \begin{cases} \textbf{subcut. AT} \\ \textbf{visceral AT} \end{cases} \end{cases}$$

Fig. 2. A CT-calibrated anthropometric three-compartment model to determine lean body mass (LBM, kg), visceral AT (kg) and subcutaneous AT (kg) from weight (W, kg), height (H, m) and sagittal recumbent trunk diameter at $L_{4\text{-}5}$ (D, cm).
Males: total AT, kg = 0.923 (1.36 · W/H – 42.0); visceral AT, kg = 0.923 (0.731 · D – 11.5).
Females: total AT, kg = 0.923 (1.61 · W/H – 38.3); visceral AT, kg = 0.923 (0.370 · D – 4.85).
Males and females: LBM, kg = BW, kg – total AT, kg. Subcutaneous AT, kg = total AT, kg – visceral AT. D is determined with spirit level and ruler of recumbent subjects. The $L_{4\text{-}5}$ level corresponds to the iliac crest level. Adapted from[19].

Prevalence of risk factors, symptoms and diseases in severely obese subjects as compared to random populations

In Table 2, the prevalence differences between obese and random subjects are illustrated by myocardial infarction in men and angina pectoris (according to Rose) in women. Depending on sex and age, various symptoms and diseases seemed to be 1.2–105 times more common among obese subjects (Table 3)[43]. The largest prevalence differences between obese and random subjects were observed at younger ages.

Table 2. Prevalence of angina pectoris and of previously experienced myocardial infarction in obese and random subjects. Adapted from ref.[43]

Age	37–42	43–47	48–52	53–57
n, obese men	125	115	102	108
n, random men			220	791
n, obese women	155	138	121	142
n, random women	372	431	398	180
Previously experienced myocardial infarction				
Obese males, %	3.2	4.3	5.9	15.7
Random males, %	—	—	0.94	3.5*
Ratio			6.3	4.5
P			<0.000	<0.000
Prevalence of angina pectoris				
Obese females, %	30	33	41	38
Random females, %	0.8	2.1	3.5	5.6
Ratio	38	16	12	6.8
P	<0.000	<0.000	<0.000	<0.000

*54- and 60-year-old men.

Table 3. Prevalence ratios (obese/random) for various symptoms and diseases in men and women

	Males	Females
Dyspnoea after two staircases	4.3	4.7–6.4
Angina pectoris	15	6.8–38
Previous myocardial infarction	4.5–6.3	(0.7/0)
Known hypertension	2.1	2.4–11
Blood pressure ≥ 155/95	1.8	1.5–5.3
Blood pressure ≥ 175/105	2.3	1.2–4.1
Known diabetes	5.2	6.6–24
Fasting blood glucose > 7.1 mmol/l	5.4	8.2–19
Stroke		(0.7/0)
Claudication	4.6	26–105
Gall bladder diseases	1.7	1.8–2.8
Back pain	2.1	1.6–1.9

Insulin, glucose, triglycerides, uric acid, ASAT and ALAT were 220, 26, 108, 11, 5 and 64 per cent higher in obese than in random men.

Corresponding figures for females were 57, 31–38, 43–73, 33–47, 16–30 and 50–90 per cent, respectively[43]. Total cholesterol was not different in obese and random males and was in fact 10 to 16 per cent lower in obese than in random females. HDL-cholesterol was 25 per cent lower in obese than random males[43] (data not available in random females). In 91 per cent of the obese males and 78 per cent of the obese females at least one of the following risk factors were observed: glucose > 7.1 mmol/l, systolic blood pressure > 160 mmHg, diastolic > 95 mmHg, total cholesterol > 7.0 mmol/l, HDL-cholesterol < 1.0 mmol/l.

Incidence calculations have not been undertaken in the SOS project since the mean follow-up time in the Intervention study is so far only 13 months.

Risk factors in relation to body composition

Using the CT-calibrated anthropometric equations given in Fig. 2 on the material presented in Table 1, we have shown that as compared to the estimated mass of subcutaneous AT, the mass of visceral AT was much more closely related to metabolic aberrations and diseases[37,38,42]. Lean body mass was never positively related to risk but tended to be negatively correlated to insulin[42].

In contrast to the possibilities with BMI and waist/hip ratio it is thus possible to separate compartments related to risk from compartments which are not by using CT calibrated anthropometry.

When taking age, LBM and subcutaneous AT into account, the estimated visceral AT was significantly related to insulin, glucose, triglycerides, systolic blood pressure and ASAT in both genders, total cholesterol, diastolic blood pressure, dyspnoea, coronary ECG, claudication and sick pension in men and to HDL-cholesterol (negative correlation), uric acid, ALAT and angina pectoris in women[37,38,42].

If both sexes were included in regressions, gender was significant in most cases when taking age and BMI or weight into account. When the estimated mass of visceral AT was taken into account as an additional factor, the importance of gender disappeared for seven of 10 tested risk variables while this was the case for only two of the 10 risk factors when waist/hip was added to the equations[37,38,42]. Similar longitudinal observations were obtained by pooling the population studies of men and women in Gothenburg[21,22]. When the incidence of myocardial infarction was examined, gender was a strong predictor. After addition of the waist/hip ratio as an additional independent variable, the contribution of sex lost its statistical significance[21,22]. These observations[21,22,37,38,42] indicate that sex differences with respect to risk factors and disease are at least partly mediated *via* differences in the size of the visceral AT depot and that this is more easily detected with CT-calibrated anthropometry than with the waist/hip ratio.

Weight changes in the Intervention study

So far (March 1991), 383 patients have been operated on and the same number of controls have been selected. At baseline, there were no significant differences between surgical cases and control cases with respect to 18 variables of predictive importance. At 1 year of follow up (n = 205 in each group) 60 per cent of the surgical cases had lost 50 per cent or more of their initial excess body weight while the corresponding figure in the control group was 3 per cent. In the surgical group, 88 per cent had lost 30 per cent or more of the excess body weight while this figure was 15 per cent in the control group. Similar results were obtained at 2 years but so far only with 45 subjects in each group (unpublished). It should be remembered, that most if not all reports on conventional weight reduction trials have been performed by groups specially interested in obesity. A 10–20 per cent short-time weight reduction has usually been obtained in these studies. In contrast to this dedicated form of treatment, the control group of the SOS project has been treated by physicians at 140 primary health care centres having an "average" interest in obesity-related problems. In many countries this kind of treatment is the one which is available for the majority of obese patients. As can be seen from the control group of the SOS project, this treatment is ineffective. The panel of a recent NIH consensus development conference has stated that obesity surgery is reasonably safe and definitely the most efficacious treatment available in severe obesity[29].

Conclusions

The morbidity and mortality of severely obese subjects is dramatically increased.

Previous inconsistencies with respect to this statement can be explained by misclassification and by conclusions drawn from small and/or short-term studies.

Obese men and women with a large visceral AT depot are at a particularly high risk.

Several sex differences with respect to risk factors and disease are at least partly mediated *via* differences in the size of the visceral AT depot.

The importance of AT distribution is detected more easily with an anthropometric estimate of visceral AT (kg) than with the waist/hip ratio. It seems warranted to move in the direction away from BMI, waist/hip and other ratios towards estimates of defined body compartments (lean body mass, subcutaneous and visceral AT, all in kg).

As compared to conventional treatment, surgical treatment of comparable obese subjects results in a much larger weight reduction. Whether the morbidity and mortality is reduced by long-term weight reduction remains to be seen.

Acknowledgements

Several co-workers have been involved in the studies reported in this chapter. CT measurements were performed by Henry Kvist, Ulla Grangård, Lars Lönn and Lars Jönsson at the Dept. of Clinical Radiology and by Badrul Chowdhury, and Per Mårin at the Dept. of Medicine, Sahlgren's Hospital, Gothenburg. The SOS material was collected by the staff at 140 primary medical care centres and 10 surgical departments in Sweden (a complete list of participants provided on request) in cooperation with Lars Backman, Dept. of Surgery, Danderyd's Hospital, Stockholm; Bo Larsson, Marianne Sullivan and Per Hallgren, Dept. of Medicine, Lars Olbe, Dept. of Surgery and Sven Lindstedt, Dept. of Clinical Chemistry, Sahlgren's Hospital, Gothenburg; Calle Bengtsson, Inst. of Primary Care, Gothenburg; Ingmar Näslund, Dept of Surgery, Örebro Hospital; Sven Dahlgren, Dept. of Surgery, Umeå Hospital; Ego Jonsson, Inst. of Medicine, Karolinska Hospital, Stockholm; Hans Wedel, Nordic Health University, Gothenburg, all in Sweden, and Claude Bouchard, Physical Activity Sciences Laboratory, Laval University, Quebec, Canada. The studies are supported by grants from the Swedish Medical Research Council (B91-19M-07852-05A, B91-19X-05239-14B, B91-19M-08338-04A), Hoffmann-La Roche and Volvo Research foundation.

References

1. Ashley, F.W., Jr. & Kannel, W.B. (1974): Relation of weight change to changes in atherogenic traits: the Framingham Study. *J. Chronic Dis.* **27**, 103-114.
2. Barrett-Connor, E.L. (1985): Obesity, atherosclerosis and coronary artery disease. *Ann. Intern. Med.* **103**, 1010-1018.
3. Bengtsson, C., Blohmé, G., Hallberg, L., Hällström, T., Isaksson, B., Korsan-Bengtsen, K., Rybo, G., Tibblin, E., Tibblin, G. & Westerberg, H. (1973): The study of women in Gothenburg 1968–1969 – a population study. General design, purpose and sampling results. *Acta Med. Scand.* **193**, 311-318.
4. *Build and Blood Pressure Study 1959* (1959): Society of Actuaries. New York: Peter F. Mallon Inc.
5. *Build Study 1979.* (1980): Society of Actuaries and Association of Life Insurance Medical Directors of America. USA: Recording and Statistical Corp.
6. Comstock, G.W., Kandrick, M.A. & Livesay, V.T. (1966): Subcutaneous fatness and mortality. *Am. J. Epidemiol.* **83**, 548-563.
7. Dustan, H.P. (1985): Obesity and hypertension. *Ann. Intern. Med.* **103**, 1047-1049.

8. Gianetta, E., Friedman, D., Adami, G.F. et al. (1985): Effect of bilio-pancreatic bypass on hypercholesterolemia and hypertriglyceridemia. *Proc. Am. Soc. Bar. Surg.* **2**, 138-142.
9. Gleysteen, J.J. & Barboriak, J.J. (1983): Improvement in heart disease risk factors after gastric bypass. *Arch. Surg.* **118**, 681-684.
10. Glueck, C.J., Taylor, H.L., Jacobs, D., Morrisson, J.A., Beaglehole, R. & Williams, O.D. (1980): Plasma high-density lipoprotein cholesterol: association with measurements of body mass. The Lipid Research Clinics Program Prevalence Study. *Circulation* **62**, (Suppl.IV), 62-69.
11. Gonen, B., Halverson, J.D. & Schonfeld, G. (1983): Lipoprotein levels in morbidly obese patients with massive surgically-induced weight loss. *Metabolism* **32**, 492-496.
12. Halvorson, J.D., Kramer, J., Cave, A. et al. (1982): Altered glucose tolerance, insulin response, and insulin sensitivity after massive weight reduction subsequent to gastric bypass. *Surgery* **92**, 235-240.
13. Herbst, C.A., Hughes, T.A., Gwynne, J.T. et al. (1984): Gastric bariatric operation in insulin-treated adults. *Surgery* **95**, 209-214.
14. Hoffmans, M.D.A.F., Kromhout, D. & de Lezenne Coulander, C. (1988): The impact of body mass index of 78,612 18-year old Dutch men on 32-year mortality from all causes. *J. Clin. Epidemiol.* **41**, 749-756.
15. Hubert, H.B., Feinleib, M., McNamara, R.M. et al. (1983): Obesity as an independent risk factor for cardiovascular disease: a 26-year follow up of participants in the Framingham Heart Study. *Circulation* **67**, 968-977.
16. Hughes, T.A., Gwynne, J.T., Switzer, B.R., et al. (1984): Effects of caloric restriction and weight loss on glycemic control, insulin release and resistance and atherosclerotic risk in obese patients with type II diabetes mellitus. *Am. J. Med.* **77**, 7-17.
17. Kannel, W.B. & Gordon, T. (1975): Some determinants of obesity and its impact as a cardiovascular risk factor. In *Recent advances in obesity research: I*, ed. A. Howard, pp. 14-24. London: Newman Publishing Ltd.
18. Keys, A. (1980): Seven Countries: *A multivariate analysis of death and coronary heart disease*. Cambridge, Mass: Havard University Press.
19. Kvist, H., Chowdhury, B., Grangård, U., Tylén, U. & Sjöström, L. (1988): Total and visceral adipose tissue volumes derived from measurements with computed tomography in adult men and women: predictive equations. *Am. J. Clin. Nutr.* **48**, 1351-1361.
20. Larsson, B. (1978): Obesity: a population study of men, with special reference to development and consequences for the health. *Dissertation*. Sweden, Gotab, Kungälv: Medical Faculty, University of Göteborg.
21. Larsson, B., Bengtsson, C., Björntorp, P., Lapidus, L., Sjöström, L., Svärdsudd, K., Tibblin, G., Welin, L. & Wilhelmsen, L. (1990): Is abdominal body fat distribution a main explanation for the male/female difference in the risk of myocardial infarction: The 6th Int. Congress on Obesity, Kobe, Oct. 21–26, 1990, Abstr. *Int. J. Obes.* **14**, Suppl. 2.
22. Larsson, B., Bengtsson, C., Björntorp, P., Lapidus, L., Sjöström, L., Svärdsudd, K., Tibblin, G., Wedel, H., Welin, L. & Wilhelmsen, L.: Is abdominal body fat distribution a main explanation for the male/female difference in the risk of myocardial infarction. *Am. J. Epidemiol.* Submitted.
23. Larsson, B., Björntorp, P. & Tibblin, G. (1981): The health consequences of moderate obesity. *Int. J. Obes.* **5**, 97-116.
24. Larsson, B., Svärdsudd, K., Welin, L., Wilhelmsen, L., Björntorp, P. & Tibblin, G. (1984): Abdominal adipose tissue distribution obesity and risk of cardiovascular diseases and death: 13 year follow up of the participants in the study of men born in 1913. *B. M. J.* **288**, 1401-1404.
25. Lew, E.A. & Garfinkel, L. (1979): Variations in mortality by weight among 750,000 men and women. *J. Chronic Dis.* **32**, 563-576.
26. Manson, J.E., Colditz, G.A., Stampfer, M.J., Willett, W.C., Rosner, B., Monson, R.R., Speizer, F.E. & Hennekens, C. (1990): A prospective study of obesity and risk of coronary heart disease in women. *N. Engl. J. Med.* **322**, 882-889.
27. Marks, H.H. (1960): Influence of obesity on morbidity and mortality. *Bull. New York Acad. Sci.* **36**, 296-312.
28. Mason, E. The impact of obesity surgery on morbidity, mortality and survival. *Abstract book of 4th Int. Symp. on Obesity Surgery*, London, August 1989.
29. National Institutes of Health Consensus Development Conference Statement. Gastrointestinal surgery for severe obesity, March 25–27, 1991. *Am J. Clin. Nutr.* (in press).

30. Paffenbarger, R.S. & Wing, A.L. (1969): Chronic disease in former college students. *Am. J. Epidemiol.* **90**, 527-536.
31. Petitti, D.B., Wingerd, J., Pellegrin, F. & Ramcharan, S. (1979): Risk of vascular disease in women. *J. Am. Med. Ass.* **242**, 1150-1154.
32. Pooling Project Reseach Group (1978): Relationship of blood pressure, serum cholesterol, smoking habit, relative weight and ECG abnormalities to incidence of major coronary events: final report of the pooling project. *J. Chronic Dis.* **31**, 201-306.
33. Rabkin, S.W., Mathewson, F.A.L. & Hsu, P.H. (1977): Relation of body weight to development of ischemic heart disease in a cohort of young North American men after a 26 year observation period: the Manitoba Study. *Am. J. Cardiol.* **39**, 452-458.
34. Rhoads, G.G. & Kagan, A. (1983): The relation of coronary disease, stroke and mortality to weight in youth and middle age. *Lancet* **i**, 492-495.
35. Rissanen, A., Heliövaara, M., Knekt, P., Aromaa, A., Reunanen, A. & Maatela, J. (1989): Weight and mortality in Finnish men. *J. Clin. Epidemiol.* **42**, 781-789.
36. Rucker, R.D., Goldenberg, F., Varco, R.L. *et al.* (1981): Lipid effects of obesity operations. *J. Surg. Res.* **30**, 229-235.
37. Sjöström, L. (1991): A CT-based multicompartment body composition technique and anthropometrlc predictions of lean body mass, total and subcutaneous adipose tissue. Speech at the Int. Symp. on Regional Fat Distribution and Morbidity. Osaka, Oct. 19-20, 1990. *Int. J. Obes.* **15**, 19-30.
38. Sjöström, I. (1991): Methods or measurement of the visceral adipose tissue volume and relationships between visceral fat: and disease in 1006 severely obese subjects. In *Progress in obesity research 1991*, eds. Y. Oomura, S. Tarui, S. Inoue & T. Shimazu, pp. 323-334. London: John Libbey.
39. Sjöström, L. (1992): Morbidity of severely obese subjects. Speech at NIH consensus development conference on gastrointestinal surgery for severe obesity. March 25–27, 1991. *Am. J. Clin. Nutr.* (in press).
40. Sjöström, L. (1992): Mortality of severely obese subjects. Speech at the NIH consensus development conference on surgical treatment of Severe Obesity. *Am. J. Clin. Nutr.* (in press).
41. Sjöström, L. (1988): SOS, en Interventionsstudie av fetma. *Lakartidningen* **85**, 636-639.
42. Sjöström, L., Backman, L., Bengtsson, C., Bouchard, C., Dahlgren, S., Jonsson, E., Larsson, B., Lindroos, A-K., Lindstedt, S., Lissner, L., Narbro, K., Näslund, I., Olbe, L., Sullivan, M. & Wedel, H: *SOS – an intervention study of obesity*. Some cardiovascular risk factors in relation to age, body composition and adipose tissue distribution in the first 1006 subjects examined. To be submitted.
43. Sjöström, L., Larsson, B., Backman, L., Bengtsson, C., Bouchard, C., Dahlgren, S., Hallgren, P., Jonsson, E., Karlsson, J., Lapidus, L., Lindroos, A-K., Lindstedt, S., Lissner, L., Narbro, K., Näslund, I., Olbe, L., Sullivan, M., Sylvan, A., Wedel, H. and Ågren, G.: *SOS – an intervention study of obesity*. Study design and a selected description of the obese state basea on the flrst 1006 subjects examined. Submitted to *Int. J. Obes.*.
44. Sjöström, L., Larsson, B., Backman, L., Bengtsson, C., Bouchard, C., Dahlgren, S., Jonsson, E., Lapidus, L., Lindstedt, S., Narbro, K., Näslund, I., Olbe, L., Sullivan, M. & Wedel, H.: *SOS – an intervention study of obesity*. The natural history of obesity as assessed from questionaries of the first 1006 subjects examined. To be submitted.
45. Sörensen, T.I.A. & Sonne-Holm, S. (1977): Mortality in extremely overweight young men. *J. Chronic Dis.* **30**, 359-367.
46. Stamler, J. (1979): Overweight, hypertension, hypercholesterolemia and coronary heart disease. In *Medical complications of obesity*, eds. M. Mancini, B. Lewis & F. Contaldo, pp. 191-216. London: Academic Press.
47. Vandenbroucke, J.P., Maurity, B.J., de Bruin, A. *et al.* (1984): Weight, smoking and mortality. *JAMA* **252**, 2859-2860.
48. VanItallie, T.B. (1985): Health implication of overweight and obesity in the United States. *Ann. Int. Med.* **103**, 983-988.
49. Waaler, H.T. (1984): Height, weight and mortality: the Norwegian experience. *Acta Med. Scand.* Suppl. 679.
50. Wannamethee, G. & Shaper, A.G. (1989): Body weight and mortality in middle aged British men: impact of smoking. *B. M. J.* **299**, 1497-1502.

Chapter 55

Psychological and Behavioural Determinants of Regional Fat Deposition

Judith RODIN
Yale University, Department of Psychology, Box 11A, Yale Station, New Haven, CT 06520-7447, USA

Abdominally localized adipose tissue appears to be an important risk factor, independent of total fat mass, for cardiovascular diseases including myocardial infarction and stroke, non-insulin dependent diabetes mellitus, essential hypertension and endometrial carcinoma[3,12,14,16,37]. Several of these conditions have risk factors in common, for example, hypertension for cardiovascular disease and stroke, insulin resistance for cardiovascular disease and non-insulin dependent diabetes. More centrally distributed fat has now been shown to be related to a variety of these major disease risk factors including elevated blood pressure, elevated lipids, including hypertriglyceridaemia, increased levels of total cholesterol and low density lipoproteins, decreased concentrations of high density lipoproteins and decreased lipoprotein lipase activity[8,17,18,27,28,38,39,40]. Regional fat distribution also appears to influence metabolic variables including decreased glucose tolerance and increased insulin resistance, and hepatic insulin extraction[6,18,19,21,28,34,35].

Several factors have been identified that regulate the distribution of body fat to different regions of the body, as shown in Table 1. Among the most important are genes, developmental changes related to growing old, being male or female, and environment or lifestyle variables[4,29]. Identifying how these determinants have their effects may lead to new understanding of the pathogenesis and treatment of the diseases that are associated with abdominal obesity. The focus of this paper is on environmental factors that may influence regional fat distributions.

Table 1. Determinants of regional fat distribution

Genes (especially gene X environment interactions)
Ageing
Sex
Environment/lifestyle
    Stress
    Dieting
    Smoking
    Alcohol use (?)

Björntorp, Rebuffé-Scrive and their colleagues first pointed to a possible role for environmental factors when they reported that glucocorticoid receptors are evident in adipose tissue throughout all femoral and abdominal regions, but that the density was highest in the deep abdominal fat[4,29]. They proposed that glucocorticoids and sex steroid hormones may regulate different regions of fat tissue. Due to the high density of glucocorticoid receptors in the internal abdominal fat, corticosteroids could play an important role in the regulation of fat metabolism in this region, in particular. This observation led to a search for a link between abdominal fat distribution and factors that elevate glucocorticoids. It has been shown for some time that Cushing patients, who have highly elevated ACTH secretion to high levels of cortisol, have an excess of abdominally distributed fat.

Stress

Stress is thought to be an important exogenous stimulus for glucocorticoid elevation. Stress triggers cortisol and other neuroendocrine secretions *via* a well described pathway (see Fig. 1). Cortisol and catecholamines both have key functions in human stress and coping processes: as sensitive indicators of the stressfulness of person–environment transactions, as regulators of vital bodily functions and under some circumstances as mediators of bodily reactions leading to disease.

Current views of how these systems are engaged by stress focus heavily, at least in humans, on *cognitive* appraisal processes. Frankenhauser and her associates, for example, suggest that the effectiveness of psychosocial factors in arousing the adrenal cortical and the adrenal medullary systems is determined by the person's cognitive appraisal of the balance between

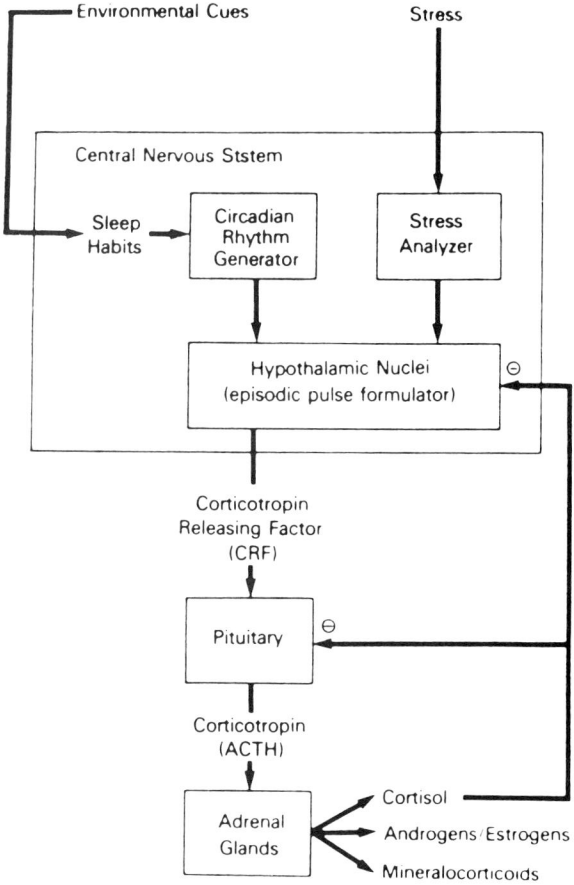

Fig. 1. Stress-induced neuroendocrine secretion pathways.

the severity of the demands of the situation on one hand and his or her coping resources on the other[10]. A basic concept, advanced by Mason, is that neuroendocrine responses to the psychosocial environment reflect its emotional impact on the individual, and that objectively different environmental conditions may evoke the same neuroendocrine responses because they have a common psychological denominator[26]. Similarly – and even more important for our present concerns – the objectively identical environmental condition may evoke different neuroendocrine responses because it provokes different psychological reactions in different individuals.

All current views of stress share the further important idea that the psychological coping response of an organism subjected to a stressful environment will play the determining role in the functioning and interactions of these biological response systems. Frankenhauser and her associates focused on two components of psychological arousal that relate to coping – effort and distress[10]. They found that these two aspects of arousal seem to be differentially associated with catecholamine and cortisol secretion, as is schematized in Fig. 2. During high

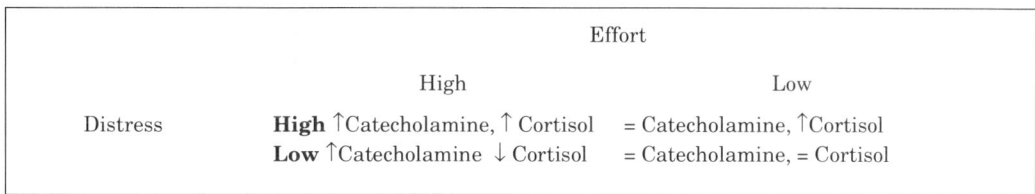

Fig. 2. Differential catecholamine and cortisol secretions in response to effort or distress.

effort (active coping), catecholamine release allows for increased cardiac output to meet heightened metabolic needs. When the individual is experiencing high distress (passive coping), the hypothalamic-pituitary-adrenocortical system acts by releasing cortisol from the adrenal cortex. I will return to the issue of control and coping more fully below.

As a first look at the stress hypothesis, Björntorp and his colleagues reanalysed data from the 1960's and 1970's population study of over 1400 women and 1000 men from Gothenburg, Sweden[22,23]. They examined previously unreported data on psychological and behavioural disturbances and personality traits. For women, more abdominal obesity was associated with what might be seen as symptoms of stress: greater impairment on a psychiatric inventory, sleeplessness, nightmares, use of tranquillizers and antidepressants and greater number of accidents and fractures. Regrettably, somewhat different data had been collected in the study of men but those with more abdominally distributed fat had a greater number of leaves from work and longer duration leaves and more psychosomatic health complaints.

Diverse as these measures are, in the aggregate they might be taken to suggest that the individuals with more abdominally distributed fat could be viewed as those who were higher in chronic arousal or stress. Shivley and Clarkson[37] had previously demonstrated that socially subordinate female macaques who have heightened adrenocortical activity were more likely than dominants to exhibit a central pattern of fat deposition. The subordinate animals were clearly in the situation where personal control was lacking.

These studies, of course, by their very nature, could not use random assignment to condition. Thus, true causal connections could not be drawn between stress responses and abdominal fat distribution. Therefore Rebuffé-Scrive and I developed an animal model to manipulate chronic uncontrollable stress, known to stimulate the pituitary adrenal axis, in order to see whether there were corresponding effects on fat accumulation, particularly in the internal fat regions[30]. We had a clear hypothesis, based on the demonstration of high receptor density for corticosteroids in internal fat in particular. Therefore we expected to see stress influence fat deposition especially in the visceral fat tissues.

We paid close attention to one deep fat region, the mesenteric, which surrounds the liver because this region drains free fatty acids directly into portal circulation. This would lead to an increased flow of FFA reaching the liver directly. High FFA concentration inhibits the hepatic uptake of insulin. This leads to hyperinsulinaemia and insulin resistance and could promote hypertension. This process might be one important reason why there is such a strong association between greater visceral fat and a number of metabolic disorders[5,9,11].

We worked with uncontrollable stressors because of the repeated demonstrations that uncontrollability in particular engages the hypothalamic-pituitary-adrenal axis leading to cortisol release. The magnitude of the effect is well demonstrated in a now classic study by Hanson, Larson, and Snowden[15] who gave animals control over a stressor and compared their cortisol responses to animals with no control and to those with no stress. Animals with control over the stressor showed only modest elevations in cortisol whereas those without control showed substantial elevations. Animals in these two groups were "yoked" so that they received the identical number of stressor exposures (see Fig. 3). Switching the conditions at time 2, so that animals with a control response had it removed and those without a control response now had one available, shows the strong impact of controllability on cortisol release. Our studies with humans show similar effects[32]. In these studies we teach stressed individuals active, control-relevant coping skills. This intervention reduces stress both immediately and up to 18 months later, as shown in Fig. 4. As Fig. 5 indicates, elevated cortisol levels decrease in the group with the coping skills intervention and remain lower over an 18 month follow-up period.

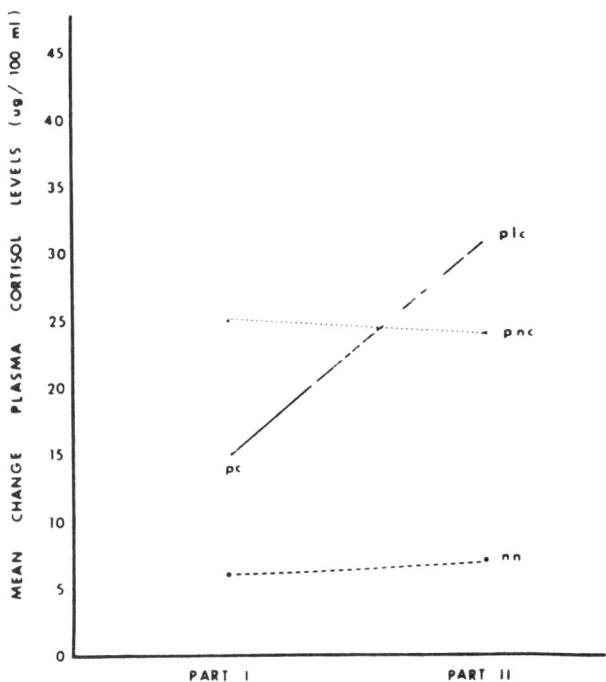

Fig. 3. Changes in cortisol levels following exposure to high intensity noise (nn = no noise; pc = control over noise; plc = loss of control over noise; pnc = no control over noise). From Hanson, Larson and Snowden, 1976, with permission.

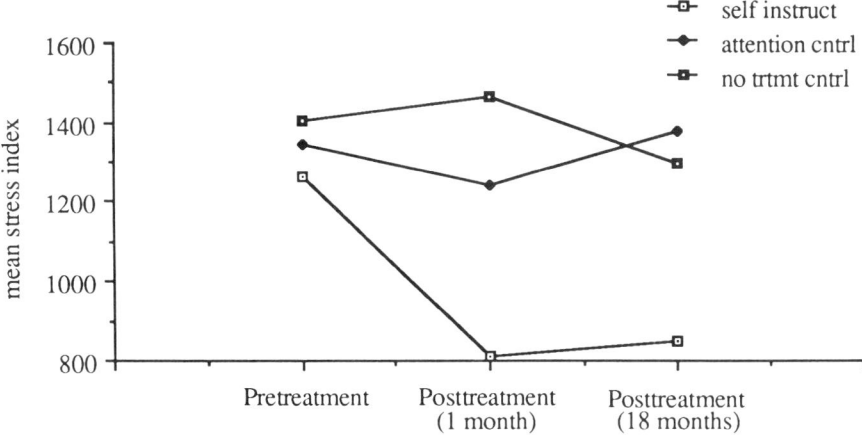

Fig. 4. Self-rated stress in response to no treatment, attention only or control-enhancing self-instructional treatment.

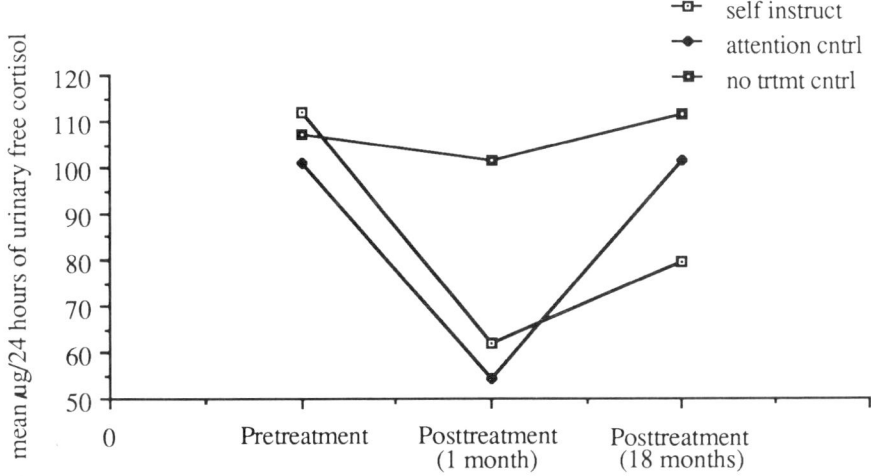

Fig. 5. Urinary free cortisol in response to no treatment, attention only or control-enhancing self-instructional treatment.

In our first study, male Sprague-Dawley rats were randomized to uncontrollable stress *vs.* no stress groups. The stress regimen lasted for 28 days, and the stressors consisted of rotation and restraint, with the regimen of stressors alternated and increased in frequency, duration and severity over time in an attempt to decrease the degree of habituation. Non-stressed and stressed animals were pairfed to control for the effect of stress on food intake and therefore on the metabolic parameters to be measured. At the end of the study, the animals were sacrificed to assess the relevant variables.

The study showed that the mesenteric (deep internal) adipose tissue seems to respond to a chronic uncontrollable stress in a different manner than other depots. The mesenteric fat pad tended to increase ($P < 0.10$) in the stressed rats in comparison with controls. This was not seen with any of the other fat pads. As shown in Fig. 6, fat cell size was significantly increased only in mesenteric fat in the stressed animals in comparison with controls ($P < 0.01$). LPL activity expressed per cell was doubled in the mesenteric fat depot of the stressed rats in comparison with controls ($P < 0.06$). No similar trends were observed in the other depots.

After 1 h in the restrainer, the stressed rats had high corticosterone values (48.4 ± 3.8 µg per cent) in comparison with normal values in the morning (2 ± 5 µg per cent) and those values remained elevated after 28 days of stress (42 ± 5.8 per cent). When corticosterone values after 28 days of stress were correlated with the weight of the various fat pads, a positive correlation was found only with the mesenteric fat depot ($P < 0.05$). No correlations were found between plasma corticosterone and fat pad weights in the control animals.

We are currently conducting studies using several different kinds of uncontrollable stressors, and the data again look quite strong for preferential effects on mesenteric fat metabolism.

To determine further whether the effects of stress on adipose tissue redistribution were due solely to changes in levels of glucocorticoids, we directly manipulated corticosterone levels in the next series of studies. First we used subcutaneous implantation of 100 mg corticosterone pellets to produce continuous administration of corticosterone for almost 2 weeks. One group of animals served as sham-operated controls, one group received two pellets (200 mg) and one group four pellets (400 mg). Figure 7 shows clear differences in plasma levels of corticosterone at day one, diminished but still remaining after 11 days. We chose the supraphysiological concentrations of corticosterone in order to exceed the animals' capacity to produce their own hormone and because we wished to fully control the amount of corticosterone in circulation. The animals were sacrificed and several organs (adrenals, spleen, thymus) sensitive to corticosterone were weighed as were all fat depots, which were also analysed for fat cell size, and LPL activity.

Even though all the rats were paired, both groups of CORT rats had significantly lower body weights than the controls. Adrenals, spleen and thymus weights were dramatically decreased in the CORT groups. In comparison with controls, the CORT rats had significantly increased fat pad weights in the mesenteric depot ($P < 0.004$). Fat cell size and LPL activity increased in all regions, but the effects were strongest in the mesenteric (all $P < 0.01$).

As a different, more phasic type of manipulation, Rebuffé-Scrive and I gave corticosterone in drinking water at several increasing concentrations (0, 100 µg, 200 µg, 400 µg) to randomly assigned groups of animals for 28 days. Corticosterone given in drinking water leads to increased hormone levels in plasma, primarily in conjunction with the night phase of the daily cycle, when drinking usually occurs. The pattern achieved in the drinking water mimics the episodic pattern of CORT release in the intact animal although the drinking water route displaces the diurnal CORT peak. Again the manipulations showed the strong effects of CORT on the adrenals and spleen indicating that the manipulation was effective. For mesenteric tissue, there was a significant linear dose-response trend for fat pad weight ($P < 0.05$). Fat cell size increased strongly in all regions, (all $P < 0.05$). LPL activity also increased in all depots with the strongest effect in the mesenteric fat pad ($P < 0.0001$).

The results from this series of studies suggest that exogenous administration of corticosterone leads to deposition of intra-abdominal fat, although it also leads less specifically to some accumulation in all depots as well. The types of stressors which activate the pituitary adrenal system endogenously have a more specific effect. Fat-pad weight and fat-cell size are significantly increased in mesenteric tissue, in particular. These effects are evident even when the animals lose weight overall. Other hormonal and neuroendocrine responses to stress may contribute to this greater specificity. For example, since catecholamines may also be elevated in these situations, they may play a modulating role as well.

We have also begun to address the stress question in humans. Eventually it will be important to follow a large cohort of people prospectively over a period of chronic uncontrollable stress.

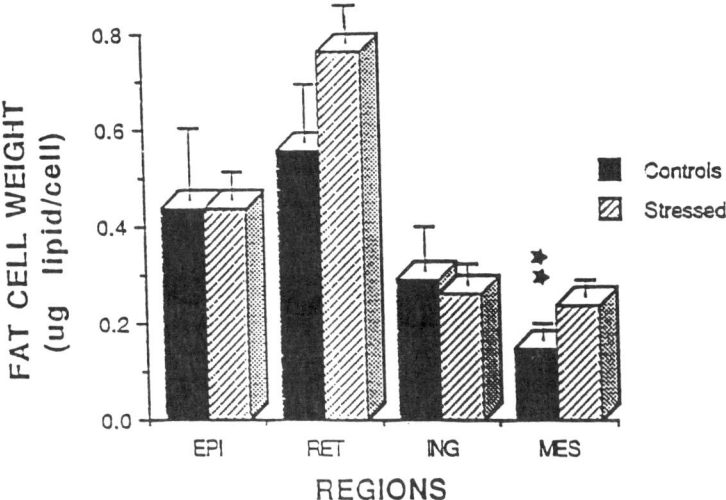

Fig. 6. Fat cell weight in four different regions as a function of uncontrollable stress or no stress (controls).

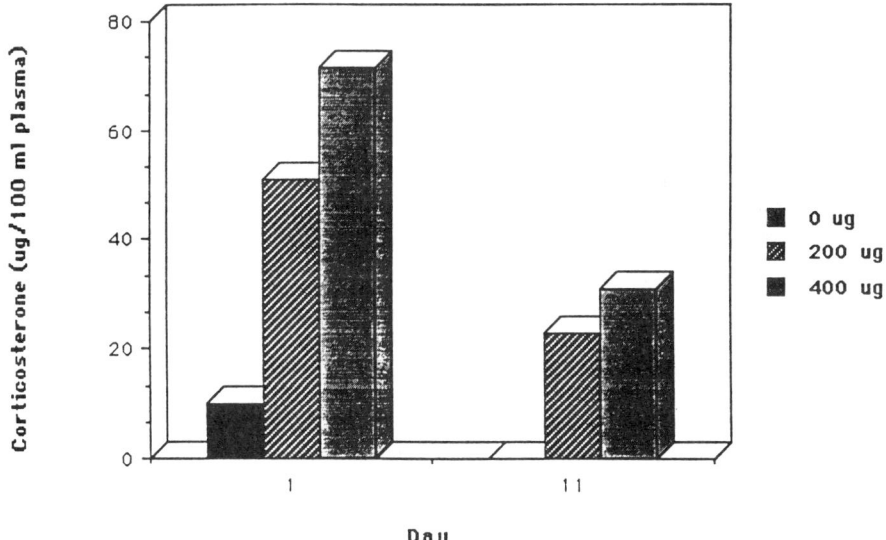

Fig. 7. Plasma levels of corticosterone with three different levels of corticosterone pellets implanted subcutaneously.

This will allow us to determine whether fat redistribution also occurs in people in response to stress. But in addition to this type of longer-term longitudinal study, one might test the same hypothesis indirectly by asking whether individuals with more abdominally distributed fat are more responsive in their corticosteroid release to uncontrollable stress. If so, we might infer that such responsiveness played some causal role in their abdominal localization. Even if such aetiology is not primary, a mechanism would at least be in place for maintaining or perhaps further increasing abdominal fat distribution.

To test this question, we recruited women between the ages of 20 and 40. They were assessed for fat deposition using the WHR. High (> 0.80) and low (≤ 0.75) abdominally distributed women were matched for age and body mass index so that the only significant variable on which they differed was fat distribution. Most were normal weight but some were overweight. They were all tested between days 5 and 12 of their menstrual cycle so that all were in the follicular phase. On two separate days, in randomized order, they either performed a number of stressful tasks or simply rested while listening to relaxing music, and salivary levels of free cortisol were measured at specific time points throughout each session. The stressor tasks included difficult mathematics problems for which a solution was not readily apparent, and learning a pattern of responses to shut off aversive noise – where again the correct response was not easily learned. These types of tasks have been shown to lead to feelings of uncontrollability although, inevitably with humans, not everyone experiences a lack of control.

On the average, the women with the more abdominal distribution had somewhat higher mean levels of cortisol at baseline and in response to stress, but the group differences were not large. However, measures of mood from the Profile of Mood States (POMS)[25] suggested that the subjects were quite variable in how strongly the stressful tasks seemed to affect them. This is crucial since, as I indicated earlier, the same stressor can lead to different levels or patterns of psychoendocrine responses including cortisol increase, suppression or no change, depending on how the stressor is perceived. We reasoned that only those subjects who were distressed and felt the stressors as uncontrollable should show increased cortisol secretion. Considering the three most relevant POMS subscales (tension, anger & depression; the others are vigour, fatigue and confusion), we looked at the correlations within each fat distribution group between the change in subscale score from prestress baseline ratings to several successive ratings taken during and after the stressors, and change in cortisol levels from baseline to the same time points.

For women with more abdominally distributed fat, the associations were strong and significant. The more negative their effect became, the more cortisol they secreted. On the control, non-stress day, as would be expected, there were no correlations between mood and cortisol release. For women with the more femoral distribution, there was no association on either stress or control days between change in negative mood and change in cortisol level.

Another way to evaluate the question is to determine how many women actually showed *large* and statistically significant stress-related increases in cortisol relative to their own baselines. Of 32 subjects tested, only five did. The others showed non-significant changes in one direction or another. In other words, only five reacted to the stress as if their coping efforts were ineffective, thus rendering the stress uncontrollable. Interestingly, of those five, four were in the abdominal distribution group and all of them showed increased negative affect. Only one subject with the more femoral distribution pattern had significantly increased cortisol secretion in response to stress and this was not associated with increased negative affect.

Putting all of these findings together suggests the following hypothesis. There are more women with abdominal than femoral fat distribution who respond to uncontrollable stress with increased dysphoric effect and increased cortisol secretion. For these women, in particular, environmental factors may be of more primary significance in their fat patterning or at least of secondary significance in its maintenance. But not every woman in the abdominal distribution group shows this effect, emphasizing other causal mechanisms as more important for this group, for example genetic factors. We are presently exploring this hypothesis with more impactful and long-term uncontrollable stressors.

Weight cycling

Another type of stressor that we have been investigating is the stress due to repeated bouts of dietary restriction and regain. The most simple way to define weight cycling is on the basis of responses to a questionnaire. Extensive validation using weight fluctuation determined from actual weights reported in medical records as the criterion has shown that the three items indicated below are the most appropriate for defining weight cyclers and noncyclers.

Noncyclers: Those who respond "no" to the question "are you a yo-yo-dieter"; "never" to "rarely" to the question about how often they diet; and who have lost 1–10 pounds no more than 5 times in their lives.

Cyclers: Those who answer "yes" to the question "are you a yo-yo-dieter," who report dieting "often" or "always" about how often they diet, and who have lost 10 pounds or more at least 10 times in their lives.

First, we simply looked to see whether there was a correlation between an individual's weight-cycling history – calculated as a composite of the number and severity of their weight loss and regain episodes – and more abdominally distributed fat. The relationship is strong and significant, controlling for BMI[33]. In other words, the more often a woman has lost and regained weight, regardless of whether she is normal weight or overweight, the higher her WHR.

After making this observation, we decided to do a more precise experimental investigation. Weight cyclers and noncyclers were matched for BMI and tested in the follicular phase for fat-cell size and LPL activity by analysing fat surgically removed from the femoral and

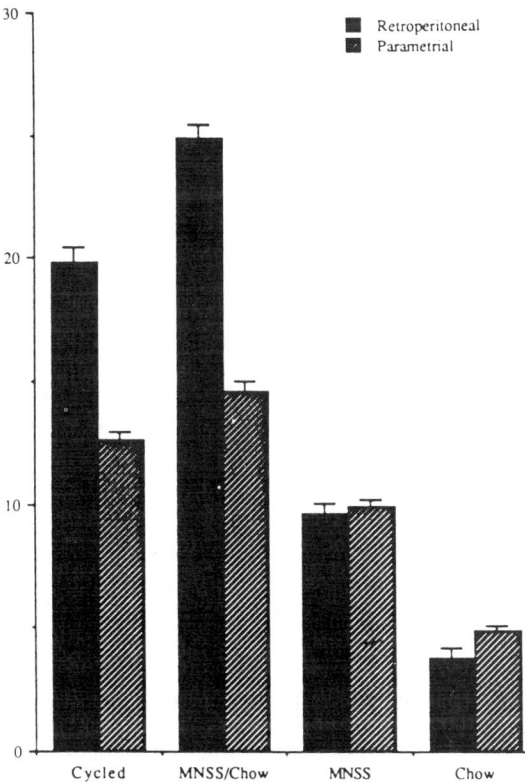

Fig. 8. Mean (± SEM) of the retroperitoneal and parametrical adipocyte depot weights for each group. From Reed et al., 1988, with permission.

abdominal regions. The data showed strong regional specificity of effects. There were no differences between groups in the femoral depots and significant differences in the abdominal, showing increased fat cell size and LPL activity for the weight cyclers ($P < 0.05$).

This observation is supported by animal studies that Danielle Reed and I conducted where rats were put on different types of cycles of dietary restriction and weight gain[31]. Despite actually being lighter in weight than controls when they were sacrificed at the end of the study, autopsy showed significantly more internal fat in the cycled animals (Fig. 8). Quite notably, when cycled animals were given their choice of macronutrients as part of the study protocol, they selected more fat at the expense of protein. Fat is the most efficient nutrient to replace body fat stores and this increased fat preference therefore provides the fuel needed to increase body fat reserves. But the data showed that they distributed these new stores preferentially to the visceral adipose tissue regions when stressed by bouts of weight cycling.

The same is true for women with more extreme weight-cycling histories. In a prospective study of pregnancy that I have been conducting for some time, we identified women prior to pregnancy as either cyclers or noncyclers. At baseline we found that both preference ratings and actual consumption of the cyclers showed increased preference for fat. Our hypothesis is that this fat is preferentially being deposited in the intra-abdominal region when it is stored. Therefore, we predict that a high fat diet coupled with the stress of weight cycling potentiates intra-abdominal fat deposition. We are currently testing this hypothesis in a series of animal studies.

Cigarette smoking

Recent data suggest other environmental stressors that may also be linked to increased abdominal fat distribution – smoking in particular. As den Tonkelaar and colleagues showed in the large Dutch breast screening sample[7], there is a positive correlation between amount of cigarette smoking and the waist/hip ratio. This increase in WHR with smoking was clear in all categories of Quetelet's index. Several other epidemiological studies have shown that, despite their lower level of fatness, smokers have higher waist/hip ratios[13,24]. Moreover Andres and his colleagues[36] have recently shown that while WHR does not actually decrease when people quit smoking, the increase in WHR associated with post-cessation weight gain is significantly smaller than expected. Further, WHR increases in those who start smoking despite their overall weight loss.

In addition to stimulating increased cortisol secretion[2,13] cigarette smoking is also known to be anti-oestrogenic[12] and to stimulate increased production of adrenal androgen[20]. All of these could be important mechanisms contributing to the effects of smoking on regional fat distribution.

Conclusions

The data are beginning to provide strongly suggestive evidence that stress and stress-related lifestyle variables such as smoking, and dieting and regaining weight, and perhaps alcohol use, are important determinants of fat distribution. In fact, in terms of deposition to the high risk site, the intra-abdominal or visceral region, it appears that the environmental factors may play the more significant factor because of the role of glucocorticoids in fat deposition in this region. In view of the implications of fat in this region for impaired insulin metabolism and elevated plasma lipid and lipoprotein levels, this relationship is extremely noteworthy.

These data suggest a new biological pathway between stress on the one hand and morbidity and mortality on the other. This pathway is based on the consequences of stress for repositioning where fat is distributed to more risk-enhancing sites.

Acknowledgements

Much of the research described here was supported by the John D. and Catherine T. MacArthur Foundation Research Program on Determinants and Consequences of Health-Promoting and Health-Damaging Behaviour.

References

1. Anonymous (1986): Anti-oestrogenic effect of cigarette smoking. *Lancet* **ii**, 1433.
2. Baer, L., & Radickerich, I. (1985): Cigarette smoking in hypertensive patients – blood pressure and endocrine response. *Am. J. Med.* **78**, 564-568.
3. Björntorp, P. (1985): Regional patterns of fat distribution. *Ann Int. Med.* **103**, 994-995.
4. Björntorp, P. (1988): Possible mechanisms relating fat distribution and metabolism. In *Fat distribution during growth and later health outcomes*, pp. 175-191. New York: John Wiley & Sons.
5. Björntorp, P. (1990): "Portal" adipose tissue as a generator of risk factors for cardiovascular disease and diabetes. *Arteriosclerosis* **10**, 493-496.
6. Bouchard, C., Tremblay, A., Després, J.P., Nadeau, A., Lupien, P.J., Thériault, G., Dussault, J., Moorjani, S., Pinault, S. & Fournier, G. (1990): The response to long-term overfeeding in identical twins. *N.Engl. J. Med.* **322**, 1477-1482.
7. den Tonkelaar, I., Seidell, J.C., van Noord, P.A.H., Baanders-van Halewijn, E.A. & Ouwehand, I.J. (1990): Fat distribution in relation to age, degree of obesity, smoking habits, parity and estrogen use: a cross-sectional study in 11 825 Dutch women participating in the DOM-project. *Int. J. Obes.* **14**, 753-761.
8. Després, J.P., Allard, C., Tremblay, A., Talbot, J. & Bouchard, C. (1985): Evidence for a regional component of body fatness in the association with serum lipids in men and women. *Metabolism* **34**, 967-973.
9. Després, J.P., Nadeau, A., Tremblay, A., Ferland, M., Moorjani, S., Lupien, P.J., Thériault, G., Pinault, S. & Bouchard, C. (1989): Role of deep abdominal fat in the association between regional adipose tissue distribution and glucose tolerance in obese women. *Diabetes* **38**, 304-309.
10. Frankenhaeuser, M. (1983): The sympathetic-adrenal and pituitary-adrenal response to challenge: comparison between the sexes. In *Karger Biobehavioral Medicine Series Vol 2, Biobehavioral bases of coronary heart disease*, eds. T.M. Dembroski, T.H. Schmidt, G. Blumchen, pp. 91-105. Basel: S. Karger.
11. Fujioka, S., Matsuzawa, Y., Tokunaga, K. & Tarui, S. (1987): Contribution of intra-abdominal fat accumulation to the impairment of glucose and lipid metabolism in human obesity. *Metabolism* **36**, 54-59.
12. Gillum, R.F. (1987): The association of body fat distribution with hypertension, hypertensive heart disease, coronary heart disease, diabetes and cardiovascular risk factors in men and women aged 19–79 years. *J. Chronic Dis.* **40**, 421-428.
13. Gossain, V.V., Shaerma, N.K., Srivastava, L., *et al.* (1986): Hormonal effects of smoking. II: Effects on plasma cortisol, growth hormone and prolactin. *Am. J. Med. Sci.* **291**, 325-327.
14. Haffner, S.M., Mitchell, B.D., Hazuda, H.P. & Stern, M.P. (1991): Greater influence of central distribution of adipose tissue on incidence of non-insulin-dependent diabetes in women than men. *Am. J. Clin. Nutr.* **53**, 1312-1317.
15. Hanson, J.D., Larson, M.E. & Snowden, C.T. (1976): The effects of control over high intensity noise or plasma cortisol levels in rhesus monkeys. *Behav. Biol.* **16**, 333.
16. Hartz, A., Grubb, B., Wild, R., Van Nort, J.J., Kuhn, E., Freedman, D. & Rimm, A. (1990): The association of waist hip ratio and angiographically determined coronary artery disease. *Int. J. Obes.* **14**, 657-665.
17. Jensen, M.D., Haymond, M.W., Rizza, R.A., Cryer, P.E. & Miles, J.M. (1989): Influence of body fat distribution on free fatty acid metabolism in obesity. *Am. Soc. Clin. Invest.* **83**, 1168-1172.
18. Kalkhoff, R.K., Hartz, A.H., Rupley, D., Kissebah, A.H. & Kelber, S. (1983): Relationship of body fat distribution to blood pressure, carbohydrate tolerance, and plasma lipids in healthy obese women. *J. Lab. Clin. Med.* **102**, 621-629.
19. Kaye, S.A., Folsom, A.R., Prineas, R.J., Potter, J.D. & Gapstur, S.M. (1990): The association of body fat distribution with lifestyle and reproductive factors in a population study of postmenopausal women. *Int. J. Obes.* **14**, 583-591.
20. Khaw, K., Tazuda, S. & Barrett-Conner, E. (1988): Cigarette smoking and levels of adrenal androgens in postmenopausal women. *N. Engl. J. Med.* **318**, 1705-1708.

21. Kissebah, A.H., Vydelingum, N., Murray, R., Evans, D.J., Hartz, A.J., Kalkhoff, R.K. & Adams, P.W. (1982): Relation of body fat distribution to metabolic complications of obesity. *J. Clin. Endocrinol. Metab.* **54**, 254-260.
22. Lapidus, L., Bengtsson, C., Hallstrom, T. & Björntorp, P. (1989): Obesity, adipose tissue distribution and health in women – results from a population study in Gothenburg, Sweden. *Appetite* **12**, 25-35.
23. Larsson, B., Seidell, J., Svardsudd, K., Welin, L., Tibblin, G., Wilhelmsen, L. & Björntorp, P. (1989): Obesity, adipose tissue distribution and health in men – the study of men born in 1913. *Appetite* **12**, 37-44.
24. Larsson, B., Svardsudd, K., Welin, L., *et al.* (1980): Obesity, adipose tissue distribution and health – the study of men born in 1913. In *Obesity in Europe 88*, eds. P. Björntorp & S. Rössner, pp. 45-50. London: John Libbey.
25. McNair, D.M., Lorr, M. & Droppleman, L.F. (1971/1981): *Profile of mood states manual.* San Diego, Educational and Industrial Testing Service.
26. Mason, J.W. (1975): Emotion as reflected in patterns of endocrine integration. In *Emotions: their parameters and measurement*, ed. L. Levi. Raven, Press: New York.
27. Peiris, A.N., Mueller, R.A., Smith, G.A., Struve, M.F. & Kissebah, A.H. (1986): Splanchnic insulin metabolism in obesity. Influence of body fat distribution. *J. Clin. Invest.* **78**, 1648-1657.
28. Pouliot, M.C., Després, J.P., Nadeau, A., Tremblay, A., Moorjani, S., Lupien, P.J., Thériault, G. & Bouchard, C. (1990): Associations between regional body fat distribution, fasting plasma free fatty acid levels and glucose tolerance in premenopausal women. *Int. J. Obes.* **14**, 293-302.
29. Rebuffé-Scrive, M. (1988): Metabolic differences in fat depots. In *Fat distribution during growth and later health outcomes*, pp. 163-173. New York: Alan R. Liss, Inc.
30. Rebuffé-Scrive, M., Walsh, U.A., McEwen, B. & Rodin, J. (Manuscript under review): Effect of chronic stress on regional distribution of fat.
31. Reed, D.R., Contreras, R.J., Maggio, C., Greenwood, M.R.C. & Rodin, J. (1988): Weight cycling in female rats increases dietary fat selection and adiposity. *Physiol. Behav.* **42**, 389-395.
32. Rodin, J. (1986): Health, control, and aging. In *Aging and control*, eds. M. Baltes & P. Baltes, pp. 139-165. Hillsdale, NJ: LEA.
33. Rodin, J., Radke-Sharpe, N., Rebuffé-Scrive, M. & Greenwood, M.R.C. (1990): Weight cycling and fat distribution. *Int. J. Obes.* **14**, 303-310.
34. Schwartz, R.S., Shuman, W.P., Bradbury, V.L., Cain, K.C., Fellingham, G.W., Beard, J.C., Kahn, S.E., Stratton, J.R., Cerqueira, M.D. & Abrass, I. (1990): Body fat distribution in healthy young and older men. *J. Geron.* **45**, 181-185.
35. Selby, J.V., Newman, B., Quesenberry, P., Fabsitz, R.R., Carmelli, D., Meaney, F.J. & Slemenda, C. (1990): Genetic and behavioral influences on body fat distribution. *Int. J. Obes.* **14**, 593-602.
36. Shimokata, H., Muller, D.C. & Andres, R. (1989): Studies in the distribution of body fat III. Effects of cigarette smoking. *JAMA* **261**, 1169-1173.
37. Shively, C.A. & Clarkson, T.B. (1988): Regional obesity and coronary artery atherosclerosis in females: a nonhuman primate model. In *Health implications of regional obesity*, eds. P. Björntorp, U. Smith & P. Lonnroth, pp. 71-78. Stockholm: Almqvist & Wiksell.
38. Troisi, R.J., Weiss, S.T., Segal, M.R., Cassano, P.A., Vokonas, P.S. & Landsberg, L. (1990): The relationship of body fat distribution to blood pressure in normotensive men: the normative aging study. *Int. J. Obes.* **14**, 515-525.
39. Williams, P.T., Fortmann, S.P., Terry, R.B., Garay, S.C., Vranizan, K.M., Ellsworth, N. & Wood, P.D. (1987): Associations of dietary fat, regional adiposity, and blood pressure in men. *JAMA* **257**, 3251-3256.
40. Zwiauer, K., Widhalm, K. & Kerbi, B. (1990): Relationship between body fat distribution and blood lipids in obese adolescents. *Int. J. Obes.* **14**, 271-277.

Chapter 56

Effect of Longterm Overfeeding on Energy Expenditure

Angelo TREMBLAY, Jean-Pierre DESPRÉS, Germain THÉRIAULT and Claude BOUCHARD
Physical Activity Sciences Laboratory, Laval University, Ste-Foy, Canada, G1K 7P4

The effect of long-term overfeeding on energy expenditure was investigated in 23 young men who were subjected to a 353 MJ excess energy intake over 100 days. The major part of this energy excess (222 MJ) was stored as body energy, which implies that the total increase in energy expenditure overfeeding corresponded to 131 MJ. The increase in energy cost of weight maintenance, integrating the increase in RMR, postprandial energy expenditure and energy cost of activities, totalled 52 MJ and was proportional to body weight gain. When this value was added to the obligatory cost of fat and lean tissue gains, we accounted for an overall increase in energy expenditure corresponding to 100 MJ. Significant correlations were observed between overfeeding-induced changes in body weight and those in energy cost of weight maintenance ($P < 0.05$). In the 12 subjects who exhibited the highest body-weight gain, the ratio of the increase in energy cost of weight maintenance on body energy was strictly similar to that observed in low-weight gainers. Thus, we conclude the following: (1) in response to long-term overfeeding in humans, the excess energy intake is mainly stored as body energy. (2) This treatment also induces a substantial increase in energy cost of weight maintenance which is proportional to body weight gain. (3) No evidence for a difference in energy efficiency was observed between high and low body weight gainers.

Introduction

Overfeeding is known to be accompanied by an increase in energy expenditure[1,6,7], which means that the resulting weight gain is lower than could be expected on the basis of the excess energy intake. This increase in expenditure is explained by the energy cost of fat and lean tissue gains as well as the increased energy cost of maintenance that results from an increase in body substance. Beyond these obligatory increases in expenditure, experimental evidence suggests that facultative diet-induced thermogenesis could contribute to the excess energy expended in response to overfeeding[5,8]. From a clinical point of view, this involves the possibility that the increase in energy expenditure induced by overfeeding would be proportionally higher than body-weight gain. As previously reviewed[3,4], there is no agreement regarding the notion that the increase in energy expenditure resulting from long-term overfeeding is out of proportion to the associated morphological changes. Therefore, it appeared relevant to take advantage of a research programme aimed at the investigation of the role of heredity on the response to overfeeding[2] to further investigate this issue.

Methods

Twenty-four sedentary young men, aged 21 ± 2 years (means ± SD), gave their written consent to participate in this study. These subjects constituted 12 pairs of identical twins who were recruited in a study designed to investigate the role of heredity in the response to long-term overfeeding[2]. However, due to technical difficulties with the measurement of energy expenditure in one subject at the end of the study, the values of 23 subjects were used to analyse the effect of overfeeding on energy expenditure.

For the duration of the study, the subjects were living on the campus of Laval University. They were housed in a closed section of a dormitory adjacent to the cafeteria where they were taking their meals. The subjects were under 24 h supervision by research assistants who were living with them. Each subject stayed in the unit for 120 days which included the following periods: a 14-day base-line observation period, 3 days for testing before overfeeding, 100 days for the period of overfeeding, and 3 days for post-feeding tests.

After the completion of the first 3-day testing period, the subjects were fed a dietary regimen containing an excess of 4.2 MJ (1000 kcal) per day over the pre-established energy cost of weight maintenance, 6 days a week for 100 days. On the remaining day of each week, there was no overfeeding, i.e. the level of energy intake corresponded to the base-line daily energy needs. The subjects were thus overfed during 84 of the 100 days, the total excess energy intake being 353 MJ (84,000 kcal). The contribution of each macronutrient to energy intake was as follows: 15 per cent protein, 35 per cent lipid, and 50 per cent carbohydrate.

Results

The overfeeding protocol induced a mean increase in body weight of 8.1 kg. The associated gain in body fat and fat-free mass corresponded to 67 and 33 per cent of the body weight gain, respectively. These morphological changes represented a considerable increase in body energy which explained 63 per cent of the total excess energy intake. As expected, a significant increase in RMR, postprandial energy expenditure, energy cost of walking, and energy cost of weight maintenance was observed following overfeeding. The difference between the excess energy intake and the gain in body energy, i.e. 131 MJ, represented the total increase in energy expenditure associated with overfeeding. On the basis of changes in the energy cost of weight maintenance and of some postulates regarding the energy cost of fat and protein gains, we could explain an increase in expenditure of 100 MJ. Therefore, these overall estimates together with body energy gain accounted for 91 per cent of the total excess energy intake.

As expected, a significant correlation was observed between the energy cost of weight maintenance and body weight or fat-free mass either before or after overfeeding ($r = 0.47$ and 0.48, respectively; $P < 0.05$). Furthermore, the slope and the level of regression lines were comparable before and after overfeeding, indicating that the changes in the energy cost of weight maintenance were proportional to those in body weight or fat-free mass.

Several characteristics of the 12 subjects who exhibited the highest weight gain were compared to those who displayed the lowest weight gain. There was no difference between the initial body weight in the two groups. As expected, body fat and body energy gain were much higher in the high- than in the low-weight gainers. The increase in energy cost of weight maintenance also tended to be higher in the high-weight gainers. However, the ratio of the change in the energy cost of weight maintenance on the change in body energy was similar in the two groups.

Discussion

During the last decades, the issue of a facultative component of energy expenditure has been very controversial. When applied in the context of the present study, the concept of facultative thermogenesis suggests that beyond the obligatory costs for the synthesis and maintenance of new body substance, thermogenesis might operate to further attenuate body energy gain. In the present study, we tried to investigate this issue by comparing regression lines of the energy cost of weight maintenance on body weight or fat-free mass before and after overfeeding. Results showed that the level and the slope of these regressions were similar before and after overfeeding, suggesting that changes in adaptive thermogenesis did not contribute significantly to energy expenditure.

The comparison of the high- and low-weight gainers also did not permit us to clearly identify a contribution of facultative thermogenesis. Indeed, if this component of energy expenditure had really played a significant role in the present study, it would be realistic to expect that the increase in energy cost of weight maintenance relative to the gain in body energy would have been higher in the low-weight gainers. As indicated above, results did not support this notion but rather showed that the ratio of these two variables was identical in the two groups. This observation thus suggests that the high weight gainers were not more energy thrifty in response to overfeeding than the low weight gainers.

In summary, results of the present study showed that the major part of a 353 MJ excess energy was stored as body energy. This overfeeding was also accompanied by a substantial increase in energy expenditure. Beyond the obligatory energy cost of fat and lean tissue gains, overfeeding induced a significant increase in energy cost of weight maintenance which was proportional to body weight gain. The sum of the costs of fat and lean tissue gains and the increase in energy cost of weight maintenance did not account for all the increase in energy expenditure induced by overfeeding. The remaining unexplained energy expenditure was likely explained by errors of measurement and errors in the assumptions made to estimate overall energy balance. Finally, results of this study did not allow us to demonstrate a role for facultative thermogenesis as a factor attenuating weight gain in response to overfeeding.

References

1. Apfelbaum, M., Bostsarron, J. & Lacatis, D. (1971): Effect of caloric restriction and excessive caloric intake on energy expenditure. *Am. J. Clin. Nutr.* **24**, 1405-1409.
2. Bouchard, C., Tremblay, A., Després. J.-P., Nadeau, A., Lupien, P.J., Thériault, G., Dussault, J., Moorjani, S., Pinault, S. & Fournier, G. (1990): The response to long-term overfeeding in identical twins. *N. Engl. J. Med.* **322**, 1477-1482.
3. Danforth, E., Burger, A.G., Goldman, R.F. & Sims, E.A.H. (1978): Thermogenesis during weight gain. In *Recent advances in obesity research 2*, ed. G. Bray, pp. 229-236. London: Newman.
4. Garrow, J. (1978): The regulation of energy expenditure in man. In *Recent advances in obesity research 2*, ed. G. Bray, pp. 200-210. London: Newman.
5. James, W.P.T. & Trayhurn, P. (1981). Thermogenesis and obesity. *Br. Med. Bull* **37**, 43-48.
6. Norgan, N.G. & Durnin, J.V.G.A. (1980): The effect of 6 weeks of overfeeding on the body weight, body composition, and energy metabolism of young men. *Am. J. Clin. Nutr.* **33**, 978-988.
7. Ravussin, E., Schutz, Y., Acheson, K.J., Dusmet, M., Bourquin, L. & Jéquier, E. (1985): Short-term, mixed-diet overfeeding in man: no evidence for "luxuskonsumption". *Am. J. Physiol.* **249**, E470-E477.
8. Rothwell, N. & Stock, M.J. (1981): Regulation of energy balance. *Annu. Rev. Nutr.* **1**, 235-256.

Chapter 57

Meal-induced Thermogenesis in Lean and Obese Prepubertal Children

Claudio MAFFEIS, Yves SCHUTZ** and Leonardo PINELLI*
Regional Centre for Juvenile Diabetes, Department of Paediatrics, *Chairman, Preventive and Social Paediatrics, University of Verona, Policlinico, 37134 Verona, Italy; **Institute of Physiology, Faculty of Medicine, University of Lausanne, Rue du Bugnon 7, 1011 Lausanne, Switzerland

The resting metabolic rate (RMR) and the thermic effect of a meal (TEM) were measured in a group of 16 prepubertal obese and 10 non-obese children. In absolute value the RMR was higher in obese than in control children (4971 ± 485 vs 4519 ± 326 kJ/d $P < 0.05$). However, when the RMR was adjusted for the effect of fat-free mass, similar values in the two groups were observed (4887 ± 389 vs 4686 ± 389 kJ/d respectively in the obese and control groups).

The thermic effect of a liquid mixed meal (TEM) was found to be significantly lower in obese than in control children: expressed as a percentage of the energy content of the meal, the TEM averaged 4.4 ± 1.2 per cent in obese vs 5.9 ± 1.7 per cent in the non-obese group ($P < 0.05$) whereas the TEM expressed as the percentage increase over premeal RMR was found to be 10.6 ± 3 per cent in the obese vs 14 ± 4.3 per cent in the non-obese group ($P < 0.05$).

Although a blunted postprandial thermogenesis may constitute a contributing factor for energy storage and weight gain in the obese children, the quantitative importance of this phenomenon in the aetiology of obesity remains to be further evaluated.

Introduction

Some studies in obese adults have supported the hypothesis that a blunted postprandial thermogenesis may play a role in the aetiology of some human obesity[1,6,7,8]. In the paediatric group little information is available on the thermic effect of a meal (TEM). Therefore the present study was undertaken to assess the magnitude of TEM in a group of prepubertal obese children and to compare the results with that of non-obese children.

Methods

Sixteen prepubertal (8.8 ± 0.3 years) obese children and 10 age-matched (8.6 ± 0.4 years) children of normal body weight were studied. As shown in Table 1 the two groups differed significantly with respect to weight and relative body fat, both being significantly higher in the obese than in the control group ($P < 0.001$). In contrast, the fat-free mass (FFM) was comparable in both groups.

Physical examination and routine laboratory tests indicated the absence of any health problems. At the time of the study, no child was taking any drug or medication. Informed consent was obtained from the parents of all children. The food intake of each child was assessed by a dietary history interview, which was conducted by a trained dietician. The day of the calorimetric test, the child arrived by car in the paediatric department at about 7.30 a.m. in post-absorptive conditions. Fasting venous blood samples were taken for plasma glucose, immunoreactive insulin (IRI) and free fatty acids concentrations. The rate of oxygen consumption and carbon dioxide production were measured by means of an open circuit computerized indirect calorimeter (Deltatrac TM, Datex Inc, Finland) using a transparent ventilated hood system. Energy expenditure was calculated by means of classical formula[3].

Respiratory gas exchange was measured continuously for a total of 225 min, i.e. 45 min during the premeal resting metabolic rate (RMR) baseline and then for 180 min after the ingestion of a mixed liquid formula (Ensure, Abott, USA) containing 17 per cent of the energy derived from protein, 53 per cent from carbohydrate and 30 per cent from fat. The energy level was calculated to cover 30 per cent of the premeal RMR extrapolated to 24 h. Due to their greater preprandial RMR, the obese received proportionally more test meal energy than the control children: 1489 ± 142 vs 1356 ± 96 kJ respectively.

Table 1. Physical characteristics and body composition of the children (X ± SD)

M/F	Obese (n=16) 8/8	Controls (n=10) 4/6	Statistical difference P
Age, yrs	8.8 ± 0.3	8.6 ± 0.4	ns
Height, cm	135 ± 8	134 ± 3	ns
Weight, kg	43.6 ± 9.2	31.0 ± 6.0	< 0.001
BMI, kg/m^2	24.3 ± 4.2	18.3 ± 1.7	< 0.001
Weight for height, %	135.1 ± 15.4	103.6 ± 4.5	< 0.001
Body fat, % weight	29.7 ± 5.3	20.6 ± 6.0	< 0.001
FFM, kg	30.3 ± 5.5	26.6 ± 4.7	ns

Results

The energy intake of the obese group was significantly higher than that of the control group (9970 ± 2309 vs 8058 ± 1971 kJ/d, $P < 0.05$). However, calculated per unit FFM the difference between the two groups vanished (329 ± 29 vs 312 ± 56 kJ/kg FFM.d in the obese and control group respectively). The post-absorptive glycaemia (4.66 ± 0.51 mmol/l) and FFA plasma concentration (643 ± 121 nmol/ml) of the obese children were similar to those of the control group (4.61 ± 0.64 mmol/l and 681 ± 237 nmol/ml).

Post-absorptive plasma IRI concentration was significantly higher in the obese than in the control children (15.5 ± 1.66 vs 11.09 ± 0.43 µu/ml, $P < 0.05$). The RMR of the obese, expressed in absolute value, was found to be higher than that of the non-obese group (4971 ± 485 vs 4519 ± 326 kJ/d, $P < 0.05$) but similar when adjusted for FFM by means of the analysis of covariance: 4887 ± 389 vs 4686 ± 389 kJ/d in obese and non-obese children respectively. Both the premeal (0.86 ± 0.03 vs 0.85 ± 0.03) and postmeal (0.90 ± 0.02 vs 0.90 ± 0.03) respiratory quotients were not different in the two groups of children.

Calculated as a per cent of the meal metabolizable energy, the TEM was found to be slightly but significantly lower in obese than in lean children averaging 4.4 ± 1.2 per cent and 5.9. ± 1.7 per cent and 10.6 ± 3.0 and 14.0 ± 4.3 per cent respectively (Fig. 1). However, the net increase in energy expenditure calculated over the 3 h postprandial period was found to be similar in obese and control children (67 ± 17 vs 79 ± 21 kJ respectively, ns) despite the fact that the size of the test meal was significantly greater in obese than in non-obese children ($P < 0.05$).

Discussion

In the prepubertal age, obesity seems to be accompanied by a reduction in postprandial

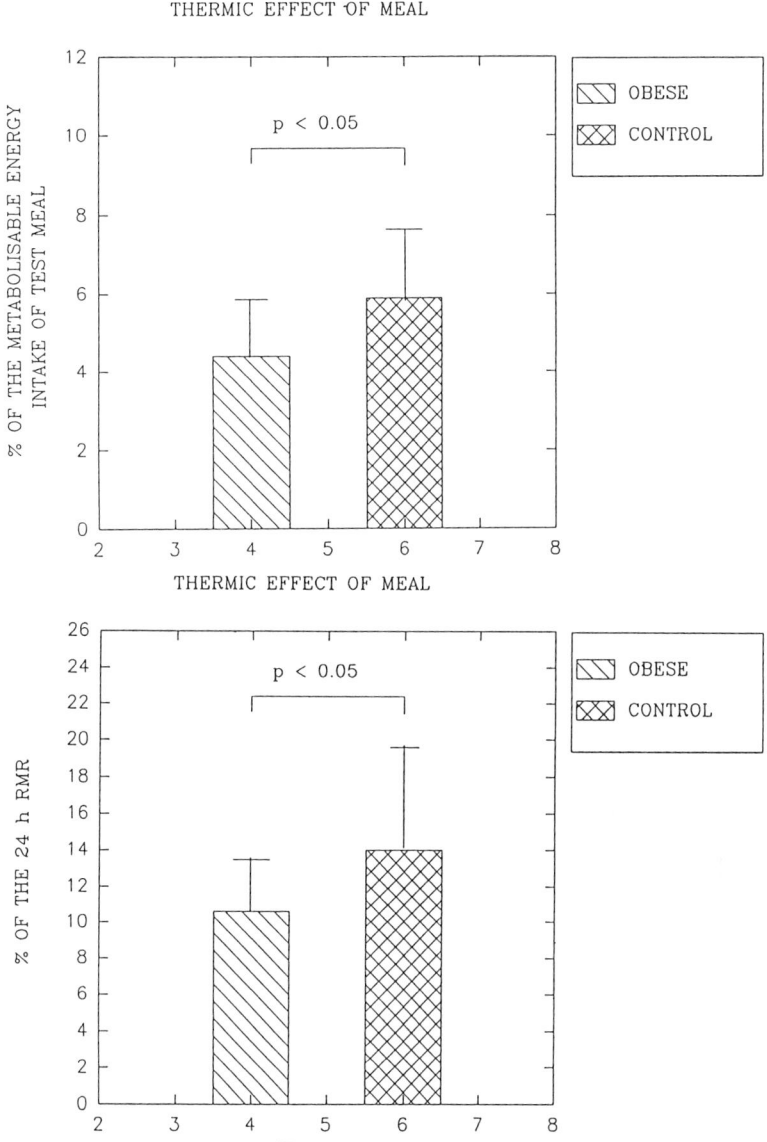

Fig. 1. Thermic effect of mixed meal ($\overline{X} \pm SD$)(expressed as a percentage of the metabolizable energy intake (upper graph) or as a percentage of the premeal RMR (lower graph) in obese and non-obese children.

thermogenesis. This confirms the observations made in some obese adults[1,6,7,8] but not in others[2] and suggests that the thermogenic defect encountered in adulthood may have already originated early in life. Whether or not the blunted TEM of the present obese children will still remain low at puberty and in the postpubertal phase up to adulthood remains the object of further prospective investigations.

The extent to which the energy saving by a reduction of TEM may contribute to body weight gain and eventually difficulties in achieving weight loss is questionable since the difference in postprandial thermogenesis (5.9 vs 4.4%) would constitute an energy saving of 150 kJ/d considering the level of energy intake observed in the present study. The real importance of the reduction of TEM on the energy balance should be evaluated together with the remaining components of the total energy expenditure, i.e. postabsorptive RMR and physical activity. In the present study the RMR, expressed in absolute value, was found to be higher in obese than in non-obese children. The extent to which the rate of physical activity is different in obese as compared to non-obese children cannot be evaluated from the present study.

In the present study the total energy intake of the obese group was 24 per cent greater than that of the non-obese children, whereas the preprandial RMR was 10 per cent more elevated and the average postprandial RMR was 6.7 per cent more elevated in obese than in non-obese children. It can be calculated that less than a quarter of the excess energy intake in the obese, as compared to the non-obese group, could be accounted for by the excess absolute RMR observed in the former group. The remaining part could be accounted for by the activity-related energy expenditure as well as the increased energy storage which must accompany the dynamic phase of obesity. From the present data it is virtually impossible to calculate the respective contribution of each of these two components to total energy expenditure. However, it is worth mentioning that when the ratio of total energy intake divided by RMR is calculated in each group, a higher value was found in the obese (1.99 x RMR) as compared to the control children (1.77 x RMR). Since for a given rate of physical activity the energy cost of exercise, expressed in absolute value, will be greater in the obese than in the non-obese children, it would be erroneous to conclude from this calculation that the rate of physical activity was similar in both groups.

Longitudinal studies in which daily food intake and total energy expenditure are accurately measured for prolonged period of time under various usual life situations are needed to throw more light on this issue. The use of either the doubly labelled water[4] and/or the heart rate methods[5] (the latter being particularly suited for studies in children) may provide more information on the total energy expenditure of obese children in free-living conditions.

Further studies in which the TEM is assessed in the same children before and after weight loss will indicate whether or not the blunted TEM observed in obese children is a primary pathogenic factor in child obesity rather than a secondary phenomenon favouring energy retention and body-weight gain.

Acknowledgements

We want to thank the children for their participation and we are indebted to the dietician, Mrs Rita Piccoli, who performed the dietetic history.

References

1. Bessard, T., Schutz, Y & Jéquier, E. (1983): Energy expenditure and postprandial thermogenesis in obese women before and after weight loss. *Am. J. Clin. Nutr.* **38**, 680-693.
2. Jéquier, E. (1974): Energy utilization in human obesity. *Ann. N. Y. Acad. Sci.* **499,** 73-78.
3. Jéquier, E., Acheson, K. & Schutz, Y. (1987): Assessment of energy expenditure and fuel utilization in man. *Ann. Rev. Nutr.* **7**, 187-208.
4. Schoeller, D.A. (1988): Measurement of energy expenditure in free-living humans by using doubly labelled water. *J. Nutr.* **118**, 1278-1289.
5. Schutz, Y. (1981): Use of non-calorimetric techniques to assess energy expenditure in man. In *Recent advances in obesity research: III*, eds. P. Björntorp, M. Cairella & A.N. Howard, pp. 153-158. London: John Libbey.
6. Schutz, Y., Bessard, T. & Jéquier, E. (1984): Diet-induced thermogenesis measured over a whole day in obese and non-obese women. *Am. J. Clin. Nutr.* **40**, 542-552.
7. Schutz, Y., Golay, A., Felber, J.P. & Jéquier, E. (1984): Decreased glucose-induced thermogenesis after weight loss in obese subjects: a predisposing factor to relapse of obesity? *Am. J. Clin. Nutr.* **39,** 380-387.
8. Shetty, P.S., Jung, R.T., James, W.P.T., Barrand, M.A. & Callingham, B.A. (1981): Postprandial thermogenesis in obesity. *Clin. Sci.* **60**, 519-525.

Chapter 58

Energy Expenditure Determines Weight Loss Independent of BMI, RMR, FFM or Nitrogen Conservation; a VLCD Study

A. COXON, S. KREITZMAN, P. JOHNSON and W. MORGAN
Howard Foundation Research and BSIA Ltd, Cambridge, England; Department of Medical Physics, Swansea University, Wales

Current obesity research focuses on resting metabolic rate (RMR) as a predictor of energy requirements, although the direct relationship to total energy expenditure in the free-living state has not been determined. The doubly labelled water technique was used to assess energy output in 11 female subjects with BMI range 22.2-42.4 dieting 11 weeks on VLCD with assessments of resting metabolic rate (RMR), and body composition by a variety of techniques including neutron activation. Weight losses were highly related to energy expenditure but not to RMR or lean body mass (FFM). The ratio of total energy expenditure to RMR was wider than that suggested by indirect estimates. Nitrogen conservation was demonstrated throughout the BMI range with this ketogenic VLCD, with no increase in nitrogen loss in those individuals with higher energy output or in those with a higher TEE/RMR ratio to justify recommendations for premature cessation of dieting or for a higher protein intake than 42 g in female dieters down to BMI 17.

Introduction

Research on energy requirements in man in the free-living state have been limited by techniques which involved predictions of resting metabolic rate from age/sex/BMI and estimates of additional output from broad description of activity. Measurements involving calorimetry in a closed environment inevitably impose restrictions on normal activity which influence the result. The advent of the doubly labelled water technique allows an accurate measurement of energy output in the normal environment[1]. This method was applied to 11 female subjects with a wide span of BMI over the first 6 weeks of an 11 week VLCD diet in which they continued their normal lives. The measurement of body composition change included neutron activation as a direct measure of total body nitrogen, to determine the relationship of protein change to energy expenditure. These findings have implications for those considering the recommendations for the composition and safety of VLCD.

Subjects and methods

Subjects

The subjects were female volunteers, aged 31.5–60.3 years (mean 46.5), BMI 22.2–43.2 (mean 32.1) at the start of the study, who were medically fit and gave informed consent to the protocol which was approved by the West Glamorgan District Ethical Committee.

Diet

All subjects were advised to remain weight stable for 3 months prior to the study. An initial period of food standardization with a formula 1600 kcal food diet containing 68 g protein for 10 days preceded measurements of body composition or energy expenditure. The VLCD was a liquid formula commercial preparation (Cambridge Diet Extra) containing 405 kcal, 42 g protein, 6.4 g nitrogen. Compliance was assured with weekly weight and urine ketone measurement.

Body composition

Body composition measurements were made at the start and end of the VLCD diet period using *in vivo* neutron activation analysis for total body nitrogen (TBN), tritiated water (total body water: TBW), dual X-ray absorptiometry (minerals) with ^{40}K at start and at day 5 (glycogen). These measures were selected to identify more accurately the components of lean body mass (FFM) change in individual subjects.

The measurement of TBN requires a knowledge of the subjects TBW. Each subject was fasted overnight but allowed a normal water intake until the start of the test. Blood and urine samples were taken immediately before an oral dose of 3.7 MBq tritiated water. The subject then had TBN measurement in which the prompt neutron gamma ray spectrum was recorded simultaneously as the patient was scanned over a vertically collumated neutron beam, with a radiation dose of 0.3 mSv. Further blood and urine samples were obtained at 4 and 5 h after the oral dose of tritiated water. The method has been validated by phantom studies and studies on normal volunteers[2]. The method achieves an accuracy and precision of ±5 per cent and ±2.5 per cent respectively.

Energy measurement

Resting metabolic rate

RMR was determined weekly in fully recumbent subjects resting for 20 min in a quiet darkened room at normal temperature. The measures used the Deltatrac ventilated hood, with 10 min readings after baseline values had been obtained. Test/retest accuracy of 25 kcal was observed.

24 h energy expenditure

Total free living energy expenditure was measured from the start of the VLCD diet period using water labelled with the stable isotopes deuterium and oxygen-18 (^{2}H$_2$ ^{18}O: doubly labelled water method: DLW). After an overnight fast urine samples were obtained from all subjects. The dose given was calculated from body weight, with 0.375 g/kg H$_2$ ^{18}O and 0.15 g/kg ^{2}H$_2$O, this dose being three times that normally used in studies of 21 days duration in normal adults. Urine samples were collected at 4 and 6 h after the dose to allow TBW measurement by ^{18}O and ^{2}H. Further urine samples were collected each morning for three days, on the seventh day, and then weekly to the end of the study. Hydrogen and oxygen isotope abundance was measured using a VG SIRA isotope ratio mass spectrometer. Duplicate urine samples were used for H/D determination by the method of Coleman, and ^{18}O/^{16}O ratios using a water/CO$_2$ calibration system. Both ratios were measured against the international standard SMOW using two different enriched standards for each ratio supplied by IAEA Vienna. For H/D analysis precision was 0.15 ppm at natural abundance and 0.40 ppm at high enrichment levels. For ^{18}O/^{16}O precision at natural abundance was 0.4 ppm and at high enrichment 2.4 ppm. Determination of TBW was by the Schoeller equation. Carbon dioxide production rates were calculated by the Lifson formula. Energy expenditure was calculated assuming a respiratory quotient for the diet of 0.85. Correction was made for water losses from a determination of TBW by bioelectrical impedance at weekly intervals. The calculation used is referred to as the "two-point method", and the measures were validated by the Dunn laboratory "multi-point method".

Results

Weight loss

A mean weight loss of 16.2 kg (SD 2.4) was achieved, final BMI 16.9–36. The weight was recorded separately at each body composition measure.

Body composition

Calculation of FFM was made from the measures obtained by:

1. assumption 33.1 gN/kg FFM

2. direct measure of the components of FFM by protein (TBN), water (TBW), minerals (DEXA), and glycogen (^{40}K).

Table 1. Body composition changes

	Initial BMI kg/m^2	Weight loss kg	TBN loss kg	FFM(1) loss kg	FFM(2) loss kg
	22.2	14.0	0.11	3.2	2.5
	25.8	13.0	0.12	3.6	2.5
	27.0	13.1	0.07	2.1	1.9
	30.6	17.3	0.18	5.6	5.5
	31.6	16.3	0.02	0.6	6.1
	32.7	16.0	0.12	3.6	1.7
	32.8	15.1	0.06	1.9	2.2
	34.4	15.9	0.20	5.9	2.2
	35.9	18.8	0.18	5.4	4.1
	36.7	20.4	0.18	5.5	6.4
	43.3	18.3	0.14	4.2	5.4
Mean	32.2	16.2	0.125	3.8	3.7
SD	5.8	2.4	0.057	1.7	1.8
% of weight loss		100	0.77*	23.5	22.8

*Mean loss of TBN 7.7 gN/kg wt loss.

The variation in calculation of FFM by the two methods in individuals is accounted for mainly by the hydration of FFM which varied between individuals but was not related to BMI. The mean measures showed close agreement, and confirmed nitrogen and FFM sparing with weight loss over 11 weeks on this ketogenic diet of 42 g protein/day.

Energy expenditure

The daily energy expenditure was determined at 6 weeks from the start of the study and validated by readings at weekly intervals from the start dose. Readings were stable for all subjects to week 5 and for eight subjects to week 6, after which enrichment levels gradually became insufficient for analysis.

The two point Schoeller analysis averaged 2424 kcal/day and the multipoint method of Coward 2393 kcal/day, r = 0.75. Analytical accuracy was assessed as 3 per cent for this study, within the range of the IDECG working group.

Table 2. Weight loss, BMI, RMR and 24 h EE

	BMI kg/m²	Wt loss kg	RMR wk 0 kcal	RMR wk 4 kcal	TEE wk 0 kcal	TEE wk 4 kcal	TEE/RMR wk 0	TEE/RMR wk 4
	22.1	13.5	1121	1011	1940	2182	1.82	2.36
	25.5	11.9	1371	1279	2462	2370	1.58	1.68
	26.3	13.3	1357	1159	2167	1978	1.58	1.39
	30.3	16.4	1303	1059	2240	1974	1.44	1.77
	31.9	17.9	1460	1310	3010	2647	1.82	2.09
	32.5	14.6	1429	1441	1809	2184	1.73	1.47
	32.5	14.0	1539	1149	2242	2678	1.41	1.81
	33.6	15.2	1251	1087	2078	1982	1.20	1.85
	35.3	19.5	1344	1331	2862	2985	2.07	2.22
	36.7	21.0	1409	1372	2874	2444	1.87	2.17
	42.8	18.0	1429	1262	2073	2496	1.73	2.04
Mean	31.8	15.9	1365	1223	2341	2356	1.66	1.90
SD	5.7	2.9	112	139	407	332	0.25	0.31

Resting metabolic rate (Table 2) showed the expected fall of 10.4 per cent in the first 2 weeks of diet, the values then remaining stable to the end of the study in spite of continued weight loss. Also as expected RMR showed close agreement with FFM (r = 0.81) (Table 4), but FFM could not be predicted from BMI (r = 0.31). Energy expenditure showed a wide variation (1809–3010 kcal/day) in individual subjects. The trend with diet varied, mean values remaining stable (Table 3). Energy expenditure was independent of RMR (r = 0.52), BMI (r = 0.42) and of FFM (r = 0.31), but was clearly related to weight loss (r = 0.82).

The ratio of RMR/TEE was higher than expected using the measured reduced values of RMR at week 4 of the diet (RMR/TEE 1.90) in this group of averagely unfit middle-aged women with active lifestyles but no formal fitness training (WHO predicted value TEE/RMR females 1.56–1.82)[3]. The variation in individual subjects was also more than expected, RMR/TEE 1.39–2.36.

Nitrogen conservation was demonstrated throughout the BMI range with no difference between the higher and lower BMI groups. There was also no increase in nitrogen loss associated with higher energy expenditure, or with higher TEE/RMR ratio, demonstrating the metabolic effectiveness of ketosis in protein conservation.

Table 3. 24 h energy expenditure during VLCD dieting

	Week 0–1	Week 0–2	Week 0–3	Week 0–4	Week 0–5	Week 0–6
Mean	2341.7	2265.7	2423.9	2379.8	2222.8	2282.5
SD	406.4	382.2	301.1	441.4	421.3	536.2
n	11	11	11	11	8	5

Table 4. Correlations of energy expenditure

r =	TEE	RMR	FFM
Weight loss	0.82	0.37	
RMR	0.52		
FFM	0.31	0.81	
BMI	0.42	0.47	0.37

Discussion

The results of this detailed study indicate that a ketogenic VLCD is associated with protein preservation during an 11 week period of weight loss across a wide range of BMI in dieting female subjects. Direct measurement of energy expenditure shows some higher values than obtained by prediction with no tendency to diminish with diet, unlike RMR which shows an initial decrease only. Nitrogen loss/kg wt. loss does not increase with the higher weight losses achieved by the more energetic individuals, indicating the efficiency of ketosis in protein sparing.

These findings are of relevance to those concerned with the adaptive physiology of body composition change with weight reduction[4]. Emphasis on the need for levels of protein intake in VLCD diet higher than 42 g/day are not justified by these data, and there is no difference demonstrable in the physiological adaptation of the relatively lean individual (down to BMI 16.9).

Equally these findings may not apply to diets with more than 4550 g carbohydrate in which sustained levels of ketosis may not be achieved[5].

References

1. Prentice, A.M. ed. (1990): The doubly-labelled water method for measuring energy expenditure. *Technical recommendations for use in humans*, Vienna: NAHRES-4 International Atomic agency.
2. Ryde, S.J.S., Morgan, W.D., Birks, J.L. *et al.* Total body nitrogen measurements in a normal population. *Clin. Physiol. Meas.* in press.
3. *Energy and protein requirements.* (1985): Report of a joint FAO/WHO/UNU expert consultation. Technical report series 724. Geneva: WHO.
4. *The use of very low calorie diets in obesity.* (1987): Report of the working group on VLCDs: Committee of Medical Aspects of Food Policy, Department of Health and Social Security: Report on health and social subjects 31. London: HMSO.
5. (1989): How ketones spare protein in starvation. *Nutr. Rev.* **3**, 80-81.
6. Diaz, E., Goldberg, G.R., Taylor, M., Savage, J.M., Sellen, D., Coward, W.A. & Prentice A.M. (1991): Effects of dietary supplementation on work performance in Gambian laborers. *Am. J. Clin. Nutr.* **53**, 803-811
7. Casper, R.C., Schoeller, D.A., Kushner, R., Hnilicka, J. & Gold, S.T. (1991): Total daily energy expenditure and activity level in anorexia nervosa. *Am. J. Clin. Nutr.* **53**, 1143-1150.

Chapter 59

Increased Energy Expenditure and Carbohydrate Oxidation in Post-obese Women on a High-carbohydrate Diet. Mediation by the Sympathetic Nervous System

A. ASTRUP[1], B. BUEMANN[1], N.J. CHRISTENSEN[2], J. MADSEN[3] and F. QUAADE[1]

[1]*Research Department of Human Nutrition, The Royal Veterinary and Agricultural University, 25 Rolighedsvej, 1958 Frederiksberg, Copenhagen;* [2]*Department of Internal Medicine and Endocrinology, Herlev Hospital, 2730 Herlev and* [3]*Institute of Medical Physiology C, 2200 N, University of Copenhagen, Denmark*

It has been shown that energy expenditure (EE) in post-obese individuals is more susceptible to the dietary ratio of carbohydrate to fat than in subjects without a predisposition to obesity. To study the mechanisms underlying the proposed enhancing effect of a high-carbohydrate/low-fat diet on EE, 24 h EE was measured in a respiratory chamber in weight-stable post-obese women and matched controls. They received a diet providing energy from 30 per cent fat, 55 per cent carbohydrate and 15 per cent protein and followed a fixed physical activity programme. Mean 24 h EE was higher in the post-obese women than in the controls (8292 *vs.* 7646 kJ/d, $P = 0.01$). The higher EE in the post-obese group was entirely covered by a 25 per cent higher carbohydrate oxidation ($P = 0.035$). Plasma concentrations of noradrenaline were greater by 50 per cent in the post-obese than in the controls ($P = 0.04$). Most of the variance (55 per cent) in 24 h EE was accounted for by group membership (post-obese *vs.* control), but when plasma levels of catecholamines were included in the analysis, noradrenaline replaced group membership and accounted for 65 per cent of the variance in 24 h EE. 24 h heart rate measured continuously by telemetry was also higher in the post-obese group than in the control group (74 bpm *vs.* 67 bpm, $P < 0.03$), and the entire group difference could be accounted for by differences in plasma noradrenaline concentrations.

We conclude that in post-obese women a high-carbohydrate/low-fat diet induces SNS hyperactivity, which is responsible for the higher levels of 24-h EE, carbohydrate oxidation and heart rate.

Introduction

There is evidence to suggest that a low energy expenditure (EE) is a risk factor for obesity. The literature on post-obese subjects is, however, conflicting, with reports of both lower[2] and normal[3-6] levels of 24 h EE in post-obese subjects (Table 1). Lean and James found that EE in post-obese women was highly susceptible to the dietary ratio of carbohydrate (CHO) to fat, and that a high dietary CHO/fat ratio increased 24 h EE above that of the matched controls[4,5]. By contrast, a diet providing a low CHO/fat ratio suppressed 24 h EE below the levels of the control group. This paper studies the mechanisms underlying the proposed enhancing effect of a high-carbohydrate/low-fat diet on 24 h EE in weight-stable post-obese women and matched controls.

Table 1. Studies on 24 h energy expenditure in post-obese subjects

Authors and reference	Diet	Body weight matching post-obese–controls (kg)	24 h deviation from controls (%)	
Geissler et al. 1987[2]	?	−1	−15	
Lean & James 1988[4,5]	High CHO	+11	+3	
Lean & James 1988[4,5]	Low CHO	+11	−3	
Goldberg et al. 1990[3]	?	+6	0	(ns)
McNeill et al. 1990[6]	?	−1	−7	(ns)

Subjects and methods

Eight post-obese women who had been weight stable for 7-25 weeks, and eight controls, matched with respect to age, height, weight and body composition, were studied in their follicular menstrual phase. The post-obese women had on an average lost about 20 kg on a conventional 4.2 MJ/d low-fat diet as outpatients at the Department. They maintained a high-carbohydrate/low-fat diet in the weight stabilization period. Body composition was estimated by the bio-impedance method. Twenty-four hour energy expenditure was measured in our two closed-circuit indirect calorimetry chambers[1] on a fixed physical programme and on a diet providing energy from 30 per cent fat, 55 per cent carbohydrate and 15 per cent protein. Heart rate and ECG were continuously monitored by a telemetry system (Dialogue 2000, Danica Electr., Denmark). After the stay in the respiratory chambers, venous blood samples were taken before, and 25 and 50 min after, a carbohydrate-rich breakfast.

Results

Mean 24-h EE was higher in the post-obese women than in the controls (8292 vs. 7646 kJ/d, $P = 0.01$), and the difference was mainly due to a higher day-time EE. The higher EE in the post-obese group was entirely covered by carbohydrate oxidation, which was about 25 per cent higher than in the control group ($P = 0.035$). By contrast the lipid and protein oxidation rates were similar in the post-obese and controls. Fasting and postprandial venous plasma concentrations of noradrenaline were greater by 50 per cent in the post-obese than in the controls ($P = 0.004$). Most of the variance (55 per cent) in 24 h EE was accounted for by group membership (post-obese vs. control), whereas a further 24 per cent was explained by differences in fat-free mass. When plasma levels of catecholamines were included in the analysis, noradrenaline replaced group membership and accounted for 65 per cent of the variance in 24 h EE. Twenty-four hour heart rate measured continuously by telemetry was also higher in the post-obese group than in the control group (74 bpm vs. 67 bpm, $P < 0.03$). Most of the variance (74 per cent) in heart rate, and the group difference, could be accounted for by differences in plasma noradrenaline concentration.

Discussion

The present results confirm those of Lean and James[4,5], who reported that a high-carbohydrate/low-fat diet in post-obese subjects increased 24 h EE above that of the control group. We further show that the increased EE was entirely covered by an increased carbohydrate oxidation, and that both these increases in the post-obese group were mediated by a SNS hyperactivity, as indicated by higher levels of plasma noradrenaline and mean 24 h heart rate. The data suggest that constitutional abnormalities in the regulation of sympathetic activity in the post-obese group make them highly sensitive to the dietary composition. Lean and James found that a low-carbohydrate/high-fat diet reduced 24 h EE in post-obese women below that of a control group, which is conceivably brought about by a suppression of SNS activity.

Our finding that the post-obese group had a 45 g/day higher carbohydrate oxidation than the control group may be central for their predisposition to obesity. Recent evidence shows that carbohydrate and fat balance are regulated separately, and that carbohydrate balance has priority over fat balance. According to the glucostatic concept of regulation of food intake, energy intake could be regulated by the rate of carbohydrate utilization and a minimal amount of carbohydrates must be ingested to maintain carbohydrate stores[7]. Consequently, ingesting a high-fat diet may, in these subjects, exert an enhancing effect on spontaneous energy intake. This hypothesis is supported by the study by Zurlo et al.[8] who found that the ratio of carbohydrate to fat oxidation was a familial trait, and that a high ratio predicted subsequent weight gain independently of EE. We conclude that post-obese women on a high-carbohydrate/low-fat diet have an enhanced sympathetic nervous system activity, which is responsible for the higher levels of 24 h EE, carbohydrate oxidation and heart rate. In post-obese women SNS activity and EE are highly susceptible to dietary composition, findings which may have implications for both the aetiology and the dietary treatment of obesity.

Acknowledgement

The work was supported by the Danish Medical Research Council (12-9537).

References

1. Astrup, A., Thorbek, G., Lind, J. & Isaksson, B. (1990): Prediction of 24-h energy expenditure and its components from physical characteristics and body composition in normal-weight humans. *Am. J. Clin. Nutr.* **52**, 777-783.
2. Geissler, C.A., Miller, D.S. & Shah M. (1987): The daily metabolic rate of the post-obese and the lean. *Am. J. Clin. Nutr.* **45**, 14-20.
3. Goldberg, G.R., Black, A.E., Prentice, A.M. & Coward, W.A. (1990): No evidence of lower energy expenditure in post-obese women. *Proc. Nutr. Soc.* **50**, 2A.
4. Lean, M.E.J. (1988): Current status of research: why do people get fat? In *Obesity – current approaches*, eds. W.P.T. James, S.W. Parker, pp. 1-12. Southampton: Duphar Medical Relations.
5. Lean, M.E.J. & James, W.P.T. (1988): Metabolic effects of isoenergetic nutrient exchange over 24 hours in relation to obesity in women. *Int. J. Obes.* **12**, 15-27.
6. McNeill, G., Bukkens, S.G.F., Morrison, D.C. & Smith, J.S. (1990): Energy intake and energy expenditure in post-obese women and weight-matched controls. *Proc. Nutr. Soc.* **49**, 14A.
7. Tremblay, A., Lavallée, N., Almeras, N., Allard, L., Despres J.-P. & Bouchard, C. (1991): Nutritional determinants of the increase in energy intake associated with a high-fat diet. *Am. J. Clin. Nutr.* **53**, 1134-1137.
8. Zurlo, F., Lillioja, S., Puente, A.E.-D., et al. (1990): Low ratio of fat to carbohydrate oxidation as predictor of weight gain: study of 24-h RQ. *Am. J. Physiol.* **259**, E650-657.

Chapter 60

Are Sex Hormones Involved in Resting Metabolic Rate and Glucose-induced Thermogenesis?

A Study in Obese Men and Women

Greet VANSANT, Luc Van GAAL and Ivo De LEEUW
University of Antwerp, Department of Endocrinology, Metabolism and Clinical Nutrition, Universiteitsplein 1, B-2610 Wilrijk-Antwerp, Belgium

The role of sex hormones in the control of energy expenditure in humans in still unclear. In this study, the impact of androgens and oestrogens on resting metabolic rate and glucose-induced thermogenesis was investigated in obese men and women. The results indicate that androgens only play a minor role in energy expenditure in humans. The importance of oestradiol needs further investigation.

Introduction

The role of sex hormones in the control of energy expenditure in humans is still unclear. In rats, it was suggested that oestradiol can influence energy expenditure[4]. In women, Contaldo observed a lower thermogenesis after ovariectomy[1]. Results of studies on the influence of the menstrual cycle show contradictory results. Webb found an increase of 9 per cent for 24 h energy expenditure during the luteal phase[5]. Weststrate did not observe any difference for both resting metabolic rate (RMR) and diet-induced thermogenesis during the cycle[6]. The influence of androgens on energy expenditure is still unknown.

This study was designed to investigate whether androgens and oestradiol may influence RMR and glucose induced thermogenesis (GIT) in obese men and women.

Patients and methods

In a first part (protocol 1), nine men and 13 women were selected in order to compare RMR, GIT and substrate oxidation rates in two groups with comparable age and BMI but with completely different androgen levels. None of the patients were taking any medication. Characteristics are given in Table 1.

In a second study 22 men and 29 women were selected of which BMI and age were comparable. All women were in the follicular phase of their menstrual cycle, according to plasma progesterone values.

Table 1. Patient characteristics: protocol 1

	Men	Women	P
n	9	13	
Age, years	40 ± 10	37 ± 7	ns
BMI, kg/m^2	37.5 ± 4.3	37.2 ± 6.2	ns
FFM, kg	68.7 ± 4.8	46.4 ± 5.5	0.0001
FM, %	43.1 ± 5.2	50.8 ± 6.8	0.007
Testosterone, nmol/l	16 ± 6	3 ± 2	0.0001
SHBG, nmol/l	41 ± 59	40 ± 48	ns
FTI	79 ± 51	10 ± 7	0.02

FFM = fat free mass; FM = fat mass; SHBG = sex hormone binding globuline; FTI = free testosterone index.

Table 2. Patient characteristics: protocol 2

	Men	Women
n	22	29
Age, years	39 ± 10	33 ± 9
BMI, kg/m^2	34.7 ± 4.2	36.1 ± 4.8
FFM, kg	66.6 ± 6.8	47.1 ± 5.8
FM, %	37.9 ± 7.3	50.0 ± 4.6
Testosterone, nmol/l	19 ± 7	3 ± 2
SHBG, nmol/l	19 ± 8	26 ± 11
FTI	112 ± 54	16 ± 17
Oestradiol, pg/ml	30 ± 6	57 ± 47

Hormone concentrations were all measured at the routine laboratory of the University Hospital, Antwerp. Resting metabolic rate and thermogenic response after ingestion of 100 g glucose were measured by continuous indirect calorimetry. Body composition was determined by bioelectrical impedance. Substrate oxidation rates were calculated with the Lusk formulas[3].

Results

Results of these studies are given in Tables 3 and 4.

In study 1, RMR was significantly higher for men (5.63 ± 0.80 kJ/min) in comparison with women (4.01 ± 0.59 kJ/min). However, after correction for fat-free mass, this difference disappeared. No differences were found for thermogenesis. Substrate oxidation rates, both basal and postprandial, were identical in the two groups.

In study 2, Pearson correlation coefficients were calculated and indicate that, both for men and women, total and free testosterone levels were not related to the measured indices of energy metabolism. Also no relationship was found with the binding protein (SHBG). Oestradiol was significantly related to RMR (r = 0.48; $P < 0.01$) and GIT (r = 0.38; $P < 0.05$) in men. For women, no relationship was found with GIT, while RMR was negatively related to oestradiol (r = –0.37; $P < 0.05$).

Chapter 60 – Are Sex Hormones Involved in Resting Metabolic Rate

Table 3. Energy expenditure and substrate oxidation rates in obese men and women: protocol 1

	Men	Women	P
RMR, kJ/min	5.63 ± 0.80	4.01 ± 0.59	0.0001
RMR/kg FFM, kJ/kg.min	0.08 ± 0.01	0.09 ± 0.01	ns
GIT 1st hour, kJ/min	0.54 ± 0.22	0.51 ± 0.39	ns
GIT 2nd hour, kJ/min	0.57 ± 0.44	0.51 ± 0.28	ns
GIT 3rd hour, kJ/min	0.19 ± 0.24	0.19 ± 0.18	ns
GIT, % above RMR	7.80 ± 4.47	10.45 ± 6.29	ns
GIT, % ME	4.64 ± 2.54	4.38 ± 2.53	ns
RQ basal	0.80 ± 0.04	0.80 ± 0.06	ns
RQ git	0.85 ± 0.04	0.88 ± 0.05	ns
Protein oxidation RMR, %	21 ± 3	22 ± 9	ns
Fat oxidation RMR, %	54 ± 13	53 ± 24	ns
CHO oxidation RMR, %	26 ± 13	28 ± 19	ns
Protein oxidation GIT, %	20 ± 5	20 ± 12	ns
Fat oxidation GIT, %	32 ± 17	28 ± 15	ns
CHO oxidation GIT, %	48 ± 13	52 ± 15	ns

RMR = resting metabolic rate; GIT = glucose-induced thermogenesis; RQ = respiratory quotient; %ME = % of ingested calories; CHO = carbohydrates.

Table 4. Correlation coefficients between parameters of energy expenditure and sex hormones in obese men (n = 22) and obese women (n = 29)

	RMR	RMR/FFM	GIT (%ME)	RQ basal	RQ git
Men					
Testosterone	−0.05	−0.03	0.08	−0.27	−0.03
SHBG	−0.22	−0.19	−0.29	−0.13	−0.06
FTI	0.15	0.08	0.27	−0.07	0.21
Oestradiol	0.48**	0.41*	0.38*	−0.09	0.01
Women					
Testosterone	−0.05	−0.02	−0.05	−0.15	−0.32*
SHBG	0.02	0.04	−0.14	0.19	−0.20
FTI	−0.06	0.02	−0.09	−0.05	0.06
Oestradiol	−0.37*	−0.47*	0.09	−0.27	−0.15

* $P < 0.05$; ** $P < 0.01$.

Discussion

The first study shows that there is no difference between men and women for the measured parameters of energy expenditure. These results already suggest that the role of androgens as a determinant of energy expenditure is limited. This was confirmed in the second part of the study. Oestradiol however, seems to be involved both in obese men and women. A positive relationship was found for men. These results were comparable with those observed previously in rats[4]. The mechanism behind them is not clear. In rats, oestradiol can influence both energy uptake and expenditure. It may be possible that the brown adipose tissue plays a role. The importance for men is not clear[2]. Another possible explanation could be that oestradiol influences the activity of the lipoprotein lipase[4]. For women, an inverse relationship was observed between EE and oestradiol levels confirming the data of Contaldo[1]. He showed an increase in RMR after ovariectomy and suggested that the fat-free mass (FFM) may play a role. After correction for FFM, in our study the relationship still exists. Most probably, there are still other factors which are important. These results indicate that androgens only play a minor role in energy expenditure in humans. The role of oestradiol needs further investigation.

References

1. Contaldo, F., Scalfi, L., Coltorti, A., Di Palo, M.R., Martinelli, P. & Guerritore, T. (1987): Reduced regulatory thermogenesis in pregnant and ovariectomized women. *Int. J. Vitam. Nutr. Res.* **57**, 299-304.
2. Jéquier, E. (1987): Energy utilization in human obesity. *Ann. NY Acad. Sci.* **499**, 73-83.
3. Lusk, G. (1924): Animal calorimetry: analysis of the oxidation of mixtures of carbohydrate and fat. *J. Biol. Chem.* **59**, 41-42.
4. Wade, G.N. (1986): Sex steroids and energy balance: sites and mechanisms of action. *Ann. NY Acad. Sci.* **474**, 389-399.
5. Webb, P. (1986): 24-hour energy expenditure and the menstrual cycle. *Am. J. Clin. Nutr.* **44**, 614-619.
6. Weststrate, J. (1989): Resting metabolic rate and diet-induced thermogenesis. PhD thesis, Wageningen.

Section X
Cellular and molecular biology in the analysis of obesity

Chapter 61

Cellular and Molecular Biology in the Analysis of Obesity

Daniel RICQUIER
Centre de Recherche sur l'Endocrinologie Moléculaire et le Développement, CNRS-UPR 1511, 9 rue Jules Hetzel, 92190 Meudon, France

Introduction

Obesity is a disease that arises through an increased number of adipocytes and an excessive lipid accumulation. Intensive studies of adipocyte biochemistry over the past 20 years have revealed much about the hormonal control of carbohydrate and lipid metabolism. In other fields intensive research was also done on the isolation of fibroblastic clones capable of adipocyte differentiation. Important information on the mechanism of differentiation of adipocytes came out from studies on preadipocyte cell-lines[1]. However the molecular basis of obesity aetiology remains poorly understood. More recently, the revolution in molecular biology has brought new opportunities and a stimulating challenge for metabolic research[3,4].

Contribution of cellular and molecular biology

Outstanding advances have been made in culturing the cells of vertebrates. The use of cell cultures has greatly unified experimental studies on one particular type of cells. What is referred to now as "molecular biology" offers the immense advantage of unifying areas of biological research that were traditionally separated such as cell biology, biochemistry, genetics, immunology and physiology (endocrinology and neurobiology)[5]. Consequently, all researchers interested in biological research can share a unitary language and a unified approach. With the tools of molecular biology, genes or cDNAs of all types of proteins can be isolated, sequenced, modified, deleted, and reintroduced in various types of cells including germ lines of organisms[5].

Generally the molecular biology approach was used to clone known proteins of interest. The obtention of a cDNA then allows researchers to (i) determine the primary structure of the protein and predict a functional organization, (ii) assay the corresponding mRNA level and the transcriptional activity of the gene and (iii) map and isolate the gene. This, in turn, permits the investigation of the *cis* and *trans* regulatory factors that govern the (tissue-specific or not) expression of the gene. In other respects, the differential screening of cDNA libraries, reverse genetics, transformation of cells by viruses, transfection of cells with genomic DNA, use of antibodies etc... led to cloning and discovery of unknown proteins playing a key role in differentiation, development or pathology.

To date, research in molecular biology has focused on the characterization of specific genes and on the processes which alter their expression. Many genes have been sequenced, their regulatory regions delineated and various mutations involved in disease processes have been described. More recently, several genes of metabolic interest have been cloned and among them are genes of which the activity is relevant to adipocytes and to lipid metabolism, and presumably to obesity.

Isolation of genes of metabolic interest

Table 1 is a non-exhaustive list of enzymes and components of metabolic interest that have been cloned as cDNA and/or genes. In fact it appears that within a short period of time, thanks to molecular cloning, scientists and clinical investigators have acquired a large number of tools. Many enzymes of the lipid and carbohydrate metabolism were cloned. Several proteins associated with adipocyte differentiation were also cloned. In addition, several regulatory proteins such as receptors for neurotransmitters and hormones and such proteins as glucose transporters were cloned.

Table 1. Cloned cDNAS or genes of potential interest for obesity research*

Enzymes of lipid metabolism	Other proteins
FA synthetase, Acyl CoA synthetase	Adipsin, aP2, pOB24, AP27, S14, C/EBP
αGPDH, ME, PEPCK	Enzyme of glycolysis, glucokinase, hexokinase
Acetyl CoA carboxylase	Cytochrome oxydase and ATPase subunits
LP lipase, HS lipase	UCP, PDH
HMG-CoA reductase	Perilipin
Receptors & related proteins	**Transporters**
Insulin, IGF1, GH	CPT
T_3, T_4-steroid hormones	Glut1–5
Catecholamines ($\alpha_{1,2}$-$\beta_{1,2,3,4}$?)	(Glut4: regulated by insulin in adipose and
Dopamine, acetylcholine	muscle cells)
LDL	
Adenyl cyclase, G proteins	

abbreviations used are:
FA = fatty acid; CoA = coenzyme A; GPDH = glycerol-phosphate-dehydrogenase; ME = malic enzyme; PEPCK = phosphoenolpyruvate carboxykinase; LP = lipoprotein; HS = hormone-sensitive; HMG = hydroxymethyl-glutaryl; IGF = insulin-like growth factor; GH = growth hormone; LDL = low-density lipoprotein; UCP = uncoupling protein; PDH = pyruvate dehydrogenase; CPT = carnitine-palmitoyl transferase.

Molecular studies on genes specifically expressed in adipocytes

Several laboratories have developed studies of regulation of genes of metabolic interest such as PEPCK, αGPDH, GAPDH and glucokinase. A small number of groups have concentrated their activity on genes that are uniquely expressed in differentiating adipocytes and especially on adipsin and aP2 genes.

The adipsin gene is an adipocyte-specific serine protease which has complement factor D activity[11]. Spiegelman and his colleagues have investigated the molecular regulation of this gene by transfection of adipsin gene constructs containing a marker gene into cultured adipocytes and also by the creation of transgenic animals. They demonstrated that sequences conferring the adipocyte-specificity of adipsin gene are contained between –114 and +35 relative to the start of transcription. Moreover, genomic elements that respond to the *db* gene lie between –950 and –114. These data indicate that 950 bases of the 5′-flanking region of the adipsin gene carry information that specifies both expression in adipose cells and a response to a signal or a gene that induces obesity[10].

The aP2 gene encodes a protein which is a homologue of myelin P2 protein and which is also partially homologous to several members of family of intracellular lipid carrier proteins. The aP2 gene is strongly expressed during adipocyte differentiation[11]. It was demonstrated that both adipsin and aP2 gene contain two elements that were termed "fat-specific elements" or FSE1 and FSE2[9]. Moreover Spiegelman and his colleagues demonstrated that the FSE2 element functions as a negative regulator in preadipocytes and is recognized by a *trans*-acting factor. Then the same group demonstrated that the FSE2 element was a target sequence for the binding of a protein complex containing the product of the c-*fos* proto-oncogene[6]. More recently it was shown that aP2 gene contains AP-1 and C/EBP binding sites[8] as well as an enhancer at −5.4 kb that functions in a differentiation-dependent fashion[7]. Thus, molecular studies on the regulation of at least one gene specifically expressed during adipocyte differentiation is highly advanced.

Prospects and perspectives of research

It may be anticipated that the use of molecular genetics and modern cellular biology will contribute to significant progress in the understanding of fundamental mechanisms that control adipose tissue growth and energetic metabolism. The future lines of research will concern (i) the genetic mechanisms that force a fibroblast-like cell to be committed as a preadipocyte, (ii) the characterization of endocrine or autocrine factors controlling the growth of adipose cells, (iii) the molecular mechanisms of insulin-resistance, (iv) the mapping of DNA segments associated with obesity syndrome in rodents and humans. Interestingly, Bell and his associates have just recently reported that a gene for non-insulin dependent diabetes mellitus is linked to DNA polymorphism on human chromosome 20q[2]. In other respects, one must not forget that significant progress in obesity research will also probably result from advances in neurobiology since it is obvious that most processes of energy storage and energy expenditure are regulated by the nervous system.

References

1. Ailhaud, G. (1990): Extracellular factors, signalling pathways and differentiation of adipose precursor cells. *Cur. Opin. Cell Biol.* **2**, 1043-1049.
2. Bell, G.I., Xiang, K.S., Newman, M.V., Wu, S.H., Wright, L.G., Fajans, S.S., Spielman, R.S. & Cox, N.J. (1991): Gene for non-insulin-dependent diabetes mellitus (maturity-onset diabetes of the young subtype) is linked to DNA polymorphism on human chromosome 20q. *Proc. Natl. Acad. Sci. USA* **88**, 1484-1488.
3. Bray, G., Ricquier, D. & Spiegelman, B. (1990): *Obesity: towards a molecular approach.* New York: Wiley-Liss.
4. Cushman, S., Londos, C., Manganiello, V. & Smith, U. (1991): *The adipose cell: a model for integration of hormone signalling in the regulation of cellular function.* New York: Wiley-Liss.
5. Darnell, J., Lodish, H. & Baltimore, D. (1986): *Molecular cell biology.* New York: Scientific American Books.
6. Distel, R.J., Ro, H.S., Rosen, B.S., Groves, D.L. & Spiegelman, B.M. (1987): Nucleoprotein complexes that regulate gene expression in adipocyte differentiation: direct participation of c-*fos*. *Cell* **49**, 835-844.
7. Graves, R.A., Tontonoz, P., Ross, S. & Spiegelman, B.M. (1991): Identification of a potent adipocyte-specific enhancer: involvement of an NF-1-like factor. *Genes Dev.* **5**, 428-437.
8 Herrera, R., Ro, H.S., Robinson, G.S., Xanthopoulos, K.G. & Spiegelman, B.M. (1989): A direct role for C/EBP and the AP-1-binding site in gene expression linked to adipocyte differentiation. *Mol. Cell Biol.* **9**, 5331-5339.
9. Hunt, C.R., Ro, J.H., Dobson, D., Min, H.Y. & Spiegelman, B.M. (1986): Adipocyte P2: developmental expression and homology of 5′-flanking sequences among fat cell-specific genes. *Proc. Natl. Acad. Sci. USA.* **83**, 3786-3790.
10. Platt, K.A., Min, H.Y., Ross, S.R. & Spiegelman, B.M. (1989): Obesity linked regulation of the adipsin gene promoter in transgenic mice. *Proc. Natl. Acad. Sci. USA* **86**, 7490-7494.
11. Spiegelman, B.M., Distel, R.J., Ro, H.S., Rosen, B. & Satterberg, B. (1988): *fos*-Protooncogene and the regulation of gene expression in adipocyte differentiation. *J. Cell Biol.* **107**, 829-832.

Chapter 62

Identification of a Marker of the Preadipose State as a Component of the Extracellular Matrix

Azeddine IBRAHIMI, Sylvie BARDON*, Bénédicte BERTRAND, Gérard AILHAUD and Christian DANI

Centre de Biochimie du CNRS (UMR 134), Université de Nice-Sophia Antipolis, UFR Sciences, Parc Valrose, 06108 Nice Cédex 2, France

We have previously described the molecular cloning of a cDNA probe which detects a 6 kb mRNA termed pOb24. pOb24 mRNA appeared to be a marker of adipose cell commitment both *in vitro* and *in vivo*. To isolate the full length pOb24 cDNA and identify the corresponding protein, a pOb24 genomic fragment was used to screen a cDNA library constructed from mRNA of preadipose Ob1771 cells. The screening yielded a new cDNA clone which detected a 3.7 kb mRNA species in addition to the 6 kb mRNA species. Both the 3.7 kb and 6 kb species emerged in parallel, increased sharply in early differentiating Ob1771 adipose cells and decreased thereafter. Tissue distribution studies showed high levels of expression in white adipose tissues, ovaries and adrenal glands and low levels of expression in brain, heart and kidney, whereas no expression was detected in liver and skeletal muscle of adult mice. From the complete nucleotide sequence of the 3.7 kb mRNA, the encoded protein showed strong similarities with the α2 chain of the human type VI collagen.

The role of collagen VI in the adipose differentiation process remains presently unknown but the binding properties of this protein may shed some light on the events required for terminal differentiation.

Introduction

The understanding of the mechanisms underlying adipose cell differentiation requires the characterization of proteins which emerge early during adipose cell commitment. We have previously described the molecular cloning, by differential screening, of a cDNA probe which detects a 6 kb mRNA named pOb24. This mRNA rose sharply in early differentiating Ob1771 adipose cells and decreased rapidly at a time when mRNAs encoding for terminal differentiation markers, such as glycerol-3-phosphate dehydrogenase (GPDH) and adipsin, were still increasing. In post-natal mice, pOb24 mRNA appeared to be preferentially expressed in non-terminally differentiated adipose cells[9]. Thus pOb24 mRNA appeared to be an early marker of adipose cell differentiation both *in vitro* and *in vivo*. The induction of pOb24 gene in confluent Ob1771 cells did not require adipogenic hormones. In contrast, growth arrest at the G_1/S boundary of the cell-cycle was sufficient to induce pOb24 gene transcription[1,9]. The pOb24 gene was regulated in a differentiation-dependent manner by the tumour necrosis factor-α (TNF-α) and the transforming growth factor-β (TGF-β). TNF-α and TGF-β decreased the pOb24 mRNA level in early differentiating Ob1771 cells, at a time when these two cytokines inhibit adipose differentiation. In contrast when terminal differentiation was underway, TNF-α and TGF-β had no effect on pOb24 gene expression[9,10]. Altogether, these results indicate that the pOb24 gene product may play an important role in the process of adipose cell differentiation.

In the present study, the molecular cloning and the identification of a pOb24-related peptide is described.

Methods

Construction and screening of genomic and cDNA libraries

A genomic library, containing inserts of approximately 20 kb from MboI partial digests of L929 DNA, constructed in the λEMBL3 cloning vector, was screened by *in situ* hybridization technique according to Benton and Davis[3]. Two positive clones from approximately 5×10^6 clones were identified by probing with the 0.35 kb HinfI-BglII fragment of pOb24 cDNA and were shown to be identical by restriction analysis; this clone was designated λg8. Phage DNA was prepared and a 2 kbp EcoR1-BglII fragment was subcloned into the pSP72 vector.

A cDNA library was prepared in the λgt10 vector. For that purpose mRNAs were prepared from 4-day post-confluent differentiating Ob1771 cells. Double-stranded cDNAs were synthesized as previously described[9]. cDNAs were methylated, ligated with EcoRl linker, cleaved with EcoR1 and subsequently ligated to EcoR1-digested, phosphatase-treated λgt10 vector DNA according to the instructions of the manufacturer (Amersham) and packaged *in vitro*. This library containing about 5×10^5–10^6 independent clones was screened using the 2.0 kb EcoR1-BglII insert of cloned genomic DNA fragment.

Ten positive clones were purified. Two non-overlapping inserts of 3.0 kbp and 1.7 kbp were subcloned into PUC18 plasmid and designated CPU18-11 and CPU18-7, respectively.

DNA sequencing and analysis

Genomic and cDNA fragments, generated by digestion with various restriction enzymes, were ligated to PUC18 and pSP72 plasmids.

Denaturated recombinant plasmid DNAs were sequenced by the dideoxy chain-termination method and the use of modified T7 DNA polymerase. Some specific oligonucleotide primers were synthesized to obtain sequences from both strands. Sequence data were decoded and examined using BISANCE sequence analysis programs (CITI 2, Paris). Nucleotide sequence and deduced amino-acid sequence of the C3-PU18-11 clone was made and homology searches in protein data bank NBRF were performed using the algorithm and programme of Pearson and Lipman[16].

Isolation and analysis of RNA and DNA

RNA was isolated from Ob1771 cells and tissues of C57 BL/6J mice, and was analysed as previously described[9]. Phage DNAs and plasmid DNAs were prepared as described in[11] and [14], respectively.

Results and discussion

Characterization of two pOb24 mRNAs

The characterization of the protein encoded by the pOb24 mRNA requires the cloning of a full-length cDNA. For that purpose, a 2 kbp EcoR1-BglII pOb24 genomic fragment was used to screen a λgt10 cDNA library constructed with mRNAs from differentiating Ob1771 preadipocytes.

Among the clones isolated, one clone, named C3-PU18-7, was shown to contain an insert of 1.7 kb in length. When used in Northern blot analysis, C3-PU18-7 cDNA revealed only the 6 kb pOb24 mRNA. Another clone, named C3-PU18-11, was found to contain a 3 kbp insert

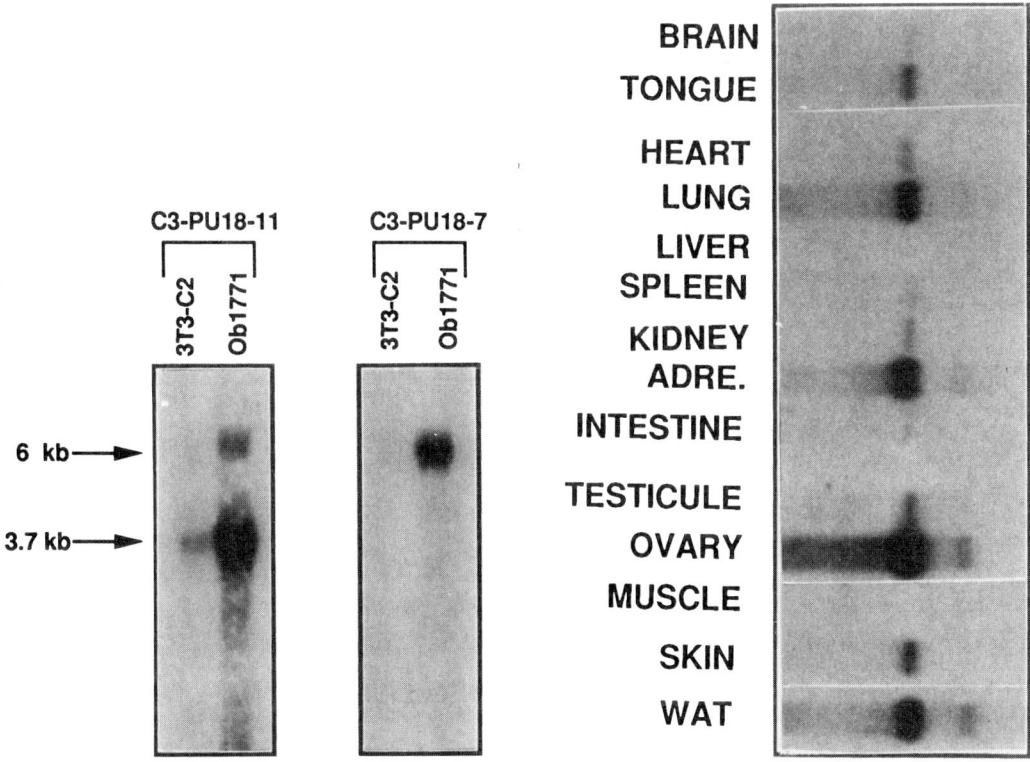

Fig. 1 (left). Expression of the 6 kb and 3.7 kb mRNAs in preadipose and non-preadipose cells. Three micrograms of oligo(dT)⁻ purified mRNAs from 3T3-C2 fibroblasts and Ob1771 preadipocyte cells were electrophoresed and blotted onto Hybond-N Amersham membranes. Filters were separately hybridized with C3-PU18-11 and C3-PU18-7 cDNAs. The size of the mRNA bands were determined from standards of ribosomal RNAs and 0.24–9.5 kb RNA ladder (Gibco/BRL, France).

Fig. 2 (right). Expression of the 3.7 kb and 6 kb mRNAs in various mouse tissues. Twenty micrograms of total RNA from each tissue of 4-month-old mice were analysed as described in Fig. 1.

which revealed two species of mRNA in Ob1771 differentiated cells, 3.7 kb and 6 kb mRNAs (Fig. 1).

Sequences of the 3' ends of the two cDNA inserts indicated that both 3.7 kb and 6 kb mRNAs were polyadenylated. In order to understand how the two mRNAs were generated we compared the sequences of the two cDNAs with that of the genomic fragment in addition to RNA mapping by RNAse protection analysis. Altogether the results indicated that alternative polyadenylation sites and alternative splicing were involved to generate both mRNA species (not shown).

Expression of the 3.7 kb and 6 kb mRNA species during differentiation of Ob1771 cells and in various mouse tissues

As previously shown for the 6 kb pOb24 mRNA[9,10], the 3.7 kb mRNA was preferentially expressed in Ob1771 preadipose cells than in 3T3-C2 non-preadipose cells (Fig. 1). This result suggested that the expression of the 3.7 kb mRNA was regulated in a differentiation-dependent manner. In agreement with this hypothesis, the emergence of the 3.7kb mRNA was examined during differentiation of Ob1771 cells and compared with that of pOb24 and adipsin mRNAs. In a separate experiment, it was found that the 3.7 kb mRNA content was absent in growing cells, attained a maximal level in early differentiating cells and decreased rapidly at a time when mRNA encoding for adipsin[8], a marker of terminal differentiation, was still increasing (not shown). Both the emergence of 3.7 kb mRNA and that of 6 kb pOb24 mRNA were superimposable, indicating that both mRNAs could be considered as early markers of adipose cell differentiation. The expression of both RNA species was further investigated in various tissues from 4-month-old mice.

As shown in Fig. 2, the 6 kb pOb24 mRNA was preferentially expressed in epididymal white adipose tissue and ovaries. A lower expression was detected in adrenal glands and lung. No expression could be detected in the other tissues. The 3.7 kb mRNA presented the same tissue-specific expression since no expression was observed in liver and muscle. However, in contrast to the 6 kb mRNA species, a low signal was detected for the 3.7 kb species in heart, kidney and skin. This observation could be due to the fact that the 3.7 kb mRNA is about 10-fold more abundant than the 6 kb mRNA and/or by a differential tissue-specific expression. The results of Table 1 seem to be in favour of the last hypothesis, but further experiments using liquid hybridization with single-stranded probes would be required to assess this point.

Table 1. Expression of the 3.7 kb and 6 kb mRNAs in 4-month-old mice

Tissues	3.7 kb mRNA	6 kb mRNA	3.7 kb/6 kb ratio
White adipose tissue	6.30	0.87	7.2
Ovaries	8.44	0.98	8.6
Adrenal glands	5.86	0.36	16.3
Lung	4.13	0.27	15.3
Tongue	1.17	UND	
Skin	1.18	UND	
Testicles	1.26	UND	
Kidney	0.5	UND	
Heart	0.61	UND	
Brain	0.24	UND	
Liver	UND	UND	
Muscle	UND	UND	

Results from Fig. 3 were quantitated by densitometry using an LKB Ultroscan laser densitometer scanning. Values were expressed in densitometry units. UND = undetectable signal.

The protein encoded by the 3.7 kb mRNA is homologous to the human α2 chain of Type VI-Collagen

In order to identify protein(s) encoded by the two mRNAs, we have sequenced the two cDNAs. As expected, the C3-PU18-7 sequence was identical to the pOb24 cDNA sequence previously cloned[9] and corresponds to the 3' untranslated region of the 6 kb mRNA. A comparison of

```
C3-PU18-11      R G P D G Y P G E A G S P G E R G D Q G
                * * * * * * * * * * * * * * * * * * * *
HA2COL6         R G P D G Y P G E A G S P G E R G D Q G
```

Fig. 3. Comparison of amino-acid sequences of peptide encoded by the 3.7 kb mRNA and human α2 chain of type VI collagen.
The accession number of the amino-acid sequence of the human α2 chain of type VI collagen (HA2COL6) is S05378 in NBRF data bank. Amino-acid sequence encoded by the 3.7 kb mRNA was obtained from the C3-PU18-11 cDNA. The open reading frame of this cDNA contained 823 amino-acids.

the sequence with those from the European Molecular Biology Laboratory (EMBL, Heidelberg, Germany) databank or the Genbank database revealed no extensive homology with any of the sequences reported therein. The same result was obtained with the 3′ end of the C3-PU18-11 cDNA, but in this case we had the possibility to sequence the near full-length cDNA and to search for homology with the amino-acid deduced sequence. Figure 3 indicates the comparison between the open reading frame of the C3-PU18-11 cDNA and amino-acid sequences reported in the National Biomedical Research Foundation database. As shown there was complete homology with the amino-acid sequence of the α2 chain of human type VI-collagen.

Type VI collagen is a protein of the extracellular-matrix of mesenchymal cells which is absent from the matrix of tumour cells[18]. The protein is a heterotrimer consisting of α1(VI), α2(VI) and α3(VI) chains which are synthesized as polypeptides with M_r of 140, 140 and 260 respectively[4,7,12,20].

The structure of the Type VI collagen was recently determined by cloning of genes encoding for the three polypeptides in human[6] and chicken[20]. This protein represents a hybrid molecule consisting of a short triple helix collagenous domain which is flanked by two large globular domains. The globular domains contribute more than 80 per cent of the molecular mass. Another characteristic of this particular type of collagen is the fact that it contains numerous Arg-Gly-Asp (RGD) sequences, some of which may be used as cell-binding sites[2]. The globular domains are composed of several homologous repeats which show a striking similarity to the collagen-binding motif described in von Willebrand factor[19]. The RGD sequence and collagen-binding motif were also found in mouse α2 chain (S. Bardon, unpublished data).

The cell-attachment *via* RGD sequences to the integrin cellular receptors and the type I collagen-binding properties of type VI collagen led some investigators to speculate that this particular collagen might serve as a unique adaptor molecule for cell adhesion[5]. The function of type VI collagen in normal and pathological processes is unknown, but the relationship between components of the extracellular-matrix and gene regulation in cell differentiation already was suggested in adipose cell differentiation[13,17] whereas it was shown recently that the occupancy of the receptors for extracellular matrix components is critical in triggering the metabolic events leading to myogenic terminal differentiation[15]. Further studies will shed some light on the function of type VI collagen during terminal differentiation of early marker-expressing preadipocyte cells.

Acknowledgements

The authors are grateful to Dr C. Sardet for providing us with a mouse genomic library. Thanks are also due to Dr. Spiegelman for the kind gift of adipsin probe. The efficient secretarial assistance of G. Oillaux is gratefully acknowledged.

This work was supported by the "Centre National de la Recherche Scientifique" (UMR 134) and the Institut National de la Santé et de la Recherche Médicale (Grant CRE 894005 to C.D.).

Abbreviations

GPDH = glycerol-3-phosphate dehydrogenase; LPL = lipoprotein lipase; RGD = Arg-Gly-Asp; TNF-α = tumour necrosis factor-α; TGF-β = transforming growth factor-β.

References

1. Amri, E., Dani, C., Doglio, A., Etienne, J., Grimaldi, P. & Ailhaud, G. (1986): Adipose cell differentiation: evidence for a two-step process in the polyamine-dependent Ob1754 clonal line. *Biochem. J.* **238**, 115-122.
2. Aumailley, M., Mann, K., von der Mark, H. & Timpl, R. (1989): Cell attachment properties of Collagen Type VI and Arg-Gly-Asp dependent binding to its α2(VI) and α3(VI) chains. *Exp. Cell Res.* **181**, 463-474.
3. Benton, W.D. & Davis, R.W. (1977): Screening λgt recombinant clones by hybridization to single plaques in situ. *Science* **196**, 180-182.
4. Bonaldo, P. & Colombani, A. (1989): The carboxyl terminus of the chicken α3 chain of Collagen VI is a unique mosaic structure with glycoprotein Ib-like, Fibronectin type III, and Kunitz modules. *J. Biol. Chem.* **264**, 20235-20239.
5. Bonaldi, P., Russo, V., Bucciotti, F., Doliana, R. & Colombatti, A. (1990): Structural and functional features of the α3 chain indicate a bridging role for chicken Collagen VI connective tissues. *Biochemistry* **29**, 1245-1254.
6. Chu, M.K., Conway, D., Pzan, T.C., Baldwin, C., Mann, K., Deutzmann, R. & Timpl, R. (1988): Amino acid sequence of the triple-helical domain of human collagen type VI. *J. Biol. Chem.* **263**, 18601-18606.
7. Colombatti, A., Bonaldo, P., Ainger, K., Bressan, G.M. & Volpin, D. (1987): Biosynthesis of chick type VI Collagen. I. Intracellular assembly and molecular structure. *J. Biol. Chem.* **262**, 14454-14460.
8. Cook, K.S., Groves, D.L., Min, H.Y. & Spiegelman, B.M. (1985): A developmentally regulated mRNA from 3T3 adipocytes encodes a novel serine protease homologue. *Proc. Natl. Acad. Sci. USA* **82**, 6480-6484.
9. Dani, C., Doglio, A., Amri, E., Bardon, S., Fort, P., Bertrand, B., Grimaldi, P. & Ailhaud, G. (1989): Cloning and regulation of a mRNA specifically expressed in the preadipose state. *J. Biol. Chem.* **264**, 10119-10125.
10. Dani, C., Amri, E., Bertrand, B., Enerback, S., Bjursell, G., Grimaldi, P. & Ailhaud, G. (1990): Expression and regulation of pOb24 and lipoprotein lipase genes during adipose conversion. *J. Cell. Biochem.* **43**, 103-110.
11. Davis, L.G., Dibner, M.D. & Battey, J.F. (1986): In *Basic methods in molecular biology*, pp. 152-156. New York: Elsevier Science Publishing.
12. Hessle, H. & Engvall, E. (1984): Type VI Collagen. Studies on its localization, structure and biosynthetic form with monoclonal antibodies. *J. Biol. Chem.* **259**, 3955-3961.
13. Kuri-Harcuch, W., Argüello, C. & Marsch-Moreno, M. (1984): Extracellular matrix production by mouse 3T3-F442A cells during adipose differentiation cell culture. *Differentiation* **28**, 173-178.
14. Maniatis, T., Fritsch, E.F. & Sambrook, J. (1982): In *Molecular cloning. A laboratory manual.* ed. Cold Spring Harbor Laboratory, pp. 227-228. New York: Cold Spring Harbor Laboratory
15. Menko, A.S. & Boettiger, D. (1987): Occupation of the extracellular matrix receptor, integrin, is a control point for myogenic differentiation. *Cell* **51**, 51-57.
16. Pearson, W.R. & Lipman, D.J. (1988): Improved tools for biological sequence comparison. *Proc. Natl. Acad. Sci. USA* **85**, 2444-2448.
17. Spiegelman, B.M. & Ginty, C.A. (1983): Fibronectin modulation of cell shape and lipogenic expression in 3T3-adipocytes. *Cell* **35**, 657-666.

18. Schreier, T., Friis, R.R., Winterhalter, K.H. & Trueb, B. (1988): Regulation of type VI collagen synthesis in transformed mesenchymal cells. *Biochem. J.* **253**, 381-386.
19. Titani, K. & Walsh, K.A. (1988): Human von Willebrand factor: the molecular glue of platelet plugs. *Trends Biochem. Sci.* **13**, 94-97.
20. Trueb, B., Schaeren-Wiemers, N., Schreier, T. & Winterhalter, K.H. (1989): Molecular cloning of chicken type VI collagen. Primary structure of the subunit α2(VI)-pepsin. *J. Biol. Chem.* **264**, 136-140.

Chapter 63

Adrenergic Regulation of Differentiation and Proliferation in Brown Adipocyte Cultures

Jan NEDERGAARD[1], Myriam NÉCHAD[1,2], Stefan REHNMARK[1], David HERRON[1], Anders JACOBSSON[1], Pertti KUUSELA[1], Pere PUIGSERVER[1,3], Josef HOUSTEK[1,4], Gennady BRONNIKOV[1,5] and Barbara CANNON[1]

[1]*The Wenner-Gren Institute, Stockholm University, S-106 91 Stockholm, Sweden;*
[2]*Université P & M Curie, Paris, France;* [3]*Universitat de les Illes Balears;*
[4]*Czechoslovakian Academy of Sciences, Prague, Czechoslovakia;* [5]*USSR Academy of Sciences, Pushchino, Russia*

Introduction

The recruitment process in brown adipose tissue consists basically of two processes which in cell biology are often considered antagonistic: cell proliferation and cell differentiation. When the tissue is recruited, as occurs around birth in all mammalian species (including humans)[25], and in adult mammals under certain other physiological conditions (e.g. during cold exposure[15] and under the influence of certain diets[33], at least in smaller animals), cell proliferation and differentiation are apparently stimulated in parallel in the animal. That these processes are initiated to a large extent by release of norepinephrine from sympathetic nerves in the tissue (just as is thermogenesis itself), has long been realized (for review see e.g.[5]).

For the study of the cell biology of these processes, the introduction of brown fat cell cultures has opened new possibilities.

Brown fat cell cultures

Although some attempts to create *immortalized* cell lines from the brown adipose tissue have been reported[9,11,17], these attempts have generally until recently met with technical difficulties. Thus, the cultures being studied are presently generally *primary cultures* originating from young rats[8,19,22,23,28] or mice[16,20,30,31]. The brown adipose tissue in the interscapular region is dissected out, and isolated cells are prepared, principally following techniques developed for the isolation of mature brown-fat cells[26]. However, for cell culture studies, the mature cells in the preparation (which, due to their lipid content, float in the test tube) are discarded, and, principally, only the undifferentiated cells are placed in the cell culture flasks[4].

For most investigations published so far, the medium used has been semi-defined, consisting of 80-90 per cent of a defined medium such as Dulbecco's modification of Eagle's Minimal Essential Medium. To this medium, 10–20 per cent foetal or newborn calf serum has been added. The addition of serum is apparently necessary for plating and for initiation of the growth of the cells, but it is probable that the serum can be removed after a few days.

The cell cultures can be analysed in several different ways: for their acquisition of adipocyte characteristics, for the presence of adrenergic pathways leading to stimulation of triglyceride break-down, for the appearance in the cell culture of the ultimate marker for brown-adipocyte differentiation – the uncoupling protein thermogenin – and for proliferation stimulation.

Acquisition of adipocyte characteristics

A very typical feature of adipocytes is the accumulation in the cells of lipid droplets[8,23]. In a morphometric study (Fig. 1) we found that during their growth in culture flasks, the cells accumulated lipid droplets, but that the size of these droplets in the brown fat cells remained smaller than the size of lipid droplets in parallely grown cells obtained as precursors from white adipose tissue depots[23].

This observation in itself thus demonstrates both that the lipogenic enzymes are being expressed in these cells (and the cells thus undergo adipocyte conversion) and that brown-fat cell clones possess inherent characteristics which even under *in vitro* conditions direct their development in a way different from that of white-fat cell precursors. Also direct enzymatic analyses have demonstrated the occurrence in such cell cultures of lipogenic enzymes and of lipoprotein lipase[6,9,10,19,20,28].

The presence of adrenergic pathway

In order for adrenergic signals to be processed by the cells, they must possess adrenergic receptors. However, although it would appear possible to investigate this by the use of the binding of radioactively labelled adrenergic ligands, the developing understanding that most adrenergic signals in brown adipose tissue are mediated by β_3 receptors[2] has invalidated such techniques, because no ligand is available for β_3 receptors.

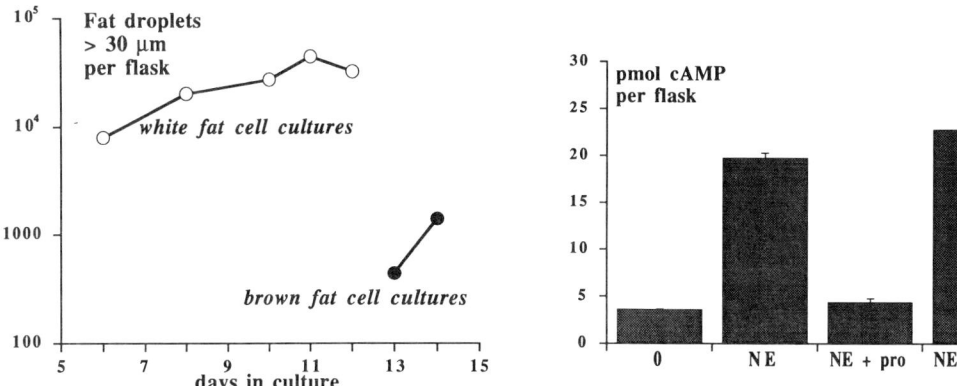

Fig. 1 (left). Appearance of very large fat droplets in cell cultures started from brown and white fat depots.
Despite the fact that these cultures proliferate in parallel and start to accumulate fat droplets at approximately the same time, it is only in the white-fat cell cultures that a high number of large fat droplets are found. Adapted from[23].
Fig. 2 (right). Effect of adrenergic stimulation on cAMP accumulation in brown-fat cell cultures. The accumulation of cAMP was investigated in 4-day-old cultures treated for 30 min with 1 µM norepinephrine (NE), 10 µM propranolol (pro) or 10 µM yohimbine (yoh). Data from[3].

Instead, it is necessary to rely on analysis of effects. Thus, the addition of norepinephrine to the brown fat cell cultures does lead to an increase in the level of cAMP in these cells[24,35], and the magnitude of this response increases with time in culture, indicating a successive appearance of β-adrenergic receptors or of their coupling to adenylate cyclase[3,24]. Further analysis of this response (Fig. 2) indicates that it is mediated via β-adrenergic receptors, in that it is inhibited by the β-blocker propranolol[3]. There is some evidence for an α_2-adrenergic component in that there is some tendency to an increase in cAMP as an effect of the α_2-blocker yohimbine. Analysis of the β-adrenergic fraction of the cAMP response seems to indicate that in the differentiated cultured cells it is mainly mediated via β_3-receptors[3]. That the entire β-adrenergic pathway is functional is evident from the fact that norepinephrine stimulation of the cells leads to lipolysis and release of fatty acids from the cells[9,18,35] (Fig. 3). In good parallelism with the effects on cAMP accumulation, the fatty acid release is blocked by propranolol but shows a tendency to a stimulation with the α-adrenergic inhibitor phentolamine, again indicating some α_2-component in the response.

The emergence in the cell cultures of the ultimate marker for brown adipocyte differentiation: the uncoupling protein thermogenin

Whereas adipocyte conversion and the emergence of lipogenic and lipolytic enzymes in white-fat cell cultures constitute evidence that the differentiation process has been completed, full differentiation in brown-fat cell cultures necessitates the further emergence of the unique brown-fat specific protein, the uncoupling protein thermogenin (UCP)[27].

With molecular biology techniques it is possible to analyse the brown fat cell cultures for the

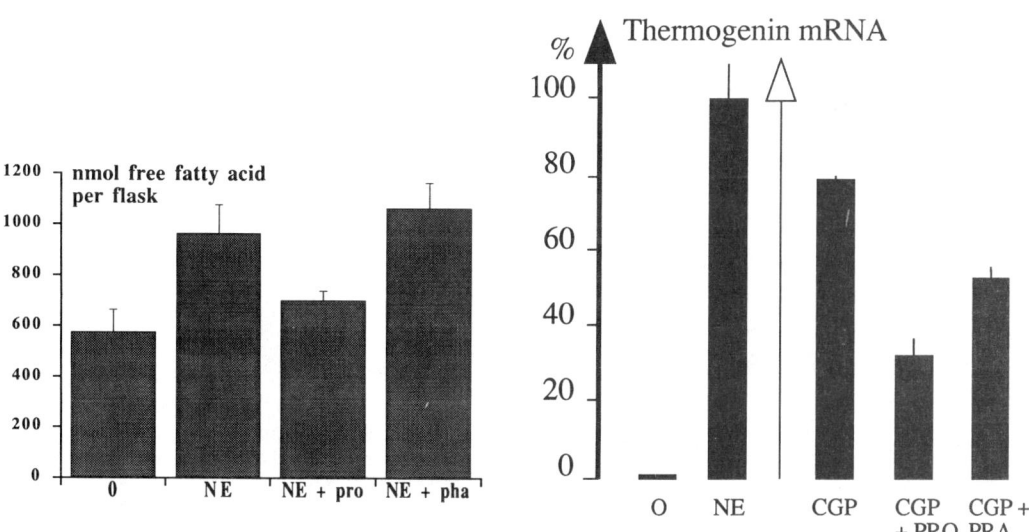

Fig. 3 (left). Effect of adrenergic stimulation on fatty acid release in brown-fat cell cultures. The amount of free fatty acids was measured in 11-day-old cultures, 2 h after stimulation with 10 μM norepinephrine (NE), 30 μM propranolol (pro) or 30 μM phentolamine (pha). Data from[18].

Fig. 4 (right). Effect of adrenergic stimulation on thermogenin mRNA levels in brown-fat cell cultures. The amount of thermogenin mRNA was measured in 6-day old cultures, 4 h after stimulation with 0.1 μM norepinephrine (NE), 0.1 μM CGP-12177 (CGP), 10 μM propranolol (PRO) or 10 μM prazosin (PRA). Data from[31].

presence of thermogenin mRNA. Although for a long time this mRNA species was elusive in the cell cultures, it has recently become evident that the brown-fat cell cultures may advance to a differentiation state in which the thermogenin gene is expressed[30,31] (Fig. 4). This expression seems virtually fully dependent upon norepinephrine stimulation of the cells, but the cell cultures in this respect are only fully sensitive to norepinephrine for a short time – some days around cell confluence.[31] It is, however, clear from these experiments that the effect of norepinephrine to promote differentiation is a direct effect on the brown-fat cells themselves.

We have analysed the adrenergic nature of the norepinephrine response. It is clear that the major part of the response is β-adrenergic, and as this part can be competently stimulated with the adrenergic agent CGP12177 (Fig. 4), it must be concluded that the effect of norepinephrine is mediated *via* β_3 receptors. This is because the agent CGP-12177 functions as an antagonist or as a very weak agonist on β_1-adrenergic receptors (which thus cannot mediate the gene expression response seen here) but as a competent agonist on β_3 receptors[13,21,34]. Also the β_3 agonist BRL-37344 can induce thermogenin gene expression.[31]

However, it would seem that stimulation of the β-adrenergic pathway by other compounds which also increase cAMP in the cells cannot fully mimic the norepinephrine response. Some of the response can also be inhibited by the α_1-antagonist prazosin. Thus, there is some evidence for an involvement of α_1-receptors in the gene expression response. This is also evident from the fact that the α-adrenergic agonist oxymethazoline can augment the thermogenin mRNA level above that induced by cAMP analogues[31].

That not only thermogenin mRNA but also thermogenin itself is induced by norepinephrine stimulation of the cultured cells has been demonstrated by immunoblotting techniques[14,16]. Significant amounts of thermogenin are measurable already after 2 h norepinephrine stimulation, but we have found that the thermogenin amount in these cultures continues to

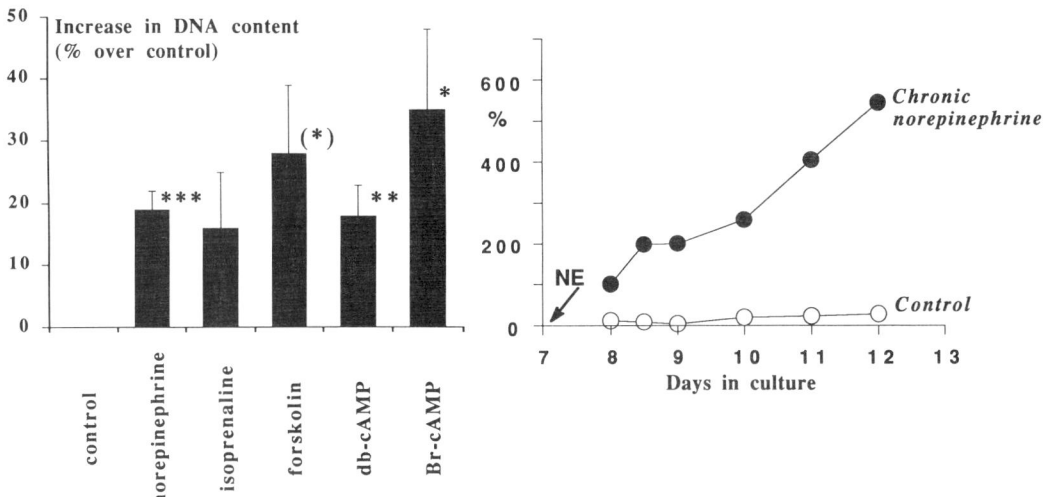

Fig. 5 (left). Effect of adrenergic stimulation on thermogenin content in brown-fat cell cultures. The total amount of thermogenin per well was measured in cultures stimulated chronically from day 7 with norepinephrine. The content in cultures stimulated for 24 h with norepinephrine was set to 100 per cent. Adapted from[29].

Fig. 6 (right). Effect of adrenergic stimulation on cell proliferation in brown-fat cell cultures. The amount of DNA was measured in 4-day-old cultures, 4 h after stimulation with the indicated agents. Based on data in[3].

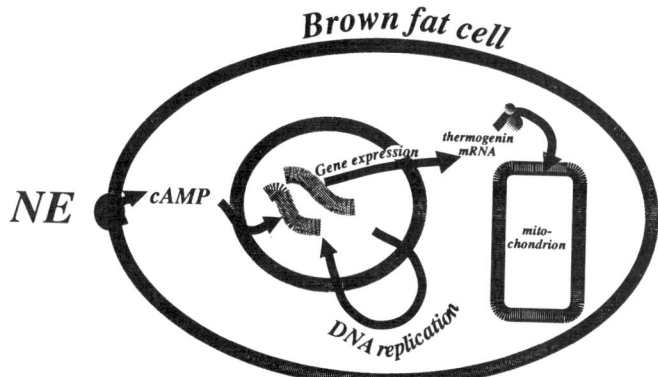

Fig. 7. Adrenergic regulation of proliferation and differentiation in brown fat cells. In brown fat cells, norepinephrine – working through β-adrenergic receptors and cAMP – stimulates both proliferation and differentiation. This is physiologically sound but poses questions concerning the cellular coordination of these processes.

increase during a 5-day treatment[29] (Fig. 5), leading to vast increases in the potential thermogenic capacity of the cells. The thermogenin synthesized is apparently both transported to and incorporated into the mitochondria[14] which is in good agreement with observations in other *in vitro* systems[7].

Proliferation stimulation

The brown-fat cell cultures divide spontaneously, with a doubling time of 1–2 days, until cell confluence is reached in the flasks; the cell division rate is then markedly decreased[3,16,23].

This cell proliferation must be considered to be an effect of the absence of contact inhibition in the flasks, combined with the effect of general cell growth stimulating agents present in the serum.

However, as there is evidence from experiments *in vivo* that norepinephrine may also have a stimulatory effect on cell proliferation[12,32], we have investigated the effect of norepinephrine on the cell cultures. We found that when norepinephrine was added to the growing cell cultures, it led to a 20–40 per cent increase in the amount of DNA measured 4 h later, as compared with untreated cells[3]. In cell cultures where contact inhibition had already developed, there was no significant effect of norepinephrine.

The effect of norepinephrine was evident already with 0.1 μM norepinephrine and was clearly also mediated *via* β-adrenergic receptors and an increase in cAMP (Fig. 6).

Cell proliferation *versus* cell differentiation

Although it is often recognized that cell proliferation and cell differentiation are antagonistic events, the data above clearly indicate that in the brown-fat cell cultures, as well as in the brown adipose tissue, these events may both be stimulated *via* the same pathway (Fig. 7). However, this does not necessary imply that the same cell responds with both a proliferative response and with an increase in degree of differentiation[1]. Rather, it would seem likely that the cells pass through different developmental stages, in which first proliferation and then differentiation may be successively stimulated, *via* β_1- and β_3-adrenergic responses respectively.[3]

References

1. Ailhaud, G. (1990): Extracellular factors, signalling pathways and differentiation of adipose precursor cells. *Curr. Opin. Cell Biol.* **2**, 1043-1049.
2. Arch, J. (1989): The brown adipocyte β-adrenoceptor. *Proc. Nutr. Soc.* **48**, 215-223.
3. Bronnikov, G., Houštek, J. & Nedergaard, J. (1992): β-Adrenergic, cAMP-mediated stimulation of proliferation of brown fat cells in primary culture. Mediation *via* β1 but not *via* β3 adrenoceptors. *J. Biol. Chem.* (in press).
4. Cannon, B. & Nedergaard, J. (1987): Adipocytes, preadipocytes, and mitochondria from brown adipose tissue. In *The biology of the adipocytes: research approaches*, eds. G.J. Hausman & R. Martin, pp. 21-51. New York: Van Nostrand Reinhold Company.
5. Cannon, B., Rehnmark, S., Néchad, M., Herron, D., Jacobsson, A., Kopecky, J., Obregon, M.J. & Nedergaard, J. (1989): Hormonal control of brown fat recruitment. In *Living in the cold II*, eds. A. Malan & B. Canguilhem, pp. 359-366. London: John Libbey.
6. Carneheim, C.M.H. (1987): Regulation of lipoprotein lipase in brown adipose tissue. Doctoral Thesis. Stockholm: University of Stockholm.
7. Casteilla, L., Blondel, O., Klaus, S., Raimbault, S., Diolez, P., Moreau, F., Bouillaud, F. & Ricquier, D. (1990): Stable expression of functional mitochondrial uncoupling protein in Chinese hamster ovary cells. *Proc. Natl. Acad. Sci. USA* **87**, 5124-5128.
8. Cigolini, M., Cinti, S., Bosello, O., Brunetti, L. & Björntorp, P. (1986): Isolation and ultrastructural features of brown adipocytes in culture. *J. Anat.* **145**, 207-216.
9. Forest, C., Doglio, A., Ricquier, D. & Ailhaud, G. (1987): A preadipocyte clonal line from mouse brown adipose tissue. Short and long-term responses to insulin and β-adrenergics. *Exp. Cell Res.* **168**, 218-232.
10. Forest, C., Doglio, A., Ricquier, D. & Ailhaud, G. (1987): Expression of the mitochondrial uncoupling protein in brown adipocytes. Absence in brown preadipocytes and BFC-l cells. Modulation by isoproterenol in adipocytes. *Exp. Cell Res.* **168**, 233-246.
11. Fox, N., Crooke, R., Hwang, L.H., Schibler, U., Knowles, B.B. & Solter, D. (1989): Metastatic hibernomas in transgenic mice expressing an alpha-amylase-SV40 T antigen hybrid gene. *Science* **244**, 460-463.
12. Geloen, A., Collet, A.J., Guay, G. & Bukowiecki, L.J. (1988): β-Adrenergic stimulation of brown adipocyte proliferation. *Am. J. Physiol.* **254**, C175-C182.
13. Granneman, J.G. & Whitty, C.J. (1991): CGP 12177A modulates brown fat adenylate cyclase activity by interacting with two distinct receptor sites. *J. Pharmacol. Exp. Therap.* **256**, 421-425.
14. Herron, D., Rehnmark, S., Néchad, M., Loncar, D., Cannon, B. & Nedergaard, J. (1990): Norepinephrine-induced synthesis of the uncoupling protein thermogenin (UCP) and its mitochondrial targeting in brown adipocytes differentiated in culture. *FEBS Lett.* **268**, 296-300.
15. Himms-Hagen, J. (1986): Brown adipose tissue and cold-acclimation. In *Brown adipose tissue*, eds. P. Trayhurn & D.G. Nicholls, pp. 214-268. London: Edward Arnold.
16. Kopecky, J., Baudysova, M., Zanotti, F., Janikova, D. & Houštek, J. (1990): Control of mitochondrial uncoupling protein content in brown adipocytes differentiated in cell culture. *J. Biol. Chem.* **265**, 22204-22209.
17. Kozak, L.P. & Kozak, U.C. (1991): Regulation of gene expression in a brown fat cell culture derived from a SV40-induced tumor. Abstract. *J. Cell. Biochem.* Supplement **15B**, 31-31.
18. Kuusela, P., Nedergaard, J. & Cannon, B. (1986): β-Adrenergic stimulation of fatty acid release from brown fat cells differentiated in monolayer culture. *Life Sci.* **38**, 589-599.
19. Lorenzo, M., Roncero, C., Fabregat, I. & Benito, M. (1988): Hormonal regulation of rat foetal lipogenesis in brown-adipocyte primary cultures. *Biochem. J.* **251**, 617-620.
20. Masuno, H., Blanchette-Mackie, E.J., Chernick, S.S. & Scow, R.O. (1990): Synthesis of inactive nonsecretable high mannose-type lipoprotein lipase by cultured brown adipocytes of combined lipase-deficient cld/cld mice. *J. Biol. Chem.* **265**, 1628-1638.
21. Mohell, N. & Dicker, A. (1989): The β-adrenergic radioligand (^{3}H)CGP-12177, generally classified as an antagonist, is a thermogenic agonist in brown adipose tissue. *Biochem. J.* **261**, 401-405.
22. Néchad, M. (1983): Development of brown fat cells in monolayer culture. II. Ultrastructural characterization of precursors, differentiating adipocytes and their mitochondria. *Exp. Cell Res.* **149**, 119-127.

23. Néchad, M., Kuusela, P., Carneheim, C., Björntorp, P., Nedergaard, J. & Cannon, B. (1983): Development of brown fat cells in monolayer culture. I. Morphological and biochemical distinction from white fat cells in culture. *Exp. Cell Res.* **149**, 105-118.
24. Néchad, M., Nedergaard, J. & Cannon, B. (1987): Noradrenergic stimulation of mitochondriogenesis in brown adipocytes differentiating in culture. *Am. J. Physiol.* **253**, C889-C894.
25. Nedergaard, J., Connolly, E. & Cannon, B. (1986): Brown adipose tissue in the mammalian neonate. In *Brown adipose tissue*, eds. P. Trayhurn & D.G. Nicholls, pp. 152-213. London: Edward Arnold.
26. Nedergaard, J. & Lindberg, O. (1982): The brown fat cell. *Int. Rev. Cytol.* **74**, 187-286.
27. Nicholls, D.G., Cunningham, S.A. & Rial, E. (1986): The bioenergetic mechanisms of brown adipose tissue thermogenesis. In *Brown adipose tissue*, eds. P. Trayhurn & D.G. Nicholls, pp. 52-85. London: Edward Arnold.
28. Poissonnet, C.M., Ouagued, M., Aron, Y., Pello, J.-Y., Swierczewski, E. & Krishnamoorthy, R. (1988): Retrieval of precursors for white-type adipose conversion in brown adipose tissue. *Biochem. J.* **255**, 849-854.
29. Puigserver, P., Herron, D., Gianotti, M., Palou, A., Cannon, B. & Nedergaard, J. (1992): Induction and degradation of the uncoupling protein thermogenin in brown adipocytes *in-vitro* and *in-vivo:* evidence for a rapidly degradable pool. *Biochem. J.* (in press).
30. Rehnmark, S., Kopecky, J., Jacobsson, A., Néchad, M., Herron, D., Nelson, B.D., Obregon, M.J., Nedergaard, J. & Cannon, B. (1989): Brown adipocytes differentiated *in-vitro* can express the gene for the uncoupling protein thermogenin. Effects of hypothyroidism and norepinephrine. *Exp. Cell Res.* **182**, 75-83.
31. Rehnmark, S., Néchad, M., Herron, D., Cannon, B. & Nedergaard, J. (1990): α- and β-adrenergic induction of the expression of the uncoupling protein thermogenin in brown adipocytes differentiated in culture. *J. Biol. Chem.* **265**, 16464-16471.
32. Rehnmark, S. & Nedergaard, J. (1989): DNA synthesis in brown adipose tissue is under β-adrenergic control. *Exp. Cell Res.* **180**, 574-579.
33. Rothwell, N.J. & Stock, M.J. (1986): Brown adipose tissue and diet-induced thermogenesis. In *Brown adipose tissue*, eds. P. Trayhurn & D.G. Nicholls, pp. 269-338. London: Edward Arnold.
34. Scarpace, P.J. & Matheny, M. (1991): Adenylate cyclase agonist properties of CGP-12177A in brown fat: evidence for atypical β-adrenergic receptors. *Am. J. Physiol.* **260**, E226-E231.
35. Sugihara, H., Miyabara, S., Yonemits, N. & Ohta, K. (1983): Hormonal sensitivity of brown fat cells of fetal rats in monolayer culture. *Exp. Clin. Endocrinol.* **82**, 309-319.

Chapter 64

The Siberian Hamster as a New Model to Study the Hormonal Regulation of Brown Adipocyte Differentiation and Uncoupling Protein Expression

Susanne KLAUS, Anne-Marie CASSARD, Martin KLINGENSPOR* and Daniel RICQUIER

*Centre de Recherche sur la Nutrition (CNRS), 9 rue Jules Hetzel, 92190 Meudon/Bellevue, France; *Fachbereich Biologie/Zoologie, Philipps Universität, 3550 Marburg, Germany*

The mammalian brown adipose tissue (BAT) produces heat during non-shivering thermogenesis and plays thus an important role in energy balance, which is due to a unique uncoupling protein (UCP) located in the inner mitochondrial membrane of brown adipocytes. Here we report first results of brown adipocyte differentiation from preadipocytes obtained from the Djungarian (Siberian) dwarf hamster *Phodopus sungorus*. In this species BAT may represent as much as 5 per cent of body weight. We obtained a high yield of brown fat fibroblastic preadipocytes which were able to differentiate in cell culture and express UCP as revealed by Northern blotting as well as immunoblotting. Growth and differentiation required the presence of foetal calf serum (FCS) as well as insulin. Basal UCP expression was very low but could be considerably increased by β-adrenergic stimulation including the novel β-adrenergic agonist D7114 (ICI pharmaceuticals). Tests with a defined, serum-free medium showed that survival of mature adipocytes required the presence of insulin and that UCP mRNA levels were considerably elevated after 24 h by the synergistic action of triiodothyronine and insulin.

Introduction

Contrary to white adipose tissue (WAT), which functions in energy storage, brown adipose tissue (BAT) plays a role in energy dissipation as the effector organ of non-shivering thermogenesis in small and newborn mammals. This function is due to the uncoupling protein UCP, uniquely expressed in BAT, which is located in the inner mitochondrial membrane[9]. Numerous *in vivo* studies have shown that acute UCP function as well as UCP gene expression are stimulated by noradrenaline and numerous β-adrenergic agents[16]. For the study of brown adipocyte development and differentiation it is necessary to have a cell culture system in which the expression of UCP, the marker protein for brown adipocytes is evident. Only recently different groups have succeeded in obtaining UCP expression in brown adipocytes of mice[11,12] or lambs[5] differentiated *in vitro*. We decided to try to develop a new animal model by using the Siberian dwarf hamster *Phodopus sungorus*. This small hamster of about 40 g body weight shows extreme adaptive abilities of cold resistance by a high capacity of non-shivering thermogenesis (NST) which is located mainly in brown adipose tissue[7]. Consequently, this animal possesses very large amounts of BAT which can make up to 5 per cent of its body weight. It has further been shown that UCP activity as well as UCP

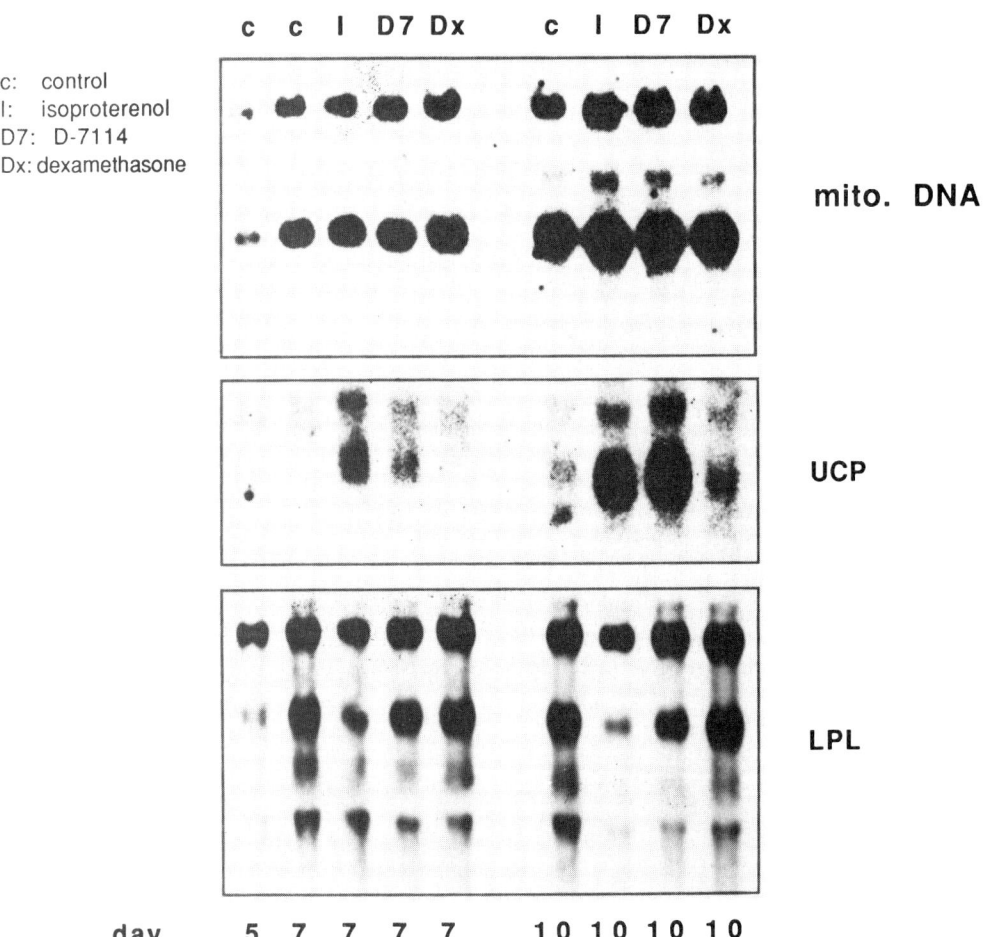

Fig. 1. Northern analysis of Phodopus sungorus *brown adipocytes differentiated in vitro at different days of culture. Each lane corresponds to 10 µg total RNA. One blot is shown which was successively hybridized with total mouse mitochondrial DNA (mito DNA), uncoupling protein cDNA (UCP) and lipoprotein lipase cDNA (LPL). At day 5 of culture the following substances were added to the culture medium: 10 µM isoproterenol (I), 1 µM D7114 (D), or 10 nM dexamethasone (Dx). c indicates cells without any addition. Cells were harvested at days 5, 7 and 10 of culture as indicated at the bottom.*

mRNA levels in BAT of *Phodopus* can be highly stimulated by cold exposure[17]. This species possesses furthermore large quantities of white adipose tissue, which allows comparative studies on white and brown adipocyte differentiation. In this study we investigated growth and differentiation of preadipocytes from brown fat of *P. sungorus* and the influence of β-adrenergic agonists including the novel atypical agonist D7114 (see article by Holloway *et al.* in this volume) on UCP expression. We furthermore found a stimulation of UCP synthesis by insulin plus triiodothyronine in a defined, serum-free medium.

Materials and methods

BAT of animals aged between 4 and 6 weeks was excised (0.6–0.8 g per animal), digested with collagenase and the stromar vascular fraction isolated. About 150,000 fibroblastic preadipocytes were inoculated in Petri dishes (10 cm diameter). Standard cell culture medium consisted of 50 per cent modified Eagle's medium (GIBCO/BRL) and 50 per cent Ham's F12 medium (GIBCO/BRL) supplemented with $NaHCO_3$ (1.2 g/l), biotin (4 mg/l), Ca panthotenate (2 mg/l), glutamine (5 mM), glucose (4.5 g/l), HEPES (pH 7.4, 15 mM), penicillin G (6.25 mg/l), streptomycin (5 mg/l), insulin (20 nM), triiodothyronine (T_3, 1 nM), and 10 per cent (v/v) foetal calf serum (FCS).

Cells were harvested at times indicated and used either for total RNA isolation[8] or isolation of mitochondria. Western blotting of mitochondria was performed as described before[4] using anti-rat UCP raised in sheep. RNA electrophoresis and Northern blotting was performed as described by Ricquier *et al.*[14]. Blots were hybridized with a ^{32}P-labelled rat UCP cDNA[14], a pBR 325 plasmid containing the total mouse mitochondrial genome[3], and a pGEM plasmid containing a mouse lipoprotein lipase cDNA insert (gift of Dr M. Schotz, UCLA). D7114 was a gift from Dr B. Holloway (ICI Pharmaceuticals, Manchester, UK).

Results and discussion

Growth and differentiation of brown adipocytes

An average of 0.7 g BAT could be dissected per animal, yielding about 1.1×10^6 fibroblastic preadipocytes per gram BAT. Confluency was reached around day 5 or 6 of culture at a density of approximately 350 cells/mm^2. Differentiation rate was highest during the 2 days following confluency and at day 10 between 40 per cent and 60 per cent of cells showed the morphology of differentiated adipocytes, i.e. a rounded shape and inclusion of lipid droplets. Mature adipocytes occurred in clusters, surrounded by non-differentiated cells. This is a typical pattern, also found in different white adipocyte cell lines[1]. Adipocyte differentiation was dependent on the presence of insulin and triiodothyronine as is the case in several adipose cell lines[1]. Lipoprotein lipase (LPL) mRNA, an early adipocyte differentiation marker[1] could already be detected around confluency (Fig. 1). Mitochondrial development followed behind cell differentiation. Mitochondrial transcription products were very low at day 5 and increased considerably until day 10 (Fig. 1). Measurement of cytochrome *c* oxidase activity showed a 20-fold increase per cell between days 5 and 10 of culture. Adipocytes differentiated in culture can be considered as true brown adipocytes, as they expressed the BAT marker protein UCP (uncoupling protein). However, UCP expression could only be detected after confluency, when first differentiated adipocytes could be observed. This supports findings in mice brown adipocyte primary culture, where UCP expression is also dependent on adipocyte differentiation[12].

Action of β-adrenergic agonists

Basal UCP expression, as detected by Northern as well as immunoblotting was very low, but could be highly increased by β-adrenergic stimulation, which is also the case in mouse brown adipocyte primary culture[12]. As can be seen in Fig. 1, UCP mRNA could be first detected at day 7, and increased considerably until day 10. β-Adrenergic stimulation by either isoproterenol or D7114, a novel atypical β-agonist (ICI Pharmaceuticals) was equally effective in increasing UCP mRNA levels. Mitochondrial transcription rate increased during cell development, but was not significantly influenced by β-adrenergic stimulation. This is consistent with findings *in vivo*, where cold exposure of *P. sungorus* also did not influence mitochondrial transcription[13]. LPL mRNA levels seemed to be slightly decreased by isoproterenol treatment. This seems surprising, as in this species LPL activity in BAT is stimulated by cold exposure[10] *in vivo*. Two explanations are possible: LPL enzyme activity might be regulated on a post-transcriptional level, or the cold response of LPL is not exclusively regulated by β-adrenergic action. The latter seems to be a possible explanation, as noradrenaline injection *in vivo* failed to increase LPL enzyme activity in BAT of *Phodopus* (Klingenspor, unpublished data).

The novel, atypical β-adrenergic agonist D7114 proved to be very effective on UCP stimulation in this culture system (Fig. 1, Table 1). Treatment of mature adipocytes with 1 μM D7114 increased UCP mRNA levels significantly after 2 h, reaching maximal levels after 8 h which stayed at this level for at least 48 h after addition. Increase of UCP, as detected by immunoblotting in the mitochondrial fraction, was apparent after 8 h, increasing still until 48 h after addition. D7114 was already effective at 10 nM with the maximal response reached at 100 nM (data not shown).

Table 1. Effect of addition of foetal calf serum (FCS, 10%), insulin (20 nM), triiodothyronine (T_3, 1 nM), and D7114 (1 μM) on UCP mRNA levels in brown adipocytes differentiated *in vitro*

FCS	Insulin	T_3	D7114	UCP mRNA*
+	/	/	/	−
+	+	+	/	0
+	+	+	+	++
/	/	/	/	−
/	+	/	/	−
/	/	+	/	0
/	+	+	/	++
/	+	+	+	+++
/	/	/	+	−

Preadipocytes were grown in the medium until a high number of differentiated cells containing lipid droplets could be observed (about three days after confluency). Cells were then washed twice with PBS and cultured for further 24 h in the standard medium with supplementations as indicated. Changes in UCP mRNA levels as compared to cells before the treatments are shown. * 0 indicates no change; − indicates an increase; + indicates an increase.

UCP expression in a serum-free medium

In vivo studies have shown that T_3 amplifies the noradrenaline stimulation of UCP gene expression[2] and that insulin is important for thermogenic action of BAT, including UCP expression[6,15]. In order to investigate the action of these hormones *in vitro*, we replaced the standard medium with a serum-free medium after mature adipocytes were visible. They could be maintained in a serum-free medium for several days in the presence of insulin. Without addition of insulin, protein content per dish decreased by over 60 per cent within 24 h which could be prevented by addition of insulin but not T_3. However, UCP mRNA levels decreased when only insulin was present, whereas addition of T_3 prevented this decrease. Interestingly, in the presence of insulin plus T_3 we also found a large increase in UCP mRNA level (Table 1). This indicates a synergistic action of insulin and T_3, which is inhibited by the presence of FCS. However, it is not yet clear if this increase is caused by an activation of UCP transcription or due to a post-transcriptional process. As can be seen in Table 1, in the absence of insulin and T_3 no β-adrenergic stimulation of UCP expression could be observed. This agrees with previous findings that in primary culture of mouse brown adipocytes the presence of either insulin or T_3 was necessary for noradrenaline-induced increase of UCP expression[12].

Conclusion

Phodopus sungorus proved to be a very suitable animal model to study brown adipocyte development and differentiation in primary cell culture. The brown adipocyte marker protein UCP was expressed and detectable in mitochondria. Its expression could be increased by β-adrenergic stimulation. The novel, atypical β-adrenergic agonist D7114 was very efficient in stimulation of UCP expression in this cell model. We could also demonstrate a stimulation of UCP expression by the combined action of insulin and T_3 in a serum-free medium, indicating for the first time an *in vitro* activation of UCP expression independent of adrenergic stimulation.

References

1. Ailhaud, G., Dani, C., Ez-Zoubir, A., Djian, P., Vannier, C., Doglio, A., Forest, C., Gaillard, D., Negrel, R. & Grimaldi, P. (1989): Coupling growth arrest and adipocyte differentiation. *Environ. Health Perspect.* **80**, 17-23.
2. Bianco, A.C., Sheng, X. & Silva, J.E. (1988): Triiodothyronine amplifies norepinephrine stimulation of uncoupling protein gene transcription by a mechanism not requiring protein synthesis. *J. Biol. Chem.* **263**, 18168-18175.
3. Bibb, M., van Etten, R., Wright, C., Walberg, M. & Clayton, D. (1981): Sequence and gene organization of mouse mitochondrial DNA. *Cell* **26**, 167
4. Casteilla, L., Blondel, O., Klaus, S., Raimbault, S., Diolez, P., Moreau, F., Bouillaud, F. & Ricquier, D. (1990): Stable expression of functional mitochondrial uncoupling protein in Chinese hamster ovary cells. *Proc. Natl. Acad. Sci. USA* **87**, 5124-5128.
5. Casteilla, L., Nougues, J., Reyne, Y. & Ricquier, D. (1991): Differentiation of ovine brown adipocyte precursor cells in a chemically defined serum-free medium. Importance of glucocorticoids and age of animals. *Eur. J. Biochem.* **198**, 195-199.
6. Geloen, A. & Trayhurn, P. (1990): Regulation of uncoupling protein in brown adipose tissue by insulin. *Am. J. Physiol.* **258**, R418-R424.
7. Heldmaier, G. & Buchberger, A. (1985): Sources of heat during nonshivering thermogenesis in Djungarian hamsters: a dominant role of brown adipose tissue during cold adaptation. *J. Comp. Physiol. B* **156**, 237-245.
8. Jacobsson, A., Stadler, U., Glotzer, M.A. & Kozak, L.P. (1985): Mitochondrial uncoupling protein from mouse brown fat. Molecular cloning, genetic mapping, and mRNA expression. *J. Biol. Chem.* **260**, 16250-16254.
9. Klaus, S., Casteilla, L., Bouillaud, F. & Ricquier, D. (1991): The uncoupling protein UCP: a membraneous mitochondrial ion carrier exclusively expressed in brown adipose tissue. *Int. J. Biochem.* **28**, 791-801.
10. Klingenspor, M., Klaus, S., Wiesinger, H. & Heldmaier, G. (1989): Activation of brown fat lipoprotein lipase by short photoperiod and cold exposure in the Djungarian hamster, *Phodopus sungorus. Am. J. Physiol.* **26**, R1123-R1127.
11. Kopecky, J., Baudysova, M., Zanotti, F., Janikova, D., Pavelka, S. & Houstek, J. (1990): Synthesis of mitochondrial uncoupling protein in brown adipocytes differentiated in cell culture. *J. Biol. Chem.* **265**, 2204-2209.
12. Rehnmark, S., Nechad, M., Herron, D., Cannon, B. & Nedergaard, J. (1990): Alpha- and beta-adrenergic induction of the expression of the uncoupling protein thermogenin in brown adipocytes differentiated in culture. *J. Biol. Chem.* **265**, 16464-16471.

13. Reiter, J.R., Klaus, S., Ebbinghaus, C., Heldmaier, G., Redlin, U., Ricquier, D., Vaughan, M.K. & Steinlechner, S. (1990): Inhibition of 5'deiodination of thryroxine suppresses the cold-induced increase in brown adipose tissue mRNA for mitochondrial uncoupling protein without influencing lipoprotein lipase activity. *Endocrinology* **126**, 2550-2554.
14. Ricquier, D., Bouillaud, F., Toumelin, P., Mory, G., Bazin, R., Arch, J. & Penicaud (1986): Expression of uncoupling protein mRNA in thermogenic or weakly thermogenic brown adipose tissue. *J. Biol. Chem.* **261**, 13905-13910.
15. Seydoux, J., Trimble, E.R., Bouillaud, F., Assimacopoulos-Jeannet, F., Bas, S., Ricquier, D., Giacobino, J.P. & Girardier, L. (1984): Modulation of beta-oxidation and proton conductance pathway of brown adipose tissue in hypo- and hyperinsulinemic states. *FEBS Lett.* **166**, 141-145.
16. Trayhurn, P. & Nicholls, D.G. (eds.) (1986): *Brown adipose tissue*. London: Edward Arnold.
17. Wiesinger, H., Klaus, S., Heldmaier, G., Champigny, O. & Ricquier, D. (1989): Increased nonshivering thermogenesis, brown fat cytochrome-*c* oxidase activity, GDP-binding, and uncoupling protein mRNA levels after short daily cold exposure of *Phodopus sungorus*. *Can. J. Physiol. Pharmacol.* **68**, 195-200.

Chapter 65

Mitochondrial DNA Variants in Relation to Body Fat

France T. DIONNE, Josée TRUCHON, Lucie TURCOTTE, Angelo TREMBLAY, Jean-Pierre DESPRÉS and Claude BOUCHARD

Physical Activity Sciences Laboratory, Laval University, Ste-Foy, Québec, Canada, G1K 7P4

Mitochondrial DNA sequence polymorphism was analysed using the restriction fragment length polymorphism technology in 12 pairs of monozygotic twins subjected to a 100-day period of overfeeding to determine whether there was a relationship between mitochondrial DNA variants and the relative changes observed in body weight, body composition and energy expenditure phenotypes in response to overfeeding. Mitochondrial DNA variants were detected with six restriction enzymes in only six pairs of twins. Three of them exhibited multiple variants while the others had only one. None of the mitochondrial DNA variants were present in a number of pairs sufficient to undertake statistical analysis. Instead, we elected to compare the lowest and highest gainers for each phenotype in terms of mitochondrial DNA variants. For more than half the phenotypes, the lowest gainer was a pair of twins carrying mitochondrial DNA variants and, for a majority of these phenotypes, the highest gainer pair was also carrier of mitochondrial DNA variants. These results suggest that mitochondrial DNA sequence polymorphism could be associated with a positive or negative influence on the response to overfeeding possibly through its impact on oxidative phosphorylation.

Introduction

A poor coupling between energy expenditure and caloric intake may cause positive or negative energy balance. Chronic positive energy balance leads to body weight and body composition alterations and ultimately to obesity. Studies of experimentally overfed subjects have shown that there were considerable inter-individual differences in the changes observed for body weight and body composition in response to an identical excess in caloric intake[2,10]. One of the main conclusions of these studies was that genetic factors are likely involved in determining the susceptibility to gain weight, alter body composition and become obese.

At the molecular level, such genetic factors will ultimately imply variation of the mitochondrial (mt) and nuclear DNA sequence. Candidate genes potentially associated with the complex multifactorial phenotype of obesity (excess mass or fat for stature) are numerous in humans. mtDNA is related to various aspects of metabolism through its contribution to the respiratory chain and oxidative phosphorylation. Indeed, mtDNA codes for 13 out of the 67 proteins involved in these metabolic pathways. In addition, mtDNA is self-replicative, it codes for 22 tRNAs and 2 rRNAs and has a region called the D-Loop which contains the origin sites of replication and transcription. The complete sequence of mtDNA which is a closed circular molecule of 16569 base pairs was first published by Anderson *et al.*[1]

In this paper, we report on the associations between mtDNA sequence polymorphism and the relative changes in body mass, body composition, subcutaneous fat distribution, resting metabolic rate (RMR) and the thermic effect of food (TEM) in 12 pairs of monozygotic twins, overfed by 4.2 MJ per day, 6 days a week, for a period of 100 days.

Methods

Subjects, anthropometric and metabolic measurements

Twelve pairs of male monozygotic twins, 19 to 27 years of age, gave their informed consent to participate in this study. Subjects were submitted to a 100-day overfeeding period in which energy intake was increased by 4.2 MJ (1000 kcal) per day over their respective baseline, 6 days a week, for a total caloric overload of 353 MJ or 84,000 kcal. A complete description of the inclusion criteria, baseline assessment and overfeeding protocol has recently been published[2]. Body weight, body mass index (BMI), body density, fat mass and fat-free mass were determined as described[2]. Skinfold thickness was measured with a Harpenden caliper on 10 sites, five on the trunk (subscapular, suprailiac, abdominal, midaxillary, and chest) and five on the extremities (biceps, triceps, front midthigh, suprapatellar, and medial calf). The ratio of trunk skinfolds to extremity skinfolds (T/E) was used as an indicator of the relative distribution of subcutaneous fat. RMR and thermic effect of a 4.2 MJ (1000 kcal) meal were determined using the ventilated hood technique[3]. For each of these variables, results were considered in terms of relative changes (in per cent) induced by the overfeeding treatment.

DNA extraction and mtDNA RFLP analysis

Total DNA (mt and nuclear) was extracted from white blood cells as described[6]. mtDNA sequence analyses were carried out using the restriction fragment length polymorphism (RFLP) technology and Southern blotting[12] using 22 restriction enzymes[6]. The size of the mtDNA fragments, visualized by hybridization with a human ^{32}P-labelled mtDNA probe[6], was then determined using size standards. Morph identification was established according to the published data on mtDNA RFLPs[4,5,7-9].

Results

Table 1 summarizes the mtDNA sequence variations found with the 22 restriction enzymes used in this study. Nine different mtDNA RFLPs were detected with six of the enzymes. For all these enzymes, except Kpn I, morph 1 corresponds to the reference sequence of Anderson et al.[1]. For Kpn I, morph 2 is the expected restriction fragment pattern based on the reference sequence. Six pairs of twins presented mtDNA sequence polymorphism. Pairs 7, 10, and 12 exhibited multiple RFLPs while the others had only one. All these RFLPs originated from the loss or the gain of restriction sites on the mtDNA genome at or near the position indicated in the table. The loci of mutation were assigned according to the report of the committee on human mtDNA[13].

Table 2 presents the mean relative changes (per cent) observed for the 12 pairs of twins after the 100-day overfeeding treatment. Morphological characteristics of the monozygotic twins changed considerably with the overfeeding protocol. The mean increase in body weight and BMI was about 14 per cent while the fat mass (in kg or per cent), the ratio of fat mass over fat-free mass and the different skinfold thicknesses were increased by 50 to 130 per cent. The mean increase in fat-free mass (kg) was much lower (5 per cent). RMR (kJ), total TEM (kJ) and TEM minus RMR (kJ) increased on the average by about 6 to 10 per cent. Interindividual differences in the response to the overfeeding protocol were observed as indicated by the high standard deviation values. However, as reported earlier by Bouchard et al.[2], the within-twin pair resemblance in response to overfeeding was significant. In other words, members of each pair were more similar in the response pattern than individuals of various pairs.

Table 1. Mitochondrial DNA RFLP analysis in 12 pairs of monozygotic twins

Twin pair number	Restriction enzyme*	Morphs number detected	Position of mutation (bp)†	Site gain (+) or loss (−)	Locus of mutation‡
12	Ava II	3	16390†	−	D-loop
10		5	8270	+	MTCO2
			16390†	−	D-loop
10, 12	Bam HI	2	16350	+	D-loop
5	BstNI	2	13705	−	MTND5
7		3	16505	+	D-loop
6	Hae II	2	9052†	−	MTATP6
10		3	4533	−	MTND2
10, 11	Kpn I	1	16133	−	D-loop
7	Pst I	3	9024	−	MTATP6

* No polymorphism was detected with the enzymes Bcl I, Dra I, Eco RI, Eco RV, Hinc II, Hind III, Hpa I, Msp I, Nci I, Nco I, Pvu II, Sac I, Sca I, Stu I, Xba I, Xho I.
† Sites identified in the reference sequence of Anderson et al.[1], which are accurate to the nucleotide. The other sites are only estimated since they have been assigned by restriction mapping.
‡ Gene loci of mutation correspond to mitochondrial (MT) subunit II of cytochrome c oxidase (MTCO2), to subunit 6 of the ATPase (MTATP6), to subunits 2 and 5 of NADH dehydrogenase (MTND2 and MTND5).

Table 2. Relative changes induced by 100 day of overfeeding in 12 pairs of twins and the pair with the lowest and highest gains

Phenotype	Relative change (%) Mean ± SD	Pair of twins	
		Lowest gainer	Highest gainer
Weight, kg	13.7 ± 43	# 12**	# 10***
BMI, kg/m^2	13.7 ± 43	# 12**	# 10***
% fat	75.2 ± 55.4	# 12**	# 3
Fat mass, kg	99.7 ± 64.5	# 12**	# 3
Fat-free mass, kg	5.3 ± 2.9	# 12**	# 1
Fat mass/fat-free mass	89.7 ± 61.4	# 12**	# 3
Σ 10 skinfolds, mm	73.0 ± 27.6	# 1	# 5*
Abdomen skin, mm	129.3 ± 63.8	# 9	# 5*
Trunk skin, mm	90.9 ± 34.6	# 1	# 5*
Extremities skin, mm	50.9 ± 22.6	# 4	# 8
T/E	38.0 ± 14	# 1	# 7**
RMR, kJ	10.1 ± 8.7	# 6*	# 10***
TEM, kJ	8.2 ± 6.9	# 4	# 9
TEM minus RMR, kJ	6.6 ± 25.7	# 4	# 7**

* Carriers of one mtDNA variant; ** carriers of two mtDNA variants; *** carrier of four mtDNA variants.

We then looked for an association between the relative changes induced by the overfeeding treatment and the presence of mtDNA variants in these pairs of twins. As none of the mtDNA variants were present in a sufficiently large number of pairs, statistical analyses could not be performed. Instead, we compared pairs of twins who were the lowest and highest gainers for each phenotype. As shown in Table 2, pair 12, carrier of two mtDNA variants in the D-Loop, had the lowest relative changes in body weight and body composition variables. For RMR, pair 6, carrier of one variant in the ATPase subunit 6 locus, was the lowest gainer. For all other phenotypes listed in this Table, non carriers of mtDNA variants exhibited the lowest response. Interestingly, the highest gainers were mainly found in the carriers of mtDNA variants. Pair 10, carrier of four mtDNA variants located in the D-Loop and the NADH subunit 2, was the highest gainer in body weight, BMI and RMR. Pair 5, carrier of one mtDNA variant in the NADH subunit 5, presented the highest relative changes in subcutaneous fat. Finally, the highest gainer for the ratio T/E and the TEM minus RMR phenotype was pair 7, carrier of two mtDNA variants located in the D-Loop and the ATPase subunit 6.

Discussion

This study attempts to identify human DNA markers associated with the response to positive energy balance. The overfeeding study involving 12 pairs of monozygotic twins provided an opportunity to look for associations between the response of body weight, body composition, metabolic rates and mtDNA variants.

Several mtRFLPs were detected in these 12 pairs of twins. These results were expected since mtDNA is known to be very polymorphic even among individual of the same ethnic group[4,5,7-9]. Even though the results presented in this paper are essentially descriptive, they suggest that mtDNA sequence variation might be important in the response to overfeeding. Indeed, lowest gainers for each phenotype were generally pairs of twins carrying one or two mtDNA variants and, perhaps even more importantly, a large majority of the highest gainers were carrying mtDNA variants in the regulatory region of the D-loop. The fact that carriers of mtDNA variants were found in both the lowest and highest gainers, suggests that mtDNA polymorphism could have a positive or negative influence on the response to overfeeding, possibly through its impact on metabolic rate. Given the small number of genotypes involved in the overfeeding experiment, it is not possible to establish yet whether the pattern observed is random or not. However, it is interesting to note that Rowe et al.[11] recently reported that carriers of a mtDNA variant exhibited a significantly higher BMI compared to non carriers.

These results have led us to undertake a study on a larger cohort of women exhibiting a wide range of BMI and adiposity. Preliminary results indicate that some mtDNA variants are indeed significantly associated with the phenotypic variance observed for body weight and body composition related variables (J. Truchon, L. Turcotte, T. Song, J.P. Després, C. Bouchard, F.T. Dionne, unpublished data).

Acknowledgement
Supported by the National Institutes of Health of the USA and the Fonds FCAR Quebec.

References

1. Anderson, S., Bankier, A.T., Barrell, B.G., De Bruijn, M.H.L., Coulson, A.R., Drouin, J., Eperon, I.C., Nierlich, D.P., Roe, B.A., Sanger, F., Schreier, P.H., Smith, A.J.H., Staden, R. & Young, I.G. (1981): Sequence and organization of the human mitochondrial genome. *Nature* **290**, 457-465.
2. Bouchard, C., Tremblay, A., Després, J.P., Nadeau, A., Lupien, P.J., Thériault, G., Dusseault, J., Moorjani, S., Pineault, S. & Fournier, G. (1990): The response to long-term overfeeding in identical twins. *N. Engl. J. Med.* **322**, 1477-1482.
3. Bouchard, C., Tremblay, A., Nadeau, A., Després, J.P., Thériault, G., Boulay, M.R., Lortie, G., Leblanc, C. & Fournier, G. (1989): Genetic effect in resting and exercise metabolic rates. *Metabolism* **38**, 364-370.

4. Brega, A., Gardella, R., Semino, O., Morpurgo, G., Astaldi Ricotti, G.B., Wallace, D.C. & Santachiara Benerecetti, A.S. (1986a): Genetic studies on the Tharu population of Nepal: restriction endonuclease polymorphisms of mitochondrial DNA. *Am. J. Hum. Genet.* **39**, 502-512.
5. Brega, A., Scozzari, R., Maccioni, L., Iodice, C., Wallace, D.C., Bianco, I., Cao, A. & Santachiara Benerecetti, A.S. (1986b): Mitochondrial DNA polymorphisms in Italy. I. Population data from Sardinia and Rome. *Ann. Hum. Genet.* **50**, 327-338.
6. Dionne, F.T., Turcotte, L., Thibault, M.C., Boulay, M.R., Skinner, J.S. & Bouchard, C. (1991): Mitochondrial DNA sequence polymorphism, VO_2max, and response to endurance training. *Med. Sci. Sports Exerc.* **23**, 177-185.
7. Gelinas, Y., Turcotte, L., Bouchard, C., Thibault, M.C. & Dionne, F.T. (1989): Mitochondrial DNA polymorphism detected with the restriction enzymes Bst NI and Bcl I in a French Canadian population. *Ann. Hum. Genet.* **53**, 319-325.
8. Horai, S., Gojobori, T. & Matsunaga, E. (1984): Mitochondrial DNA polymorphism in Japanese. I. Analysis with restriction enzymes of six base pair recognition. *Hum. Genet.* **68**, 324-332.
9. Johnson, M.J., Wallace, D.C., Ferris, S.D., Rattazzi, M.C. & Cavalli-Sforza, L.L. (1983): Radiation of human mitochondria DNA types analysed by restriction endonuclease cleavage patterns. *J. Mol. Evol.* **19**, 255-271.
10. Poehlman, E.T., Tremblay, A., Després, J.P., Fontaine, E., Pérusse, L., Thériault, G. & Bouchard, C. (1986): Genotype-controlled changes in body composition and fat morphology following overfeeding in twins. *Am. J. Clin. Nut.* **43**, 723-731.
11. Rowe, M., Bremm, G., Cooper, J. & Perry, J. (1991): Mitochondrial DNA polymorphism in inherited increased BMI. *FASEB J.* **5**, abstract 708.
12. Southern, E.M. (1975): Detection of specific sequences among DNA fragments separated by gel electrophoresis. *J. Mol. Biol.* **98**, 503-517.
13. Wallace, D.C. (1989): Report of the committee on human mitochondrial DNA. *Cytogenet. Cell Genet.* **51**, 612-621.

Section XI
Adipose tissue metabolism and regional distribution

Chapter 66

Psychosocial Factors and Fat Distribution

Per BJÖRNTORP
Department of Medicine 1, Sahlgren's Hospital, University of Gothenburg, Sweden

Clinical observations have shown that conditions with high cortisol secretion and low sex-steroid-hormone production are associated with visceral fat accumulation. Appropriate interventions to correct these aberrations seem to be followed by a diminution of visceral fat mass.

The regulatory factors of regional fat distribution include sex steroid hormones in combination with nervous and circulatory factors. The regional effects of the former are probably mediated *via* specific receptors for these hormones. The glucocorticoid and androgen receptors probably have a high density in visceral fat. The glucocorticoid receptor seems to express the activity of mainly fat accumulating enzymes, counteracted by progesterone in competition over this receptor. The density of the androgen receptor is upregulated by testosterone and this receptor expresses lipolytic β-adrenergic receptors. An elevated cortisol secretion particularly in combination with low sex-steroid-hormone secretions, would therefore presumably result in visceral fat accumulation, in excellent agreement with the clinical observations.

Subjects with visceral fat accumulation without obvious, known endocrine disorders, have signs of an increased sensitivity of the hypothalamo-adrenal cortex axis, and increased cortisol production under "field" conditions. They also have decreased sex steroid hormone productions, particularly of testosterone (men) and progesterone (women). The latter phenomenon might be secondary to an inhibition by corticotrophin-releasing factor of gonadotropin-releasing hormone. This would mean a functional hypercortisolism, and the similarities of the syndrome of visceral fat accumulation with Cushing's syndrome, although less dramatic, then becomes obvious. In addition, there is evidence emerging of the regulation of central haemodynamics by stress similar to that seen in defeat situations.

This set of endocrine and circulatory signs of hypothalamic arousal is reminiscent of systematization of stress responses in the defence or defeat reactions, well described in experimental animals. Men and women with visceral fat accumulation often suffer from psycho-social handicaps with psychosomatic and psychiatric disease expressions, which might be signs of a stressful environment to which they react with insufficient coping and a defeat reaction. If this turns out to be correct, the neuroendocrine, endocrine and circulatory abnormalities, as well as visceral fat accumulation, might be explained along these lines. Recent work in the experimental animal suggests that this is indeed the correct interpretation, because both primates and rats react with such endocrine aberrations, followed by metabolic derangement, hypertension, visceral accumulation of fat, as well as coronary atherosclerosis and decreased glucose tolerance with insulin resistance, a picture identical to that already reported in humans with abdominal obesity.

Introduction

The clinical importance of accumulation of body fat in visceral adipose depots has recently been documented. There are statistical correlations, not only to diabetes and cardio-cerebrovascular disease, but also to established risk factors for these diseases (for review, see[2]). Intensive research during the past few years has attempted to find out potential explanations to these statistical associations. Different alternatives seem plausible, as outlined schemati-

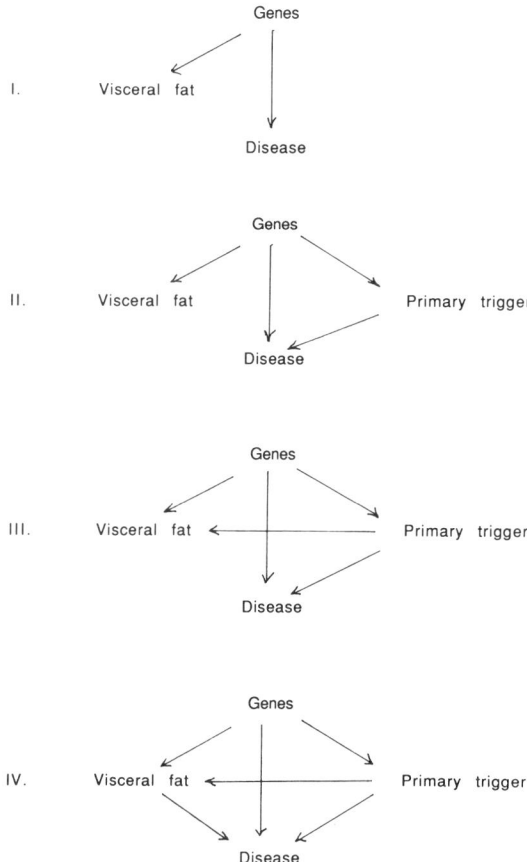

Fig. 1. *Principal possibilities of disease-generating mechanisms involving genetic predisposition for visceral fat accumulation involving an intermediary, primary trigger factor. These factors might act separately, in combination or by amplification as outlined in different alternatives (for details see text).*

cally in Fig. 1. Similar to most other clinical situations there is a genetic background to the expression of the syndrome in question, most likely at several points, as the diseases in question are no doubt polygenic. Genetic predispositions may then, as a first alternative in Fig. 1, act separately on the mechanisms for visceral fat accumulation and disease expression. Another alternative (II) is involvement of a primary trigger of disease, which might also be involved in the accumulation of visceral fat (III). Finally, visceral fat may be the disease-generating factor itself, or amplify the mechanisms leading to disease triggered by a primary factor (IV). There is currently evidence for all these alternatives, and they may well contribute to the syndrome with combined effects (for review, see[2]).

Although the predisposition to the expression of these various phenomena has a genetic base, there is no doubt that environmental factors also play important roles, and interfere at different points in these schemes. In the present overview, the influence of environmental factors on visceral fat accumulation will be placed in focus. This is of obvious importance, whatever the correct alternative turns out to be in the putative cause–effect chains, because visceral fat accumulation may either be an indicator of disease (Fig. 1, alts. I-III) and/or be directly involved in the mechanisms precipitating disease (alt. IV).

What causes visceral fat accumulation?

As in many other situations, clinical observations provide a good start for generation of hypotheses. Cushing's syndrome provides the most dramatic expression of visceral fat accumulation. This phenomenon is specifically reversible with successful treatment of the excess cortisol production, as observed with computerized tomography (CT) techniques[36]. These observations show that increased cortisol production is involved in this syndrome. This is supported by other studies of regional distribution of fat after exogenous administration of corticosteroids, for therapeutic purposes utilizing measurements of fat-cell size as an instrument[23]. Conditions with functional hypercortisolism such as alcohol consumption and tobacco smoking are also associated with visceral fat accumulation, providing further evidence along this line[7,14].

There are, also, additional clinical and physiological situations strongly suggesting that fat distribution is also regulated by sex steroid hormones. Ageing with relative hypogonadism in men, as well as menopause in women are associated with visceral fat accumulation. Intervention with substitution of testosterone seems to be followed by diminution of visceral fat masses in hypogonadal men[28]. Women on replacement therapy after menopause have less visceral fat, and similar to young women, have characteristics of peripheral adipose tissue, directing storage fat to these depots.[31] These intervention studies then strongly suggest that the sex steroid hormones are also involved in the distribution of body fat. In contrast to cortisol, sex steroid hormone effects are preventing visceral fat accumulation and/or directing depot fat into peripheral adipose tissue regions. Taken together these observations include several well-defined endocrinological situations, where the hormonal secretions that are associated with visceral fat accumulation are well characterized and counteracted by appropriate interventions. In summary, these observations strongly suggest that glucocorticoids direct depot fat to visceral adipose tissues while the sex steroid hormones exert opposite effects.

Factors that regulate fat accumulation in adipose tissue regions

The size of an adipose tissue depot is dependent on the triglyceride contents of its adipocytes. This in turn is the end-result of the balance between rates of lipid input and mobilization from the fat cells. The main source of adipocyte triglyceride in man is probably exogenous lipid, arriving at the adipocyte *via* the capillary system and its lipoprotein lipase (LPL) trap, where it is hydrolysed and accumulated in the cells. The main rate-limiting steps here seem to be substrate availability and LPL activity. The former factor is dependent on the concentration of triglyceride in the capillary circulation in the adipose tissue region in question. Probably this seldom reaches concentrations where LPL activity is rate limiting. The distribution of exogenous fat in different adipose tissue regions is thus dependent on the distribution of the triglycerides in the adipose tissue capillaries in different regions, in combination with a sufficient activation of LPL. In summary, regional blood flow and sufficient LPL activity seem to be the main regulatory factors for regional triglyceride uptake.

Lipid mobilization is regulated in an analogous way. A first step requires hydrolysis of stored triglyceride. This is occurring *via* another lipase system, dependent on activation of adrenergic receptors at the cell surface. In man, the sympathetic nervous system seems to be the main provider of signals through these receptors. The adrenergic receptors are of the β- (stimulatory) or α_2 (inhibitory) subtypes. Sufficient blood flow is also of major importance for this regulation; accumulation of the lipolytic product of free fatty acids (FFA) tends to inhibit the lipolytic machinery by feedback mechanisms. Insulin plays an important role in the inhibition of the lipolytic activity. The regional aspects of this regulation then include mainly the sympathetic nervous system and circulatory factors, including insulin.

The next question, then, is how these factors provide their regulation in different regions, focusing mainly on visceral fat. Lipid uptake is considerably higher in visceral adipose tissue than subcutaneous depots, measured in man *in vivo*[27]. This is not necessarily dependent on a rate-limiting effect of LPL, but may well depend primarily on a high blood flow through this tissue[37]. To maintain a steady state of visceral adipose tissue mass, lipid mobilization must be equally, proportionally elevated, and both *in vivo*[6] and *in vitro*[30] measurements have shown this to be the case. This includes the antilipolytic effect of insulin which is less marked in visceral than subcutaneous depots. The main regulators of the high lipolytic activity and fat mobilization in visceral adipose tissue seem to be a high blood flow[37], and an abundance of sympathetic nerve endings[29] exerting their effects *via* a high density of β-adrenergic receptors[1]. The blunted antilipolytic effect of insulin also contributes importantly to the potential of lipid mobilization of visceral adipose tissues[4].

The next question then is, how do the steroid hormones influence these rate-limiting steps of triglyceride mass balance, particularly in visceral fat? This area has recently been reviewed[3] and the reader may find detailed references in that review. A brief outline will be given in the following. The effects of these hormones are mediated *via* specific receptors. A difference in density of these receptors in different adipose regions would presumably regulate the impact of steroid hormone effects. It seems likely that the glucocorticoid and androgen receptors have a particularly high density in visceral fat. The net result of this would be a high turnover of visceral fat, because cortisol expresses LPL activity while testosterone expresses lipolytically active β-adrenergic receptors. This is probably amplified by the ability of testosterone to "upregulate" the androgen receptor density[9]. It is noteworthy that an imbalance between these hormonal effects with cortisol secretion and low testosterone secretion would tend to give visceral fat accumulation. Progesterone competes for the glucocorticoid receptor, and thus would be expected to protect from glucocorticoid effects. Again, an imbalance between cortisol and progesterone, to the advantage of the former, would give mainly cortisol-dominating net effects, *viz* fat accumulation, particularly in visceral fat with high glucocorticoid-receptor density.

There is thus evidence at the cellular and molecular level that cortisol secretion, not balanced by appropriate secretions of male or female sex steroid hormones, would result in visceral fat accumulation. This, then, provides an explanation to the clinical and physiological findings of visceral fat accumulation with this endocrine imbalance, correctable with appropriate interventions as reviewed in a preceding section.

Several important pieces of information are, however, missing, and more definite conclusions cannot be arrived at before this knowledge becomes available. Very little is known about potential effects of steroid hormones on blood flow and innervation in adipose tissue, particularly potential regional differences in such actions. Both these factors play major roles for both lipid accumulation and mobilization as reviewed above. It should be noted in this context that corticosteroids[11] as well as testosterone[39] exert "permissive" effects on catecholamine-stimulated lipolysis. The dense catecholaminergic supply to visceral adipose tissue[29] may in this way increase the efficiency of lipid mobilization from it, under the influence of cortisol and/or testosterone. Another area of incomplete knowledge is the regional regulation of insulin receptors by steroid hormones, although it is known that insulin receptors have a low density in visceral fat[4].

It should be noted that although blood flow and innervation factors are of obvious importance, the regulatory mechanisms at the cellular level also play significant roles. Cortisol-induced variations in LPL activity are one of the determining factors, and provided blood flow does not vary with cortisol exposure, it would be the sole regulator even if substrate is provided below saturation limits. Similarly, the density of the cellular adrenoreceptors is an important, independent regulatory factor of lipolysis. The integrated system regulating regional distribution of body fat is thus complex, and current information is insufficient to understand its details. The net results are, however, seen in physiological and clinical conditions with the different balances between cortisol and sex steroid hormones described above. The intervention studies introducing changes in the balance of these hormones are particularly helpful towards understanding them. These observations indicate that cortisol directs accumulation of storage triglycerides to visceral fat, while sex steroid hormones counteract this, and may instead facilitate storage in peripheral depots. The information available at the cellular and molecular level of adipose tissue provides a possible mechanism for this to occur, although much more information is needed to understand fully the details involved.

The endocrine characteristics associated with visceral fat accumulation

With this background it becomes important to decide whether endocrine aberrations follow subjects with a preponderance of visceral fat, who have no defined endocrinological disease such as Cushing's syndrome. In other words what is the endocrine status of obese (or non-obese) subjects in the general population who have an increased proportion of adipose tissue triglyceride in visceral depots? Of particular interest here is obviously whether one might trace similarities to the cortisol-sex steroid hormone imbalance, described above, in such persons. As will be reviewed in the following this seems indeed to be the case.

Cortisol

Starting with cortisol, previous studies have suggested that urinary output of metabolites of adrenal corticosteroids and androgens is increased[24]. We have during the past few years devoted much work to this important question. Urinary output of free cortisol shows a moderate increase with increased central obesity. It should be noted that this is not immediately apparent and requires large materials and studies under "field" conditions. In other words, the increased output may not be detectable under steady state conditions, but requires an influence of the daily activities of the subjects examined. This increased secretion is much more clear when challenged with stimuli at different levels of the corticotrophin releasing factor (CRF)-adrenocorticotrophin hormone (ACTH)-cortisol axis. ACTH-stimulation tests give a clearly elevated response in subjects with central obesity as compared with peripheral obesity. Dexamethasone inhibition tests are, however, normal. Furthermore, laboratory stress-tests also reveal increased responsiveness along the CRF-ACTH-cortisol axis, including both mental and physical stressors. Taken together this information indicates an increased sensitivity or readiness of the hypothalamo-CRF-ACTH-cortisol axis in subjects with abdominal depot fat accumulation[8].

It is of considerable interest that recent work in the obese *(fa/fa)* rat has shown almost identical results. Such rats have an increased corticosterone excretion, sensitive to stimuli at the adrenal and central, hypothalamic levels, normally inhibited by dexamethasone[15]. In addition to obesity these rats, like abdominal obese humans, have derangements in lipid and carbohydrate metabolism as well as hypertension. This whole syndrome can be totally abolished by adrenalectomy ([15] and refs. therein) providing evidence that hyperactivity along the hypothalamo-adrenal axis might be the origin of this condition. Our recent data suggest that the human condition may indeed be explained by a similar mechanism.

Sex steroid hormones

Sex-steroid-hormone secretions are also deranged in human abdominal obesity. In men, free testosterone levels are low, and sex-hormone-binding globulin levels elevated. Interestingly enough, this seems to be the case even if obesity is not pronounced[27,34].

Female sex-steroid-hormone secretions are also abnormal. Although oestrogen concentrations appear normal, menstrual irregularities, as well as amenorrhea followed by low progesterone secretion, have been reported[17]. Although not examined, these abnormalities of sex-steroid-hormone secretions are probably mainly due to aberrations in the balance of gonadotrophin secretions.

It has recently been reported that increased CRF production is inhibiting the secretion of gonadotrophin-releasing hormone and thereby the gonadotrophins[33]. The interesting possibility is thus apparent that the combined secretory abnormalities along the hypothalamo-CRF-ACTH axis and the gonadotrophin axis may indeed be due to hyperactivity in the former. In other words, an increased activity along the hypothalamo-adrenal axis in subjects with visceral preponderance of body fat might be a primary factor in the multiple endocrine aberrations seen in this condition.

Evidence is thus now available indicating that subjects in the population with abdominal preponderance of body fat have an endocrine aberration with a "functional" oversecretion of cortisol, and a low secretion of particularly testosterone and progesterone. This would be a situation of an imbalance of the secretions of cortisol (elevated) and sex steroid hormones (diminished), typical for other conditions with visceral fat accumulation, as reviewed in a preceding section. Although less dramatic the analogies with the Cushing's syndrome are rather obvious. It is therefore suggested that these endocrine aberrations actually direct depot fat to visceral depots, and that the basic cause of visceral obesity is of hypothalamo-adrenal origin. Returning back to Fig. 1, the factor labelled the primary trigger might at least partly consist of this hypothalamo-adrenal endocrine aberration.

Circulatory regulation

Recent studies have also shown that circulatory factors are related to obesity and body fat distribution. In young normobesive men examined for central haemodynamics at rest and during standardized mental stress, obesity, measured as the BMI, was followed by increased cardiac output and stroke volume at rest, augmented during mental stress where blood pressure rose and peripheral resistance decreased. In contrast, abdominal distribution of body fat was inversely related to cardiac output and stroke volume, again amplified with stress when peripheral resistance rose with blood pressure increase, and there was a tendency to decreased heart rate. This meant that the blood pressure rise following obesity was dependent mainly on increased cardiac output, but with abdominal fat distribution this rise was accomplished mainly by an elevated peripheral resistance[21]. Recent echocardiographic studies show a concentric cardiac hypertrophy in subjects with elevated WHR, an expected consequence of the mentioned haemodynamic reaction[38].

The response of central dynamics to stress were thus completely different when obesity and abdominal fat distribution were compared. With obesity, cardiac output-dependent pressor responses were dominating, which is the classic defence response in both man and experimental animals[5,12]. The increased stroke volume might be related either to increased blood volume, or increased heart volume[38]. In contrast, abdominal distribution was followed by a vasoconstrictor type of response with a depressed reaction of central haemodynamics. Interestingly, this type of response has previously been observed in rats after short-term immobilization stress, eliciting a defeat type of stress reaction[16]. This reaction is far less defined from a haemodynamic point of view than the defence reaction but includes peripheral vasoconstriction in combination with downregulation of central haemodynamics, as well as increased vagal activity with peptic ulcer formation[12].

Other recent studies have shown that response to stress is different during physiological hyperinsulinaemia, where a cardiac-output dependent pressor response was changed to a vasoconstriction type of response[20] similar to that seen in relation to abdominal distribution of body fat. Insulin levels did not correlate with the vasoconstriction response in the young men with abdominal fat distribution, however[21].

The vasoconstriction type of stress response is thus found in association with abdominal fat distribution and with hyperinsulinaemia. Furthermore, under defined stress resulting in a defeat type of stress reaction this is seen, as well as a compensatory downregulation of central haemodynamics, similar to that found with abdominal fat distribution. The mechanisms behind this reaction pattern might be central or peripheral, but they are clearly distinct from the normal, classical type of response by mainly augmentation of central haemodynamics. The central haemodynamics associated with abdominal fat are thus similar to those seen as a defeat reaction to stress.

What is the cause of the endocrine and circulatory aberrations in visceral obesity?

These new data then suggest that central haemodynamics react differently to mental stress. A defence reaction to stress is typical of obesity, while a defeat type of reaction is seen with abdominal fat distribution. Furthermore, as reviewed in a preceding section abdominal obesity is followed by a neuroendocrine stress reaction *via* the hypothalamo-adrenal axis.

This set of observations is reminiscent of arousal reactions at the level of hypothalamus, which are well described in the experimental animal. There are two typical endocrine and circulatory responses elicited *via* neuroendrocrine mechanisms. One has been called the defence reaction and is characterized by an arousal of the central sympathetic nervous system, while the defeat reaction leads to an endocrine arousal over the hypothalamo-adrenal axis with low steroid hormone secretions. In circulation this is followed by a vasoconstrictor response in combination with depressed central haemodynamics. These are the reactions to perceived stimuli to various types of stressful environmental factors[19]. They are often mixed or alter from one type of response to another[18]. Humans also respond principally in this way, although isolated responses of one specific type are probably seldom seen[13] and the reactions are probably mixed. It is of interest that both alcohol and tobacco smoking elicit neuroendocrine reactions over the hypothalamo-adrenal axis, in other words the same as the defeat reaction.

It is apparent then that abdominal fat distribution is followed by the defeat type of reaction, both in the neuroendocrine, hypothalamo-adrenal axis, as well as in central haemodynamics. Obesity without regional distinction then seems to be different. In haemodynamic variables the response seems to be mainly that of the classical defence reaction. Such reaction pattern has been suggested to be a precursor to primary hypertension[22], based on a rather firm body of observations, including sensitivity to stress factors, which produce central sympathetic arousal in subjects with early primary hypertension[10].

A clinical counterpart to the defeat type of reaction has, however, never been identified. It seems possible that the syndrome of visceral obesity might be such a condition. A mixed reaction would embrace visceral obesity with hypertension.

If this is the correct alternative one would expect stress-reactions of mainly a defeat type to be typical for subjects with visceral distribution of body fat. In the following, recent observations will be presented which give evidence that this might indeed be the case.

In population studies psychosocial factors have recently been analysed in relation to distribution of body fat to abdominal areas[25,26]. It was then found that men with such characteristics belong to a low social class, have a low degree of education and a poorly paid, physical type of job. They are often sick and absent from work. Psychosomatic diseases such as peptic ulcer are frequently seen, as well as tobacco smoking and alcohol overconsumption.

These observations might be interpreted to mean that these men were pressurized by environmental, socio-economic factors with which they had difficulties in coping. The result may well be absenteeism, poor health and increased use of stimulants. The high prevalence of peptic ulcers is noteworthy because this has specifically been linked to the defeat reaction[12,16]. Specific professions could not be traced directly, but this seems to be a group belonging to a low social class with unskilled labour.

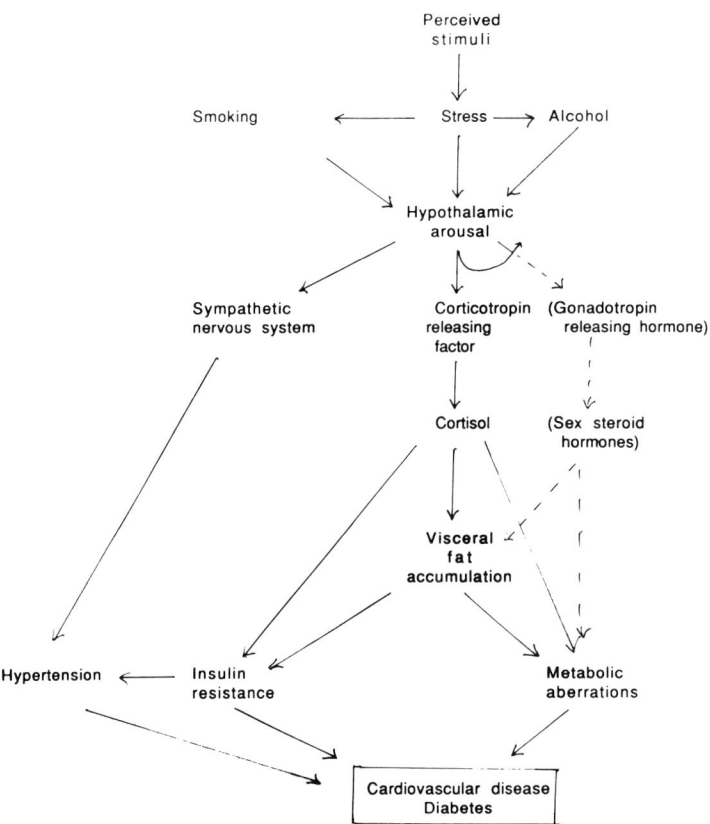

Fig. 2. A cause–effect chain explaining the statistical association between visceral fat accumulation and disease. Stress, smoking and alcohol (level 1) express a hypothalamic arousal syndrome (2) with neuroendocrine disturbances (3), endocrine aberrations (4), visceral fat accumulation (5), disease risk factors (triggers) (6) and disease (7).

The observations in women were partly parallel, but showed some interesting differences. First, social class did not play such a dominant role. Instead women with abdominal accumulation of body fat had psychological characteristics typical of the sensation-seeking personality with high scores in extroversion and affiliation. This might lead such women into frustration and strain, leading to a chronic arousal (stress) syndrome. They also often had peptic ulcer and signs of anxiety and depressive disorders. Infections and accidents as well as use of tobacco and alcohol were also frequently reported among these women. All these phenomena might be the consequences of a chronic stress reaction of a mixed defence-defeat type, dependent on an inability to cope with environmental pressures. A woman with these characteristics may be exposed to strains either in a pressurized home environment and/or in a professional environment with high demands, such as might be experienced by some women in responsible executive positions. Recent observations indicate that both alternatives might indeed be valid.

The observations reviewed might well provide a combination of psychosocial factors leading to external pressures in certain type of personalities who are prone to react with responses of the defeat type in particular. By neuroendocrine mechanisms they may therefore frequently develop an arousal along the hypothalamo-adrenal cortex axis with visceral fat

Chapter 66 – Psychosocial Factors and Fat Distribution

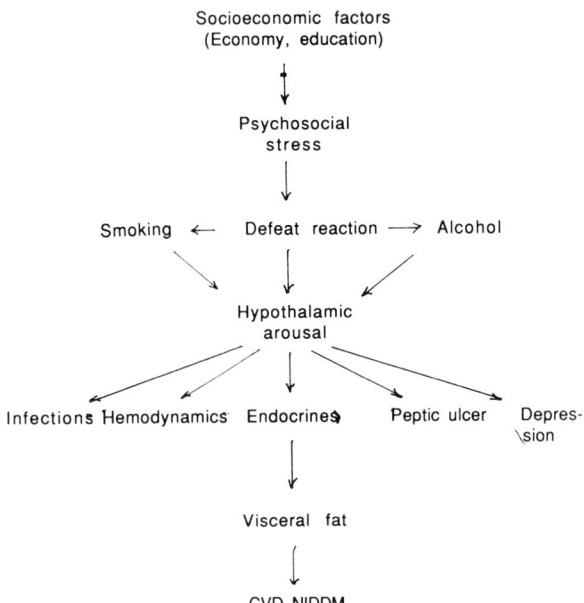

Fig. 3. Putative connections between psychosocial factors eliciting a defeat reaction with a number of consequences in various functional systems, all found associated with visceral fat accumulation. Factors within circles have been observed in recent studies (for references, see text).

accumulation, combined with metabolic derangement. They may also have a specific vasoconstriction type of haemodynamic reaction, and their proneness to develop infections and ulcers might be another less well-defined part of a neuroendocrine activity[12,16,25]. This possibility is actually supported on each point of the chain linking visceral fat accumulation with endocrine disturbances, hypertension, psychosomatic disease and metabolic aberrations. This kind of mechanism may also provide the missing link between psychosocial factors and cardio-cerebrovascular disease. Further research along these lines may therefore be rewarding.

Recent work in the experimental animal provides strong support that the suggested mechanisms are indeed correct. In primates, standardized, psychosocial stress actually produces reactions which are identical to those seen in humans with visceral fat accumulation. Such animals actually react with neuroendocrine responses of a similar type, followed by increased secretion of corticosteroids, low sex-steroid-hormone production, hypertension and deranged carbohydrate-lipid metabolism, as well as coronary atherosclerosis. They also develop central fat accumulation[35]. Furthermore, rats subjected to uncontrollable stress specifically increase the size of the mesenteric (visceral) fat depot with an increased LPL activity, parallel to increased corticosterone production[32]. These data are closely similar to those already reported in humans[25,26], and suggest that the interpretation of the observations in humans put forward above are indeed correct.

The presumed chain of events reviewed here, coupling visceral fat accumulation with primary reactions to perceived stress, followed by endocrine aberrations and generation of disease risk factors is summarized in Fig. 2.

The putative correlations between psychosocial factors, the defeat reaction and its consequences are depicted in more detail in a summary in Fig. 3.

References

1. Arner, P. (1989): Regulation of lipolysis in different regions of human adipose tissue. In *Obesity in Europe*, eds. P. Björntorp & S. Rossner, pp. 201-208. London: John Libbey.
2. Björntorp, P. (1990): Obesity and diabetes. *Diabetes Annu.* **5**, 373-395.
3. Björntorp, P., Ottosson, M., Rebuffé-Scrive & Xu, X. (1990): Regional obesity and steroid hormone interactions in human adipose tissue. In *Obesity: towards a molecular approach*, UCLA Symposia on Molecular and Cellular Biology, eds. G.A. Bray, D. Ricquier & B. Spiegelman, Vol. 132, pp. 147-157. New York: Wiley-Liss.
4. Bolinder, J., Kager, L., Östman, J. & Arner, P. (1983): Differences at the receptor and postreceptor levels between human omental and subcutaneous adipose tissue in the action of insulin on lipolysis. *Diabetes* **32**, 117-123.
5. Brod, J. (1960): Essential hypertension: haemodynamic observations with a bearing on its pathogenesis. *Lancet* **ii**, 773-778.
6. Chowdury, B., Kvist, H., Sjöström, L., Andersson, B. & Björntorp, P. (1990): Multiscan CT-determined changes in adipose tissue distribution during a small weight reduction of obese males. *Am. J. Clin. Nutr.* in print.
7. Cicero, T.J. (1982): Alcohol-induced deficits in the hypothalamic luteinizing hormone axis in the male. *Alcohol. Clin. Exper. Res.* **6**, 207-229.
8. Darin, N., Amemeya, T., Andersson, P., Mårin, P., Jern, S. & Björntorp, P. (1991): Cortisol secretion in relation to body fat distribution in obese premenopausal women. Submitted.
9. De Pergola, G., Xu, X., Yang, S., Giorgino, P. & Björntorp, P. (1990): Up regulation of androgren-receptor binding in male rat adipose precursor cells exposed to testosterone: study in a whole cell assay system. *J. Steroid Biochem.* **37**, 553-558.
10. Eliasson, K., Hjelmdahl, P. & Kahan, T. (1983): Circulatory and sympathoadrenal responses to stress in borderline and established hypertension. *J. Hypertens.* **1**, 131-139.
11. Fain, J.N., Kovacev, V.P. & Scow, R.O. (1965): Effects of growth hormone and dexamethasone on lipolysis and metabolism in isolated fat cells of the rat. *J. Biol. Chem.* **240**, 3522-3528.
12. Folkow, B. (1987): Physiology of behaviour and blood pressure regulation in animals. In *Handbook of hypertension: behavioral factors in hypertension*, vol. 9, eds. S. Julius & D.R. Bassett, pp. 1-18. Amsterdam: Elsevier.
13. Frankenhaeuser, M. (1983): The sympathetic-adrenal and pituitary-adrenal responses to challenge: comparisons between the sexes. In *Bio-behavioural bases of coronary heart disease, human psychophysiology*, Biobehavioral Medicine Series, vol. 2, eds. T.M. Dombrowski, T.H. Schmidt & G. Blümchen, pp. 91-105. Basel: Karger.
14. Friedman, A.J., Raoniker, V.A. & Barbieri, R.L. (1987): Serum steroid hormone profiles in postmenopausal smokers and non-smokers. *Fertil. Steril.* **47**, 398-401.
15. Guillaume-Gentil, C., Rohner-Jeaunrenaud, F., Abramo, F., Bestetti, G.E., Rossi, G.L. & Jeanrenaud, B. (1990): Abnormal regulation of the hypothalamo-pituitary-adrenal axis in the genetically obese fa/fa rat. *Endocrinology* **126**, 1873-1879.
16. Hallbäck, M., Magnusson, G. & Weiss, L. (1974): Stress-induced ulcer in spontaneously hypertensive rats. *Acta Physiol. Scand.* **91**, 617.
17. Hartz, A.J., Rupley, D.C. & Rimm, A.A. (1984): The association of girth measurements with disease in 32,856 women. *Am. J. Epidemiol.* **119**, 71-79.
18. Henry, J. & Grim, C.E. (1990): Psychosocial mechanisms in primary hypertension. *J. Hypertens.* **8**, 783-793.
19. Henry, J. & Stephens, P.M. (1977): Stress, health and social environment. *A sociobiological approach to medicine*. New York: Springer.
20. Jern, S. (1991): Effects of acute carbohydrate administration on central and peripheral hemodynamic responses to mental stress. *Hypertension* (in press).
21. Jern, S., Bergbrant, A., Björntorp, P. & Hansson, L. (1991): Relation of central hemodynamics at rest and during mental stress to obesity and body fat distribution. Submitted.
22. Julius, S., Esler, M.D. & Randall, O.S. (1975): Role of the autonomic nervous systems in mild human hypertension. *Clin. Sci. Mol. Med.* **48**, 243s-252s.

23. Krotkiewski, M., Blohmé, G., Lindholm, N. & Björntorp, P. (1986): The effects of adrenal corticosteroids on regional adipocyte size in man. *J. Clin. Endocrinol. Metab.* **42**, 91-97.
24. Krotkiewski, M., Butruk, E. & Zembrzuska, Z. (1966): Les fonctions cortico-surrenales dans les divers types morphologiques d'obesite. *Diabète* **19**, 229-233.
25. Lapidus, L., Bengtsson, C., Hällström, T. & Björntorp, P. (1989): Obesity adipose tissue distribution and health in women. Results from a population study in Gothenburg, Sweden. *Appetite* **12**, 25-35.
26. Larsson, B., Seidell, J. Svärdsudd, K., Welin, L., Tibblin, G., Wilhelmsen, L. & Björntorp, P. (1989): Obesity, adipose tissue distribution and health in men – the study of men born in 1913. *Appetite* **13**, 37-44.
27. Mårin, P., Andersson, B., Svedberg, J., Jönsson, L., Olbe, L. & Björntorp, P. (1990): Uptake of triglyceride fatty acids in total and visceral adipose tissue *in vivo* in man. *Int. J. Obes.* **14** (suppl. 2), 79.
28. Mårin, P. & Björntorp, P. (1990): Glucose tolerance, insulin sensitivity and fat distribution after androgen treatment of middle aged, obese men. Submitted.
29. Rebuffé-Scrive, M. (1991): Personal communication.
30. Rebuffé-Scrive, M., Andersson, B., Olbe, L. & Björntorp, P. (1989): Metabolism of adipose tissue in intraabdominal depots in non-obese men and women. *Metabolism* **38**, 453-458.
31. Rebuffé-Scrive, M. & Björntorp, P. (1985): Regional adipose tissue metabolism in man. In *Metabolic complications of human obesities*, eds. J. Vague., et al., pp. 149-159. Amsterdam: Excerpta Medica.
32. Rebuffé-Scrive, M., Walsh, U.A., McEwen, B. & Rodin, J. (1991): Effect of chronic stress on regional distribution of fat. Submitted.
33. Rivier, C. & Vale, W. (1989): Influence of coricotrophin-releasing factor on reproductive functions in the rat. *Endocrinology* **114**, 914-921.
34. Seidell, J.C., Björntorp, P., Sjöström, L., Kvist, H. & Sannerstedt, R. (1990): Visceral fat accumulation in men is positively associated with insulin, glucose, and C-peptide levels but negatively with testosterone levels. *Metabolism* **39**, 897-901.
35. Shively, C.A., Clarkson, T.B., Miller, C. & Weingard, K.W. (1987): Body fat distribution as a risk factor for coronary artery atherosclerosis in female *Cynomolgus* monkeys. *Atherosclerosis* **7**, 226-231.
36. Sjöström, L. (1991): Methods for measurement of the total and visceral adipose tissue volume, and relationships between visceral fat and disease in 1006 severely obese subjects. In *Progress in obesity research 1990*, eds. Y. Oomura, S. Tarui, S. Inoue & T. Shimazu. London: John Libbey.
37. West, D.B., Prinz, W.A. & Greenwood, M.R.C. (1989): Regional changes in adipose tissue blood flow and metabolism in rats after a meal. *Am. J. Physiol.* **257**, R711-R716.
38. Wikstrand, J., Pettersson, P. & Björntorp, P. (1991): In preparation.
39. Xu, X., de Pergola, G. & Björntorp, P. (1990): The effects of androgens on the regulation of lipolysis in adipose precursor cells. *Endocrinology* **12**, 1229-1234.

Chapter 67

Plasma Glucagon Levels in Upper Body Obesity. Glucagon–lipid Interactions

Luc Van GAAL, Greet VANSANT and Ivo De LEEUW
University of Antwerp, (UIA), Department of Endocrinology, Metabolic Diseases and Clinical Nutrition, Universiteitsplein 1, B-2610 Antwerp, Belgium

Introduction

Although glucagon behaviour in obesity remains controversial, hyperglucagonaemia has been reported in obese patients especially in those subjects with fatty liver and hypertriglyceridaemia[7]. The role of glucagon in obesity was studied initially about one decade ago and is not so clear. Normal, elevated and decreased levels have been reported under various conditions. Wise and co-workers reported that glucagon levels were reduced in overall obesity[9]. Kalkhoff on the contrary, using arginine as the glucagon secretagogue, reported elevated glucagon secretion in obesity[5]. These differences could have been explained by different quantities of CHO ingestion prior to the tests and by differences in methodology of glucagon measurements. Gossain et al. showed that glucagon responses to arginine were exaggerated in diabetic patients who represented states of relative or absolute hypoinsulinaemia as well as in obese nondiabetic subjects who manifested hyperinsulinaemia[3].

Since the accumulation of abdominal fat may reflect differences in metabolic and hormonal responsiveness of adipose tissue, we evaluated glucagon levels in obese men with upper and lower body obesity.

Patients and methods

Seventy-two obese men (mean age ± SD, 35.3 ± 10.4 years) attending the out-patient obesity clinic, were recruited for this study protocol. They were not taking any medication known to interfere with glucose tolerance. Patients taking lipid-lowering drugs were excluded from this study. In order to avoid the interference of the age effect, two age- and BMI-matched groups were formed, based on age distribution. In this group of 56 men, age varied from 22 to 46 years (mean 35.8 ± 6.8 years).

A 75 g oral glucose tolerance test was performed with determination of plasma glucose, insulin, C-peptide, glucagon and free fatty acids. Total area responses to glucose and pancreatic hormones were calculated as the incremental area under the 3 h curves. Differences of body fat distribution were measured using the waist-to-hip circumference ratio (WHR).

Results

Table 1 shows the clinical characteristics of all patients. Only WHR and percentage body fat were significantly different between both groups of 28 patients.

Table 1. Clinical and anthropometric characteristics (mean ± SD) of the 56 patients subdivided in upper (AO) and lower (GFO) body obesity

	AO (n = 28)	GFO (n = 28)
Age, years	37.2 ± 6.0	34.4 ± 7.4
BMI, kg/m^2	35.5 ± 4.1	35.2 ± 5.2
WHR	1.04 ± 0.04	0.95 ± 0.04*
SSF, mm	39.4 ± 11.9	38.0 ± 13.4
FFM, kg	68.0 ± 6.6	67.7 ± 5.7
FM, %	37.2 ± 5.5	40.3 ± 4.8**

*$P < 0.00001$; **$P < 0.05$.

No basal parameters of glucose metabolism are significantly higher in upper body obesity. However, cumulative parameters of glucose, insulin, C-peptide and glucagon were significantly higher in men with upper body obesity, most prominently for serum C-peptide levels ($P < 0.002$).

Figure 1 shows basal and cumulative glucagon values in both groups of patients. Fasting glucagon was significantly ($P < 0.04$) higher in upper (AO) *versus* lower (GFO) obesity: fasting levels reached 173 ± 66 *vs.* 142 ± 38 pg/ml in AO and GFO obesity, respectively. Cumulative glucagon values during GTT were 3239 ± 1318 and 2745 ± 704 ($P = 0.12$) in AO and GFO respectively.

Pearson correlation coefficients between age, obesity variables and insulin (n = 56) are given in Table 2.

Sex hormones are only related to free fatty acids; free testosterone index is significantly related to fasting and integrated free fatty acids whereas SHBG is negatively related to fasting and cumulative free fatty acids.

Table 3 shows the relationship between insulin and glucagon parameters and different lipid parameters.

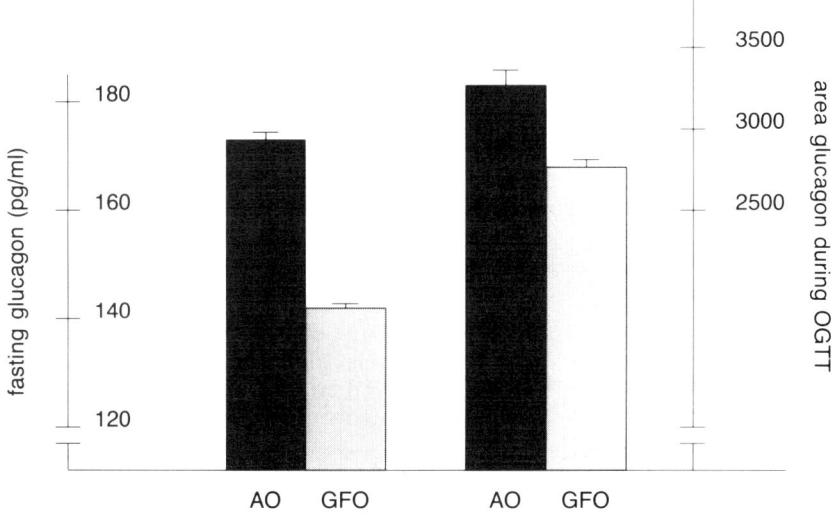

Fig. 1. Fasting and cumulative glucagon values (mean ± SEM) in obese men with upper (AO) and lower (GFO) body obesity.

Table 2. Simple Pearson's correlation coefficients between age, obesity variables (BMI, WHR), fasting (F) and area (a) insulin and glucagon parameters in 56 obese men

	Age	BMI	WHR
BMI	0.10	–	–0.02
WHR	0.25	–0.02	–
F insulin	–0.19	0.26**	0.02
F glucagon	0.01	0.10	0.42*
F FFA	0.06	0.02	0.27**
a insulin	–0.18	0.28**	0.16
a glucagon	0.07	0.06	0.41*
a FFA	0.05	0.13	0.39*

*$P < 0.003$; **$P < 0.01$.

Table 3. Relationship of fasting insulin, C-peptide, glucagon and free fatty acids with different lipids and lipoproteins (mg/dl). Highly significant correlations are found among all variables

	Insulin	C-peptide	cp/ins ratio	FFA	Glucagon
HDL	–0.41*	–0.42*	0.49*	–0.34*	–0.26†
HDL2	–0.28**	–0.19	0.43*	–0.18	0.33**
TG	0.11	0.23†	0.04	0.54*	0.58*
AI	0.22†	0.26**	–0.21	0.55*	0.64*
apo A1	–0.32**	–0.19	0.36‡	–0.25†	–0.17

*$P < 0.001$; **$P < 0.02$; †$P < 0.05$; ‡$P < 0.004$.

Discussion

In recent years it has indeed become quite clear that the adipose tissue is not a homogeneous organ with respect to hormonal responsiveness and metabolism. Hyperinsulinaemia is a well-recognized factor of simple and morbid obesity, a feature of upper body obesity in particular[8]. Since upper body fat predominance is associated with alterations in metabolic and hormonal responsiveness of adipose tissue, not only insulin but also glucagon has to be considered.

In this study of obese, but otherwise healthy men, abdominal obesity was associated with overall higher values (significant or as a major trend) of cumulative serum glucose, insulin, C-peptide and glucagon levels during OGTT.

An interesting finding is the relationship between body distribution of fat and glucagon levels. Glucagon levels seem to be higher in upper body obesity and both fasting and integrated glucagon levels during GTT correlate significantly with WHR.

This finding of increased glucagon levels in men with AO is intriguing and the origin of this finding remains to be determined. Since the most important site of glucagon degradation is probably the kidney and not the liver[6], increased glucagon secretion rather than reduced catabolism probably accounts for this hormonal imbalance.

Two possible pathways could be considered. First, a nervous vagus mediated glucagon secretion induced by central imbalance and stimuli could be the initial mechanism[1]; since glucagon is a potent lipolytic hormone, elevated plasma levels could subsequently contribute to increased plasma FFA concentrations, especially from the lipolytic sensitive abdominal fat cells. A second possibility comprises noradrenaline which can be at the origin of increased plasma concentrations of glucagon. It is however speculative to accept that a higher adrenergic drive exists in patients with upper body obesity.

Although glucagon behaviour in obesity remains controversial, hyperglucagonaemia has been reported in obese patients, especially in those subjects with fatty liver and hypertriglyceridaemia[7]. Whether fatty livers with hypertriglyceridaemia may modulate glucagon dynamics remains unclear although it was shown that mechanisms of hepatic glucagon extraction exist[4]. Glucagon resistance may be the hormonal basis for endogenous hyperlipaemia[2], especially in men with upper body fat; this relationship of glucagon with lipid and lipoprotein fractions has also been shown in our results.

Data of our OGTT results indicate that suppression of glucagon levels following glucose administration is clearly diminished in AO which suggests that in upper body obesity an insensitivity of plasma glucagon exists to variations in plasma glucose concentrations. In respect to the findings of Gossain[3] and Starke[7], patients with upper body fat and characterized by IGT and/or hyperinsulinaemia, may most probably show some degree of glucagon resistance, which can consequently contribute to lipid abnormalities and a premature atherosclerosis.

References

1. Bloom, S., Vaughan, N.J. & Russell, R. (1974): Vagal control of glucagon release in man. *Lancet* **ii**, 546-549.
2. Eaton, P. & Schade, D. (1973): Glucagon resistance as a hormonal basis for endogenous hyperlipemia. *Lancet* **i**, 973-974.
3. Gossain, V.V., Matute, M.L. & Kalkhoff, R.K. (1974): Relative influence of obesity and diabetes on plasma alfa-cell glucagon. *J. Clin. Endocrinol. Metab.* **38**, 238-243.
4. Jaspan, J.B., Ruddick, J. & Rayfield, E. (1984): Transhepatic glucagon gradients in man: evidence for glucagon extraction by human liver. *J. Clin. Endocrinol. Metab.* **58**, 287-292.
5. Kalkhoff, R.K., Gossain, V.V. & Matute, M.L. (1973): Plasma glucagon in obesity. Response to arginine, glucose and protein administration. *N. Engl. J. Med.* **30**, 465-467.
6. Sherwin, R.S., Fischer, M., Bessoff J., Snyder N., Hendler, R., Conn, H.O. & Felig, P. (1978): Hyperglucagonemia in cirrhosis: altered secretion and sensitivity to glucagon. *Gastroenterology* **74**, 1224-1228.
7. Starke, A., Erhardt, G., Berger, M. & Zimmerman, H. (1984): Elevated pancreatic glucagon in obesity. *Diabetes* **33**, 277-280.
8. Van Gaal, L., Vansant, G., Van Acker, K. & De Leeuw, I. (1991): Decreased hepatic insulin extraction in upper body obesity. Relationship to unbound androgens and sex hormone binding globulin. *Diab. Res. Clin. Pract.* **12**, 99-106.
9. Wise, J., Hendler, R. & Felig, P. (1973): Evaluation of alpha-cell function by infusion of alanine in normal, diabetic and obese subjects. *N. Engl. J. Med.* **288**, 487-490.

Chapter 68

Changed Adipose Tissue Distribution After Treatment of Cushing's Syndrome

Lars LÖNN[1], Henry KVIST[1], Lars SJÖSTRÖM[2] and I. ERNEST[2]

Department of Diagnostic Radiology[1] and Medicine[2], Sahlgren Hospital, University of Göteborg, S-413 45 Göteborg, Sweden

Introduction

Cushing's syndrome is characterized by a preponderance of abdominal and neck adipose tissue. The volume of adipose tissue, muscles and visceral organs can be defined directly by computed tomography (CT)[2,3,7]. The multiscan method is probably the most reproducible and accurate body composition technique available today. Furthermore, information about regional adipose tissue distribution can be obtained by CT. These body composition facilities have been utilized in this study which examines patients with Cushing's syndrome before and after treatment.

Study design and material

We have currently examined 6 females with Cushing's syndrome. They were analysed with a multiscan CT-technique using 22 scans. Examinations were performed preoperatively and 8 months postoperatively. Body weight (BW), body mass index (BMI) and urine-cortisol were determined on both occasions (Table 1). Four patients had pituitary adenomas and two had adrenal adenomas. All patients had an operation on the pituitary gland or the adrenals, respectively. One patient with a pituitary adenoma had a residual adenoma after initial improvement. She was nevertheless included in the material.

Table 1. Detals of six females with Cushing's syndrome before and after treatment

	Before	After	P
Age, years	32 ± 10	33 ± 10	
Body weight, kg	78.5 ± 16.8	67.4 ± 12.0	0.044
Height, m	1.66 ± 0.05		
BMI, kg/m^2	28.3 ± 6.0	24.2 ± 4.0	0.049
Urine cortisol	1555 ± 975	124 ± 213	0.017

Methods

Examinations were performed with a Philips Tomoscan 310 CT-scanner at 120 kV with a slice thickness of 12 mm. Exposure and scan times were 1.2 and 4.8 s, respectively. Image reconstruction was made with convolution filter no 4, i.e. a smoothing filter designed for soft tissue studies. The total adipose tissue area of each scan was determined as the area of picture elements (pixels) within the attenuation interval from −190 to −30 HU. Visceral adipose tissue was determined in the same way by circumscribing the visceral region in the muscle/bone wall of the trunk with the cursor. Muscles and visceral organs were determined with a similar cursor technique using the attenuation interval from −29 to +151 HU[6]. Area determinations of tissues were performed and the volumes of subcutaneous and visceral adipose tissue, muscles and internal organs were determined according to the formula:

$$V = \sum_{1}^{i=23} \frac{a_i (b_i + c_i)}{2}$$

where a_i = distance between two adjacent scans; b_i and c_i = tissue areas of scans.

The sum of 23 partial body composition volumes constitute the total volume of the tissue involved. Volumes of adipose tissue was multiplied by 0.923 in order to obtain the adipose tissue weight. Muscles and internal organs were converted to weight by using a density of 1.05.

Statistics

The significance of absolute changes was tested by Student's t-test and relative changes by Wilcoxon's non-parametric test.

Results and discussion

The mean body weight (BW) was 78.5 kg preoperatively and 67.4 kg postoperatively. The body mass index (BMI) was reduced from 28.3 to 24.2 kg/m². The urine-cortisol level was also significantly reduced (Table 1).

The body weight reduction was entirely due to the reduction of adipose tissue. The small reductions of muscle mass and visceral organs were not significant (Fig. 1). The subcutaneous AT volume was reduced with 5.5 l and the visceral AT volume with 2.1 l (Table 2). The latter reduction could approximately be divided into retro- and intra-abdominal volumes of 0.5 and 1.6 l, respectively. In relative terms the adipose tissue of the retroperitoneal and visceral depots were reduced with 43% and 38%, respectively. Other adipose tissue regions showed smaller relative reductions. Following weight loss, a reduction of visceral and subcutaneous AT areas in the lumbar region has previously been described. However, changed AT areas of single scans do not prove a changed AT distribution. The evidence for a changed distribution requires regional and total determinations and assessments of relative changes as shown in Fig. 2. This proves that different adipose tissue depots respond differently to cortisol withdrawal.

Table 2. Adipose tissue depot changes before and after treatment of Cushing's syndrome

	Before (litres)	After (% change)	P
Subcutaneous trunk	−5.5	−28	0.01
Legs	−1.6	−16	ns
Viscera	−2.1	−38	0.05
Arms	−0.5	−21	0.01
Neck	−0.3	−36	0.05

Chapter 68 – Changed Adipose Tissue Distribution After Treatment of Cushing's Syndrome

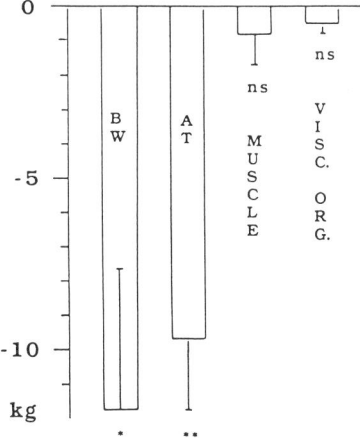

Fig. 1. The body weight reduction of 11.1 kg postoperatively (P < 0.05) corresponded to an AT reduction of 9.2 kg (P < 0.01). The reduction of muscle mass and visceral organs were of no significance (copyrights reserved).

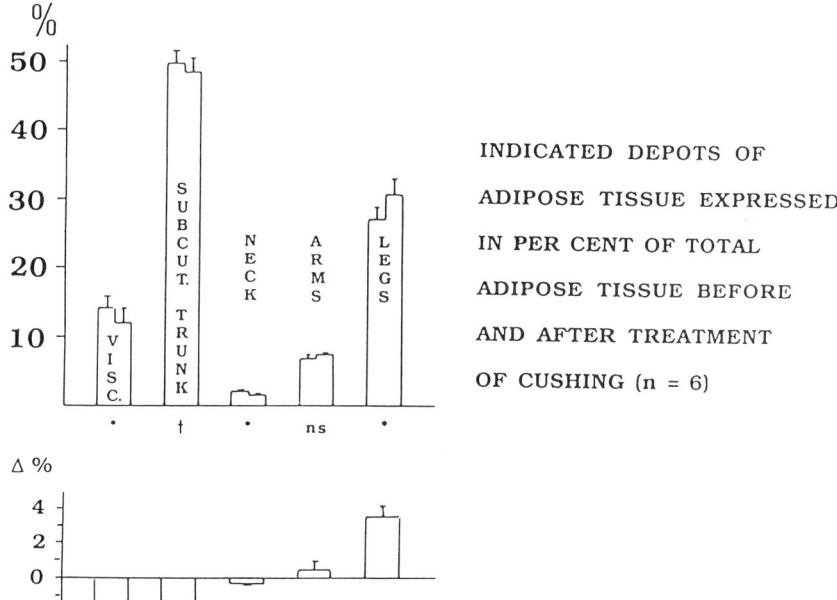

Fig. 2. (upper). Preoperatively the patients had 14.2 per cent of their AT volume in the visceral depot. Postoperatively this was reduced to 12.0 per cent (P < 0.05). Corresponding figures for subcutaneous AT were 50.0 and 48.5 per cent, respectively (P < 0.06). On the other hand, the percentage of AT in arms and legs increased, in legs by 3.6 per cent (P < 0.05).
(lower). A significant decrease in the visceral, subcutaneous and head and neck regions is counterbalanced by a relative increase in arms and legs (copyright reserved).

Biochemistry

The background to cortisol-induced visceral adipose tissue accumulation has recently been at least partly clarified at the molecular biology level[1]. Thus cortisol increases the excretion of lipoproteinlipase preferentially in visceral fat cells. This mechanism is inhibited by sex steroid hormones In men, abdominal obesity is then increased in subjects with low testosterone levels[4]. Our body composition studies before and after withdrawal of excess cortisol provides clinical evidence to previous molecular biological studies.

Conclusions

The sensitivity for cortisol is different for different adipose tissue depots. Weight reduction after treatment of Cushing's syndrome is entirely due to a reduction of adipose tissue. The visceral adipose tissue depot and the head and neck region are most sensitive to reduced cortisol levels.

Acknowledgements

U. Grangård, Department of Radiology, University of Göteborg, Sweden for her skilful technical assistance. This study was supported by grants from the Swedish Medical Research Council (19X-5239) and Hoffman-La Roche. Financial support for the radiological assessments has been received from Göteborg Medical Society and Swedish Society of Medical Radiology.

References

1. Björntorp, P. (1990): "Portal" adipose tissue as a generator of risk factors for cardiovascular disease and diabetes. *Arteriosclerosis* **10**, 493-496.
2. Kvist, H., Chowdhury, B., Sjöström, L., Tylén, U. & Cederblad, Å. (1988): Adipose tissue volume determinations in males by computed tomography and ^{40}K. *Int. J. Obes.* **12**, 249-266.
3. Kvist, H., Sjöström, L. & Tylén, U. (1986): Adipose tissue volume determinations in women by computed tomography: technical considerations. *Int. J. Obes.* **10**, 53-67.
4. Seidell, J.C., Björntorp, P., Sjöström, L., Kvist, H. & Sannerstedt, R. (1990): Visceral fat accumulation in men is positively associated with insulin glucose and c-peptide levels, but negatively with testosterone levels. *Metabolism* **39**, 897-901.
5. Seidell, J.C., Oosterlee, A., Thijssen, A., M.A.O., *et al.* (1987): Assessment of intraabdominal and subcutaneous abdominal fat relation between anthropometry and computed tomography. *Am. J. Clin. Nutr.* **45**, 7-13.
6. Sjöström, L. (1991): A computed tomography based multicompartment body composition technique and anthropometric predictions of lean body mass, total and subcutaneous adipose tissue. *Int. J. Obes.* (in press).
7. Sjöström, L., Kvist, H., Cederblad, Å. & Tylén, U. (1986): Determinations of total adipose tissue volume and body fat in women by CT, ^{40}K and tritium. *Am. J. Phys.* **250**, E736-E745.

Chapter 69

Lactate Production in Subcutaneous Adipose Tissue in Lean and Obese Man

P.-A. JANSSON, U. SMITH and P. LÖNNROTH
Department of Medicine II, Sahlgren's Hospital, University of Gothenburg, S-413 45 Gothenburg, Sweden

Measurements of interstitial subcutaneous lactate concentrations combined with determinations of the blood flow rate support the view that adipose tissue is a significant source of lactate production. Consequently, lactate production is increased in obese subjects due to their larger body fat mass. The physiological significance of this finding in terms of the enhanced supply of the gluconeogenic precursor in obesity remains to be established.

Introduction

It is well-known that obesity is associated with insulin resistance and non-insulin dependent diabetes (NIDDM). One important reason for the fasting hyperglycaemia in diabetes is an increased hepatic glucose production. Moreover, in the post-absorptive state gluconeogenesis may account for most of the excess hepatic glucose output in NIDDM[3]. Furthermore, in a recent study it was shown the subjects with NIDDM had an increased substrate flux to the liver as well as an increased intrahepatic substrate conversion to glucose in the basal state as compared to lean non-diabetic individuals[4]. Therefore, the tissues responsible for the supply of lactate and alanine need to be identified. Since skeletal muscle was not identified as the major source of gluconeogenic precursors in NIDDM[4], other production sites have been discussed[2], especially for lactate, the most important gluconeogenic substrate.

In this paper we present data to show that adipose tissue is a significant source of lactate production. In addition, results are presented to suggest that obesity is characterized by considerable lactate formation.

Measurements *in vivo*

More than 20 years ago Doar *et al.* reported that mean fasting blood lactate levels were higher in obese than non-obese subjects, irrespective of whether the glucose tolerance was normal or impaired[6]. The elevated lactate levels were considered to be due to an increased production rather than a reduced utilization[6]. However, the source of lactate was not discussed.

In contrast, Kreisberg *et al.*[13] found an increased lactate turn-over in lean compared to obese subjects. However, that study was hampered by the limited number of subjects studied and by the known drawbacks of the isotopic dilution technique, which might at least partly explain the conflicting data. To our knowledge these are the only studies of lactate turnover in obesity in man.

Recently, Lovejoy *et al.*[14] found an association between the postabsorptive blood lactate levels and the degree of obesity in men. It was suggested that this association may reflect an increased lactate production from enlarged adipocytes and an increased fat mass[14]. In addition, there was an inverse correlation between the increase in lactate levels following an oral glucose ingestion and degree of obesity. Since the obese individuals had higher glucose levels this finding was interpreted to indicate a decreased ability of adipose tissue to convert glucose to lactate[14].

Measurements *in vitro*

Previous investigations aimed at studying different mechanisms of insulin resistance in isolated human adipocytes *in vitro*, showed that ≈60 per cent of the total glucose utilized under maximally insulin-stimulated conditions was converted to lactate. This was demonstrated in cells obtained from both healthy subjects and individuals with NIDDM[12].

Similar data have been obtained with isolated rat adipocytes *in vitro*[5]. In that study lactate accounted for 10–15 per cent of the glucose metabolized by small fat cells under "basal" incubation conditions, whereas 40 per cent of the glucose utilized by large fat cells at glucose concentrations greater than 6 mM was converted to lactate. Hence, it was concluded that lactate was a major metabolite of glucose in adipocytes, particularly in the large fat cells.

Further investigations from the same laboratory have demonstrated that mesenteric fat cells from lean and obese rats metabolized significantly more glucose per cell and converted more glucose to lactate than cells from other fat depots, suggesting regional differences in adipocyte lactate production from glucose[18]. Moreover, streptozotocin-induced diabetes in male Wistar rats was associated with an increased relative conversion of glucose to lactate by fat cells[19]. However, it was also demonstrated in that study that adipose cells from obese diabetic rats produced significantly more lactate from glucose than cells from lean diabetic rats, both in the absence and presence of insulin.

In another investigation, Mårin *et al.* studied the uptake of radioactive oral glucose by adipose tissue *in vivo* in man. Glucose uptake conversion to triglyceride by adipose tissue was less than 4 per cent of ingested glucose. However, when glucose conversion to lactate *in vitro* was considered, total glucose uptake by the adipose tissue may well be quantitatively important, accounting for a maximal uptake of ≈30–50 per cent of an oral glucose load in obese subjects. In addition, abdominal adipocytes produced more lactate from glucose *in vitro* than femoral adipocytes[17].

Measurements *in situ*

In 1987, we described a microdialysis technique enabling sampling and characterization of the interstitial water of the subcutaneous adipose tissue in man[15]. By using our newly developed calibration procedure the concentration of any small molecular compound can be estimated[15]. Using this procedure we have found that glycerol levels are higher in the adipose tissue than in the blood[11], whereas adenosine levels are similar[16]. Furthermore, it was shown that glucose could be drained from the interstitial space by the catheters, unless appropriate cautions were taken, indicating that microdialysis enables studies of the tissue water space[9].

By using microdialysis we have demonstrated that abdominal subcutaneous adipose tissue in lean subjects produces lactate both in the postabsorptive state and after an oral glucose load[10]. Similar results have been reported by Hagström *et al.* using another microdialysis probe[8] as well as from Frayn *et al.* by cannulating the epigastric vein[7].

In order to estimate the lactate released by the subcutaneous tissue we recently conducted a study (to be published) where the interstitial lactate concentrations were measured both before and after an oral glucose load, concomitant with recordings of the blood flow[1]. The data from two representative subjects are shown in Table 1, indicating that the obese subject had increased tissue lactate as well as arterial lactate concentrations compared to the lean individual. In the fasting state, adipose tissue blood flow was lower in both sites in obesity and, furthermore, after an oral glucose load the increase in blood flow was blunted in the obese volunteer (Table 2). Taken together, basal lactate release from the adipose tissue was enhanced in obese subjects, whereas this difference was not obvious after an oral glucose load due to the blunted response of the blood flow.

Table 1 (a). Clinical characteristics

	Age, years	BW, kg	BMI, kg/m^2	BF, kg	WHR	Haematocrit, %
Lean	32	80	22.3	9	0.81	40
Obese	29	130	43.1	42	1.11	43

BW = body weight; BMI = body mass index; BF = body fat; WHR = waist/hip circumference ratio

Table 1(b). Metabolic data before and after an oral glucose tolerance test

	Abdominal interstitial lactate (µM)	Femoral interstitial lactate (µM)	Plasma lactate (µM)	Plasma insulin (mU/l)	Plasma glucose (mM)
Lean					
0 min	1196	995	635	5	4.5
120 min	1774	1410	924	32	6.8
Obese					
0 min	1470	1742	854	11	4.9
120 min	1634	1930	1047	80	8.3

Table 2. Adipose tissue blood flow (ATBF) before and after an oral glucose tolerance test

	ATBF abdominal subcutaneous tissue (ml/min x 100 g)	ATBF femoral subcutaneous tissue (ml/min x 100 g)
Lean		
0 min	3.1	2.3
120 min	5.0	5.1
Obese		
0 min	1.6	1.4
120 min	1.8	2.4

In conclusion, the results imply that a substantial amount of lactate is produced in the subcutaneous tissue in obese subjects, probably due to their large adipose tissue mass. Thus, adipose tissue cannot be disregarded from playing a role in glucose homeostasis in man.

Acknowledgements

This work was supported by grants from the Swedish Medical Research Council, Svenska Sällskapet för Medicinsk Forskning, the Swedish Society of Medicine, Göteborg Läkaresällskap och "Förenade Liv" Mutual Group Life Insurance Company, Stockholm, Sweden. We wish to thank Helle Persson for technical assistance.

References

1. Andree Larsen, O., Lassen, N.A. & Quaade, F. (1966): Blood flow through human adipose determined with radioactive xenon. *Acta Physiol. Scand.* **66**, 337-345.
2. Buchalter, S.E., Crain, M.R. & Kreisberg, R. (1989): Regulation of lactate metabolism *in vivo*. *Diab. Metab. Rev.* **5**, 379-391.
3. Consoli, A., Nurjhan, N., Capani, F. & Gerich, J. (1989): Predominant role of gluconeogenesis in increased hepatic glucose production in NIDDM. *Diabetes* **38**, 550-557.
4. Consoli, A., Nurjhan, N., Reilly, J.J., Bier, D.M. & Gerich, J.E. (1990): Mechanism of increased gluconeogenesis in noninsulin-dependent diabetes mellitus. *J. Clin. Invest.* **86**, 2038-2045.
5. Crandall, D.L., Freid, S.K., Francendese, A.A., Nickel, M. & DiGirolamo, M. (1983): Lactate release from isolated rat adipocytes: influence of cell size, glucose concentration, insulin and epinephrine. *Horm. Metab. Res.* **15**, 326-329.
6. Doar, J.W.H. & Cramp, D.G. (1970): The effects of obesity and maturity-onset diabetes mellitus on L(+) lactic acid metabolism. *Clin. Sci.* **39**, 271-279.
7. Fayn, K.N., Coppack, S.W., Humphreys, S.M. & Whyte, P.L. (1989): Metabolic characteristics of human adipose tissue *in vivo*. *Clin. Sci.* **76**, 509-516.
8. Hagström, E., Arner, P., Ungerstedt, U. & Bolinder, J. (1990): Subcutaneous adipose tissue: a source of lactate production after glucose ingestion in humans. *Am. J. Physiol.* **258**, E888-E893.
9. Jansson, P.-A., Fowelin, J., Smith, U. & Lönnroth, P. (1988): Characterization by microdialysis of intercellular glucose level in subcutaneous tissue in humans. *Am. J. Physiol.* **255**, E218-E220.
10. Jansson, P.-A., Smith, U. & Lönnroth, P. (1990): Evidence for lactate production by human adipose tissue *in vivo*. *Diabetologia* **33**, 253-256.
11. Jansson, P.-A., Smith, U. & Lönnroth, P. (1990): Interstitial glycerol concentrations measured by microdialysis in two subcutaneous regions in humans. *Am. J. Physiol.* **258**, E918-E922.
12. Kashiwagi, A., Verso, M.A., Andrews, J., Vasquez, B., Reaven, G. & Foley, J.E. (1983): *In vitro* insulin resistance of human adipocytes isolated from subjects with noninsulin-dependent diabetes mellitus. *J. Clin. Invest.* **72**, 1246-1254.
13. Kreisberg, R.A., Pennington, L.F. & Boshell, B.R. (1970): Lactate turnover and gluconeogenesis in normal and obese humans. *Diabetes* **19**, 53-63.
14. Lovejoy, J., Mellen, B. & DiGirolamo, M. (1990): Lactate generation following glucose ingestion: relation to obesity, carbohydrate tolerance and insulin sensitivity. *Int. J. Obes.* **14**, 843-855.
15. Lönnroth, P., Jansson, P.-A. & Smith, U. (1987): A microdialysis method allowing characterization of intercellular water space in humans. *Am. J. Physiol.* **253**, E228-E231.
16. Lönnroth, P., Jansson, P.-A., Fredholm, B.B. & Smith, U. (1989): Microdialysis of intercellular adenosine concentration in subcutaneous tissue in humans. *Am. J. Physiol.* **256**, E250-E255.
17. Mårin, P., Rebuffé-Scrive, M., Smith, U. & Björntorp, P. (1987): Glucose uptake in human adipose tissue. *Metabolism* **36**, 1154-1160.
18. Newby, F.D., Sykes, M.N. & DiGirolamo, M. (1988): Regional differences in adipocyte lactate production from glucose. *Am. J. Physiol.* **255**, E716-E722.
19. Newby, F.D., Bayo, F., Thacker, S.V. Sykes, M. & DiGirolamo, M. (989): Effects of streptozocin-induced diabetes on glucose metabolism and lactate release by isolated fat cells from young lean and older, moderately obese rats. *Diabetes* **38**, 237-243.

Chapter 70

Epinephrine-Induced Glycerol Release in Subcutaneous Adipose Tissue Measured by Microdialysis in Patients With Android Obesity

Herwig H. DITSCHUNEIT, Marion FLECHTNER-MORS and Hans DITSCHUNEIT

Department of Medicine, University of Ulm, Robert-Koch-Straße 8, D-7900 Ulm, Germany

The results of the present study show that there are regional differences of lipolysis rate in women with android obesity. Epinephrine is more effective in stimulating glycerol release in the abdominal than in the femoral adipose tissue. These findings may be of pathogenetic importance for the development of android obesity.

Introduction

Prospective studies have shown that obesity is a risk factor for premature atherosclerosis, but several studies have reported that excess abdominal adipose tissue means a higher risk than obesity itself,[4,12,13] confirming the early observations of Vague that the site of fat predominance is an important factor in the association of obesity with metabolic diseases[19,20]. Abdominal fat accumulation is associated with impaired glucose tolerance[10] and diabetes mellitus[6] and hypertriglyceridaemia[3,9]. The underlying mechanisms are not well understood. An increased lipolysis rate associated with an increased abdominal fat mass in the aetiology of the metabolic disorders has been suggested[15] and abdominal adipose tissue lipolysis has been shown to contribute significantly to the plasma insulin and triglyceride levels[17]. The factors regulating the fat distribution in the upper or lower parts of the body and the factors important for accumulating fat mass preferentially in the abdominal region are unknown. Differences in the control of lipolysis in the different regions of the body may play a role. Therefore we investigated basal and epinephrine stimulated lipolysis rate *in situ* in the intact subcutaneous adipose tissue in patients with the android type of obesity.

Methods

Subjects. We investigated six obese women with the android type of obesity. All subjects were without medication and their body weight had been stable in the previous 3 months. They were asked to maintain their habitual diet and physical activity 3 days before investigation. The clinical characteristics are given in Table 1. The waist/hip ratio was measured without clothes in the erect position, around the waist through a point one-third of the distance between the xiphoid process and the umbilicus and around the hips through a point 4 cm below the superior anterior iliac spine. The patients gave their informed consent and the study had been approved by the Ethical Committee of the University of Ulm.

Table 1. Clinical characteristics

	Age years	Body weight kg	Height cm	BMI kg/m^2	Waist/hip ratio cm
	49	99.0	158	40.0	1.15
	47	102.2	168	36.0	0.90
	42	144.0	162	57.0	0.86
	31	129.3	164	48.0	0.92
	35	104.0	171	36.0	1.00
	30	145.0	169	49.5	0.87
Mean	39	120.6	165.3	44.1	0.95
± SD	8.2	21.4	4.9	8.5	0.10

Experimental protocol

The patients fasted overnight and were studied at rest in the supine position. Experiments started at 8 a.m. and were done in a room temperature at 25°C. With a guide cannula (diameter 1.1 mm) a microdialysis tube (0.3 x 30 mm, Cuprophane B 4 AH, 3000 MW cut-off, Cobe, Denver, Co., glued to a nylon tube and sterilized) was placed in the periumbilical (5 cm lateral and 5 cm caudal of the umbilicus) and in the ventral femoral subcutaneous fat tissue (10 cm below the inguinal ligamentum); no local anaesthetics were given. The inlet of the nylon tubing was connected to a precision pump (Perfusor VI, Braun Melsungen, FRG) and perfused with isotonic saline at a rate of 2.5 µl/min. After an equilibration period of 60 min, the dialysate was collected in 15 min fractions from the outlet of the nylon tube. With the subcutaneous microdialysis calibration technique described in detail by Lönnroth[14] the calculation of the interstitial glycerol can be measured and also the percentage recovery of the interstitial glycerol concentration in the dialysate. In the present study at a perfusion rate of 2.5 µl/min the recovery of glycerol in the interstitial adipose tissue was 38 ± 4 per cent.

For stimulation of glycerol release epinephrine in isotonic saline was used. The microdialysis tubing was perfused at a rate of 2.5 µl/min for 30 min, and epinephrine concentration in the perfusate was 0.2 µg/µl. Total epinephrine perfused amounted to 15.0 µg.

Analysis of glycerol. 10 µl of tissue dialysate were used for the analysis of glycerol, using an ultrasensitive kinetic bioluminescence assay using an ultrasensitive luminescence analyser (Berthold LB 950 CL)[9]. All enzymes and coenzymes used for conversion of glycerol and for luminescence were obtained from Boehringer Mannheim, FRG.

Statistical analysis. Values given are means ± SE. Statistical significance was tested with Student's *t*-test for paired data.

Results

Four microdialysis tubes were used in each patient, on the right and on the left side lateral to the umbilicus and on both ventral sides of each thigh. Isotonic saline was used as the dialysis solvent. The glycerol concentrations in the outlet of the mirodialysis tubings were measured for up to 5 h at 10 min intervals and they remained constant (data not shown). The addition of epinephrine to the perfusate resulted in a rapid and marked increase in the adipose tissue dialysate glycerol concentration (Fig. 1). In the abdominal adipose tissue the mean glycerol concentration in the dialysate increased up to 200 per cent from basal within 15 min and in the dialysate collected between 15 and 30 min it increased up to 300 per cent. After 30 min only saline was perfused, glycerol concentration in the dialysate increased further and glycerol concentration in the fraction collected between 30 and 45 min reached

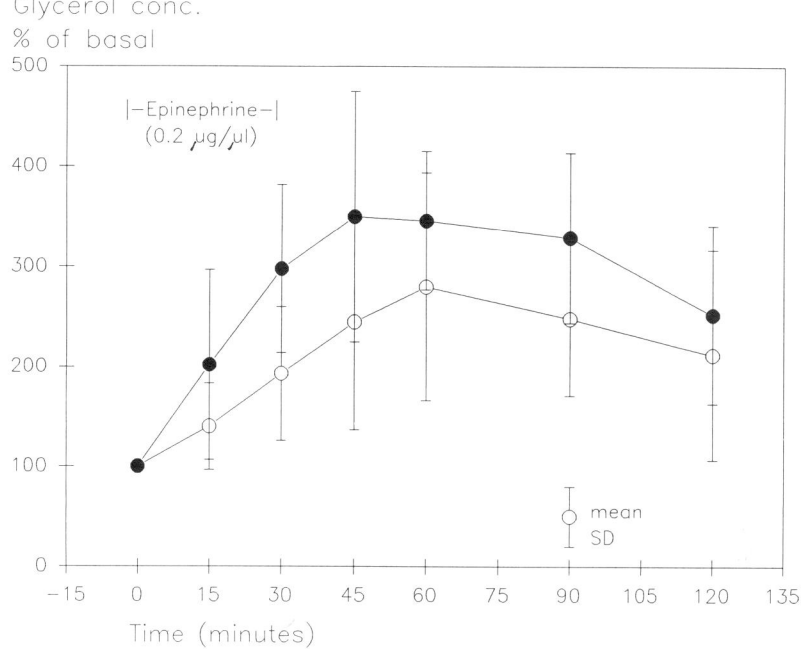

Fig. 1. Glycerol release (per cent from basal) in abdominal (filled circle symbols) and in femoral (open circle symbols) subcutaneous adipose tissue, stimulated by locally administered epinephrine (0.2 µg/µl for 30 min at a perfusion rate of 2.5 µl/min) in six women with android obesity.

its maximum of 350 per cent from basal. Thereafter glycerol release slowed down, but remained high even in the fraction which was collected from 105 to 120 min. In the dialysate of the femoral adipose tissue, the increase of glycerol concentration was significantly lower, and the highest concentration was achieved in the fraction collected between 45 and 60 min. At any time interval the glycerol concentration in the dialysate of femoral adipose tissue was lower than in the dialysate of abdominal adipose tissue.

Discussion

The regulation of lipolysis has been studied extensively in the last few years using *in vitro* methods. But the *in vivo* situation may be different because isolated fat cells or adipose tissue pieces are removed from their natural surroundings and disconnected from nerve innervation and from blood supply. Now there is a method available for the investigation of lipolysis *in situ* in human adipose tissue using microdialysis[1,14]. The data obtained with this new method demonstrate that glycerol release of abdominal adipose tissue into intercellular space is stimulated by epinephrine, and stimulation is enhanced as compared to the glycerol release of femoral adipose tissue. This confirms data obtained by isolated fat cells from different regions *in vitro*[8,18,19]. A different lipolysis rate in different adipose tissue regions have also been reported by Jansson et al.[7] for obese persons and by Arner et al.[2] for non-obese persons. The mechanisms underlying these regional differences are not known. It has been suggested that the α_2-/β-adrenergic receptor status may be important[16]. Regional differences also have been shown in the response of fat cells to other hormones[11]. These findings of regional differences of fat cells may be of importance with regard to different rates of metabolic disorders. A significant association between abdominal adipose cell lipolysis and metabolic disorders, particularly plasma insulin and triglyceride levels, in premenopausal women has been shown by Mauriege et al.[17]. Increased lipolysis response to epinephrine of abdominal fat cells may increase the concentrations of free fatty acids in plasma. The increased concentration of free fatty acids leads to impaired glucose disposal and in consequence to hyperinsulinaemia and to the development of an insulin-resistant state.

References

1. Arner, P., Bolinder, J., Eliasson, A., Lundin, A. & Ungerstedt, U. (1988): Microdialysis of adipose tissue and blood for *in vivo* lipolysis studies. *Am. J. Physiol.* **255 E**, 737-742.
2. Arner, P., Kriegholm, E., Engfeldt, P. & Bolinder, J. (1990): Adrenergic regulation of lipolysis *in situ* at rest and during exercise. *J. Clin. Invest.* **85**, 893-898.
3. Després, J.P., Allard, C., Tremblay, A., Talbot, J. & Bouchard, C. (1985): Evidence for a regional component of body mass fatness in the association with serum lipids in men and women. *Metabolism* **34**, 967-973.
4. Ducimetière, P., Richard, J. & Cambien, F. (1986): The pattern of subcutaneous fat distribution in middle-aged men and the risk of coronary heart disease: the Paris prospective study. *Int. J. Obes.* **10**, 229-240.
5. Haffner, S.M., Stern, M.P., Hazuda, H.P., Pugh, J. & Patterson, J.K. (1987): Do upper-body and centralized adiposity measure different aspects of regional body fat distribution? Relationship to non-insulin dependent diabetes mellitus, lipids and lipoproteins. *Diabetes* **36**, 43-51.
6. Hartz, A.J., Rupley, D.C., Kalkhoff, R.D. & Rimm, A.A. (1983): Relationship of obesity to diabetes: influence of obesity and body fat distribution. *Prev. Med.* **12**, 351-357.
7. Jansson, P.-A., Smith, U. & Lönnroth, P. (1990): Interstitial glycerol concentration measured by microdialysis in two subcutaneous regions in man. *Am. J. Physiol.* **258 E**, 918-922.
8. Kather, H., Zöllig, K., Simon, B. & Schlierf, G. (1977): Human fat cell adenylate cyclase: regional differences in adrenaline responsiveness. *Eur. J. Clin. Invest.* **7**, 595-597.
9. Kather, H., Schröder, F. & Simon, B. (1982): Microdetermination of glycerol using bacterial NADH-linked luciferase. *Clin. Chim. Acta* **120**, 295-300.
10. Kissebah, A., Vydelingum, N., Murray, R,. Evans,D.E., Hartz,A.J., Kalkhoff, P.W. & Adams, P.W. (1982): Relation of body fat composition to metabolic complications of obesity. *J. Clin. Endocrinol. Metab.* **54**, 254-260.
11. Krotkiewski, M. & Björntorp, P. (1976): The effect of progesterone and of insulin administration on regional adipose tissue cellularity in the rat. *Acta Physiol. Scand.* **96**, 122-128.
12. Lapidus, L., Bengstsson, C., Larsson, B., Pennert, K., Rybo, E. & Sjöström, L. (1984): Distribution of adipose tissue and risk of cardiovascular disease and death. *B. M. J.* **289**, 1257-1261.
13. Larsson, B., Svärdsudd, K., Welin, L., Wilhelmsen, L., Björntorp, P. & Tibblin, G. (1984): Abdominal adipose tissue distribution, obesity and risk of cardiovascular disease and death. *B. M. J.* **288**, 1401-1404.
14. Lönnroth, P., Jansson, P.-A. & Smith, U. (1987): A microdialysis method allowing characterization of the intercellular water space in humans. *Am. J. Physiol.* **253 E**, 228-231.
15. Lönnroth, P. (1988): Potential role of adipose tissue for the development of insulin resistence in obesity. *Acta Med. Scand.* **723** (Suppl), 91-94.
16. Mauriège, P., Galitzki, J., Berlan, M. & Lafontan, M. (1987): Heterogenous distribution of beta and alpha2-adrenoceptor binding sites in human fat cells from various deposits: functional consequences. *Eur. J. Clin. Invest.* **17**, 156-165.
17. Mauriège, P., Després, J.P., Marcotte, M., Ferland, M., Tremblay, A., Nadeau, A., Moorjani, S., Lupie, J., Theriault, G. & Bouchard, C. (1990): Abdominal fat cell lipolysis, body fat distribution, and metabolic variables in premenopausal women. *J. Clin. Endocrinol. Metab.* **71**, 1028-1035.
18. Östman, J., Arner, P., Engfeldt, P. & Kager, L. (1979): Regional differences in the control of lipolysis in human adipose tissue. *Metabolism* **28**, 1198-1205.
19. Smith, U. (1985). Regional differences in adipocyte metabolism and possible consequences *in vivo*. *Int. J. Obes.* **9** (Suppl. I), 145-148.
20. Vague, J. (1950): Differenciation semelle et repartition graisseuse. *Semin. Hop. Paris.* **26**, 1157-1175.
21. Vague, J. (1956): The degree of masculine differentiation of obesities: a factor determining predisposition to diabetes, atherosclerosis, gout and uric calculus disease. *Am. J. Clin. Nutr.* **4**, 20-34.

Chapter 71

Vasoactive Substances in Human Adipose Tissue Biopsies

D.L. CRANDALL[1,3], H.E. HERZLINGER[3], P. CERVONI[3], T.M. SCALEA[2] and J.G. KRAL[2]

Departments of Medicine[1] and Surgery[2], SUNY HSC Brooklyn, NY and Cardiovascular Research, American Cyanamid Co.[3], Pearl River, NY, USA

Most of the metabolic and haemodynamic complications of obesity are associated with the accumulation of fat in intra-abdominal adipose tissue depots. Interdepot variations in storage and release of lipids from adipose tissue correlate with regional differences in catecholamine sensitivity and receptor density. We investigated the existence of novel vasoactive factors with haemodynamic and angiogenic properties in human adipose tissue biopsies. In seven severely obese patients (BMI = 48 ± 6) undergoing anti-obesity surgery, subcutaneous, omental and mesenteric adipose tissue biopsies were homogenized prior to differential centrifugation to yield highly purified microsomal preparations. Angiotensin-converting enzyme (ACE), endothelin-1 and transforming growth factor alpha were analysed using RIA with appropriately radiolabelled polyclonal antibodies. Fat cell size, protein content and wet weight were used as references for all analyses.

Significant concentrations of each substance were found in all depots. Endothelin-1 and transforming growth factor alpha values ranged from 5–50 pg/g adipose tissue wet weight, with significantly greater quantities in mesenteric fat whether expressed per unit wet weight, per 10^6 fat cells or per mg protein. ACE was also elevated in mesenteric adipose tissue per unit wet weight, with values ranging from 150–300 units/g wet weight in all depots, but was not elevated in this depot when expressed in terms of protein or fat cells. Our results indicate that vasoactive substances are detectable in human fat with higher concentrations of endothelin-1 and transforming growth factor alpha in the mesenteric depot. These findings could have implications for both adipose tissue growth and cardiovascular homeostasis.

Introduction

Adipose tissue is the second largest tissue in normal-weight subjects and the largest in obese patients. Adipocyte hyperplasia is characteristic of increasing body weight and is predominantly combined with hypertrophy of fat cells in clinically significant obesity. Although it is well recognized that obesity is associated with prevalent co-morbidity, with the exception of conditions caused mainly by excess body weight *per se* (such as osteoarthritis and possibly respiratory failure) it is not clear whether the increase in adipose tissue mass of itself is deleterious or contributory to the co-morbidity. Most co-morbidity is found with adipocyte hypertrophy[2] and recently "visceral" or intra-abdominal location of adipose tissue has been shown to be associated with the majority of complications of obesity[9].

Studies of adipose tissue have mainly focused on regulation of storage and release of lipid or, to a lesser degree, on development and growth of the tissue to accommodate (excess) substrate. The hyperdynamic circulation of obesity[1] and obesity-related hypertension[13] are less well studied and are poorly understood. The relatively few studies of regional adipose tissue blood flow are confined to rodents in varying nutritional states (review[4]) and have virtually neglected haemodynamic regulation.

Recently novel vasoactive substances implicated in normal regulation and pathophysiological states have been identified in the systemic circulation and in specific tissues[3]. Interestingly, factors initially believed to solely regulate haemodynamics have also been shown to influence angiogenesis and tissue growth[14]. In this study, for the first time we demonstrate the existence of vasoactive substances in biopsies of human adipose tissue from different depots.

Patients and methods

Seven patients (six women), clinically severely obese (mean BMI = 48 ± 6, sem), aged 30–43 years (mean 36 ± 1.7) undergoing surgical treatment for obesity had adipose tissue biopsies performed at the time of surgery. Written informed consent was obtained from all patients and the protocol was approved by the Institutional Review Board. All patients were normotensive, none were diabetic and none were taking haemodynamically active medications. The women were pre-menopausal and were not taking oral contraceptives.

After an overnight fast, but with a 5 per cent glucose solution administered intravenously at a rate of 125 ml/h, under general anaesthesia maintained by nitrous oxide and phentanyl, knife biopsies of 1–5 g of adipose tissue were taken immediately upon entering the abdomen through an upper midline incision. Samples were taken in the epigastric subcutaneous fat, the peripheral omentum and mesenteric fat close to the wall of the terminal ileum. The tissue was finely cut into normal saline at 23°C, transported to the laboratory and processed within 2 h.

The tissue was placed on laboratory film, minced, and transferred to a 50 ml plastic test-tube containing 10 ml of cold TRIS HCl buffer, then immediately homogenized using a Brinkmann polytron with 2 x 10 s bursts and 1 x 30 s burst at the highest setting. The resulting white, viscous homogenate was centrifuged at 1500 **g** for 10 min in a Sorvall 28S refrigerated centrifuge maintained at 4°C. This initial centrifugation resulted in an upper layer of caked lipid, a clear infranatant, and a coarse pellet containing fibrous elements. After decanting the lipid, the infranatant was suctioned through polyethylene tubing into a syringe without disturbing the pellet, and immediately spun at 8500 **g** for 10 min. The resulting supernatant was subjected to a third and final centrifugation at 100,000 **g** for 30 min yielding mainly stroma-vascular elements. The final pellets were resuspended in 1 ml of the TRIS buffer, and either assayed immediately or stored at –75°C.

Adipose tissue cellularity

Aliquots of freshly obtained tissue were placed in a solution of Kreb's Ringer bicarbonate (KRB) buffer, pH 7.4, containing 6 mM glucose, 4 per cent albumin and collagenase at a concentration of 2 mg/ml. Following gassing with 95 per cent O_2, the cells were placed in a shaking incubator and maintained at 37°C, while being shaken at 60 strokes per minute for 1 h. Lipid content was determined and cell sizing was performed by microscopic analysis yielding total cell number[7].

Biochemical assays

Angiotensin converting enzyme (ACE) activity was assayed using acylated tripeptide as a substrate for the enzymatic release of hippuric acid (Ventrex Corporation, Portland, ME) in 50 µl of the 100,000 **g** resuspended pellets. Captopril in a final concentration of 10^{-7} M was used to further verify the presence of the enzyme. One activity unit was equivalent to the amount of angiotensin converting enzyme required to hydrolyse the substrate at an initial rate of 1 per cent per minute at 37°C. Control samples provided by the commercial supplier were always assayed with the vascular preparations, and were consistently within the range denoted on the label.

Transforming growth factor-1, the 50 amino acid peptide also called TGF-alpha, and endothelin-1 were assayed in the 100,000 **g** pellet using commercially available iodinated radioimmunoassay systems (Peninsula Laboratories, Inc., Belmont, CA). Samples were removed from –75°C, thawed in an ice bath, 500 KIU of aprotinin was added in a 20 µl total volume, and the sample further diluted 1:1 with buffer supplied with the system. Standards were assayed at the same time, and binding curves generated from these values served for calculating the concentration of unknown.

Protein analysis was performed by the method of Lowry[11]. Results are expressed as mean ±SEM, and are considered significantly different at $P < 0.05$ using Student's t-test.

Results

There were no statistically significant differences between sites in percentage lipid content (65–67 per cent), water content (31–33 per cent) or fat cell weight (0.53–0.57 µg/g). However, the protein content of mesenteric adipose tissue (241 ± 57 µg/g) was statistically significantly greater than in the omental (172 ± 22) and subcutaneous (141 ± 13) depots ($P < 0.05$).

The mesenteric depot contained significantly more angiotensin-converting enzyme (ACE) per g wet weight 262.3 ± 90.5, vs 141.8 ± 27.9 in the omental and 134.2 ± 32.6 units/g in the subcutaneous ($P < 0.05$) depots, with no differences when expressed per mg protein or 10^6 fat cells.

Table 1 presents levels of transforming growth factor alpha and endothelin-1, both of which were significantly higher in the mesenteric than in the omental or subcutaneous depots regardless of the method of expression.

Table 1. Transforming growth factor alpha (TGF alpha) and endothelin-1 (ET-1) in adipose tissue homogenates from subcutaneous (SQ) omental (OM) and mesenteric (MES) depots in seven severely obese patients (mean ± SEM)

	SQ	OM	MES
TGF alpha			
pg/g wet weight	2.66 ± 3.20	9.34 ± 3.42	37.57 ± 13.02*
pg/mg protein	36 ± 12	44 ± 20	160 ± 70*
pg/10^6 fat cells	3.88 ± 0.11	5.12 ± 0.19	25.2 ± 7.2*
ET-1			
pg/g wet weight	9.50 ± 2.54	7.68 ± 1.82	48.5 ± 12.2**
pg/mg protein	69 ± 16	38 ± 7	245 ± 83**
pg/10^6 fat cells	8.18 ± 1.98	5.96 ± 1.28	35.5 ± 9.2**

* $P < 0.05$ vs OM and SQ; ** $P < 0.01$ vs OM and SQ.

Discussion

This is the first demonstration of ACE, TGF alpha and endothelin-1 in homogenates of human adipose tissue from different depots. ACE is an endothelial cell marker that catalyses the conversion of angiotensin I to the potent vasoconstrictor angiotensin II. Angiotensin II has recently been shown to also stimulate growth of smooth muscle cells[14]. The finding of higher levels of ACE in the mesenteric depot than in the other two when expressed per gram wet weight, may reflect increased vascularity of this depot, also evident in the higher protein content.

Endothelin-1, as the name indicates, is derived from vascular endothelium and is also a powerful vasoconstrictor. The peptide releases epinephrine, vasopressin and atrial natriuretic peptide, all of which have potent haemodynamic effects. Elevated levels of endothelin in the systemic circulation have been shown to occur in essential hypertension[6] and other hypertensive clinical conditions[15,10]. Contrary to the findings with ACE, endothelin was elevated in mesenteric tissue regardless of the mode of expression.

Transforming growth factor alpha belongs to a class of growth factors that stimulate endothelial cell proliferation and promote angiogenesis. The peptide has been ascribed an autocrine role in several growth processes including liver regeneration[12], though it has not previously been studied in adipose tissue. Recently TGF alpha has also been shown to stimulate regional arterial blood flow *in vivo* and is presumed to have a persistent regulatory role in control of vascular tone[8].

Our findings of vasoactive and angiogenic factors in human adipose tissue homogenates, though potentially of great importance for understanding adipose tissue growth, substrate partitioning and haemodynamic regulation, require further investigation. Three issues need further study, namely identifying the components of adipose tissue containing the factors (stroma-vascular *vs* adipocyte), determining the origin of the substances within adipose tissue (synthesis *vs* binding), and comparing adipose tissue levels with those of other tissues, particularly with variations in clinically relevant conditions such as hypertension and obesity.

We have recently reported detectable levels of vasoactive substances in separated adipocyte and stroma-vascular elements of rat adipose tissue[5] though the preparation of human tissue in this study is mainly stroma-vascular. Studies of mRNA are in progress to elucidate whether these factors are synthesized in adipose tissue. Further studies are warranted to determine the role, if any, of these vasoactive substances in haemodynamic regulation and adipose tissue growth in obesity.

Acknowledgements

Brian Saunders and Rebecca Zolotor provided excellent technical assistance, for which we are grateful.

References

1. Alexander, J.K., Dennis, E.W., Smith, W.G., *et al.* (1962–63): Blood volume, cardiac output, and distribution of systemic blood flow in extreme obesity. *Cardiovascular Research Center Bulletin* **1**, 39-44.
2. Björntorp, P., Bengtsson, C., Blohme, G., *et al.* (1971): Adipose tissue fat cell size and number in relation to metabolism in randomly selected middle-aged men and women. *Metabolism* **20**, 927-935.
3. Campbell, D.J. (1987): Circulating and tissue angiotensin systems. *J. Clin. Invest.* **79**, 1-6.
4. Crandall, D.L. & DiGirolamo, M. (1990): Hemodynamic and metabolic correlates in adipose tissue: pathophysiologic considerations. *FASEB J.* **4**, 141-147.
5. Crandall, D.L., Herzlinger, H.R., Cervoni. P. & Kral, J.G. (1991): Transforming growth factor alpha (TFG alpha) in adipocyte and stromal-vascular fractions of rat adipose tissue. *FASEB J.* **5(5)**, A904.
6. Davenport, A.P., Ashby, M.J., Easton, P., *et al.* (1990): A sensitive radioimmunoassay measuring endothelin-like immunoreactivity in human plasma: comparison of levels in patients with essential hypertension and normotensive control subjects. *Clin. Sci.* **78**, 261-264.
7. DiGirolamo, M., Mendlinger, S. & Fertig, J. (1971): A simple method to determine fat cell size and number in four mammalian species. *Am. J. Physiol.* **221**, 850-858.
8. Gan, B.S., Hollenberg, K.L., MacCannell, K. *et al.* (1987): Distinct vascular actions of epidermal growth factor-urogastrone and transforming growth factor alpha. *J. Pharmacol. Exp. Ther.* **242**, 331-337.
9. Gillum, R.F. (1987): The association of body fat distribution with hypertension, hypertensive heart disease, coronary heart disease, diabetes and cardiovascular risk factors in men and women aged 18–79 years. *J. Chronic Dis.* **40**, 421-428.
10. Hirata, Y., Itoh, K., Ando, K., *et al.* (1989): Plasma endothelin levels during surgery. *NEJM* **321**, 1686.

11. Lowry, O.H., Rosebrough, N.J., Farr, A.L. & Randall, R.J. (1951): Protein measurement with the Folin phenol reagent. *J. Biol. Chem.* **193**, 265-275.
12. Mead, J.E. & Fausto, N. (1989): Transforming growth factor may be a physiological regulator of liver regeneration by means of an autocrine mechanism. *Proc. Natl. Acad. Sci. USA* **86**, 1558-1562.
13. Messerli, F.H., Ventura, H.O., Reisin, E., *et al.* (1982): Borderline hypertension and obesity: two prehypertensive states with elevated cardiac output. *Circulation* **66**, 55-60.
14. Naftilan, A.J., Pratt, R.E. & Dzau, V.J. (1989): Induction of platelet-derived growth factor A-chain and c-myc gene expressions by angiotensin II in cultured rat vascular smooth muscle cells. *J. Clin. Invest.* **83**, 1419-1424.
15. Shichiri, M., Hirata, Y., Ando, K., *et al.* (1990): Postural change and volume expansion affect plasma endothelin levels. *JAMA* **263**, 661.

Chapter 72

Site Differences in the Regulation of Adipose Tissue Lipolysis in Men

P. MAURIÈGE, J.P. DESPRÉS, D. PRUD'HOMME, M.C. POULIOT, A. TREMBLAY and C. BOUCHARD

Physical Activity Sciences Laboratory, Laval University, Ste-Foy, Québec, Canada, G1K 7P4

We have investigated the adrenergic control of lipolysis in subcutaneous abdominal and femoral adipose cells from lean and obese men. In abdominal adipocytes from obese individuals, epinephrine promoted an inhibition of lipolysis at low concentrations, this effect being completely reversed at higher doses, whereas the physiological amine was only lipolytic in lean subjects. Moreover, clonidine-induced antilipolysis was more pronounced in abdominal adipocytes from obese men compared to lean controls whereas such difference was not observed in femoral adipose cells. There was also no variation among adipose sites, nor between lean and obese men when lipolysis was stimulated with isoproterenol. In addition, epinephrine- and clonidine-induced maximal antilipolyses of abdominal adipocytes were both positively associated with various indices of total body fatness and fat distribution. This study suggests that, in men, variations in the abdominal adipose cell lipolytic response to catecholamines appear to involve differences in the functional balance between α_2- and β-adrenoceptors.

Introduction

Since the pioneering works of Vague[22,23], it is has been well established that body fat distribution is a significant correlate of variables related to the health status and that abdominal obesity is closely associated with various metabolic complications, whereas peripheral adiposity appears to be rather benign[4,5,8,9,24]. It has become thus evident that human adipose tissue is heterogeneous regarding its metabolic activity. More recently, sex- and site-differences in adipose cell lipolytic response to catecholamines have been extensively described[11]. It has also been proposed that alterations in the functional balance between α_2- and β-adrenoceptor components may account for the regional variations in lipolysis particularly observed in obesity[1], but the mechanisms underlying such site differences remain partly unknown. Furthermore, as most studies published so far have been conducted in women, we have therefore investigated the regional variation in the regulation of adipose tissue lipolysis in obese and lean men.

Material and methods

Fifty-four healthy and sedentary men, aged 36 ± 3 years (mean ± SD) (32 obese and 22 lean) participated in this study. None of them had recent illness or endocrine abnormalities. Total body fatness was estimated by the body mass index (BMI), and derived from the measurement of body density[20] obtained by hydrostatic weighing technique[3]. Abdominal (L4-L5) and femoral (mid-thigh) subcutaneous fat areas were determined by computed tomography (CT)[21]. After an overnight fast, participants were subjected to biopsies of subcutaneous fat performed at both abdominal and femoral sites, and about 200 mg of adipose tissue were surgically removed from the two depots. After collagenase digestion[19], the isolated adipocytes were used for lipolysis measurements. At the end of the incubation procedure (2 h, 37°C), glycerol release was determined according to a sensitive bioluminescent technique[7].

Results and discussion

Obese men differed significantly from lean subjects for BMI and percentage of body fat. The wide range of BMI indicated that our sample included lean (19 kg/m^2) to moderately obese individuals (34 kg/m^2). Abdominal and femoral subcutaneous fat areas assessed by CT were also greater in obese men than in lean controls.

There were marked regional variations between obese and lean subjects as well as among adipose sites in the lipolytic effects of catecholamines, as summarized in Table 1.

Table 1. Hormone-induced lipolysis in obese (Ob) and lean (Le) men

	EPI Ob	EPI Le	CLO Ob	CLO Le	ISO Ob	ISO Le
ABD	– – –/+	+ +	– –	–	+ +	+ +
FEM	– –/+	– +	– –	–	+ +	+ +

– antilipolysis; + lipolysis.

In femoral adipocytes from both groups, epinephrine, a dual α_2- and β-adrenergic agonist, inhibited lipolysis at low concentrations (10^{-9} to 10^{-7} M), and exerted a lipolytic action at higher doses (10^{-6} to 10^{-5} M). The complexity of the hormone responsiveness probably reflects the differential recruitment of α_2-, followed by β-adrenoceptors[12]. In abdominal adipocytes from obese men, epinephrine initiated a similar biphasic responsiveness (with a stronger antilipolysis as compared to femoral adipose cells) whereas in lean subjects, the physiological amine acted as an exclusive lipolytic agent, thus suggesting either a weaker α_2-adrenoceptor activity or its complete counteraction by a β-stimulation. It thus seems reasonable to assume that the functional balance between α_2- and β-adrenoceptors is mainly responsible for the regional differences in subcutaneous lipolysis[12,25]. Several investigations have already pointed out that the lipolytic effect of catecholamines is much more pronounced in abdominal than in femoral fat cells[16]. Moreover, regional differences in lipolysis seem to involve some early steps in catecholamine action[6,10,14].

Clonidine, an α_2-agonist, inhibited lipolysis in both adipose depots and groups. The maximal antilipolytic effect in obese individuals was, however, more pronounced in abdominal than in femoral adipocytes, whereas this regional difference was not found in lean men. Moreover, maximal antilipolysis was also greater in obese than in lean men for abdominal adipocytes, suggesting a stronger α_2-inhibitory component. Sensitivity to clonidine estimated as the half-maximal antilipolytic response was similar in both adipose sites and groups. These results indicate that obesity enhances the antilipolytic effect of epinephrine in men, and thus, the α_2-adrenergic component. A relatively greater α_2-antilipolytic response of abdominal adipose tissue in obese men may contribute to their tendency to accumulate excess fat in the abdominal area[10]. The lower α_2-effect in abdominal adipocytes of lean men is also consistent with the exclusive lipolytic response of epinephrine in these cells.

A similar comparison of the lipolytic effects of isoproterenol, a selective β-agonist, revealed neither regional variation, nor group difference, suggesting an unaltered hormone responsiveness. However, the lower EC_{50} (i.e. the concentration of isoproterenol required for half-maximal stimulation of lipolysis) in abdominal adipocytes from obese men may reflect a greater β-adrenoceptor sensitivity which could be one determinant of the regional differences in catecholamine action[25]. This result is concordant with a sensitivity to isoprotere-

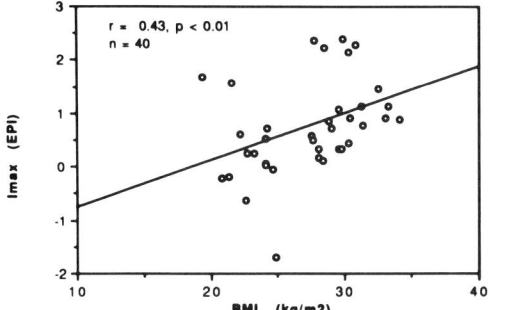 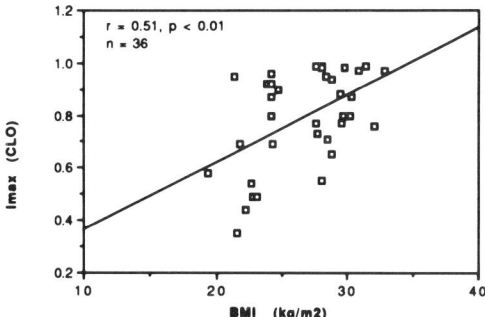

Fig. 1. Relationships between the maximal abdominal antilipolytic effects of epinephrine (EPI) and clonidine (CLO) and the body mass index (BMI). Maximal inhibition (Imax) of lipolysis at 10^{-7} M of each agent is expressed as the ratio: (ADA minus agent / ADA minus basal), where ADA represents adenosine deaminase stimulated lipolysis. The number of subjects (n) is indicated on the figure.

nol higher in abdominal than in gluteal or femoral adipose cells of obese men, which has been reported not only in obese women[10], but also in healthy men and women[16,18]. Recently, a greater β-adrenergic lipolytic response has also been documented in abdominal adipose tissue from obese as compared to lean premenopausal women[13]. As only a few available α_2- and β-adrenoceptors need to be occupied to obtain a maximal effect in human fat cells[2], changes in sensitivity reflect alterations in hormone action which are rather located at or near the receptor level whereas alterations in responsiveness usually reflect changes in hormone action at further intracellular steps in the pathway of the signal.

On the other hand, maximal antilipolyses induced by both epinephrine and clonidine in abdominal adipocytes were positively associated with various indicators of total body fatness and adipose tissue distribution such as the percentage of fat and the amount of subcutaneous abdominal fat measured by CT (results not shown). Relationships between the BMI and the maximal antilipolytic responses of both agents are illustrated in Fig. 1. In contrast, the maximal antilipolytic responses of femoral adipose cells to epinephrine and clonidine were related neither to the BMI, the percentage of fat, nor to the CT-derived subcutaneous femoral fat area (data not shown). Finally, it is however difficult to draw any firm conclusion on the physiological function of the α_2-adrenoceptor, as correlational analyses cannot clarify whether a high α_2-adrenergic component increases the risk of fat accumulation or whether a great α_2-adrenergic activity reflects the consequence (rather than a cause) of an obese state.

Conclusion

Results of our investigation suggest that variations in the abdominal lipolytic response to catecholamines involve differences in the ratio of α_2- to β-adrenoceptors probably related to the density of α_2-adrenergic receptors. Sex steroids and glucocorticoid hormones may affect adipose tissue metabolism and lipolysis, via specific hormonal receptors[15,17]. Further research is clearly needed to identify the mechanisms underlying such regional differences.

Acknowledgements. The authors wish to express their gratitude to Judith Maheux, Martine Marcotte and Claude Leblanc for their excellent collaboration at various stages of the study. The subjects and the staff of the Physical Activity Sciences Laboratory are also gratefully acknowledged. Supported by the Fonds de la Recherche en Santé du Québec (FRSQ), the Fonds FCAR-Québec, and the Medical Research Council of Canada. J.P. Després is a FRSQ scholar, whereas M.C. Pouliot is a FRSQ fellow.

References

1. Arner, P. (1988): Control of lipolysis and its relevance to development of obesity in man. *Diabetes Metab. Rev.* **4**, 507-515.
2. Arner, P., Hellmer, J., Wennlund, A., Ostman, J. & Engfeldt, P. (1988): Adrenoceptor occupancy in isolated fat cells and its relationship with lipolysis rate. *Eur. J. Pharmacol.* **146**, 45-56.
3. Behnke, A.R. & Wilmore, J.H. (1974): *Evaluation and regulation of body build and composition*, pp. 20-37. Englewood Cliffs, NJ: Prentice-Hall.
4. Björntorp, P. (1988): Possible mechanisms relating fat distribution and metabolism. In *Fat distribution during growth and later health outcomes. Current topics in nutrition and disease*, eds. C. Bouchard & F.E. Johnston, pp. 175-191. New York: Alan R. Liss.
5. Després, J.P., Moorjani, S., Lupien, P.J., Tremblay, A., Nadeau, A. & Bouchard, C. (1990): Regional distribution of body fat, plasma lipoproteins, and cardiovascular disease. *Arteriosclerosis* **10**, 497-511.
6. Kather H., Zöllin, K., Simon, B. & Schlierf, G. (1977): Human fat cell adenylate cyclase: regional differences in adrenaline responsiveness. *Eur. J. Clin. Invest.* **7**, 595-597.
7. Kather, H., Schroder, F. & Simon, B. (1982): Microdetermination of glycerol using bacterial NADH-linked luciferase. *Clin. Chim. Acta* **120**, 295-300.
8. Kissebah, A.H., Vydelingum, N., Murray, R., Evans, D.J., Hartz, A.J., Kalkhoff, R.K. & Adams, P.W. (1982): Relation of body fat distribution to metabolic complications of obesity. *J. Clin. Endocrinol. Metab.* **54**, 254-260.
9. Krotkiewski, M., Björntorp, P., Sjöström, L. & Smith, U. (1983): Impact of obesity on metabolism in men and women. Importance of regional adipose tissue distribution. *J. Clin. Invest.* **72**, 1150-1162.
10. Leibel, R.L. & Hirsch, J. (1987): Site- and sex-related differences in adrenoceptor status of human adipose tissue. *J. Clin. Endocrinol. Metab.* **64**, 1205-1210.
11. Leibel, R.L., Edens, N.K. & Fried, S.K. (1989): Physiologic basis for the control of body fat distribution in humans. *Annu. Rev. Nutr.* **9**, 417-443.
12. Mauriège, P., Galitzky, J., Berlan, M. & Lafontan, M. (1987): Heterogeneous distribution of beta- and alpha2-adrenoceptor binding sites in human fat cells from various deposits: functional consequences. *Eur. J. Clin. Invest.* **17**, 156-165.
13. Mauriège, P., Després, J.P., Marcotte, M., Ferland, M., Tremblay, A., Nadeau, A., Moorjani, S., Lupien, P.J., Thériault, G & Bouchard, C. (1990): Abdominal fat cell lipolysis, body fat distribution, and metabolic variables in premenopausal women. *J. Clin. Endocrinol. Metab.* **71**, 1028-1035.
14. Ostman, J., Arner, P., Engfeldt, P. & Kager, L. (1979): Regional differences in the control of lipolysis in human adipose tissue. *Metabolism* **28**, 1198-1205.
15. Rebuffé-Scrive, M., Lundholm, K. & Björntorp, P. (1985): Glucocorticoid binding of human adipose tissue. *Eur. J. Clin. Invest.* **15**, 267-272.
16. Rebuffé-Scrive, M., Lönnroth, P., Marin, P., Wesslau, C., Björntorp, P. & Smith, U. (1987): Regional adipose tissue metabolism in men and postmenopausal women. *Int. J. Obes.* **11**, 347-355.
17. Rebuffé-Scrive, M., Brönnegard, M., Nilsson, A., Eldh, J., Gustafsson, J.A. & Björntorp, P. (1990): Steroid hormone receptors in human adipose tissues. *J. Clin. Endocrinol. Metab.* **71**, 1215-1219.
18. Richelsen, B. (1986): Increased alpha2- but similar beta-adrenergic receptor activities in subcutaneous gluteal adipocytes from females compared with males. *Eur. J. Clin. Invest.* **16**, 302-309.
19. Rodbell, M. (1964): Metabolism of isolated fat cells. I-Effects of hormones on glucose metabolism and lipolysis. *J. Biol. Chem.* **239**, 375-380.
20. Siri, W.E. (1956): The gross composition of body fat. *Adv. Biol. Med. Phys.* **4**, 239-280.
21. Sjöström, L., Kvist, H., Cederblad, Å. & Tylén, U. (1986): Determination of total adipose tissue and body fat in women by computed tomography, ^{40}K, and tritium. *Am. J. Physiol.* **250**, E736-E745.
22. Vague, J. (1947): La differenciation sexuelle, facteur determinant des formes de l'obesité. *La Presse Médicale* **30**, 339-340.
23. Vague, J. (1956): The degree of masculine differentiation of obesities: a factor determining predisposition to diabetes, atherosclerosis, gout and uric calculous disease. *Am. J. Clin. Nutr.* **4**, 20-38.
24. Vague, J., Björntorp, P., Guy-Grand, B., Rebuffé-Scrive, M. & Vague, P. (1985): *Metabolic complications of human obesities*. Amsterdam: Elsevier Science Publishers.
25. Wahrenberg, H., Lonnqvist, F. & Arner P. (1989): Mechanisms underlying regional differences in lipolysis in human adipose tissue. *J. Clin. Invest.* **84**, 458-467.

Section XII
Psychosocial aspects of human obesity

Chapter 73

Psychosocial Aspects of Obesity Pathogenetic and Therapeutic Importance

B. GUY-GRAND and M. LE BARZIC
Service de Médecine et Nutrition, Hôtel Dieu, Place du Parvis Notre Dame, 75181 Paris cedex 04, France

The psychosocial aspects of obesity probably have a much larger clinical importance than could be derived from the place that they commonly have in scientific meetings.

It is now increasingly recognized that body fatness is a heterogeneous symptom of multifactorial origin. This concept implies that it is the consequence of the subtle interplay of different interactive factors – constitutional somatic factors either inherited or acquired, environmental factors and psychological factors – constituting a complex system which results in innumerable sets of individually specific situations. Each of these factors may have predisposing, starting, expending and/or maintaining effects on body weight setting, depending upon the subject, his past and present history and his situational context; each of them can be viewed in a kaleidoscopic way giving rise to what could be considered either as a chaos or as a determinism.

The psychosocial factors associated with obesity can be described from three different points of view: as consequences of body fatness, as factors of possible aetiological importance and, in any case, as features affecting the outcome of the treatment.

Psychosocial consequences of obesity

The negative psychosocial consequences of being fat are largely documented[16,19], albeit not commonly listed among the risks of obesity.

There is no doubt that obese or overweight people are placed in an hostile cultural context generating adverse reactions. Fear of fatness and worship of slimness are characteristics of Western countries and largely fill magazines and mass media; the recognition of the somatic hazards of obesity has contributed. The stigmatization of the obese is in evidence if we consider the negative words which dress them up: cheating, dirtiness, forgetfulness, laziness, dishonesty, stupidity, sloppiness and so on are associated with fatness in the mind of the general population and of the obese themselves and have been shown to be present as early as in preschool children. Last but not least, the same is true in a majority of health care professionals, including physicians[7].

Social and professional prejudice against obese subjects is also documented[1], showing that they are much less acceptable and paid less for the same job than the average.

Finally it is clear that obese people are socially rejected and submitted to some antifat racism. Social rejection may have important psychological consequences and must be considered as a major stressor: although secondary to obesity it is often a maintaining and/or a reinforcing factor of obesity itself, feeding one of the numerous vicious circle of obesity. It may induce or amplify disparagement of body image which is one of the psychological disturbances most often observed, especially in obese young women and adolescents[14]. It reinforces the lack of confidence and esteem, generates guilt, shame and depression, the frequency of which is differently appreciated among obese people according to whether or not denied depression (not evaluated with the conventional tests) is taken into account[15]. Also, unsuccessful dieting and restraint behaviour are stressors[9] generating the yo-yo syndrome and setting the obese in a situation of failure contributing to reinforce guilt, shame and depression.

We have thus to take care that some injunctions to lose weight or to lose more weight that is reasonably possible for a given individual could be deleterious. This is typically the case when a slim mother asks her child to diet for losing weight: for the child the message could well be understood as: because I love you, I ask you to be different that you are, I don't accept you, thus I don't love you. This is a typical "paradoxical attitude" that was pointed out long ago by Hilde Bruch[2].

Psychosocial factors of pathogenetic importance

Since obesity basically results from an imbalance between energy expenditure and food intake, some psychosocial factors affecting one or both of these terms may have a crucial importance as promoting weight gain or making it more severe.

Food intake

There is little doubt that both quantitative and qualitative aspects of food intake, particularly food choices, are strongly influenced by social variables: availability, variety, palatability, eating together, have stimulatory functions and modern society provides us with large amounts of pleasant foods and promotes their consumption through advertising (with strong advice to be as slim as possible). An increase in the proportion of fat calories parallels the economic development and favours energy storage.

The socio-economic status is a well-known factor influencing the prevalence of obesity[13]. In Western countries there is an inverse relationship between social class and prevalence of obesity, more marked in women than in men. By contrast, in developing countries the relationship is a direct one. It has been recently shown in a large sample of French people[10] that men and women of the lowest socio-economic class (containing two to four times more obese people) ate significantly more than those from the upper class, even if chronic restraint and/or underreporting was apparent in the fattest women. This culturally determined relative hyperphagia has probably a permissive effect on the phenotypic expression of the genetic background that is likely to be shared by both upper and lower class, thus allowing the appearance of more obesity in the lower class. In developing countries, only the upper class have enough food to pass beyond the threshold permitting the phenotypic expression of obesity.

Another possible impact of psychosocial factors on food intake is maladjusted eating behavior which is present in a vast majority of obese people[3]. Snacking and between meals intake – either nibbling, craving or both – are present in some 60 per cent of outpatient obese women, leading to a very significant hyperphagia. Depending on their type and on the patients themselves, these feeding patterns have different psychological functions, particularly antidepressive, anxiety sedation and non-verbal communication[18]. These compensatory attitudes are facilitated by social stress, the so-called "consumer society", food prohibition and taboos and dietary restraint.

Energy expenditure

Modern transport and conveniences, television, shame of the obese body etc... reduce physical exercise, increase sedentariness, and contribute to decreased energy expenditure; they are, at least, processes facilitating weight gain in predisposed subjects.

Food efficiency

The question that is raised in this section is: are traumatic life events able to induce modifications of food efficiency? In other words are some obese people affected by psychosomatic mechanisms in a way similar to that described in psychosomatic diseases such as asthma or duodenal ulcer[6]? Psychosomatic patients are characterized by some traits that can be recognized on projective tests; such as the Rorschach test or with psychological investigation. "Pensée opératoire"[8], alexythymia[12], emotional and affective constraint, over-investment of social conformity, prevalence of denial as a defence mechanism, defining a psychosomatic personality, have been shown to be quite frequent among obese subjects[5,17] and significantly more common than in matched controls (Le Barzic et al., unpublished data). Subjects with such types of mental functioning are thought to be more likely to develop somatic dysfunction in response to stress. As reviewed by J. Rodin (Chapter 55), stress situations are able to induce marked changes in hormones and autonomic nervous system that are compatible with changes in energy metabolism, more particularly *via* insulin secretion[4], able to lead to weight gain without detectable hyperphagia.

Psychosocial aspects of treatment

The outcome of most treatments of obesity is far from satisfactory. The search for predictors of success and reasons for failure and relapse is a developing field. Among other psychosocial factors that must be taken into account are: irrealistic weight loss expectation, short-term strategies, excessive dietary restraint, poor account of the irrational aspects of food intake and body image, even if data documenting these points are largely lacking. Systematic and stereotyped therapeutic responses to a multifactorial and heterogeneous problem can be expected to be non-adapted for many patients. Research in this field will be promising only if the classic linear model of casuality is left for the benefit of multifactorial models. As shown recently by Schlundt et al.[11], dietary slips prediction is dependent upon three domains: the socially determined situational context, the affective state and the physiological state. All these domains interact to elicit numerous specific stimulus situations predicting dietary slips, the occurrence of which, in turn, may modify the balance of the whole system. Assessing the individual's current environment as well as identifying the problem situations are needed and are probably prerequisites for helping to maintain weight loss.

In conclusion the psychosocial factors represent important pieces of the puzzle. Accounting for them may lead to re-evaluation of the targets and of the methods of management.

References

1. Allon, N. (1982): The stigma of overweight in everyday life. In *Psychological aspects of obesity*, ed. B. Wolman, pp. 130-174. New York: Van Nostrand Reinhold Co.
2. Bruch, H. (1957): The mental development of obese children. In *The importance of overweight*, pp. 165-187. New York: Norton & Co.
3. Craplet, C., Brillant, M., Gibert, M., Sudrot, C. & Vergne, C. (1988): Consommations alimentaires chez la femme obèse. Etude systematique chez 278 consultantes. In *Dietetics in the 90's*, ed. M.F. Moyal, pp. 51-54. London: John Libbey.
4. Jeanrenaud, B. (1990): Neuroendocrinology and evolutionary aspects of experimental obesity. In *Progress in obesity research 1990*, eds. Y. Oomura, S. Tarui, S. Inoue & T.S. Shimazu, pp. 409-421. London: John Libbey.
5. Legorreta, G., Bull, R.H. & Kiely, M.C. (1988): Alexithymia and symbolic function in the obese. *Psychother. Psychosom.* **50**, 88-94.
6. Long, R., Lamont, J.N., Whipple, B., Bandler, L., Blon, G., Burgin, L. & Fessner, L. (1958): A psychosomatic study of allergic and emotional factors in children with asthma. *Am. J. Psychiatr.* **11**, 880-893.

7. Maddox, G.L. & Leiderman, V.R. (1969): Overweight as a social disability with medical implications. *J. Med. Educat.* **44**, 214-220.
8. Marty, P. & De M'uzan, M. (1963): La pensée opératoire. *Rev. Fr. Psychanal.* **27**, 345-355.
9. Polivy, J., Heatherton, T.F. & Herman C.P. (1988): Self esteem, restraint and eating behaviour. *J. Abnorm. Psychol.* **97**, 354-356.
10. Rolland-Cachera, M.F., Bellisle, F., Tichet, J., Chantrel, A.M., Guilloud-Bataille, M., Vol, S. & Pequignot, G. (1990): Relationship between adiposity and food intake: an example of pseudo contradictory results obtained in case-control *versus* between-population studies. *Int. J. Epidemiol.* **19**, 571-577.
11. Schlundt, D.G., Sbrocco, T. & Bell, C. (1989): Identification of high risk situation in a behaviour weight loss program: application of the relapse prevention model. *Int. J. Obes.* **13**, 223-234.
12. Sifneos, P. (1973): The prevalence of alexithymile characteristics in psychosomatic patients. *Psychother. Psychosom.* **22**, 255-262.
13. Sobal, J. & Stunkard, A.J. (1989): Socioeconomic status and obesity: a review of the literature. *Psychol. Bull.* **105**, 260-275.
14. Stunkard, A.J. & Rush, J. (1967): Obesity and the body image: age of the onset of disturbances in the body image. *Am. J. Psychiatr.* **123**, 1443-1447.
15. Stunkard, A. & Rush, J. (1984): Dieting and depression reexamined: a critical review of untoward responses during weight reduction for obesity. *Ann. Int. Med.* **81**, 526-533.
16. Wadden, T.A. & Stunkard, A.J. (1987): Psychopathology and obesity In Human obesity, *Ann. NY Acad. Sci.* **499,** 55-65.
17. Waysfeld, B., Le Barzic, M., Aimez, P. & Guy-Grand, B. (1977): "Pensée opératoire" in Obesity. *Psychother-Psychosom.* **28**, 127-132.
18. Waysfeld, B., Le Barzic, M. & Guy-Grand, B. (1979): Resistances pschologiques a l'amaigrissement. *Médecine et Hygiène* **37**, 1397-1399.
19. Wooley, S.C. (1987): Psychological and social aspects of obesity. In *Body weight control. The physiology, clinical treatment and prevention of obesity*, eds. A.E. Bender & L.J. Brookes, pp. 81-89. New York: Churchill Livingstone.

Chapter 74

Body Size, Age, Ethnicity, Attitudes and Weight Loss

Pippa CRAIG and Ian CATERSON
Department of Endocrinology, Royal Prince Alfred Hospital, Missenden Road, Camperdown, NSW 2050, Australia

Eighty-eight women attending a weight control programme were surveyed for their attitudes to body size, perceptions of community attitudes to the overweight and factors which influenced weight gain, maintenance and loss. The women overestimated their own body size (actual BMI 33.9 ± 7.1, perceived 38.4 ± 6.1, mean ± SD). Those with greater BMIs were less satisfied, as were the younger. There was a general perception of discrimination against the overweight (82 per cent of respondents), particularly against women. More discrimination was perceived by those of Anglo-Saxon origin than those of Southern European descent. However, this ethnic difference was not apparent for the younger women. The causes of weight gain were seen as largely beyond the individual's control, weight loss was seen as being achieved by a regime of diet and exercise, whilst "luck" was important in weight maintenance. These findings have implications for the design of weight-reduction programmes.

Introduction

Obesity is seen as a major health problem in Western societies. There is epidemiological evidence of associations between obesity and several non-communicable diseases, and of other disease states being complicated by the presence of obesity[1,2,3]. Consequently, medical and other health professionals recommend weight reduction by the obese members of society. In addition to its medical consequences, there is a strong cultural prejudice against obesity[13] particularly in women, and evidence that this prejudice has affected medical standards of acceptable sizes for females[11].

However, despite the pervasive emphasis on the benefits of slimness, obesity remains a refractory disorder[1,3], and attempts at weight reduction exhibit extremely high failure rates[13].

The aims of this study were to determine the attitudes of a group of obese women to their own and ideal body sizes; their perceptions of community attitudes towards overweight persons; and to identify factors which may influence weight gain and inhibit weight loss.

Methods

A tool for the objective measurement of attitudes towards body image was developed, based on the distorting photograph technique[10] for quantifying cultural ideals. The procedure has been described elsewhere[4].

Two series of photographs, covering an even range from BMIs from 15–45 for females, and from 17.5–47.5 for males, were used. Subjects were asked to indicate the body size which best represented their own and preferred body size, and healthy and attractive body sizes for both females and males. In addition, they were asked open-ended questions on their perceptions of how the community treated its overweight and underweight members; what they saw as the causes of weight gain, how weight was maintained by those whose weight does not change, and how weight was lost; and the ways in which they felt their current body weight affected their lives. Responses to these questions were recorded by an interviewer.

Subjects' actual height and weight, sex, age, ethnicity, education level, age of onset of weight, number of attempts to lose weight, and whether they completed the 10-week weight-reduction programme, were available from other records.

Body mass index (BMI = W/H^2) was calculated from weight and height data. The ratio of preferred:perceived size was also calculated, to measure satisfaction with current body size. The lower the satisfaction score, the less satisfied the respondent.

Content analysis was carried out on the responses to the open-ended questions. How respondents perceived the community treated the overweight were graded into one of four predetermined categories, based on the degree of discrimination (see Table 1). If a respondent gave more than one category, the score was taken as the more discriminatory category, for the purposes of further analysis. How subjects' weight affected their health, work, family and social lives were similarly graded with increasing effect.

Table 1. Perceived community attitudes to the overweight

1. Not treated differently.
2. Passively discriminated against, e.g. not accepted; shouldn't be like that; seen as a handicap; pressure to conform.
3. Actively discriminated against by omission, e.g. treated as second class citizen; don't want to include them; avoided socially; treated as invisible.
4. Actively discriminated against, verbally or physically, e.g. laughed at; jeered at; ridiculed; discriminated against at work; criticized for the way they dress, how and what they eat.

Multivariate analysis of perceived community attitudes and effects on lifestyle, using the elaboration technique[7], was conducted, to allow fuller description and understanding of the ordinal data. Significant associations between the ordinal variable and other variables were selected, and the relationship examined in more detail, under the conditions of added variables.

Responses to the questions on causes of weight gain, how weight is maintained, and how to lose weight were categorized by two raters, and interrater agreement measured using the Kappa statistic[9], corrected for chance expected agreement[6]. All Kappa values were ≥ 0.46 (ranging from good to excellent), using Landis and Koch's classification[8]. These categories were then considered adequate for further analysis.

The five categories and examples of each appear in Table 2. Those relating to *food* and *exercise* are self-explanatory. Those relating to *feelings* acknowledge some emotional causes which effect food habits; i.e. eating too much was a secondary problem. Responses relating to *luck* were seen as inevitable, unchangeable and beyond the individual's control. Those relating to *vigilance* were concerned with making conscious decisions to change lifestyle. In the case of weight gain, there was a perceived inability to resist those pressures, a lack of vigilance. An SPSSX package (SPSSX Inc, 1988, release 3.0), was used for the statistical analysis.

Table 2. Categories given for analysis of responses on causes of weight gain, maintenance and loss

A Food related responses
Weight gain: eating too much; eating the wrong foods.
Maintenance: eating carefully; not overeating.
Weight loss: eating a balanced diet; regular meals; dieting

B Exercise related responses
Weight gain: lack of exercise; accept increased weight with age.
Maintenance: regular exercise; nervy, so burn it off.
Weight loss: exercising

C Responses related to feelings, emotions
Weight gain: eating from boredom, loneliness, unhappiness, as a comfort; depressed; eating as a weapon; defiance.
Maintenance: react to stress differently; doing more.
Weight loss: treating problem behind gain, e.g. stress; being motivated; having the right attitude.

D Responses related to luck
Weight gain: established bad eating habits; lifestyle changes e.g. childbirth, menopause; metabolism; ill health.
Maintenance: good metabolism: hereditary; being brought up with good eating habits; being healthy.
Weight loss: metabolism; ill health; stress.

E Responses related to vigilance
Weight gain: blame availability of food; social pressure to eat.
Maintenance: look after themselves; have a routine; in tune with body's needs; self-discipline; work at it.
Weight loss: consciously changing bad eating habits; will power; self-discipline; enlisting other's help, e.g. attend a clinic, take pills, surgery, jaw wiring.

Results and discussion

Eighty-eight overweight women from Sydney, Australia, participated in the study. The mean age of the respondents was 43.5 ± 14.9 and mean BMI was 33.9 ± 7.1. Education ranged from primary school only to university level. (Level of education is considered a good indicator of socio-economic status, particularly in women[5].) The subjects were mostly of Anglo-Saxon origin (68 per cent were Australian or English born); 23 per cent were of Southern European origin (Italian, Greek, Spanish, Portuguese); the remaining 9 per cent being of mixed ethnic origin. These two ethnic groupings (Anglo-Saxon, Southern European), were used in further analyses.

Age and BMI were not correlated. There was no significant difference in age, BMI or educational status between the two major ethnic groupings. The younger subjects tended to be more educated ($\chi^2 = 6.1$; d.f. = 1; $P = 0.01$).

Perception of self and ideal sizes

Although the average BMI was 33.9 ± 7.1 (mean ± SD), subjects saw themselves as having a BMI of 38.4 ± 6.1 (mean ± SD). Their preferred BMI was 23.9 ± 4.4. Such differences have been described previously and in other countries[7,13]. The mean preferred sizes were 22.5 ± 4.1 and 21.4 ± 3.5 for healthy and attractive females respectively; and 23 ± 3.8 and 23.3 ± 3.5 for healthy and attractive males respectively. Thus ideal sizes for females were lower than for males, with attractive ideals being slightly lower than healthy ideals, although the differences were not significant.

Larger subjects were less satisfied with their size (Pearson's r = –0.44, P = 0.000); but so also were the younger women (Pearson's r = 0.23, P = 0.02), although they were not necessarily the largest. Older subjects were not only more satisfied with their own current body size, but also nominated larger target sizes for themselves (Pearson's r = 0.35, P = 0.0000); and chose larger ideal sizes for attractive females (Pearson's r = 0.20, P = 0.03), and healthy females (Pearson's r = 0.26, P = 0.02). These differences suggest that messages about smaller body size have had a major effect on the younger generation, whilst the older generation accept larger sizes.

Community attitudes to overweight and underweight

Respondents felt that there was more discrimination against overweight (82 per cent) than underweight (51 per cent) members of the Australian community, with active discrimination against weight groups felt to be far greater against the overweight (66 per cent) compared to the underweight (5 per cent). While 55 per cent felt that the sex of the individual was not a factor in how society treated an overweight person, a significant minority felt that women were treated far worse than men (42 per cent compared to 3 per cent).

Anglo-Saxons were more likely to state that the overweight were treated differently (χ^2 = 4.06, d.f. = 1, P = 0.04) compared with those of Southern European origin. This difference between the ethnic groups was significant for the older subjects (P = 0.02), for those less satisfied with own body size (P = 0.02) and those who had gained weight as adults (P = 0.003).

Contrary to expectation, a higher BMI was not significantly associated with more perceived health problems (χ^2 = 2.64, d.f. = 1, P = 0.10), although there was a significant relationship between BMI and health effects among the less educated (P = 0.05) and those who had gained weight as adults (P = 0.05)

Heavier subjects felt more effect of weight on their work lives (χ^2 = 5.80, d.f. = 1, P = 0.02); in particular the Anglo-Saxons (P = 0.01), and those less satisfied with their own body size (P = 0.007).

Subjects less than 45 years old felt more of an effect of their body size on family life (χ^2 = 4.52, d.f. = 1, P = 0.03). Age and effect on family life was significantly associated for those subjects with a higher educational status (P = 0.04); and those of Anglo-Saxon origin (P = 0.03).

Causes of weight gain, maintenance and loss

Responses to these three questions drew out some interesting differences (Table 3).

Table 3. Reasons for gaining, maintaining and losing weight given by 88 obese subjects attending a weight loss clinic

Categories	Gaining (n)	Maintaining (n)	Losing (n)
Food	53	30	80
Exercise	26	25	54
Feelings	59	6	13
Luck	49	63	16
Vigilance	10	22	23

Reasons for gaining weight were attributed to emotional causes (67 per cent); eating too much or the wrong foods (60 per cent); or bad luck (56 per cent) – i.e. being brought up with bad habits or inheriting 'bad' genes; with exercise and vigilance rating much lower (30 per cent and 11 per cent respectively). Some respondents found it difficult to separate emotional causes from food-related causes, since they perceived that they ate too much for emotional reasons.

Ways of maintaining weight were attributed mainly to luck – the "right" metabolism, having good eating habits (72 per cent); although active involvement in weight maintenance – by eating well, exercising and vigilance – were each acknowledged by about a third of respondents. The general impression was that weight maintainers were perceived as being in control of themselves and their lives, and generally different from weight gainers.

Weight loss is seen to be achieved largely by eating correctly (91 per cent) and exercising (61 per cent) – reflecting the focus of legitimate weight control programmes. Vigilance was mentioned by only one quarter of respondents. Despite the fact that emotional causes and lack of luck were acknowledged as the major causes of weight gain, only a fraction of the respondents mentioned dealing with these problems in an effort to lose weight (15 per cent and 18 per cent respectively).

General discussion

This group of overweight women perceived more pressure on females to be slim, which is borne out by the differing perceived norms and satisfaction levels of women as compared to men, whether overweight or not[4]. The younger, and those of higher socio-economic status are less satisfied, and chose more stringent ideals, implying they felt stronger pressure to be slim. Those of Anglo-Saxon origin tended to feel more discrimination against the overweight, and more effect on work and family life. It seems those of Southern European origin may accept increasing body size with increasing age, although the younger migrants appear to have accepted the cultural norms of the wider Australian community.

The striking mismatch between perceived causes of weight gain and ways of losing weight, is highlighted by this study. By focusing on energy balance, current weight control programmes do not deal with the perceived causes of weight gain, which were seen as very legitimate by these respondents. The constant social pressure to be slim, together with the obvious lack of long-term success exhibited by most of those attending such programmes, profoundly effects attenders' self-esteem. Differing attitudes of those of different age, and ethnic and educational status, suggest that different groups may respond more readily to approaches targeted specifically to their needs in attempting to tackle the problem of obesity. Most important, however, is dealing with community acceptance of an increasingly unrealistic and unattainable slim ideal for women, without evidence that such an ideal is beneficial to health.

References

1. Black, D., James, W.P.T. & Besser, G.M. *et al.* (1983): Obesity: a report of the Royal College of Physicians. *J. R. Coll. Physicians Lond.* **17**, 5-65.
2. Bray, G.A. & Bray, D.S. (1988): Obesity. Part 1 – Pathogenesis. *West. J. Med.* **149**, 429-441.
3. Brownell, K.D. (1982): Obesity: understanding and treating a serious, prevalent, and refractory disorder. *J. Consult. Clin. Psychol.*. **50**, 820-840.
4. Craig, P.L. and Caterson, I.D. (1990): Weight and perceptions of body image in women and men in a Sydney sample. *Community Health Stud.* **14**, 373-383.
5. Daniel, A. (1985): The measurement of social class. *Community Health Stud.* **8**, 218.
6. Fleiss, J.L. (1981): The measure of interrater agreement. In *Statistical methods for rates and proportions*, 2nd edn, pp. 212-236. New York: John Wiley and Sons.
7. Jendrick, M.P. (1985): *Through the maze: statistics with computer applications*, pp. 123-138. Belmont: Wadsworth Publishing Company.

8. Landis, J.R. & Koch, G.G. (1977): The measurement of observer agreement for categorical data. *Biometrics* **33,** 59-174. Cited in *Statistical methods for rates and proportions*. 2nd edn, ed. J.L. Fleiss, p. 218. New York: John Wiley and Sons.
9. Maclure, M. & Willett, W.C. (1987): Misinterpretation and misuse of the Kappa statistic. *Am. J. Epidemiol.* **126**, 161-169.
10. Massara, E.B. & Stunkard, A.J. (1979): A method of quantifying cultural ideals of beauty and the obese. *Int. J. Obes.* **3**, 149-152.
11. Ritenbaugh, C. (1982): Obesity as a culture-bound syndrome. *Cult. Med. Psychiatry* **6**, 347-361.
12. Thompson, J.K. & Thompson, C.M. (1986): Body size distortion and self esteem in asymptomatic, normal weight males and females. *Int. J. Eating Disorders* **5**, 1061-1068.
13. Wooley, S.C. & Wooley, O.W. (1980): Eating disorders: obesity and anorexia. In *Women and psychotherapy*, eds. A.M. Brodsky & R. Hare-Mustin, pp. 135-158. New York: Guildford Press.

Chapter 75

Fear and Loathing of Obesity: the Rise of Dieting in Childhood

Andrew J. HILL
BioPsychology Group, Department of Psychiatry, Leeds University, Leeds LS2 9LT

The pressures on women to avoid overweight and to seek slimness can be seen in the number of adolescent girls who diet. But what is the evolution of this dieting behaviour? A series of studies have been described which have revealed the presence of dieting motivation in a section of 9-year-old girls, their dissatisfactions with body weight and appearance, and their consequent behaviour. Early dieting concerns and behaviour are not innocuous and are linked with clinical eating disorders. The ways in which children respond to the stereotypes of thinness and obesity and the practice of dieting need to be understood as they have serious health implications.

Introduction

Physical appearance continues to be a dominating force in our social fabric. For women in particular, body weight or shape is among the most important determinants of appearance. The opposites of slimness and obesity are laden with symbolism concerning quality of life, personality characteristics, even an implied life course. Slimness is the desired state, equated with beauty, femininity, control, success, good health and longevity. Conversely, to be obese is to be self-indulgent, greedy, lazy, unintelligent, ugly and in poor health. Given these alternatives, the desire for slimness is all pervasive. Weight loss is advertized and adopted as a panacea which will create a new person with new life circumstances. Against this background, the prevalence of weight loss practices, particularly dieting, seems entirely reasonable. Some periodic restriction of eating as a means of losing weight or at least preventing further weight gain is the norm for adult and adolescent women. Dieting has become an affordable and acceptable form of nutritional cosmetic surgery.

Adolescent unhappiness with body shape, and dieting as a mechanism for change, are not new phenomena. Dwyer *et al.* in 1967[1] reported that 60 per cent of adolescent girls had been on weight loss diets, figures similar to those more recently reported. But what is now emerging is that dieting concerns and behaviour are being expressed by younger age groups. One study, for example, found it difficult to distinguish 12-year-olds from much older girls solely in terms of their motivation to diet[9]. But at what age does dieting become a salient feature of a child's world? And what is at the root of early dieting concerns?

The inception of dieting

The emergence of dieting was investigated by comparing a school year group of 84 9-year-old girls with a school year group of 86 14-year-olds attending the same institution on a measure of 'dietary restraint'[4]. Dietary restraint is an individual's dieting resolve or motivation. It is evaluated by questionnaire responses and has been shown to be a powerful predictor of behaviour in several carefully controlled experimental investigations[3]. These children's re-

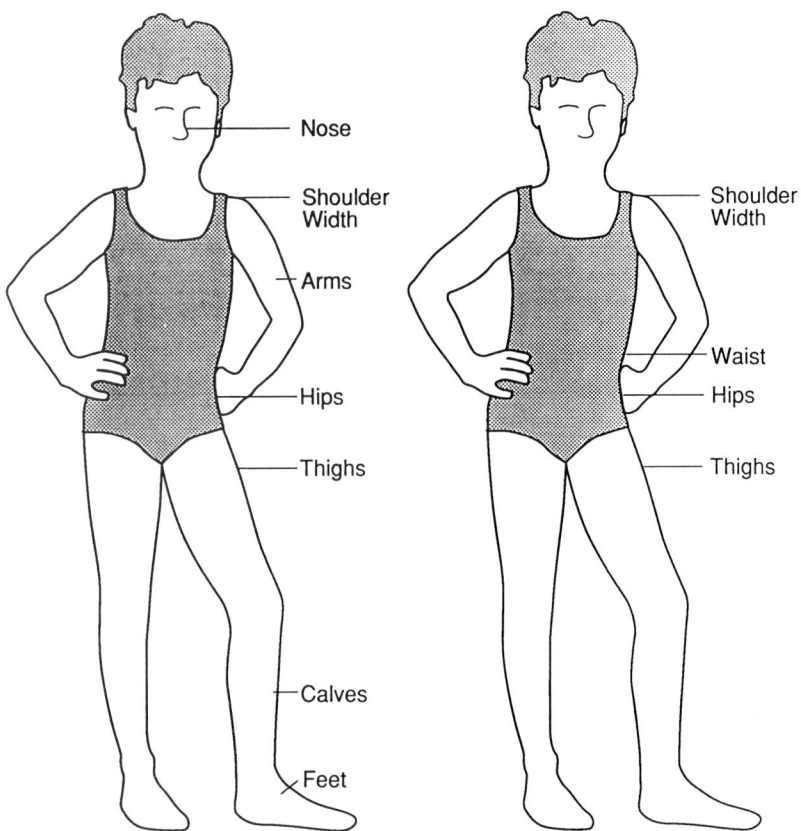

Fig. 1. A summary of the effects of age and dietary restraint on dissatisfaction with discrete body part.

sponses showed that while there was a difference in the overall shape of the distribution of restraint scores, there were representatives of each age group in every category of dieting motivation. In other words, there were girls who expressed high levels of dietary restraint even in the 9-year-old group.

The question of whether these dieting concerns are accompanied by body dissatisfactions was addressed by comparing those girls who fell in the upper and lower quartiles of the restraint distribution on several measures of body esteem and satisfaction. The older girls showed generally higher levels of body dissatisfaction, and with certain body regions in particular (Fig. 1). However, independent of these age-related effects, the highly restrained girls expressed significantly lower body-esteem and greater overall body-dissatisfaction. In particular, these girls were more dissatisfied with their shoulder width, and the size of their waist, hips and thighs. Furthermore, the girls' choice of body shape from a graded scale of silhouettes showed the restrained girls' perception of their current shape to be a significant distance from their ideal shape. Not only did they desire to be significantly thinner, but their ideal was set slimmer than that of the unrestrained and probably represented an unrealistic target shape.

An examination of the girls' actual weight status did reveal a number of overweight girls in the high restraint category. Their behaviour and concerns may therefore have some legitimacy. But what is most revealing is that nearly half of the highly restrained group were within normal weight limits for their age. It appears therefore that for some of these girls, their motivation to diet has little to do with their actual body weight. Rather, it is how they feel about their body and its perceived shape or size which is crucial.

Early dieting concerns and behaviour

There is bound to be scepticism in assessing the functionality of dieting motivation in children aged 9/10 years old. This is entirely appropriate as many people know from personal experience that it is one thing to be dissatisfied with one's weight or figure and be motivated to lose weight, but it is quite another to put these concerns into action. However, two further studies give substance to the relationship between dieting motivation and dieting behaviour in childhood and early adolescence.

In the first, another group of 9-year-old girls recorded their eating behaviour in food intake diaries for a period of 7 days[5]. Again, the high scorers were compared with the low scorers on the restraint scale. The highly restrained girls were found to consume 15 per cent less daily energy than the unrestrained girls, and 11 per cent less than the recommended daily amount for their age. They also showed a tendency to miss meals, particularly breakfast, and rated their feelings of hunger at a significantly higher level than the unrestrained. These changes in recorded behaviour and subjective experience are similar to those observed in adult dieters, and indicate that these girls' dieting concerns do have a functional effect on their behaviour.

Unfortunately, real-life dieting is not synonymous with a rigorous restriction over intake. Diet breaking or perceived lapses are frequently encountered by adult dieters. The second study investigated the susceptibility of a group of 12- and 14-year-old girls in a situation known to lead to this form of lapse in young adults[6]. The experimental procedure invited participants to eat freely from a large quantity of food while they were alone and making a series of sensory evaluations of the food. Normally, a negative association would be expected between dietary restraint and food intake, with the dieters successfully imposing their restriction over eating. However, in this case prior exposure to palatable food stimuli led to a significant positive correlation between restraint and intake, with the highly restrained girls eating substantially more than the unrestrained. This finding of disinhibition, or loss of inhibition over eating, is in complete accord with research in young adult dieters. Regardless of age therefore, dieting is associated with both a limiting of intake and episodes of non-restrained eating.

Health implications

The potential consequences of self-imposed dietary restriction during childhood are those of malnutrition. Stunted growth and delayed puberty have been observed as a result[8], but these are extreme and rare cases. Instead, it is likely that early dieting concerns and their effects will have more subtle implications for health and well-being. The preceding series of studies has characterized a number of 9- to 12-year-old girls who display an active dislike of overweight, express major body dissatisfactions, set unrealistic body shape targets, are concerned about dieting and behave accordingly, and experience control failures. Some of these girls probably face a lifetime of dispute and discontent with their physical appearance and eating behaviour. Alternatively, for some this portrayal may represent the start of a slow progression to a clinical eating disorder.

In the minds of some adults, taking personal responsibility for one's appearance and food choice is appropriate for a maturing child seeking independence and autonomy. But there is a fine line between eating for a lean weight and appearance and the health risks attached to early dieting. The importance of adolescent dieting to the emergence of eating disorders is clear. In one recent study for example, 15-year-old dieters were at eight times the relative risk of having an eating disorder 12 months later compared with non-dieters[7]. The risk attached to dieting at 9 is unknown, but may be considerable.

The urgency for weight loss is increasing. On the one hand, the ideal female shape has been getting measurably slimmer over the last 40 years. On the other, the Western world is getting heavier. Recent governmental data show the number of obese women in the UK to have almost doubled in the last decade[2]. Even if the slim stereotype gets no thinner than it already is, more and more people will find themselves further away from the ideal. The disparity between personal circumstance and cultural ideal is growing. Dissatisfaction with body size and shape is growing in both the number of people who experience it, and in the distance they are from the ideal.

Children are not immune to the stereotypes which dominate the adult world. They too feel pulled towards the effigy of thinness and pushed away from the monster of obesity. In many ways children are more responsive to stereotypes than adults, as the simple depictions they convey are easy to comprehend and the emphasis on conformity is often high during childhood. As professional researchers and practitioners in the field of obesity, we have a duty to communicate accurately the health risks associated with overweight. If there is no evidence of mild overweight causing poor health in adults, this should be clearly stated. If the imperative is for 'healthy eating', then this message should be clearly separated from considerations of overweight. Health should not become another weapon, in addition to aesthetics, with which to unreasonably beat the overweight but not obese adult and child.

References

1. Dwyer, J.T., Feldman, J.J. & Mayer, J.M. (1967): Adolescent dieters: who are they? *Am. J. Clin. Nutr.* **20**, 1045-1056.
2. Gregory, J., Foster, K., Tyler, H. & Wiseman, M. (1990): *The dietary and nutritional survey of British adults*. London: HMSO.
3. Herman, C.P. & Polivy, J. (1980): Restrained eating. In *Obesity*, ed. A.J. Stunkard, pp. 208-225. Philadelphia: Saunders.
4. Hill, A.J., Oliver, S. & Rogers, P.J. (1992): Eating in the adult world: the rise of dieting in childhood and adolescence. *Br. J. Clin. Psychol.* (in press).
5. Hill, A.J. & Robinson, A. (1991): Dieting concerns have a functional effect on the behaviour of nine-year-old girls. *Br. J. Clin. Psychol.* **30,** 265-267.
6. Hill, A.J., Rogers, P.J. & Blundell, J.E. (1989): Dietary restraint in young adolescent girls: a functional analysis. *Br. J. Clin. Psychol.* **28**, 165-176.
7. Patton, G.C., Johnson-Sabine, E., Wood, K., Mann, A.H. & Wakeling, A. (1990): Abnormal eating attitudes in London schoolgirls – a prospective epidemiological study: outcome at twelve month followup. *Psychol. Med.* **20**, 383-394.
8. Pugliese, H.T., Lifshitz, F., Grad, G., Fort, P. & Marks-Katz, M. (1983): Fear of obesity: a cause of short stature and delayed puberty. *N. Engl. J. Med.* **309**, 513-518.
9. Wardle, J. & Beales, S. (1986): Restraint, body image and food attitudes in children from 12 to 18 years. *Appetite* **7**, 209-217.

Chapter 76

Counterregulation as a Function of Cognitive Restraint?

M.S. WESTERTERP-PLANTENGA, E. VAN DEN HEUVEL, L. WOUTERS and F. TEN HOOR

Open University, P.O. Box 2960, 6401 DL Heerlen, The Netherlands; Limburg State University, Maastricht, The Netherlands

During an experimental period of 4 months four-course solid-food lunches, twice preceded by preloads, were served to the subject types: normal weight-restrained and unrestrained, overweight restrained, and overweight restrained on a controlled diet. The subjects completed the two different restrained-eating questionnaires several times during this period[3,8]. The overweight restrained eaters on the diet, had a constant energy intake at lunchtime (1908 ± 252 kJ), notwithstanding preloads of 660 or 420 kJ. They compensated for the preloads in the evenings, and their daily energy intake never exceeded 4200 kJ during this dieting period. The normal weight unrestrained eaters compensated partly for the preload energy intake, during the main course of the lunch, namely by 53 per cent; range 48–58 per cent. Counterregulation after preloads did not occur in normal weight restrained eaters and in overweight restrained eaters with the counselled diet, probably due to the within-boundary preload sizes, and to the unchallenging type of preload.

Introduction

A phenomenon like counterregulation – which is the regulation of the amount of food intake depending on the size of a preload in restrained eaters, compared to unrestrained eaters – elucidates eating behaviour during the meal, with regard to the amount eaten. Counterregulation has been shown in restrained eaters who were given a preload. Eating this preload was perceived as overeating and led to a successive deliberate increased intake. Consequently, disinhibition led to increased food intake, which was positively correlated with preload size[1].

Herman and Polivy[2] proposed that biological pressures maintain consumption within a certain range between the boundaries of hunger and satiety, which they call the range of 'biological indifference'. Within this range psychological factors would have their greatest impact on the regulation of food intake. The boundary model postulates that the zone of biological indifference is wider in dieters than in non-dieters (Fig. 1). Dieters are said to have lower hunger boundaries and higher satiety boundaries than non-dieters. Also, dieters have a third, self-imposed 'diet' boundary, located between hunger and satiety boundaries, marking their maximum desired consumption. Herman and Polivy[2] suggest that once restrained eaters transgress this diet boundary, they eat until they reach the satiety boundary. This has been called the disinhibition which explains the phenomenon of counterregulation in restrained eaters: when the self-control of restrained eaters is disrupted, overeating ensues. The perception of having overeaten disinhibits restrained eaters[5,7].

Consequently, if a preload is given within the diet boundary, counterregulation does not have to occur. Low and high caloric preload effects on food intake were measured. The subjects

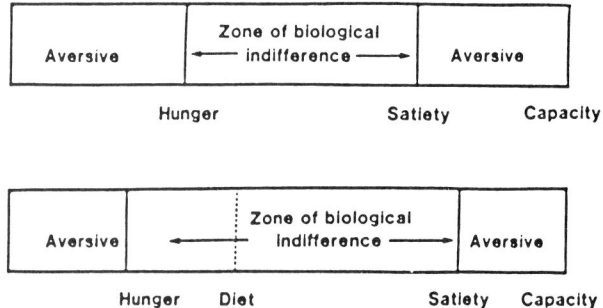

Fig.1. The boundary model of Herman & Polivy[2,4]
(above: non-dieter; below: dieter).

were invited for lunch to the laboratory about once a fortnight. In two of the seven lunches the preload experiments were conducted.

Methods: subjects

Healthy female subjects were recruited via a local newspaper from the general population in the south of the Netherlands as well as from university students and employees of the Limburg State University. From 124 respondents, 80 subjects, age 20-45 years, were selected in four categories: 20 *normal weight unrestrained eaters* (BMI < 25; scores on the TFEQ[8] F1 < 9, F2 < 9; scores on the Herman–Polivy restraint questionnaire < 15; 9 and 15 being the median in formerly studied groups[9,10]. 20 *normal weight restrained eaters* (BMI < 25; F1 > 9 or H-P > 15); 40 overweight restrained eaters (BMI > 25; F1 > 9 or H-P > 15). From the overweight restrained group 20 subjects had followed a weight-reduction programme recently, and 20 subjects were selected to follow a weight reduction programme, run by our dietician. These subjects were instructed how to keep a 1000 kcal (4200 kJ) diet of their own compositions, and with sufficient variation. They were also instructed how to keep a dietary record. The four selected groups were as homogeneous as possible, considering age and weight. Informed consent was obtained.

Methods: procedure

Data presented here are based on a series of seven lunches, which took place at the same time of the day, on the same day of the week, with a 2- or 3-week interval. Intake was monitored via an electronic weighing scale built into the table under the plate and connected to a digital computer. This set-up is similar to "the universal eating monitor" developed by Kissileff *et al.*[6]. All subjects were aware of this procedure and were assured that all data would be kept in strict confidence. The meals consisted of four courses, which were all theoretically rated as attractive (palatability ratings 7–8 on a scale of 6–10, where 6 = palatable). The courses consisted of the following components: (1) vegetable soup (150 g; 5.4 kJ/g); (2) rice (200 g; 6.3 kJ/g) and sauce (400 g; 3.6 kJ/g); (3) cucumber (50 g; 0.8 kJ/g); (4) mango (100 g; 1.8 kJ/g). Three courses (1, 3 and 4) were small to normal portions, so that the amount eaten was fixed. The second course consisted of an ample portion, of a size which previously was considered not to limit intake. Some of course 2 was always left over. Subjects were instructed to eat no solid food in the 3 h preceding a test meal. Subjects then rated their degree of hunger on a 100 mm line, which they repeated after every course. One and a half hours prior to the third and fifth lunch, subjects were given a fruit yoghurt preload, a high caloric one (150 g; 4.4 kJ/g, resulting in 660 kJ) or a low caloric one (150 g; 2.8 kJ/g, resulting in 420 kJ) at random.

Table 1. Subject characteristics (body mass index, body fat %, age, Herman–Polivy restraint score, cognitive restraint, disinhibition, hunger are given for the four subgroups split according to weight and restraint*, and to whether on a controlled diet or not, for four times during the controlled dieting period of the concerned group. *criteria for restraint: F1 > 9 or H-P > 15)

		Normal weight (BMI < 25)				Overweight (BMI > 25)			
		Non-restraint n = 20		Restraint n = 20		Restraint n = 20 (controlled diet)		Restraint n = 20	
	Week	Mean ± SD		Mean ± SD		Mean ± SD		Mean ± SD	
BMI		20.1	1.8	21.3	1.9	24.4	4.1	32.4	3.6
Age, years		32.8	8.4	33.8	9.7	36.1	7.3	37.0	9.3
		Median; range		Median; range		Median; range		Median; range	
Body fat, %		22.6	20.3-24.9	23.4	21.0-25.8	41.7	38.3-45.1	40.5	36.4-44.6
H-P		9	7–12	16	15–17	21	18–24	24	20–28
F1	0	4	2–6	10	9–12	8	5–11	11	6–16
	6–14	4	2–6	11	9–13	15	12–18	11	7–15
F2	0	4	2–6	5	3–8	10	7–13	7	4–10
	6–14	4	2–6	6	3–8	8	5–11	7	4–9
F3		4	2–6	3	1–5	6	3–10	6	4–7

BMI, age, H-P scores, F1 and F2 scores were all positively correlated, two by two (Spearman's rho: $0.3 < r < 0.9$; $P < 0.01$.

Table 2. Meal parameters (amount eaten and eating rate, given for the four subgroups split according to weight and restraint and according to being on a controlled diet or not)

		Normal weight (BMI < 25)		Overweight (BMI > 25)	
		Non-restraint n = 20	Restraint n = 20	Restraint n = 20 (Controlled diet)	Restraint n = 20
	Week	Mean ± SD	Mean ± SD	Mean ± SD	Mean ± SD
Amount eaten, g	0–2	692 139	633 133	485 66	689 159
	6–8*	624 142	631 130	482 84	718 152
	12–14*	637 145	630 131	498 78	732 157
Eating rate, g/s	0–18	0.7 0.07	0.7 0.08	0.7 0.07	0.7 0.08

*Week 6–8 high caloric preload; week 12–14 low caloric preload. The high and low caloric preloads were offered randomly, but the data are presented within these weeks.

Table 3. Hunger state (median and range of hunger state (0-100 mm scores) before the meal and after each one course, for the meals with and without preloads, in the four subject groups)

	Before the meal	After course 1	After course 2	After course 3	After course 4
Normal weight Non-restraint (n=20)					
Without preload	99; 98–100	85; 82–88	30; 24–36	15; 11–19	1; 0–2
With preload	90; 88–92	78; 76–80	29; 26–32	12; 10–14	1; 0–2
Normal weight Restraint (n=20)					
Without preload	93; 91–95	86; 82–90	45; 38–52	21; 16–26	8; 6–10
With preload	92; 89–95	87; 84–90	43; 38–48	23; 16–30	9; 6–12
Overweight Restraint (n=20) Controlled diet					
Without preload	93; 91–95	76; 73–79	36; 32–40	17; 14–20	7; 5–9
With preload	92; 89–95	78; 74–82	39; 34–44	18; 16–20	7; 4–10
Overweight Restraint (n=20)					
Without preload	91; 88–94	81; 79–83	40; 36–44	19; 16–23	6; 3–9
With preload	96; 93–99	85; 82–88	42; 40–44	18; 14–22	6; 4–8

Results

Amount eaten did not change after preloads in the normal weight restrained eaters and in the overweight restrained eaters with controlled diet (Table 2). The latter compensated as was concluded from their food intake diaries (on preload days their food intake did not seem to exceed 4200 kJ too, according to the dietary record). The normal weight unrestrained eaters compensated during the main course, with 53 per cent; range 48–58 per cent, of the energy content of the preload, irrespective of being a high or low caloric preload. The overweight restrained eaters without controlled diet showed a slight increase in the amount eaten after the preloads (table 2). Subjects were always hungry when they arrived for the meal tests, and always satiated when they left. Subjects felt they had eaten slightly more (12 per cent; range 6–18 per cent) than in their normal lunch but they felt comfortable (84 per cent; range 79–89 per cent). Subjects scored the preloads as uninterestingly (22 per cent; range 17–28 per cent). Hunger declined gradually after each course, mostly after course 2, the *ad lib* main course. (Table 3). Apart from in the normal weight unrestrained eaters the decline in hunger was the same irrespective of the preloads. In the normal weight unrestrained eaters hunger declined significantly more ($P < 0.05$) before and after course 1 in the preload situation, but the decline was the same after course 2, 3 and 4, compared to the non-preload situation.

Discussion

With regard to restraint x preload interactions, the boundary model by Herman & Polivy[2,4] was supported by data from this study, in so far that unrestrained eaters regulated food intake to a certain extent, and overweight restrained eaters without a controlled diet seemed to counterregulate. The energy contents of, and the interest in the preloads were such that the normal weight restrained eaters did not perceive to have overeaten, and the overweight restrained eaters with the controlled diet knew that they were able not to exceed their daily intake. In these groups no challenge was experienced, so self-control was not disrupted and disinhibition and subsequently counterregulation did not occur. This was was supported by the relative decreased F2 (disinhibition) score at that time (Table 1). In the restrained eaters there was no significant difference in decrease of hunger state during the meal between the preload and non-preload situation, but in the unrestrained eaters before and after course 1 hunger was decreased significantly more during the preload situation. This might already be related to the reduced subsequent food intake. Resuming consideration of the boundary model[2,4] helps in understanding whether regulation or counterregulation is likely to be observed in restrained eaters.

References

1. Herman, C.P. & Mack, D. (1975): Restrained and unrestrained eating. *J. Pers.* **43**, 647-660.
2. Herman, C.P. & Polivy, J. (1984): A boundary model for the regulation of eating. In *Eating and its disorders*, eds. A.J. Stunkard & E. Stellar, pp. 141-156. New York: Raven Press.
3. Herman, C.P. & Polivy, J. (1980): Restrained eating. In *Obesity*, ed. A.J. Stunkard, pp. 208-225. Philadelphia: Saunders.
4. Herman, C.P., Polivy, J. & Esses, V. (1987): The illusion of counterregulation. *Appetite* **9**, 161-169.
5. Hibscher, J.A. & Herman, C.P. (1977): Obesity, dieting and the expression of 'obese' characteristics. *J. Comp. Physiol. Psychol.* **91**, 374-380.
6. Kissileff, H.R., Klingsberg, G., VanItallie, T.B. (1980): Universal eating monitor for continuous recording of solid or liquid consumption in man. *Am. J. Physiol.* **238**, 14-22.
7. Ruderman, A. J. (1986): Dietary restraint: a theoretical and emperical review. *Psychol. Bull.* **99** (2), 247-262.
8. Stunkard, A.J. & Messick, S. (1985): The three-factor eating questionnaire to measure dietary restraint and hunger. *J. Psychosom. Res.* **29**, 71-83.
9. Westerterp-Plantenga, M.S., Westerterp, K.R., Nicolson, N. A., Mordant, A., Schoffelen, P.F.M. & ten Hoor, F. (1990): The shape of the cumulative food intake curve in humans, during basic and manipulated meals. *Physiol. Behav.* **47**, 569-576.
10. Westerterp-Plantenga, M.S., van den Heuvel, E., Wouters, L. & ten Hoor, F. (1990): Deceleration in cumulative food intake curves, changes in body temperature, and diet-induced thermogenesis. *Physiol. Behav.* **48**, 831-836.

Chapter 77

Cognitive Control of Eating Behaviour Disinhibition of Control, and Successful Weight Reduction

Joachim WESTENHOEFER and Volker PUDEL
University of Goettingen, Department of Psychiatry, von-Siebold-Str. 5, D-3400 Goettingen, Germany

Adequate cognitive control of eating behaviour is one of the major goals of most behavioural weight reduction programmes. On the other hand, there is well established evidence that cognitively restrained eating may be associated with the disinhibition of control. In a study of 46,525 participants of a computer-assisted weight reduction programme, the subjects filled out the Three-Factor Eating Questionnaire[4,5] at the beginning of the programme. A subsample of 7246 subjects did so again 1 year after the beginning. The results show a complex relationship between body weight and restrained eating and the disinhibition of control, higher cognitive control being associated with lower body weight and higher disinhibition with higher body weight. Successful weight reduction was also associated with higher cognitive control and lower disinhibiton. Successful participants were able to increase their cognitive control and decrease their tendency towards disinhibition.

Introduction

Restrained eating[1,2] refers to the tendency to restrict food intake in order to control body weight[6]. There is well-established evidence that dietary restraint may be causally involved in severe disturbances of eating behaviour, e.g. binge eating as is seen in patients with bulimia nervosa[3,7]. One important process in this causal relationship might be the disinhibition of control through various situational or emotional stimuli. On the other hand, adequate cognitively controlled eating behaviour may be considered as one of the major goals of most behavioural weight reduction programmes. The present study was conducted to investigate the relationship between dietary restraint, disinhibition, body weight, and weight reduction.

Methods

The sample consisted of 46,525 participants in the *Vier-Jahreszeiten-Kur* (Four-Seasons-Programme), a computer-assisted programme for weight reduction in Germany that is supported by the Federal Association of Local Health Insurances. This programme aims at the modification of eating behaviour on the basis of behavioural principles. It is implemented as a postal dialogue with the participants over 1 year. Therefore all available data are self-reported. The participants fill out the German version of the Three-Factor Eating Questionnaire TFEQ[5] (German version[4]) as a part of the initial assessment, approximately 2 months after the beginning of the programme. The TFEQ measures (1) restrained eating or the cognitive control of eating behaviour, (2) the disinhibition of control, and (3) perceived hunger.

During the initial phase of the programme, an individual target weight is proposed for each participant, based on the personally desired weight reduction, the actual degree of overweight and realistic possibilities. A maximum weight reduction of 13 kg during the first 6 months is proposed. An attempt is made to stabilize the weight reduction achieved during the last 6 months. The relative success of each participant at the end of the programme after 1 year was categorized as (a) too much weight loss, if weight reduction was higher than proposed, (b) very successful, if the target weight was reached within ± 1 kg, (c) successful, if weight reduction was 5 kg or more, but the target weight was not reached, (d) little weight loss, if weight reduction was less than 5 kg, (e) no change, if weight was within ± 1 kg of the initial weight, or (f) weight gain, if weight was higher than starting weight. A subsample of 7246 participants filled out the TFEQ again after 1 year at the end of the programme.

To investigate the relationship between the restraint, disinhibition, and body weight or weight reduction, the sample was divided in 5 x 5 subgroups according to the scores on the restraint and disinhibition scale of the TFEQ. The limits for this subgroup division were chosen to be the respective quintiles of the frequency distributions. For the restraint scale, the resulting group ranges were 0 to 9 (n = 12,353), 10 to 13 (n = 11,604), 14 and 15 (n = 7174), 16 and 17 (n = 7682), and 18 to 21 (n = 7712). For the disinhibition scale, the ranges were scores 0 to 4 (n = 7848), 5 and 6 (7876), 7 and 8 (n = 8715), 9 to 11 (n = 12,131), and 12 to 16 (n = 9955).

Results

The subjects' characteristics are detailed in Table 1, which also presents the mean scores on the three TFEQ scales separately for men and women. A comparison with the average values from the general population (Westenhoefer, in preparation: restraint 8.8 for women, 5.3 for men; disinhibition 5.5 for women, 4.8 for men) shows that the present sample has elevated values on the restraint scale and on the disinhibition scale of the TFEQ.

Table 1. Age and body mass index (BMI) of the participants and scores on TFEQ scales (means ± SD)

	Women (n = 39,034)	Men (n = 7491)
Age, years	42.9 ± 12.5	45.3 ± 12.0
BMI, kg/m^2	28.2 ± 3.9	29.4 ± 3.3
TFEQ scales:		
Dietary restraint	13.1 ± 4.6	10.6 ± 4.7
Disinhibition	8.5 ± 3.6	7.2 ± 3.3
Hunger	6.3 ± 3.5	5.8 ± 3.4

For each of the 5 x 5 subgroups, the mean body mass index (BMI, kg/m^2) was calculated. An ANOVA reveals significant effects of the restraint factor ($F[4/46,500] = 31.48$; $P < 0.001$), of the disinhibition factor ($F[4/46,500] = 47.92$; $P < 0.001$), and a significant interaction ($F[16/46,500] = 6.34$; $P < 0.001$). The results show (see Fig. 1) that increasing disinhibition is associated with a slightly higher body weight, if restraint is low. On the other hand, increasing restraint is associated with a slightly lower body weight, if disinhibition scores are high. However, these effects, corresponding to an average difference of 5 kg, cannot be considered to be very large.

Next, restraint and disinhibition were related to the average weight reduction during the first two months. There was a significant effect of the restraint factor ($F[4/46,500] = 123.14$; $P < 0.001$), and of the disinhibition factor ($F[4/46,500] = 161.90$; $P < 0.001$). The interaction was not significant ($F[16/56,500] = 0.97$). Higher restraint is associated with higher weight loss, while higher disinhibition is related to lower weight loss.

Chapter 77 – Cognitive Control of Eating Behaviour

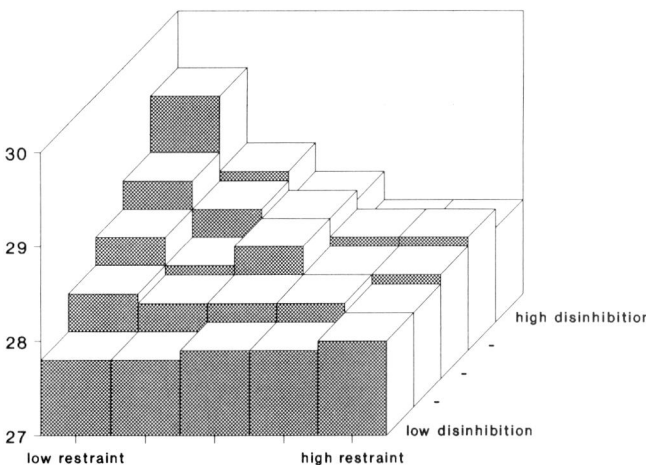

Fig. 1. Mean body mass index (BMI) for subgroups with different levels of dietary restraint and disinhibition of control.

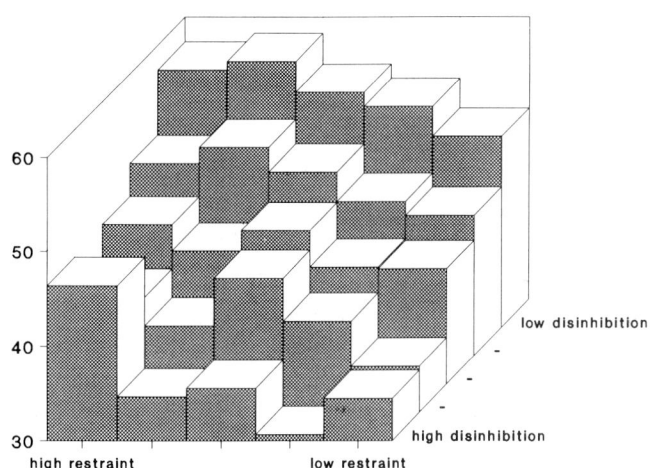

Fig. 2. Percentage of subjects with "very successful" weight reduction within subgroups with different levels of dietary restraint and disinhibition of control.

This pattern of relations between restraint, disinhibition and weight reduction is still persistent after 1 year at the end of the training programme. In Fig. 2, the percentage of participants within each subgroup is illustrated that fulfils the criteria of "very successful" weight reduction. High restraint and low disinhibition correspond with a high percentage of successful weight reduction.

From the subsample of participants who filled out the TFEQ at the end of the programme, average scores of the restraint and disinhibition scale were computed within each success category (Table 2). Participants with successful weight reduction started with higher scores on the restraint scale and still increased restraint during the programme, while they started with lower scores on disinhibition and managed to further decrease their disinhibition. Unsuccessful participants started with lower restraint and higher disinhibition and showed no significant changes of these scores during the 1 year programme.

Table 2. Means of dietary restraint and disinhibition at the beginning (pre) and at the end (post) of the weight reduction programme within the different success categories

	N	Restraint			Disinhibition		
		Pre	Post	Sign.	Pre	Post	Sign.
Too much weight loss	889	14.1	16.1	**	6.7	4.4	**
Very successful	2729	14.3	16.1	**	6.6	4.7	**
Successful	2247	13.6	15.5	**	7.7	6.3	**
Little weight loss	1054	13.3	14.3	**	7.9	7.1	**
No change	280	13.2	13.8	*	8.5	8.2	*
Weight gain	67	12.4	12.5		9.4	9.3	

Pre–post differences: $*P < 0.05$; $**P < 0.001$.

Discussion

The findings of the present study show that restrained eating and disinhibition of control are important psychological variables with regard to the regulation of body weight. However, there was only a small influence on actual body weight, if the results are compared with those reported by Westenhoefer et al.[9] for a sample of women's magazine readers. However, both variables were found to have high prognostic value for the future success of overweight subjects in reducing their body weight. Both a high level of cognitive control (i.e. dietary restraint) and a low level of disinhibition seem to be advantageous characteristics in the long-term control of body weight. This interpretation is further supported by the finding that successful weight reduction is associated with an increase of cognitive control and a decrease of disinhibition. Thus, a training of adequate cognitively controlled eating behaviour seems to be a powerful strategy for weight reduction programmes. As Westenhoefer[8] has shown, such an adequate control might be described as *flexible control* of eating behaviour which takes into account situational circumstances and personal needs, and which is associated with lower tendencies towards disinhibition.

References

1. Herman, C.P. & Mack, D. (1975). Restrained and unrestrained eating. *J. Pers.* **43**, 647-660.
2. Herman, C.P. & Polivy, J. (1975). Anxiety, restraint, and eating behavior. *J. Abnorm. Psychol.* **84**, 666-672.
3. Polivy, J. & Herman, C.P. (1985). Dieting and binging: a causal analysis. *Am. Psychol.* **40**, 193-201.
4. Pudel, V. & Westenhoefer, J. (1989): *Fragebogen zum Eßverhalten – FEV. Handanweisung*, pp. 38. Gottingen: Hogrefe.
5. Stunkard, A.J. & Messick, S. (1985): The Three-Factor Eating Questionnaire to measure dietary restraint, disinhibition and hunger. *J. Psychosom. Res.* **29**, 71-83.
6. Tuschl, R.J. (l990a). From dietary restraint to binge eating: some theoretical considerations. *Appetite* **14**, 105-109.
7. Wardle, J. (1987). Compulsive eating and dietary restraint. *B. J. Clin. Psychol.* **26**, 47-55.
8. Westenhoefer, J. (1991): Dietary restraint and disinhibition: is restraint a homogeneous construct? *Appetite* **16**, 45-55.
9. Westenhoefer, J., Pudel, V. & Maus, N. (1990): Some restrictions on dietary restraint. *Appetite* **14**, 137-141.

Chapter 78

Lipolytic Regulation During Mental Stress

Anders WENNLUND, Hans WAHRENBERG, Jan BOLINDER and Peter ARNER

Department of Medicine and Research Center, Huddinge Hospital, S-141 86 Huddinge, Sweden

There may be regional variations in lipolysis regulation. This was explored by investigating the sympathetic nervous response to mental stress. Lipolysis in the abdominal and gluteal regions of subcutaneous adipose tissue was continuously monitored in non-obese healthy subjects, using microdialysis. The glycerol concentration (lipolysis index) in adipose tissue increased markedly during a period of standardized mental stress and decreased in the post-stress period. A similar dynamic pattern was observed in blood. In women the lipolytic response to stress was much more pronounced in the abdominal than in the gluteal site; no such regional variation was observed in men.

Introduction

It is increasingly apparent that human adipose tissue is a heterogenous metabolic organ[4]. In particular, lipid mobilization from adipose tissue during lipolysis in fat cells shows considerable regional variations[1]. These site differences may be of importance for the development of regional forms of obesity[13,14]. Regional adipose tissue metabolism has above all been investigated *in vitro*. In a recent study, however, it was shown *in vivo* that lipolysis is more pronounced in abdominal as compared to gluteal subcutaneous adipose tissue during physical exercise[3]. Whether there is regional variation in lipolysis *in vivo* during other forms of sympathetic nervous activation is unknown so far. During mental stress there is a marked elevation in circulating free fatty acids and glycerol due to activation of lipolysis in adipose tissue[9]. We have recently developed a technique for directly studying the regulation of adipocyte lipolysis *in situ* by using microdialysis of the extracellular space in subcutaneous adipose tissue[3]. This method allows continuous monitoring of glycerol (lipolysis index) in adipose tissue *in vivo*. In the present study we investigated the effect of a standardized mental stress test on lipolysis in the adipose tissue of non-obese healthy men and women with the aid of microdialysis. Abdominal and gluteal subcutaneous adipose tissues were investigated simultaneously.

Material and methods

Subjects

The study group comprised 13 men and 15 women. All were healthy non-obese drug-free volunteers. The age (mean ± SE) was 30 ± 3 years in men and 40 ± 2 years in women ($P < 0.01$). The women were investigated in the middle of the menstrual cycle; none of them were menopausal and none had taken oral contraceptives for the last 6 months. Body mass index ranged between 19 and 27 kg/m^2 in men and between 19 and 27 kg/m^2 in women. However, the percentage of body fat, when calculated from calliper measurements, was higher in women than in men; 31.9 ± 1.4 per cent and 20.3 ± 1.4 per cent, respectively ($P < 0.001$). The waist/hip ratio was 0.94 ± 0.01 in men and 0.87 ± 0.02 in women ($P < 0.001$). The study was approved by the Ethics Committee at the Karolinska Institute.

Microdialysis probe

The microdialysis probe (CMA/Microdialysis AB, Stockholm, Sweden) has been described in detail previously[15]. A dialysis tubing (10 x 0.5 mm, 20,000 mol.wt. cut-off) is glued to the end of a double steel cannula. The perfusion solvent enters the probe through an inner cannula. It streams down to the tip of the probe and then upwards in the space between the inner cannula and the dialysis membrane. Thereafter the solvent leaves the probe through an outer cannula from which it is collected.

Experiment protocol

The experiments were performed with the subject at rest, sitting up in a bed at 8 a.m. after an overnight fast. One dialysis probe was inserted percutaneously, using a guide cannula (diameter 1.4 mm) without anaesthesia into the subcutaneous adipose layer to the right of the umbilicus. Another probe was inserted into the upper lateral part of the gluteal region. The inlet tubing of each probe was connected to a microinjection pump (CMA/Microdialysis AB, Stockholm, Sweden) and was continuously perfused (5 µl/min) with Ringer's solution. Fractions of the outgoing dialysate were collected at 5-min intervals for the analysis of glycerol. The first three fractions were deleted, since earlier studies[5] showed a transient rise in ATP concentration in the outgoing dialysate during the first 15 min of dialysis, reflecting the initial trauma caused by insertion of the dialysis probe. *In vitro* recovery experiments, performed as described previously[3], showed that the recovery of glycerol was about 17 per cent. During the dialysis experiments venous blood samples were simultaneously drawn at 15-min intervals from an indwelling polyethylene catheter placed in a cubital vein for the determinations of plasma catecholamines[7] and glycerol. The pulse rate was also recorded during the experiment, using continuous electrocardiographic recordings. In methodological experiments published elsewhere[3], the coefficient of variation for the glycerol values between two probes was only 6 per cent.

Mental stress test

Following the insertion of the dialysis probes and the intravenous catheter, the subjects rested in the sitting position for 30 min. The mean of the glycerol levels in the three last dialysate fractions preceeding CWT was determined and formed the baseline adipose tissue glycerol value. During the resting period the test procedure was explained to the participant. A modified filmed version of Stroop's[14] colour-word conflict test (CWT) was used as a test model. It has been described in detail previously[6]. In brief, colour-words are shown on a TV screen in different colours, the combination of words and colours being incongruent. The subject's task is to ignore the word and name the colour of the print. In addition, there is a simultaneous auditory presentation of conflicting colour-words, which also has to be ignored. The duration of visually-presented colour-words varies randomly between 0.4 and 1.0 s and that of auditorily-presented words between 0.7–1.8 s. The mental stress test lasted 30 min. Thereafter the subjects rested for a further 30 min. During the pre-stress, stress and post-stress periods, the pulse rate was recorded and blood and dialysis samples were taken as indicated.

Analysis of glycerol

For the analysis of glycerol 25 µl of plasma or tissue dialysate were used. Glycerol was determined by an automated ultrasensitive kinetic bioluminescence assay[8], using a luminescence analyser (LKB-Wallace, Helsinki, Finland).

Statistical analysis

Values are means ± SE. The coefficient of variation in duplicate determinations was

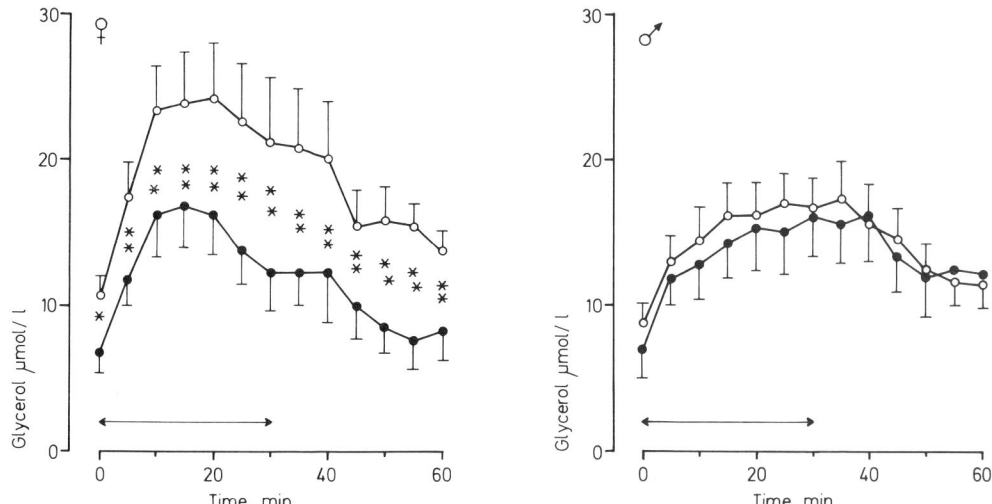

Fig. 1. Glycerol levels during mental stress in dialysate of abdominal (open circles) and gluteal (filled circles) subcutaneous adipose tissue of eight women (left) and 8 men (right). The experiments were conducted as described in Material and Methods using Ringer's solution. Two probes were used simultaneously. One probe was inserted in the abdominal area and one in the gluteal area of each subject. The subjects rested for 30 min. Then they underwent a mental stress test for 30 min. Thereafter they rested for a further 30 min. After a 15-min equilibrium period dialysate was collected at 5 min intervals. The mean glycerol level in the first four fractions preceding exercise was determined (time 0) and represents the baseline glycerol level. The stress period is indicated by an arrow. The results with abdominal and gluteal adipose tissue were statistically analysed using Student's paired t-test. Individual values and the area under the curve were compared. Both tests gave essentially the same results. The results of individual comparison are given in the figure (*= P < 0.05; **= P < 0.02).

calculated as the standard deviation divided by the mean. The area under the glycerol curve was determined by addition of the trapezoid parts of the area under the curve. The Student's paired t-test was used for statistical comparison of the values.

Results

The changes in glycerol in abdominal and gluteal subcutaneous adipose tissues during and after CWT are shown in Fig. 1. The level of dialysate glycerol at rest during the 15 min preceding CWT was constant (data not shown). CWT was accompanied by a marked increase ($P < 0.01$) in the adipose tissue dialysate glycerol. After CWT there was a gradual decline in the dialysate glycerol level. In men a similar change in the glycerol concentration during CWT and after CWT was observed in both adipose regions. In women, the increase in the dialysate glycerol level during CWT was significantly more pronounced in the abdominal than in the gluteal adipose tissues. In the former region glycerol peaked to a 50 per cent higher level than in the gluteal area during CWT ($P < 0.01$). In women, the baseline adipose tissue dialysate glycerol level was significantly higher in the abdominal than in the gluteal region. However, the changes in the glycerol level of adipose tissue above the baseline value during CWT were also more pronounced in the abdominal than in the gluteal site of women, using the area under the curve for the statistical analysis ($P < 0.05$).

Venous plasma levels of catecholamines and glycerol, as well as the pulse rate during and after CWT, were also determined (figure not shown). Plasma glycerol showed a similar dynamic pattern as adipose tissue glycerol. In both sexes it peaked during 15–20 min of CWT at a level that was twice as high as the starting level ($P < 0.01$); then it declined towards baseline values. Plasma noradrenaline increased about 50 per cent ($P < 0.05$) during CWT. The stress-induced increase in plasma noradrenaline was not different in men as compared to women. The adrenaline concentration increased about fourfold during CWT in both sexes ($P < 0.01$). At no time point did the plasma adrenaline levels differ between men and women. The heart rate was similar in both sexes before stress (about 60 beats/min). It increased 20–25 beats/min in women and men during CWT. The number of correct answers during CWT differed between the sexes. In men it was 349 ± 43 and in women 207 ± 29 ($P < 0.01$).

The women were 10 years older than the males ($P < 0.01$), which might influence the results since lipolysis regulation *in vitro* is dependent upon age[10,12]. However, neither plasma glycerol (area under the curve) nor adipose tissue glycerol (area under the curve) during mental stress were correlated with age ($r < 0.2$). In order to further evaluate a possible influence of age men and women were divided into younger (men < 30 years; seven subjects and women < 35 years; six subjects) and older (remaining subjects) groups. However, the findings regarding regional differences in adipose tissue glycerol during CWT were not different between younger and elderly subjects of either sex. On the basis of these finding it is concluded that the difference in age between the sexes has no important influence upon the results.

Discussion

In this study, the peripheral sympathetic response to mental stress has been investigated *in situ* for the first time. This was done using continuous monitoring of lipolysis in adipose tissue with microdialysis.

In women, the stress-induced increase of lipolysis *in situ* was much more pronounced in the abdominal than in the gluteal area, whereas in men both regions had a similar lipolytic response to mental stress. The mechanisms underlying regional differences in stress-induced lipolysis in women are not known at present. However, a recent *in vitro* study has shown that abdominal cells are more responsive than gluteal adipocytes to catecholamine stimulation and these site variations are significantly more apparent in women than in men[16]. Thus, regional variations in hormone sensitivity may at least in part explain the site variations in lipolysis during mental stress in women. The variations in lipolytic activity in different fat depots may have pathophysiological implications to stress-related disorders in women. It has been speculated[4,13] that increased delivery of lipolytic metabolites, such as free fatty acids, from central fat depots might be involved in the development of glucose intolerance and hypertriglyceridaemia, which are two well-known risk factors for coronary heart disease.

It should be stressed that the absolute levels of glycerol in adipose tissue were not determined in the present experiments. Therefore, no attempts were made to directly compare the dialysate glycerol levels between men and women. It is possible, using a calibration technique, to indirectly estimate the true level of a metabolite in the extracellular space with microdialysis during steady state conditions[11]. Unfortunately, calibration experiments cannot be performed at the same time as the present CWT experiments. First, the calibration experiments are very time-consuming. Secondly, they necessitate a local exposure of adipose tissue to very high concentrations of glycerol. The latter may artificially alter the following CWT experiment.

It appears from the present results that the *in vivo* response to mental stress was similar in both sexes. Thus, the pulse rate and the plasma levels of catecholamines and glycerol rose to the same extent in either sex during CWT. However, women produced fewer correct answers during CWT than men. More detailed investigations are necessary for complete understanding of the reason underlying the latter sex difference. One reason could be that the stress "dose" was higher in women. This, however, hardly explains the sex differences in the regional variations in lipolysis.

In summary, the present study shows that the lipolytic response to mental stress is marked in adipose tissue. There is also a regional variation in the lipolysis of subcutaneous adipose tissue during mental stress in women, but not in men.

References

1. Arner, P. (1988): Control of lipolysis and its relevance to development of obesity in man. *Diab. Metab. Rev.* **4**, 507-515.
2. Arner, P., Kriegholm, E. & Engfeldt, P. (1990): *In situ* studies of catecholamine-induced lipolysis in human adipose tissue using microdialysis. *J. Pharm. Exp. Ther.* **254**, 284-288.
3. Arner, P., Kriegholm, E., Engfeldt, P. & Bolinder, J. (1990): Adrenergic regulation of lipolysis *in situ* at rest and during exercise. *J. Clin. Invest.* **85**, 893-898.
4. Björntorp, P. (1987): Fat cell distribution and metabolism. *Ann N.Y. Acad. Sci.* **499**, 66-72.
5. Bolinder, J., Hagström, E., Ungerstedt, U. & P. Arner. (1989): Microdialysis of subcutaneous adipose tissue *in vivo* for continuous glucose monitoring in man. *Scand. J. Clin. Lab. Invest.* **49**, 465-474.
6. Frankenhaeuser, M., Mellis, I., Rissler, A., Björkvall, C. & P. Pälkai. (1968): Catecholamine excretion as related to cognitive and emotional reaction patterns. *Psychosom. Med.* **30**, 109-120.
7. Hallman, H., Farnebo, L.E., Hamberg, B. & Jonsson, G. (1978): A sensitive method for determination of plasma catecholamines using liquid chromatography with electrochemical detection. *Life Sci.* **23**, 1049-1052.
8. Hellmer, J., Arner, P. & Lundin, A (1989): Automatic luminometric kinetic assay of glycerol for lipolysis studies. *Anal. Biochem.* **177**, 132-137.
9. Linde, B., Hjelmdahl, P., Freyschuss, U. & Juhlin-Dannfelt, A. (1989): Adipose tissue and skeletal muscle blood flow during mental stress. *Am. J. Physiol.* **256**, E12-E18.
10. Lönnqvist, F., Nyberg, B., Wahrenberg, H. & Arner, P. (1990): Catecholamine-induced lipolysis in adipose tissue of the elderly. *J. Clin. Invest.* **85**, 1614-1621.
11. Lönnroth, P., Jansson, P.A. & Smith, U. (1987): A microdialysis method allowing characterization of intracellular water space in humans. *Am. J. Physiol.* **253**, E228-E231.
12. Marcus, C., Karpe, B., Bolme, P., Sonnenfeld, T. & Arner, P. (1987): Changes in catecholamine-induced lipolysis in isolated human fat cells during the first year of life. *J. Clin. Invest.* **79**, 1812-1818.
13. Smith, U.(1985): Regional differences in adipocyte metabolism and possible consequences *in vivo*. *Int .J. Obes.* **9** (Suppl 1) 145-148.
14. Stroop, J.R. (1935): Interference in serial verbal reactions. *J. Exp. Psychol.* **18**, 643-650.
15. Tossman, U. & Ungerstedt, U. (1986): Microdialysis in the study of extracellular levels of amino acids in the rat brain. *Acta Physiol. Scand.* **128**, 914.
16. Wahrenberg, H., Lönnqvist, F. & Arner, P. (1989): Mechanisms underlying regional differences in lipolysis in human adipose tissue. *J. Clin. Invest.* **84**, 458-467.

Author Index

AALTO, T.	221
AGOU, Karen	273
AILHAUD, Gérard	1, 277, 347
ALARANTA, H.	221
ARDOUIN, Bernadette	95
ARNER, Peter	281, 441
ASSIMACOPOULOS-JEANNET, F.	233
ASTRUP, A.	333
ATEF, Nadia	263
ATTALI, J.R.	213
BARDON, Sylvie	347
BAZIN, R.	101
BECK, B.	51
BERLAN, Michel	141
BERNARBÉ, J.	237
BERTRAND, Bénédicte	347
BESSEY, D.	67
BJÖRNTORP, Per	188, 377
BLONDELL, O.	289
BLUM, I.	255
BLUNDELL, John E.	63
BOILLOT, J.	237
BOLINDER, Jan	441
BORRELLI, Renato	125
BOUCHARD, Claude	7, 81, 177, 319, 369, 411
BRIQUET-LAUGIER, Véronique	95
BRISCOE, M.G.	289
BRONDEL, Laurent	249
BRONNIKOV, Gennady	355
BUEMANN, B.	333
BUGLIONE, Gelsomina	125
BURCKHARDT, P.	183
BURLET, C.	51
BURLEY, Victoria J.	63
BURNOL, Anne Françoise	273
BURNS, C.M.	167
BUSBY, M.	213
CAMPFIELD, L. Arthur	47
CANNON, Barbara	355
CARPENE, Christian	141
CASSARD, Anne-Marie	363
CASSUTO, D.	227
CASTILLO, M.	201
CATERSON, Ian	167, 421
CAVIEZEL, F.	217
CERVONI, P.	405
CHAMPIGNY, O.	289
CHARRAUD, A.	113
CHARZEWSKA, J.	135
CHRISTENSEN, N.J.	333
CIGOLINI, M.	135
COGAN, Uri	35
COLE, T.J.	113
COLLEDGE, Nicola	163
COMBES, M.E.	213
CONTALDO, Franco	125, 135
COOKSON, John	71
COUSIN, Béatrice	273
COXON, A.	327
CRAIG, Pippa	421
CRANDALL, D.L.	405
CREMONA, Franco	125
CUSIN, I.	233
DANI, Christian	347
DAUZATS, Michèle	277
DAVIAUD, Danielle	277
DE FILIPPO, Emilia	125
De LEEUW, Ivo	337, 389
DESLYPERE, J.P.	135
DESPRÉS, Jean-Pierre	81, 177, 319, 369, 411
DIAMOND, P.	241
DIONNE, France T.	369
DITSCHUNEIT, H.	191
DITSCHUNEIT, Hans	401
DITSCHUNEIT, Herwig H.	401
DON, R.	255
DORE, M.F.	227
DOSIO, F.	217
DUGAIL, Isabelle	95
DUHAULT, Jacques	55
DUPUY, F.	101
DUTTA-ROY, Asim K.	293

ELIAS, Nizar	35	KLAUS, Susanne	363
ELLIOTT, R.	269	KLINGENSPOR, Martin	363
ELLSINGER, B.M.	135	KOLANOWSKI, J.	207
ERLANSON-ALBERTSSON, Charlotte	41	KOPELMAN, Peter G.	89
ERNEST, I.	393	KORKEILA, M.	129
ESPINAL, Joseph	55	KOSKENVUO, M.	129
FÜCKER, K.	29	KRAL, J.G.	405
FANTINO, Marc	249	KREITZMAN, S.	327
FISCHER, S.	29	KTORZA, Alain	263
FLECHTNER-MORS, Marion	401	KUNEŠOVÁ, M.	23
FLETCHER, J.	269	KUUSELA, Pertti	355
GAILLARD, Danielle	277	KVIST, Henry	393
GALITZKY, Jean	141	LÉONET, J.	207
GIANOLLI, L.	217	LÖNN, Lars	393
GIRARD, Jean	273	LÖNNROTH, P.	397
GOODALL, Elizabeth	71	LACOUR, Francoise	55
GRAFF, E.	255	LAFONTAN, Max	141, 277
GRAVES, Reed A.	155	LANGIN, Dominique	141
GRIGGIO, M.	241	LARROUY, Dominique	141
GROSSKOPF, Y.	255	LARUE-ACHAGIOTIS, C.	237
GUIGUET, Michel	249	LAURENT-JACCARD, A.	183
GUILLAUME-GENTIL, C.	233	LAVAU, Marcelle	95
GUY-GRAND, B.	227, 417	LE BARZIC, M.	417
HÁJEK, M.	23	LE LIEPVRE, Xavier	95
HAINER, V.	23	LEBLANC, J.	241
HANEFELD, M.	29	LEEDS, A.R.	67
HARSAT, A.	255	LEFEBVRE, P.J.	201
HEIKKILÄ, K.	129	LEONHARDT, W.	29
HEITMANN, Berit Lilienthal	121	LETURQUE, Armelle	273
HERRON, David	355	LEVY, Yishai	35
HERZLINGER, H.E.	405	LOUIS-SYLVESTRE, J.	237
HILL, Andrew J.	427	LUPIEN, Paul J.	81
HITMAN, Graham A.	89	MADSEN, J.	333
HOLLOWAY, B.R.	289	MÅRIN, Per	188
HOLMÄNG, Sten	188	MAFFEIS, Claudio	323
HOLM, Göran	188	MARIE, V.	101
HOLST, Claus	85	MARKS, V.	269
HORSKÁ, A.	23	MARONE, Achille	125
HOUSTEK, Josef	355	MAURIÈGE, P.	411
HRDINA, J.	23	MAX, J.P.	51
HUANG, Yiming	293	MAYERS, R.M.	289
IBRAHIMI, Azeddine	347	MEI, Jie	41
JÖNSSON, Lars	188	MEIJER, G.A.L.	17
JACOBSSON, Anders	355	MICHEL, A.	237
JANDRAIN, B.	201	MOORJANI, Sital	81
JANSSON, P.-A.	397	MORGAN, L.	269
JAYET, A.	183	MORGAN, W.	327
JEANRENAUD, B.	233	MOYER, A.	259
JEQUIER, Eric	173	MUNRO, John F.	163
JOHNSON, P.	327	NÉCHAD, Myriam	355
KAPRIO, J.	129	NÉGREL, Raymond	277
KARST, H.	29	NADEAU, André	81, 241
KERDELHUÉ, Bernard	55	NEDERGAARD, Jan	355

Author Index

NICOLAS, J.P.	51
NOACK, R.	29
OBEN, J.	269
ORVOEN-FRIJA, E.	227
PALAIA, Raffaele	125
PAOLISSO, G.	201
PARISI, Valerio	125
PENICAUD, Luc	263, 273
PICON, Luc	263
PINELLI, Leonardo	323
PORTILLO, Maria	141
POULIOT, M.C.	411
POZZA, G.	217
PRUD'HOMME, Denis	177, 411
PUDEL, Volker	437
PUIGSERVER, Pere	355
QUAADE, F.	333
QUIGNARD-BOULANGE, Annie	95
RAISON, J.	227
RAVEL, Denis	55
RAZl, O.	255
REBUFFÉ-SCRIVE, M.	259
REHNMARK, Stefan	355
RICHARD, D.	241
RICHMAN, R.	167
ICQUIER, Daniel	289, 343, 363
RISSANEN, A.	129
ROCHEMAURE, J.	227
RODIN, Judith	259, 307
ROHNER-JEANRENAUD, F.	233
ROLLAND-CACHERA, M.F.	113
RÖNNEMAA, T.	221
ROSS, Susan R.	155
ROSSIGNOL, C.	113
RUFFOLO, Fulvio	125
SAIBENE, A.	217
SALVATORE, Marco	125
SASSANO, Mary Lisa	47
SAULNIER-BLACHE, Jean-Sébastien	141, 277
SCALEA, T.M.	405
SCALFI, Luca	125
SCHEEN, A.J.	201
SCHUTZ, Yves	173, 323
SCOGNAMIGLIO, Francesco	125
SEIDELL, J.C.	109, 135
SEMPÉ, M.	113
SILVERSTONE, Trevor	71
SJÖSTRÖM, Lars	299, 393
SMITH, Francoise J.	47
SMITH, U.	397
SØRENSEN, Thorkild I.A.	85
SPIEGELMAN, Bruce M.	155
STEINBECK, K.	167
ŠTICH, V.	23
STRICKER-KRONGRAD, A.	51
STUNKARD, Albert J.	85
SUTER, Paolo M.	173
TEN HOOR, F.	17, 431
TERRETTAZ, J.	233
THÉRIAULT, Germain	81, 319
TICHET, J.	113
TONTONOZ, Peter	155
TRAYHURN, Paul	77, 293
TREMBLAY, Angelo	81, 177, 319, 369, 411
TRUCHON, Josée	369
TURCOTTE, Lucie	369
TURNBULL, W.H.	67
VAILLANT, Geneviève	249
VALENSI, P.	213
VAN DEN HEUVEL, E.	431
Van GAAL, Luc	337, 389
VANSANT, Greet	337, 389
VERBOEKET-VAN de VENNE, W.P.H.G.	17
VERED, Y.	255
VĚTVICKA, J.	23
WAHRENBERG, Huns	441
WALTON, J.	67
WEAVER, Jolanta U.	89
WECK, M.	29
WENNLUND, Anders	441
WESTENHOEFER, Joachim	437
WESTERTERP, K.R.	17
WESTERTERP-PLANTENGA, M.S.	431
WHITTLE, Mary	71
WOUTERS, L.	431
WYSS, C.	183
YESHURUN, Daniel	35
ZAMBELLI, L.	135
ZENTI, M.G.	135
ZILLI, F.	217

Subject Index

α_2 chain	350-2
α_2-adrenergic mediated antilipolysis	277-9
α_2-adrenergic receptor	159, 357
α_2-adrenoceptors	141, 411, 412, 413
α_2-AR	277, 278, 279
α-adrenergic receptors	146, 147-9
abdominal	
adipocytes	411
adipose tissue	81-2, 307, 314, 401, 413, 443
fat	314
obesity	396
cardiovascular disease	125
coronary heart disease risk	179-80
exercise, low intensity	177-80
males	188
measures	122, 123
subcutaneous fat	412, 413
aborigines	79
ACE *see* angiotensin converting enzyme	
ACTH *see* adrenocorticotropin hormone	
activity intervention	18
adenomas	393
adenosine triphosphate (ATP) and very low calorie diet	25
adipocytes	1-4, 411
characteristics	356
differentiation of hamster preadipocytes	277-9
genes	344-5
isolated	274
adipose	
specific enhancer	155-60
tissue	1-4
abdominal	81-2, 307, 314, 401, 413, 443
biopsies, human	405-8
blood flow (ATBF)	399
cellularity	406, 413
distribution, changed	393-6
enzymatic and metabolic regulation	269-96
explants, animals	271
gluteal	443
hyperplasia	405
hypertrophy	405
intraabdominal	313, 405
lipolysis	30-3, 411-13
Na$^+$/K$^+$-ATPase	31
mesenteric	310, 312, 407
metabolism	
gut hormones	269-72
in situ	281-5
regional distribution	377-413
omental	270
perirenal	290
regions, fat accumulation	379-81
subcutaneous	303, 395, 401-4
lactate production	397-9
visceral	259-61, 303, 395, 396
see also white adipose; brown adipose	
adipsin	2, 79, 344, 345
adoption studies	78, 89
adrenalectomy	235
adrenergic	
pathway	356-7
receptors	143-9, 379
fat cell	141-51
regulation	355-9
stimulation	358
system and pharmacological strategies	149-51
adrenoceptors	142, 145, 149, 150
animal fat cell	143-7
human fat cell	142-3
adrenocortical androgen secretion	207-11
adrenocorticotropin hormone (ACTH)	207, 208, 209, 210, 211, 381, 382
ageing rat	60
see also plasma ACTH	
AER *see* albumin excretion rate	
aerobic exercise	23
long term (100 days)	82
low intensity	179-80
plasma lipoproteins	81-2
short term (22 days)	81-2
age	81, 421-5

451

body mass index	113, 115, 118	β_3 receptors	356, 358
energy intake	115, 116	β-adrenergic agonists	365-6, 380
nutritional status	117	β-adrenergic receptors	143-7, 159, 356, 359, 377, 402
recessive inheritance	85, 87	adipocyte differentiation	277
weight change	130, 131, 132	β-adrenoceptors	141, 411, 412, 413
age-standardized percentiles	110, 111	β-endorphin	59, 60
ageing	55, 60, 307, 379	Bardet-Biedl syndrome	78
agricultural species	77-8	BAT *see* brown adipose tissue	
albumin *see* albumin excretion rate; urinary albumin excretion rate		Beck Depression Questionnaire (BDI)	168
		behavioural determinants of regional fat distribution	307-16
albumin excretion rate (AER)	217, 218	Belgium	109, 111, 136
alcohol	8, 379, 383, 384	bilateral subdiaphragmatic vagotomy	264
amino acid peptide *see* transforming growth factor-alpha		bingeing	164, 165
		bioenergetics, muscle	23-7
amino acid sequences	350-1	biological indifference	431
anaemia	186	biology, cellular and molecular	343-5
androgen		bladder disease	167
levels, baseline	208	blood glucose	56, 57
receptors	377, 380	ageing rat	60
secretion, adrenocortical	207-11	fasting	208, 302
android obesity	191, 193, 194, 401-4	blood lipids	
androstenedione	210	fasting plasma insulin	135-7
angina pectoris	121, 302, 303	fat distribution	121-4
angiogenesis	406, 408	blood pressure	110
angiotensin converting enzyme (ACE)	405, 406, 408	blood lipid levels	121
angiotensin I and II	407	Europe and obesity	112
animals		prevalence ratios	302
adipose tissue explants	271	*see also* diastolic; systolic	
agricultural	77-8	BMI *see* body mass index	
fat cell adrenoceptors	143-7	body	
laboratory	78	composition	328, 329
models	89, 310	body mass index (BMI)	12
obesity genetics	77-9	risk factors	303
wild	77	energy content phototypes	13
antagonists	142, 143	fat	
anthropometry blood lipids	135-7	content	32
very low calorie diet	24	distribution/metabolism	178-9
anti-obesity action of ICI D7114	289-91	genetic basis	13
antilipolysis	277-9, 411, 412	mitochondrial DNA variants	369-72
a-adrenergic mediated	277-9	total losses	81-2
AO *see* upper body obesity		mass index (BMI)	327-31
AP1 site	156	age	113, 115, 118
aP2	2	body composition	12
appetite	63-5, 67	clonidine (CLO)	413
arachidonic acid	2-3, 293, 295, 296	energy intake/energy expenditure	19, 20
arginine	389	epinephrine	413
arteriosclerosis	196-8	genetics	85, 86, 87
arteriovenous cannulation	282-3	major affectors	11
ATBF *see* adipose tissue blood flow		risk factors (38 year old men)	111
atherosclerosis	385, 392, 401	triglyceridaemia	196
attitudes	421-5	variations (France 0-87 years)	113-19
Australia	79, 167, 423, 424, 425	weight change	130, 131, 132

Subject Index

size	421-5
weight grading	191-2
weight, initial	130
boundary model *see* Herman and Polivy	
breast cancer and fat distribution	125-7
breast diseases, benign	125, 126, 127
Britain	90, 109, 115, 116, 117
non-absorbable fat	63
pharmacotherapy	165
BRL 37344	103, 144, 145, 146, 147, 358
brown	
adipocytes	
cultures	355-9
differentiation	357-8, 363-7
adipose cells	3-4
adipose tissue	1-4, 355-6
cultures	355-9
in dogs	289-91
rats	293-6
Zucker rats, young	101-4
bulimia nervosa	437
buspirone	71-3
butterfly effect	8
C-EBP binding site	155-60
C-peptide	389, 391
calcaneal periostitis	223
calcaneal spurs	223, 224
calf muscle	23, 26
caloric	
compensation, complete absence	47-50
intake	369
regulation in liver-transplanted rats	237-9
Cambridge Diet	166, 328
candidate gene and glucose transporter (Glut 1)	89-93
cannulation, arteriovenous	282-3
carbohydrate oxidation and energy expenditure	333-5
cardiovascular disease	110, 125, 177
adipose specific enhancer	159
blood lipid levels	121
breast cancer	125
cerebrovasucular	385
osteoarthrosis	221
weight control programme	167
see also coronary heart disease	
Carpenter's syndrome	78
CAT *see* chloramphenicol acetyl transferase	
catecholamines	308, 309, 380, 411, 412, 413
adrenoceptors	142
arteriovenous cannulation	282
lipolysis	150, 277
cDNA	291, 343
cloned	344

libraries	348
cell proliferation/differentiation	359
cellular biology	343-5
central nervous system (CNS)	90, 256, 383
periphery relationships	233-65
pharmacotherapy	165
central obesity	191
cephalic postprandial thermogenesis and insulin	249-52
cephalic thermogenic phase	241-7
cerebrovascular disease	385
CGP	142
12177	143, 144, 145, 358
20712A	142, 143, 147
chaos	7-13
CHD *see* coronary heart disease	
chicken	351
children	192
body weight/height grading	191
dieting	427-30
prepubertal (lean and obese)	323-6
Chinese Meishan	78
chloramphenicol acetyl transferase (CAT)	155-60
CHMI *see* cyclohexyl-2-mercapto-imidazole	
CHO ingestion	389
cholesterol *see* HDL; LDL	
cholesterol crystals	197, 198
chronic energy deficiency (CED)	118, 119
circulatory aberrations	383-5
circulatory regulation	382-3
clonidine (CLO)	143, 148, 411, 412
body mass index	413
CNS *see* central nervous system	
cognitive	
control and eating behaviour	437-40
restraint	431-5
therapy	165
Cohen's syndrome	78
cold exposure/stress	103, 235, 355, 366
colipase	41, 42, 43, 44
colour-word conflict test (CWT)	442, 443, 444
community attitudes	
overweight	422
overweight/underweight	424
comorbidity	405
concepts, realistic and weight loss	164
consumption, prospective	69
control, disinhibition of	437-40
coronary heart disease (CHD)	81, 178
abdominal obesity	179-80
France and obesity	118
microalbuminuria	213, 215
CORT rats	312

453

corticosteroid release	313, 385	cephalic postprandial thermogenesis	250, 251, 252
corticosterone	312	drugs	166
hypercorticosteronaemia	235, 236	experimental	195
visceral adipose tissue	260	microalbuminuria	215
see also plasma corticosterone		prevalence ratios	302
corticotropin-releasing factor		streptozotocin-induced	398
(CRF)	235, 377, 381, 382	see also non-insulin dependent	
cortisol	308, 313, 314, 381, 382, 396	diabetes mellitus	198, 401
levels	311, 380	Europe and obesity	112
secretion	309, 310, 377	proteinuria	219, 220
see also plasma cortisol		type II	164, 166
counterregulation and cognitive restraint	431-5	energy metabolism	195, 196
countries comparison and body mass index	115-18	diastolic blood pressure	111, 218, 219
CPU18-11	348, 349, 350, 351	proteinuria	220
CPU18-7	348, 349, 350, 351	testosterone	188
craving	71	visceral adipose tissue	303
CRF see corticotropin-releasing factor		diet/dietary	328, 355
cross-sectional changes	115	boundary	431
Cushing's syndrome	259, 261, 301, 308, 381, 382, 393-6	Cambridge	166, 328
		childhood	427-30
fat distribution	377, 379	early and behaviour	429
CV	229	high-carbohdyrate	333-5
CWT see colour-word conflict test		high-fat	78
cyanopindolol (CYP)	142, 143, 144, 147	inception	427-9
cyclers	315	Japanese	41
cyclic AMP	3, 142, 356, 357, 358, 359	low-fat	333-5
adipose specific enhancer	155	restraint	427, 428, 429, 439, 440
levels	149	restriction	165
lipolysis	146	zero calorie	36, 37
phosphorylation	277	differentiation of brown adipocyte cultures	355-9
responsiveness	159	differentiation-specific markers in vivo	2
cyclohexyl-2-mercapto-imidazole (CHMI)		digestion, fat	41-4
	241, 242, 244, 245, 246	dihydroalprenolol (DHA)	142, 143
CYP see cyanopindolol		disease and visceral fat accumulation	384
		disorders and obesity	191-9
D7114	364, 365, 366, 367	DNA	291
d-fenfluramine	55-60, 165	extraction	370
DA see dopamine		fragment	156
dark phase and mild deprivation	47-50	glucose transporter	89, 91
dehydroepiandrosterone (DHEA)	207, 208, 209, 210, 211	isolation/analysis	348
		mitochondrial	369-72
dehydroepiandrosterone sulphate (DHEA-S)	207, 211	mobility shift binding	157, 160
Denmark	109, 121, 122	polymorphism	345
Adoption Study	85-7	sequences	9, 13, 348
deprivation	47-50, 79	variants, mitochondrial	369-72
desire to eat	69, 72	see also cDNA	
determinism	7-13	dogs	241, 242, 245
dexamethasone suppression test	235, 381	arteriovenous cannulation	282
DHA see dihydroalprenolol		brown adipose tissue	289-91
DHEA see dehydroepiandrosterone		dopamine (DA)	242, 244, 246
DHEA-S see dehydroepiandrosterone sulphate		doubly labelled water	17-22
diabetes	78, 79, 178, 281, 389	DPH	35, 36
adipose specific enhancer	159	dyslipoproteinaemia	177, 197, 199, 281

Subject Index

eating behaviour and cognitive control	437-40
EE *see* energy expenditure	
EI *see* energy intake	
elaboration technique	422
electrical impedance	122
electrochemical sensors	283-4
ELISA method	41, 42
emotions	422-5
endocrine and visceral obesity	381-5
endothelin (ET)	408
endothelin-1 (ET-1)	405, 407
energy balance	18-19, 369
genetics	77
content phototypes	13
expenditure	18, 299-340, 369, 418
24 hour	328, 334
adrenergic system	149
body mass	19, 20
carbohydrate oxidation	333-5
chaos/determinism	8, 9, 11
genetics	77, 78, 79
metabolic efficiency	29
and overfeeding, longterm	319-21
sex hormones	339
substrate oxidation rates	339
and weight loss	327-31
intake	17-22, 63-5, 70, 73
age	115, 116
body mass	19, 20
chaos/determinism	8, 9, 10, 11
genetics	77
males, lean and healthy	63-5
measurement	328
metabolism	32
glucose and free fatty acids	194-6
measurements	30
enhancer, adipose specific	155-60
enterostatin	41, 43, 45
immunoreactive	44
properties	42
environment and regional fat deposition	307, 308, 378, 383
enzymatic regulation of adipose tissue	269-96
enzyme activity, lipogenic	95-8
epidemiology observations	109-12
epinephrine	148, 411, 412
adipocyte differentiation	278
adrenoceptors	141
body mass index	413
induced glycerol release	401-4
induced lipolysis	193
ERV *see* expiratory reserve volume	
erythrocyte	
and HepG2-type glucose transporter (Glut 1)	91
membrane function	35-7
sodium/potassium ATPase	30
estradiol	338, 339, 340
ET *see* endothelin	
ethnicity	421-5
Europe and obesity	109-12
European Fat Distribution Study	136
exercise	26, 424
aerobic	81-2
long term	82
low intensity	179-80
short term	81-2
body fat distribution/metabolism	178-9
protocol	24
related responses	422
see also aerobic exercise	
values	25
very low calorie diet	23-7
expiratory reserve volume (ERV)	227, 228, 229
extracellular	
fluid sampling	283
matrix	347-52
space monitoring	283
extremity joints and osteoarthrosis	221-5
5-HT	71
FABP *see* fatty acid-binding protein	
family	89, 78, 424
fasting	195
blood glucose	208, 302
glucose	188
hyperinsulinaemia	92
insulin	90, 389, 391
insulinaemia	208, 209, 311
plasma insulin	135-7
fat	
abdominal	314
accumulation	379-81
visceral	378, 379
disease	384
endocrine characteristics	381-3
psychosocial factors	385
cell	
adrenergic receptors	141-51
adrenoceptors, animal	143-7
adrenoceptors, human	142-3
cultures, brown	355-6
size	192-4
deposition, regional	307-16
digestion	41-4
distribution	90-1

blood lipid levels	121-4	intake	41-73, 418
breast cancer	125-7	females	71-3
psychosocial factors	377-85	neuro-endocrine regulation	41-73
free mass (FFM)	19, 323, 324, 327-31, 340	stimulation	51-3
intake	41-4	related responses	422
non-absorbable	63-5	forced-expiratory volume (FEV1)	227, 228
subcutaneous abdominal	412, 413	Framingham study	121, 127
see also body fat		France	109, 113-19
fatty acid		FRC	228, 229, 230
analysis	294	free fatty acids	390, 391, 403
binding protein (FABP)	293-6	concentration and turnover	193
omental adipose tissue	270	glucose	194-6
oxidation, preferential	198	VLDL-TG synthesis	194
FCS see foetal calf serum		fullness	69
fear	427-30	functional hypercortisolism	377, 379
feedback inhibition, normal and		*Fusarium graminearum*	67
insulin secretion	201-4		
feeding intervention	18	gastric	
feelings/emotions	422-3, 424, 425	banding	300
females		inhibitory polypeptide (GIP)	269, 272
adipose tissue distribution	393-6	bypass	300
android obesity	401-4	reduction	166
body fat distribution and breast cancer	125-7	gender	81
fasting plasma insulin	136	body mass index	113
food intake	71-3	differences	169
myco-protein	68	influence	135-7
obese hirsute	207-11	and nutritional status	117
post-obese		recessive inheritance	85, 87
high-carbohydrate diet	333-5	regional fat deposition	307
weight relapse	173-5	weight change	131
sex hormones	337-40	genes	343
femoral adipose cells	413	isolation	344
femoral subcutaneous fat	412	machine	8
fenfluramine	71, 165, 166	molecular studies	344-5
see also d-fenfluramine		regional fat deposition	307
fenoterol	278	genetics	85, 86, 87
FEV1 see forced-expiratory volume		in animals and humans	77-9
FFM see fat-free mass		determinism	12-13
FI see fasting insulin		predisposition	78, 79
Finland	109, 116, 129-32	genomic libraries	348
fitness, metabolic	177-80	Germany	109
fluid mosaic model	35	GFO see lower body obesity	
fluid sampling, extracellular	283	GIP see gastric inhibitory polypeptide	
fluorescence assay	294	GIT see glucose-induced thermogenesis	
fluoxetine	166	glomerular filtration rate	219
foetal calf serum (FCS)	2, 96, 97, 98, 278, 363, 366	GLP see glucagon-like polypeptide	
brown fat cell cultures	355	glucagon	389, 391
follicular phase	71, 313	glucagon-like polypeptide (GLP)	269, 270
food	424, 255-7	glucagon-lipid interactions	389-92
consumption and myco-protein	67-70	glucocorticoid	
craving	71	differentiation specific markers	3
deprivation	79	feedback inhibition	60
efficiency	419	hormones	259-61, 413

receptors	308, 377, 380
glucoreceptor neurones (GRN)	89
glucose	
consumption (GC)	95, 96, 97
fasting	188, 208, 302
free fatty acids	194-6
handling *in vivo*	233-4
induced thermogenesis	337-40
intolerance	198
low intensity exercise	177
metabolic clearance rate (MCR)	203
metabolism	112, 275
sensitive neurones (GSN)	89
tolerance	55
impaired	401
test	299, 399
transporter	
Glut 1	89-93
Glut 4	234, 275
quantification	274
utilization index	234, 235, 236
visceral adipose tissue	303
see also blood; fasting; plasma	
glucosensor system	90
gluteal adipose tissue	443
gluteal-femoral obesity	125
glycaemia	214
glycerol	
analysis	442
levels and mental stress	443
release, epinephrine induced	401-4
release and metabolic efficiency	30, 31, 33
goal weight	169
gonadotropin releasing hormone	377, 382
Gothenburg	121
growth hormone	79
gut hormones and adipose tissue	
metabolism	269-72
gut measurement	271
gynoid obesity	191, 192, 194
hamster	2, 146, 148
preadipocytes	277-9
Siberian	363-7
hand joints	222, 223
HDL-cholesterol	82, 111, 302, 303
blood lipid levels	121, 122, 123
fasting plasma insulin	135, 137
lipolysis	198
health implications	429-30
health problems	424
heart rate	25
height grading	191-2
Henderson-Hasselbach formula	24
Herman & Polivy boundary model	431, 432, 433, 434
hibernation	77
high-carbohydrate diet	333-5
high-fat feeding	42, 43, 44, 78
hip joints	222, 223
hirsutism, idiopathic	209
homeostatic model of assessment (HOMA)	89, 92
homozygous obesity	87
hormones	259-61, 413
lipoprotein lipase activity	270
regulation	363-7
requirements, minimal	3
see also sex hormones	
humans	
adipose tissue biopsies	405-8
cephalic postprandial thermogenesis	249-52
cephalic thermogenic phase	241, 245
collagen VI	2
fat cell adrenoceptors	143-7
fatty-acid-binding protein (FABP)	293
obesity	7-13
chaos or determinism	7-13
genetics	77-9
multifaceted aspects	17-37
studies and feeding	242, 243-4
type VI-Collagen	351
hunger	72
and myco-protein	67-70
state	434
hydroxyprogesterone (17)	209
hyperandrogenism	207
hypercholesterolaemia	167
hypercorticism	236
hypercorticosteronaemia	234-6
hyperglucagonaemia	389, 392
hyperglycaemia	195, 397
hyperinsulinaemia	55, 95, 207-11, 389, 391, 403
adipose tissue metabolism	269
breast cancer	125
brown adipose tissue	103
energy metabolism	195
fasting	92
genetics	78
glucose handling	234, 235
insulin secretion	201, 202, 203, 204
islet blood flow	263, 264, 265
low intensity exercise	177
physiological	382
regional fat deposition	310
hyperlipidaemia	164
hyperphagia	78, 95, 418
adipose tissue metabolism	269

brown adipose tissue	103	glucose handling	233-4
menstrual cycle	71	glucose transport	98
MSG	51, 53	lactate production	397-8
hyperplasia	192, 405	lipolysis	402
hypertension	111, 164, 217, 405	Ob 24	347
essential	213, 408	peripheral model	257
low intensity exercise	177	triglycerides	198
microalbuminuria	214, 215	Indian origin	301
prevalence ratios	302	INSEE see National Institute for	
proteinuria	219, 220	Statistics and Economic Studies	
regional fat deposition	310	insulin	365, 366, 367, 379
weight control programme	167	assay	90
hypertriglyceridaemia	55, 198, 389, 392, 401	cephalic postprandial thermogenesis	249-52
hypertrophy	192, 382, 405	concentrations	208
hyperuricaemia	221	differentiation specific markers	3
hypogonadism	78, 379	effectors, multiple	273-5
hypoinsulinaemia	198, 389	fasting	90, 389, 391
hypothyroidism	26	fasting plasma	135-7
hypoventilatory syndrome	229	receptor kinase activity	273, 274
		resistance	92
ICI 118551	142, 143, 147	genetics	78
ICI D7114	289-91	low intensity exercise	177
Iceland	109	rats	233-6
ideal shape/size	170, 423-4	regional fat deposition	310
IGF-I	3	secretion	92, 201-4
in situ		visceral adipose tissue	303
adipose tissue metabolism	281-5	see also plasma insulin	
lactate production	398-9	insulinaemia	102, 103, 208, 209, 311
lipolysis	402	insulinization in rats	233-4
subcutaneous deposits	150	integrated plasma insulin (IPI)	195
in vitro	2	integrated plasma-glucose (IPG)	195
α_2-antagonists	150	intervention study	
adipocyte model	277	chaos/determinism	9, 11
adipose tissue metabolism	281, 282	hormone balance	381
androgen secretion	207	Swedish obese subjects	299-304
dialysis	284	intestinal contents in man	42, 44
glucose transport	98	intraabdominal adipose tissue	313, 405
ICI D7114	290	intracerebroventricular injection	
lactate production	398	(monosodium glutamate)	51-3
lipolysis	402	IPG see integrated plasma glucose	
morbid obesity	193	IPI see integrated plasma insulin	
Ob24	347	ischaemic heart disease	111, 112
terminal differentiation	4	isolated adipocytes	274
in vivo		isoproterenol	144, 145, 146, 411, 412
α_2-AR expression	277	adipocyte differentiation	278
adipocytes	95	Italy	92, 111, 112, 125-7, 136, 137
adipose tissue	156, 281, 282	ITO-matrix method	86
androgen secretion	207		
cultured cell system	159	Japan	41, 92
Cushing's syndrome	259	jaw wiring	166
dialysis	284	joints	223, 224
differentiation-specific markers	2	juveniles and body weight/height grading	191
fatty-acid-binding protein (FABP)	293		

Subject Index

Kappa statistic	422
kidney failure, chronic	213
knee arthrosis	224, 225
knee joints	222, 223
lactate production	397-9
lambs	4
Landis and Koch classification	422
Landrace	78
LBM	26
LDL-cholesterol	82, 111
blood lipid levels	121, 122, 123
fasting plasma insulin	135, 137
low intensity exercise	178
lean and obese comparison	18
Li and Sacks ITO-matrix method	86
life style factors	174
lipase	41, 43, 44
lipid	124
see also glucagon-lipid interactions	
lipodystropy	159
lipogenesis, *de novo*	233, 234
lipogenic enzyme activity	95-8
lipolysis	198, 401, 402, 403
adipose tissue	30-3, 411-13
adrenergic regulation	285
catecholamine	150, 277
cyclic AMP	146
epinephrine-induced	193
hormone-induced	412
intensified	192-4, 196-8
metabolic efficiency	29, 30
regulation and mental stress	441-5
lipoprotein lipase (LPL)	
	79, 259, 260, 271, 272, 379, 380
activity	270
adipocyte characteristics	356
plasma	81-2
Siberian hamster	365, 366
liver regeneration	408
liver-transplanted rats in caloric regulation	237-9
loathing	427-30
Locus of Control Questionnaire (LOC)	168
longitudinal studies	9, 115, 127, 198
meal-induced thermogenesis	326
regional fat deposition	313
visceral adipose tissue	303
low-fat feeding	42, 43, 44, 333-5
lower body obesity	390
LPL *see* lipoprotein lipase	
luck	423, 424, 425
luteal phase	71, 72
macronutrients	8, 11, 70, 315
macroproteinuria	213
males	
abdominal obesity	188
adipose tissue lipolysis	411-13
fasting plasma insulin	136
lean and lactate production	397-9
lean/healthy	63-5
obesity genetics	78-9
sex hormones	337-40
malnutrition	113, 429
management of obesity	141-88
management objectives	163-4
markers, differentiation-specific	2
massive obesity	213
matrix, extracellular	347-52
meal composition	255-7
membrane function	35-7
Mendelian inheritance	78, 85
menopause	379
menstrual cycle and buspirone/food intake	71-3
menstrual irregularities	381
mental stress	382
and lipolytic regulation	441-5
test	442
mesenteric adipose tissue	310, 312, 407
metabolic/metabolism	
adipose tissue	269-72
clearance rate, reduced	201-4
disorders	192-4, 402-3
efficiency, increased	29-33
energy	30
exercise	178-9
fitness	177-80
rate, basal	77
rate, resting and sex hormones	337-40
regulation of adipose tissue	269-96
risk factors	174
metabolites	282
metatarsophalangeal joints	222, 224
mice	2
brown adipocyte	365
feeding	242, 244
genetically obese (ob/ob)	78, 79, 269-72
KK	78
lean	269-72
post-natal	347
spiny	77
microalbuminuria	213-15, 217, 218
microdialysis	284-5, 401-4
probe	442
studies	150
migration, seasonal	77

mild deprivation	47-50	adipocyte differentiation	278
mitochondrial DNA variants	369-72	adrenoceptors	141
mitochondrial protein content	290	brown adipose tissue	101
molecular approaches	141-51	brown fat cell cultures	355, 356, 357, 358, 359
molecular biology	79, 343-5	caloric regulation	238, 239
molecular studies and genes	344-5	heart and BAT	245
MONICA populations	109, 110, 111, 122	meal composition	255-7
monosodium glutamate	51-3	metabolic efficiency	29, 30, 31
morbid obesity	35-7, 217, 391	normoglycaemia	89
osteoarthrosis	225	Norway	109, 121
surgical treatment	183, 186	NST see non-shivering thermogenesis	
mortality ratio	113	Nuclear Magnetic Resonance Study (NMR)	282
motivation and weight loss	164	31-P	23-7
mRNA	234, 343, 347, 348, 349-52, 408	nutrient content	68
C/EPB	155	nutrition	
differentiation specific markers	2, 3, 4	intervention	17
glucocorticoid hormone receptors	259	risk factors	174
probe	143	status	117, 118-19
MSG see monosodium glutamate			
muscle bioenergetics	23-7	Ob1771	3, 347, 348, 350
muscle, calf	23, 26	Ob17	3, 4
myco-protein	67-70	obesity	
myocardial infarction	121, 302, 303, 307	grading, insufficient	191-2
		and recessive inheritance of major gene	85-7
NA see norepinephrine accumulation		risk	299
Na/K see sodium/potassium-ATPase		oestrogen	381
National Heart Foundation (NHF)	167	OGTT	391, 392
National Institute for Statistics and		olestra	63-5
Economic Studies (INSEE)	113, 114	omental adipose tissue	270
NE see norepinephrine		osteoarthritis	405
nephropathy	213, 215, 219, 220	osteoarthrosis, radiological	221-5
nephrotic syndrome	217	overeating/feeding	
Netherlands	109, 111, 112, 115, 117, 136, 137, 432	chaos or determinism	9-12
neuroendocrine regulation/responses		longterm and energy expenditure	319-21
	41-73, 55-60, 383, 385	and stress	55-60
neuropeptide Y	79	overweight and community attitudes	422, 424
NF-1 family	160	oxidation, preferential	198
NHF see National Heart Foundation		oxygen consumption	243
NIDDM see non-insulin-diabetes mellitus		heart rate	25
nitrogen conservation	327-31	see also VO_2	
NMR see Nucelar Magnetic Resonance Study		oxymethazoline	78, 79
non-absorbable fat	63-5		
non-diabetic obesity and microalbuminuria	213-15	P2 gene	155, 156, 157, 158, 159, 344, 345
non-insulin-dependent diabetes mellitus (NIDDM)		palatability, subjective rating of	244
	213-15, 217, 307, 345, 397, 398	pancreatic islet blood flow, increased	263-5
ageing rat	55	parasympathetic system	89
glucose transporter	92	pathogenetic importance	417-19
weight control programme	167	PCr/Pi see phosphocreatine/inorganic phosphate ratio	
non-shivering thermogenesis (NST)	295, 363	Pearson correlation coefficients	
noncyclers	314		32, 338, 390, 391, 423
noradrenaline	103, 144, 145, 363, 366, 367	fasting insulin	136, 137
norepinephrine (NE)	243, 257, 260	metabolic efficiency	30, 31
accumulation	242, 244, 246, 247	peptic ulcer	382, 383, 384

percentiles	116, 117
breast cancer	126
Europe and obesity	109, 110, 111
French population	113, 114, 115, 118
recessive inheritance	85, 86, 87
periostitis, calcaneal	223
peripheral obesity	191
perirenal adipose tissue	290
permanency of change and weight loss	164-5
pharmacological strategies	149-51
pharmacotherapy	165-6
phentermine	166
pheochromocytoma	4
Phodopus sungorus see hamster, Siberian	
phosphocreatine/inorganic phosphate ratio (PCr/Pi)	
	23-7
phosphodiesters (PDE)	25, 26
physical characteristics	30
physiopathology	233-6
Pietrain	7
pigs	1, 77, 293
Pima Indians	9, 196
plasma	
ACTH	58, 235
adrenaline	150
b-endorphin	59
C-peptide levels	202, 203, 204
cholesterol	178
corticosterone	57-8
cortisol	209
GIP	271
glucagon	243, 392
caloric regulation	238
levels	389-92
glucose	252, 257, 264
integrated	195
insulin	56-7, 252, 257, 264, 403
ageing rat	60
exercise	82
fasting	135-7
integrated	195
insulinaemia	238
lipoproteins	81-2
noradrenaline	150
serotinin and meal composition	255-7
testosterone	207
tGLP-1	271, 272
platelet-poor plasma (PPP)	255, 256, 257
pOb24	2, 3, 347, 348, 350, 351
Poland	111, 136, 137
Portugal	111, 136
post-obese women	
high-carbohydrate diet	333-5

weight relapse	173-5
postprandial thermogenesis	30, 32, 33, 242
cephalic thermogenic phase	
	241, 243, 245, 246, 249-52
metabolic efficiency	29, 33
Na^+/K^+-ATPase	31
PPP *see* platelet-poor plasma	
PPT *see* postprandial thermogenesis	
Prader-Willi syndrome	78, 79
prazosin	358
preadipocytes	1
cell lines	143-7
dormant	1-4
hamster	277-9
signalling pathways	2-3
preadipose state marker	347-52
preferential fatty acid oxidation	198
pregnancy	315
premenopause	403, 413
premenstrual syndrome (PMS)	71, 72
progesterone	377, 380, 381, 382
proliferation of brown adipocyte cultures	355-9
propranolol	242, 246, 357
protein content, mitochondrial	290
protein expression	363-7
proteinuria	217-20
psychological	
determinants of regional fat	
distribution	307-16
risk factors	174
psychosocial	
aspects of obesity	417-19
factors	
fat distribution	377-85
treatment	419
visceral fat accumulation	385
questionnaire	170
Quetelet's index	315
Quorn *see* myco-protein	
rabbit	146, 148
radical therapy	166
radiological osteoarthrosis	221-5
rats	148
adult male	238
ageing	55-60, 90
brown adipose tissue	293-6
cephalic thermogenic phase	245
CORT	312
fa fa	95, 96, 146, 234, 236
insulin resistance	233-6
insulinization	233-4

lean female	47-50
liver-transplanted	237-9
Long-Evans	51-3
NA turnover	242
Osborne-Mendel	78
sand	77
Sprague-Dawley	41, 43, 47-50, 55-60, 260, 312
VMH-lesioned	89, 273-5
Wistar	264, 273, 398
Zucker	78, 79, 263-5
brown adipose tissue	101-4
multiple insulin effectors	275
pancreatic islet blood flow	263-5
white adipocytes	95-8
rauwolscine	143, 147, 148, 149
receptor kinase activity	275
see also insulin receptor kinase activity	
recessive inheritance of major gene	85-7
red blood cells	32, 33
REE *see* resting energy expenditure	
regional fat distribution/deposition	377-413
behavioural determinants	307-16
environment	307, 308, 378, 383
residual volume (RV)	227, 228
respiratory	
failure	405
function disturbances	227-30
quotient (RQ)	
energy expenditure	18
overfeeding	9
resting	173-5
resting	
energy expenditure (REE)	30, 33
metabolic rate (RMR)	
	324, 325, 326, 327-31, 370, 372
chaos/determinism	8, 9, 11
very low calorie diet	23-7
restraint, cognitive	431-5
restriction fragment length	
polymerization (RFLP)	91, 370, 371
risk factors and weight relapse	174
risk and obesity	299
RMR *see* resting metabolic rate	
RNA	291
isolation/analysis	348
see also mRNA	
rodents	89, 149, 150
see also rats	
RQ *see* respiratory quotient	
RV *see* residual volume	
RX821002	143, 148, 149, 278, 279
6 kb	349-50

salt *see* sodium chloride	
satiety	63, 65
centre	89
and myco-protein	67-70
signal	41-4
self-perception	423-4
self-reported intake	17-22
serotinin (5-HT)	257
serum	
cholesterol	121, 188
insulin	111
lipid profiles	112
triglycerides	110
severe obesity and osteoarthrosis	221-5
sex *see* gender	
sex hormones	71, 381-2, 390, 396
energy expenditure	339
fat distribution	377, 379, 380, 385
and metabolic rate, resting	337-40
regional fat deposition	308
SHBG	390
signalling pathways and preadipocytes	2-3
single fluid meal	44
single meal and enterostatin	42
size	170, 421-5
sleep apnoea	167
small-bowel bypass	166
smoking	111, 315, 379, 383, 384
SNS *see* sympathetic nervous system	
sodium chloride (NaCl)	57, 58, 59
sodium/potassium-ATPase	31, 32, 33, 35
of erythrocytes	30
metabolic efficiency	29
specific treatment options	165
squirrel, Richardson's ground	77
stress	308-14, 384
overeating	56
reaction	383
see also mental stress	
stroke	302, 307
subcutaneous abdominal fat	412, 413
subcutaneous adipose tissue	303, 395, 397-9, 401-4
subcutaneous fat	12
submaximal ergometry test	25
substrate oxidation rates	339
superobesity	185, 186
surgical treatment	183-6, 301, 304
Sweden	109, 111, 136, 137, 301
longitudinal study	127
Obese Subjects (SOS)	299-304
regional fat deposition	309
Switzerland	109

Subject Index

sympathetic nervous system (SNS) 89, 101, 149, 150, 242, 246, 247
   brown fat cell cultures 355
   fat distribution 379, 380
   hyperactivity 334, 335
   mediation 333-5
systolic blood pressure 111, 219
   proteinuria 218, 220
   visceral adipose tissue 303

T3 101, 103, 104, 366, 367
3.7 kb 349-52
tail pinch 55-60
talocrural joints 222, 224
terminal differentiation of preadipocytes 2-3
testosterone 125, 188, 210, 339, 390, 396
   fat distribution 377, 379, 380, 382
TFEQ *see* Three-Factor Eating Questionnaire
TG *see* triglyceride
TGF *see* transforming growth factor therapy
   importance 417-19
   radical 166
   strategies 141-51
therapy, cognitive 165
thermic effect of a meal (TEM) 323, 325, 326, 370, 372
thermogenesis
   adaptative 149
   cephalic 241-7
   cephalic postprandial 249-52
   chaos/determinism 11
   facultative 101
   fatty-acid-binding protein (FABP) 294
   glucose-induced 337-40
   longerm overfeeding 320, 321
   meal-induced 323-6
   metabolic efficiency 30
   see also postprandial; non-shivering thermogenin 356, 357, 358
   see also uncoupling protein thermogenin (UCP)
Three-Factor Eating Questionnaire (TFEQ) 437, 438, 439
thrifty genotype 78, 79
thyroid hormones 101
thyroxine 5′Monodeiodinase activity 101-4
TLC *see* total lung capacity
TLV 230
TNF-a 347
total cholesterol 121, 123
   fasting plasma insulin 135
   regional fat deposition 307

visceral adipose tissue 303
total lung capacity (TLC) 227, 228, 229, 230
TP *see* tail pinch
transforming growth factor 347, 405, 407, 408
triacylglycerol 1
triglyceridaemia 196
triglycerides 355, 379, 380, 381, 403
   concentrations 121, 122, 123
   fasting plasma insulin 135
   in vivo 198
   levels 82
   visceral adipose tissue 303
   see also VLDL-triglyceride
triglyceridesynthesis 196-8
triiodothyronine 365
twins
   Finnish 129-132
   genetics 78
   glucose transporter 89
   monozygotic 81-2, 319, 369-72
   overfeeding 9, 10
   recessive inheritance 85
type VI-collagen 350-2

UAER *see* urinary albumin excretion rate
UK14304 143, 148, 278
uncoupling protein (UCP) 4, 289, 291, 294, 363, 364, 365, 366
   brown fat cell cultures 356
   serum free medium 366-7
   thermogenin 357-8
underweight 424
United States 115, 116, 127, 165
upper body obesity 389-92
urinary albumin excretion rate (UAER) 213, 214, 215
vagotomy 264
vasoactive substances 405-8
VBG *see* vertical banded gastroplasty
VC *see* vital capacity
vertical banded gastroplasty 183-6, 300
very low calorie diet 165, 166, 198
   adenosine triphosphate 25
   anthropometric data 24
   energy expenditure 330
   muscle bioenergetics 23-7
   oxygen consumption/heart rate 25
   study 327-31
vigilance 423, 424
visceral
   adipose tissue 303, 395, 396
      metabolism 259-61
   fat accumulation 377, 378, 379
      disease 384

endocrine characteristics	381-5
psychosocial factors	385
obesity	405
endocrine/circulatory aberrations	383-5
vital capacity (VC)	227, 228, 229, 230
VLCD *see* very low calorie diet	
VLDL-apo B	197
VLDL-cholesterol	121, 122, 123
VLDL-TG synthesis	194
VLDL-triglyceride	196
VMH-lesioned rats	273-5
VO_2	81, 249, 250, 251
low intensity exercise	177, 178
waist/hip ratio (WHR)	315, 389, 391
blood lipid levels	121
Europe and obesity	110, 111
glucose transporter	91
WAT *see* white adipose tissue	
water, doubly labelled	17-22
weight	
change	170
age	130, 131, 132
body mass index	130, 131, 132
Finland	129-32
gender	131
intervention study	303-4
control programme and completion/attrition	167-71
cycling	314
gain causes	422-3, 424-5
grading	191-2
initial	130
loss	329, 421-5
disinhibtion of control	437-40
energy expenditure	327-31
erythrocyte membrane function	35-7
general principles	164
maintenance	422-3, 424-5
relapse	173-5
white	
adipocytes	95-8
adipose cells	3-4, 357
adipose tissue	1-4, 356, 365
fatty-acid-binding protein (FABP)	293, 295
insulin effectors, multiple	273-5,
WHR *see* waist/hip ratio	
wild animals	77
work lives	424
yohimbine	143, 147, 148, 149, 150, 357
zero calorie diet	36, 37